Revision Surgery in Otolaryngology

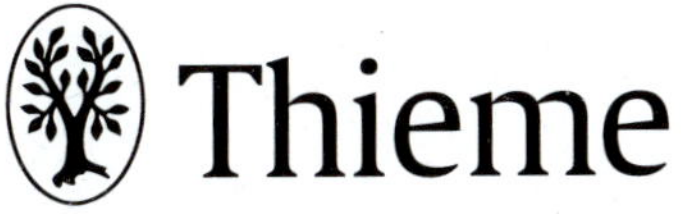

Revision Surgery in Otolaryngology

David R. Edelstein, MD, FACS
Clinical Professor of Otorhinolaryngology
Weill Medical College of Cornell University
Chairman of Otolaryngology–Head and Neck Surgery
Manhattan Eye, Ear and Throat Hospital
New York, New York

Dennis H. Kraus, MD
Professor of Otorhinolaryngology
Department of Otorhinolaryngology
Weill Medical College of Cornell University
Attending Surgeon
Department of Head and Neck Surgery
Memorial Sloan-Kettering Cancer Center
New York, New York

Norman J. Pastorek, MD
Clinical Professor of Facial Plastic Surgery
Department of Otolaryngology
Weill Medical College of Cornell University
New York Presbyterian Hospital
New York, New York

Samuel H. Selesnick, MD
Professor and Vice-Chairman
Department of Otorhinolaryngology
Weill Medical College of Cornell University
New York, New York

Robert F. Ward, MD
Division Chief of Pediatric Otolaryngology
Weill Medical College of Cornell University
New York Presbyterian Hospital
New York, New York

Thieme
New York · Stuttgart

Thieme Medical Publishers, Inc.
333 Seventh Ave.
New York, NY 10001

Consulting Medical Editor: Esther Gumpert
Managing Editor: J. Owen Zurhellen
Editorial Assistants: Dominic Pucek, Adriana di Giorgio, Cristina Baptista
Vice President, Production and Electronic Publishing: Anne T. Vinnicombe
Production Editor: Heidi Pongratz, Maryland Composition
Vice President, International Marketing and Sales: Cornelia Schulze
Chief Financial Officer: Peter van Woerden
President: Brian D. Scanlan
Medical Illustrator: Stacie Walker
Compositor: Thomson Digital
Printer: Everbest Printing Co.

Library of Congress Cataloging-in-Publication Data

Revision surgery in otolaryngology / [edited by] David R. Edelstein.
   p. ; cm.
 Includes bibliographical references and index.
 ISBN 978-1-58890-369-3
 1. Otolaryngology, Operative. 2. Head—Reoperation. 3. Neck—Reoperation. I. Edelstein, David R.
 [DNLM: 1. Otorhinolaryngologic Surgical Procedures. 2. Reoperation. WV 168 R454 2009]
 RF51.R43 2009
 617.5'1059—dc22

                                                  2008015459

Important note: Medical knowledge is ever-changing. As new research and clinical experience broaden our knowledge, changes in treatment and drug therapy may be required. The authors and editors of the material herein have consulted sources believed to be reliable in their efforts to provide information that is complete and in accord with the standards accepted at the time of publication. However, in view of the possibility of human error by the authors, editors, or publisher of the work herein or changes in medical knowledge, neither the authors, editors, nor publisher, nor any other party who has been involved in the preparation of this work, warrants that the information contained herein is in every respect accurate or complete, and they are not responsible for any errors or omissions or for the results obtained from use of such information. Readers are encouraged to confirm the information contained herein with other sources. For example, readers are advised to check the product information sheet included in the package of each drug they plan to administer to be certain that the information contained in this publication is accurate and that changes have not been made in the recommended dose or in the contraindications for administration. This recommendation is of particular importance in connection with new or infrequently used drugs.

Some of the product names, patents, and registered designs referred to in this book are in fact registered trademarks or proprietary names even though specific reference to this fact is not always made in the text. Therefore, the appearance of a name without designation as proprietary is not to be construed as a representation by the publisher that it is in the public domain.

Printed in China

5 4 3 2 1

ISBN 978-1-58890-369-3

I dedicate this book to my lovely wife Eve
and my wonderful children Jennifer, Hilary, and Matthew.

—David R. Edelstein

Contents

Foreword

With this book, the otolaryngologist–head and neck surgeon finally has a unique resource prior to embarking on a complicated and sometimes dangerous mission, revision surgery. Flying by the proverbial "seat of the pants" is not the ideal preparation for a surgical procedure, particularly a revision case. There was previously no single source of wisdom and guidance on managing this considerable challenge.

During my otolaryngology residency, my mentors at Boston University School of Medicine stressed a systematic and somewhat skeptical approach to the management of the patient who required additional surgery for a recurrence or persistence of pathology. A time-honored algorithm dictates review of everything such as prior radiographs, laboratory data, and surgical reports. I was taught to review the outside pathology slides with an expert pathologist and to distrust the "black and white report": on occasion these slides were sent to other national authorities. The prior X-rays were carefully reviewed with a trusted, experienced radiologist prior to ordering new studies. The surgeon must take time to carefully review the medical records, with particular attention to the prior operative reports. If possible, direct communication with the prior surgeon should take place, in order to review the preoperative presentation and surgical findings. The dictum was, assume nothing and start a new workup. The only logical assumption prior to a revision surgery is that there will be altered anatomy complicated by scar tissue, demanding careful preoperative planning regarding choice of incision, exposure, and wound closure. Planning should include the potential need for the participation of other skilled colleagues in disciplines such as neurosurgery, reconstructive surgery, and oral maxillofacial surgery.

A new medical textbook is valuable to the reader if it provides new information lacking in any one source and if it is authoritative, as this one is. *Revision Surgery in Otolaryngology*, ably edited by David R. Edelstein, contains invaluable information in every subspecialty of otolaryngology–head and neck surgery. The chapters are clearly written and nicely illustrated. The contributors are well-known experts who share their extensive experience in how to approach revision surgery unique to their subspecialty. Additionally, this text points out pitfalls in decision-making that may lead to unsuccessful surgery and will prove to be valuable to avoid complications in the first place.

When I was first asked to write a foreword for this text, I thought the book would be most valuable for the experienced university-based otolaryngologist likely to be referred cases requiring revision surgery. In fact, this book will be very useful for any otolaryngologist since it gives insight into the pitfalls of surgery in every subspecialty area and lessons learned about the avoidance of complications. This very valuable resource should be on the bookshelf of every otolaryngologist regardless of their level of experience and would be very useful as well for residents in training. My congratulations to Dr. Edelstein for putting together this worthwhile text.

Stanley M. Shapshay, MD, FACS
Professor of Otolaryngology–Head and Neck Surgery
Albany Medical College
Albany, New York

Preface

Recently, a patient came to my office with the usual signs of complex, chronic sinusitis-related problems. She had a distressed look on her face and was weighed down by several folders of CT scans. As I entered the examination room, I checked my watch, since these consultations usually take more than the average amount of time, and I also wanted to pace myself and direct her comments in a timely fashion. The patient had undergone four separate sinus procedures performed by different surgeons over the past 5 years. Listening to her rendition of the story, I realized how limited was her understanding of her disease, although her desire for a cure was great. As I often am, unfortunately, I was disappointed that her previous physicians had not better informed her about the nature of her disease and also saddened that, even after 5 years, she had not yet had a complete workup for sinusitis and all of its forms. When the patient finally allowed me to examine her, with the proviso that she was very sensitive after so many endoscopies, I discovered that she had undergone a rather confused set of surgeries along the way, with each side of her nose offering different challenges to correct. In addition, her CT scans showed disease in a variety of cells with different problems facing the maxillary, ethmoid, sphenoid, and frontal sinuses. This was going to be a long day!

How many of us have faced a problem like this in our office during the past week? I suspect most of us. Some physicians have more experience in head and neck surgery, others in rhinology, many in facial plastic surgery, and some in otology or neurotology. Each of us approaches patients who have recurrent disease with a variety of techniques and a spectrum of compassion. Some of us readily identify our limitations and, though we may start the arduous process with these patients, refer them quickly to more experienced otolaryngologists. Unfortunately, others of us do not accept readily either our surgical limitations or our brief experience and hold onto these patients long after this is prudent.

My own chiefs included experts in a variety of areas, including Hugh Biller, MD, a luminary in head and neck surgery; Simon Parisier, MD, a visionary in mastoid and cochlear implantation surgery; and M. Stuart Strong, MD, a pioneer in laser surgery. Although each one has a different personality, they all have a commanding respect for the diseases that they treat, a unique insight into the surgeries that they perform, and a healthy disdain for incompetence. All three taught me to accept my limitations and to appreciate the nature of the diseases I treat. All three urged me to master the variety of procedures available to the surgeon and to treat revision cases with extreme care.

The recurrent themes posed by my teachers and the daily bombardment of recidivistic disease gave me the inspiration for this book. When I sat down to review all of the major otolaryngology texts in my office, I became amazed at how little was written on revision surgery. Most existing texts are very good at describing basic surgical techniques and the anatomy, physiology, and pathology of disease. Few books, however, provide any decision trees for surgeons to follow and they almost uniformly focus on virginal cases, without addressing any of the challenges posed by recurrent surgery. Indeed, the farther along the patient is in having recidivistic disease, the less the standard otolaryngology texts give any direction.

During morning rounds at Manhattan Eye, Ear, and Throat Hospital, we used to go over all of the cases from the previous day with our residents and try to anticipate the surgical problems facing our surgeons that morning. Uniformly, the young doctors were much better able to explain the surgical choices for primary cases than to discuss the alternatives applicable to revision cases. When does one use the same incision? How does one identify obliterated landmarks in the ear? Where have the major vessels migrated in revision neck dissections? How close is the facial nerve to the skin flap in a revision parotidectomy? Where is the base of the skull in a revision endoscopic ethmoid surgery? How does one choose to perform an external rhinoplasty and should one use cartilage grafts or artificial material in a revision saddle nose deformity? The list of questions for revision cases is as endless as the disease processes and the types of surgeries available to the primary surgeon. These are the questions that this book is dedicated to begin to answer.

David R. Edelstein, MD, FACS

Acknowledgments

I would like to acknowledge my four coeditors, who worked diligently to finish this book. The good humor and encouragement of Dr. Samuel Selesnick kept my spirits up at every turn, Dr. Dennis Kraus proved invaluable in helping to edit the final chapters, Dr. Norman Pastorek somehow found time during his very busy teaching and operating schedule to cajole his friends to write for this text, and Dr. Bob Ward helped recruit the best people in the small subspecialty of pediatric otolaryngology to participate in this project. All of the contributing authors earned my gratitude with their willingness to undertake the thought and effort required to write their chapters on revision surgery. Most found this experience to be stimulating and challenging, since few of us had ever written on this subject before.

I am also extremely grateful to the editorial staff at Thieme Medical Publishers for their enthusiastic support throughout the entire process. Many thanks to Esther Gumpert, Birgitta Brandenburg, Marta Bladek, Janet Rogers, and J. Owen Zurhellen IV. I am also indebted to my office manager, Seva Karambasis, for all of her help and support along the way and to my former audiologist, Patti Brinskelle, who helped the contributing authors.

I would particularly like to thank all who were involved in the creation of this book for their support and sympathetic understanding when problems at my institution and the needs of my patients, staff, and residents caused unexpected delays in the timing of bringing this project to completion.

As a medical student, I was lucky to work with Stanley Shapshay, MD, who, at the time, was a junior attending at Boston University School of Medicine and Chief of the Otolaryngology Service at the VA in Boston. Little did I know then that I would be only one of many students, residents, and fellow otolaryngologists whom he would inspire. His sage advice and counsel over the years has been as much appreciated as his review of this book. I am very grateful for his help in my career and for his foreword for this book. Most importantly, I am eternally grateful to my wife Eve and my three children Jennifer, Hilary, and Matthew who encouraged me at every step in the production of this book. My wife helped build an office for me in our apartment so that I could at least be closer to my family on weekends. My children helped to collate the chapters. Their love and inspiration are what keeps me, like most doctors, going. In addition, I would like to acknowledge my parents, Alan and Sybil, who put me through school and who have given me the fortitude to finish this book.

Contributors

E. Fred Aguilar, MD
Clinical Assistant Professor of Plastic Surgery
Department of Otolaryngology
The University of Texas Health Science Center
Private Practice
Houston, Texas

Peter E. Andersen, MD
Associate Professor of Otolaryngology–Head
   and Neck Surgery
Department of Otolaryngology–Head and Neck Surgery
Oregon Health & Science University
Portland, Oregon

Richard L. Anderson, MD
Medical Director
Center for Facial Appearances
Salt Lake City, Utah

Benjamin A. Bassichis, MD
Clinical Assistant Professor of Otolaryngology
Department of Otolaryngology–Head and Neck Surgery
University of Texas–Southwestern
   Medical Center
Private Practice
Advanced Facial Plastic Surgery Center
Dallas, Texas

William E. Bolger, MD
Private Practice
Maryland Sinus Center
Bethesda, Maryland

Patrick J. Byrne, MD
Associate Professor of Otolaryngology–Head
   and Neck Surgery
Director of Facial Plastic and Reconstructive
Department of Otolaryngology–Head and Neck Surgery
The Johns Hopkins University
Baltimore, Maryland

John F. Carew, MD
Adjunct Assistant Professor of Otolaryngology
Department of Otolaryngology
Mount Sinai School of Medicine
New York, New York

Paul J. Carniol, MD, FACS
Clinical Associate Professor of Otolaryngology
Department of Otolaryngology
University of Medicine and Dentistry of New Jersey
Private Practice
Newark, New Jersey

Seth H. Dailey, MD
Assistant Professor of Otolaryngology–Head
   and Neck Surgery
Division of Otolaryngology–Head and Neck Surgery
University of Wisconsin Hospital and Clinics
Madison, Wisconsin

Lianne M. de Serres, MD
Associate Professor of Otolaryngology
Department of Pediatric Otolaryngology–Head
   and Neck Surgery
New York Presbyterian Hospital-Columbia Campus
New York, New York

Joseph J. Disa, MD
Associate Attending Surgeon
Department of Plastic and Reconstructive Surgery
Memorial Sloan-Kettering Cancer Center
New York, New York

Colin L. W. Driscoll, MD
Associate Professor of Otolaryngology
Department of Otolaryngology
Mayo Clinic
Rochester, Minnesota

David R. Edelstein, MD, FACS
Clinical Professor of Otorhinolaryngology
Weill Medical College of Cornell University
Chairman of Otolaryngology–Head and Neck Surgery
Manhattan Eye, Ear and Throat Hospital
New York, New York

Simon Ellul, MBBS, FRACS
Department of Otolaryngology–Head and Neck Surgery
Royal Victorian Eye and Ear Hospital
Melbourne, Victoria, Australia

Jeffrey S. Epstein, MD, FACS
Clinical Voluntary Instructor of Otolaryngology
Department of Otolaryngology–Head and Neck Surgery
University of Miami
Private Practice
Miami Florida

Jose N. Fayad, MD
Attending Surgeon of Otolaryngology–Head
   and Neck Surgery
St. Vincent Medical Center
Associate, House Ear Clinic
Los Angeles, California

Frank P. Fechner, MD
Clinical Instructor of Otolaryngology
Department of Otolaryngology
Harvard Medical School
Massachusetts Eye and Ear Infirmary
Private Practice
Worcester, Massachusetts

Berrylin J. Ferguson, MD
Associate Professor of Otolaryngology
Department of Otolaryngology
University of Pittsburgh School of Medicine
Pittsburgh, Pennsylvania

Marvin P. Fried, MD
Professor of Otorhinolaryngology
Department of Otorhinolaryngology–Head
   and Neck Surgery
Montefiore Medical Center
Albert Einstein College of Medicine
Bronx, New York

Gerry F. Funk, MD
Professor of Otolaryngology–Head and Neck Surgery
Department of Otolaryngology–Head and Neck Surgery
University of Iowa Hospitals and Clinics
Iowa City, Iowa

Dee Anna Glaser, MD
Professor and Vice Chairman of Dermatology
Department of Dermatology
Saint Louis University
St. Louis, Missouri

Robert A. Goldenberg, MD
Professor and Chief of Otolaryngology
Department of Surgery
Wright State University
Dayton, Ohio

Henry T. Hoffman, MD
Professor of Otolaryngology–Head and Neck Surgery
Department of Otolaryngology–Head and Neck Surgery
University of Iowa Hospitals and Clinics
Iowa City, Iowa

Albert Hornblass, MD, FACS[†]
Attending Surgeon of Ophthalmic Plastic
   and Reconstructive Surgery
The New York Eye and Ear Infirmary
New York, New York

Robert K. Jackler, MD
Sewall Professor and Chair
Department of Otolaryngology–Head and Neck Surgery
Professor, Departments of Neurosurgery and Surgery
Associate Dean, Continuing Medical Education
Stanford University School of Medicine
Stanford, California

Stephanie A. Joe, MD
Director, The Sinus and Allergy Center
Department of Otolaryngology–Head and Neck Surgery
University of Illinois at Chicago
Chicago, Illinois

[†]deceased

Jacqueline E. Jones, MD
Private Practice
Park Avenue ENT
New York, New York

Ashutosh Kacker, MD, FACS
Associate Professor of Otorhinolaryngology
Department of Otorhinolaryngology
Weill Medical College of Cornell University
New York, New York

Paul A. Kedeshian, MD
Associate Clinical Professor of Surgery
Department of Surgery–Head
   and Neck Surgery
UCLA Medical Center
Los Angeles, California

Robert M. Kellman, MD
Professor and Chair of Otolaryngology–Head
   and Neck Surgery
Department of Otolaryngology–Head and Neck Surgery
SUNY Upstate Medical University
Syracuse, New York

Eugene B. Kern, MD
George M. and Edna B. Endicott Professor
   of Medicine, Emeritus
Professor Rhinology and Facial Plastic Surgery,
   Emeritus
Mayo Foundation
Mayo Clinic School of Medicine
Rochester, Minnesota

Nissim Khabie, MD
Private Practice
Ear, Nose, and Throat Specialty Care
Minneapolis, Minnesota

David W. Kim, MD
Associate Professor of Otolaryngology
Chief of Facial Plastic Surgery
Department of Otolaryngology–Head and Neck Surgery
University of California, San Francisco
San Francisco, California

Michael K. Kim, MD, FACS
Director of Facial Cosmetic Surgery
M.Y. Facial Cosmetic Surgery Center
Los Alamitos, California

Charles P. Kimmelman, MD, FACS
Clinical Associate Professor of Otolaryngology
Department of Otolaryngology
Weill Medical College of Cornell University
Chief of Smell and Taste Disorders
Manhattan Eye, Ear and Throat Hospital
Director of New York City Ear, Nose and Throat Center
New York, New York

Arnold Komisar, MD, DDS, MS
Clinical Professor of Otolaryngology
Department of Otolaryngology
New York University School of Medicine
New York, New York

Dennis H. Kraus, MD
Professor of Otolaryngology
Department of Otorhinolaryngology
Weill Medical College of Cornell University
Attending Surgeon
Department of Head and Neck Surgery
Memorial Sloan-Kettering Cancer Center
New York, New York

Paul R. Lambert, MD, FACS
Professor and Chair of Otolaryngology–Head
   and Neck Surgery
Department of Otolaryngology–Head
   and Neck Surgery
Medical University of South Carolina
Charleston, South Carolina

Pierre Lavertu, MD, FRCSC, FACS
Director and Professor of Head and Neck Surgery
   and Oncology
Department of Surgery
Case Western University
University Hospitals of Cleveland
Cleveland, Ohio

William Lawson, MD, DDS
Professor of Otolaryngology
Department of Otolaryngology
Mount Sinai Medical Center
New York, New York

John P. Leonetti, MD
Professor of Otolaryngology and Neurological Surgery
Department of Otolaryngology–Head and Neck Surgery
Program Director of Cranial Base Surgery
Loyola University Medical Center
Maywood, Illinois

Boaz J. Lissauer, MD
Clinical Assistant Professor
New York University School of Medicine
Head, Oculofacial Plastic Surgery Clinic
Manhattan Eye, Ear and Throat Hospital
New York, New York

Rodney P. Lusk, MD
Director of Ear, Nose, and Throat Institute
Boys Town National Research Hospital
Omaha, Nebraska

Daniel D. Lydiatt, DDS, MD, FACS
Professor of Otolaryngology–Head and Neck Surgery
Department of Otolaryngology–Head and Neck Surgery
University of Nebraska Medical Center
Director of Methodist Cancer Center
Omaha, Nebraska

William M. Lydiatt, MD
Professor of Otolaryngology–Head and Neck Surgery
Department of Otolaryngology–Head and Neck Surgery
University of Nebraska Medical Center
Director of Head and Neck Surgical Oncology Center
Omaha, Nebraska

Dimitrios P. Mastorakos, MD
Surgery Department
General Air Force Hospital
Athens, Greece

Ralph B. Metson, MD
Clinical Professor of Otolaryngology
Department of Otolaryngology
Harvard Medical School
Boston, Massachusetts

Edwin M. Monsell, MD, PhD
Professor of Otolaryngology–Head and Neck Surgery
Department of Otolaryngology–Head and Neck Surgery
Wayne State University School of Medicine
Southfield, Michigan

Brian A. Moore, MD
Clinical Assistant Professor of Otolaryngology–Head
   and Neck Surgery
Department of Otolaryngology–Head and Neck Surgery
Tulane University School of Medicine
Eglin Air Force Base, Florida

Shervin Naderi, MD
Private Practice
The Naderi Center for Cosmetic Surgery and Skin Care
Herndon, Virginia

James L. Netterville, MD
Mark C. Smith Professor of Otolaryngology–Head
   and Neck Surgery
Department of Otolaryngology–Head and Neck Surgery
Director, Head and Neck Surgery
Vanderbilt University Medical Center
Nashville, Tennessee

Richard Nicollas, MD, PhD
Department of Pediatric Otolaryngology–Head
   and Neck Surgery
University of Aix-Marseille
Hôpital de la Timone
Marseille, France

Simon C. Parisier, MD
Professor of Otolaryngology
Department of Otolaryngology
New York Eye and Ear Infirmary
New York Medical College
New York, New York

Norman J. Pastorek, MD
Clinical Professor of Facial Plastic Surgery
Department of Otolaryngology
Weill Medical College of Cornell University
New York Presbyterian Hospital
New York, New York

Stephen W. Perkins, MD
Clinical Associate Professor of Facial Plastic
   and Reconstructive Surgery
Department of Otolaryngology–Head and Neck Surgery
Indiana University School of Medicine
Private Practice
Meridian Plastic Surgery Center
Indianapolis, Indiana

Mukesh Prasad, MD
Assistant Professor of Otorhinolaryngology
Department of Otorhinolaryngology
Weill Medical College of Cornell University
New York, New York

Stephen Prendiville, MD
Private Practice
Facial Plastic Surgery Associates
Fort Myers, Florida

Douglas Reh, MD
Assistant Professor of Otolaryngology–Head
   and Neck Surgery
Department of Otolaryngology–Head and Neck Surgery
The Johns Hopkins University
Baltimore, Maryland

Jay T. Rubinstein, MD, PhD
Virginia Merrill Bloedel Professor and Director
Departments of Otolaryngology
 and Bioengineering
University of Washington
Seattle, Washington

Mark Samaha, MD
Assistant Professor of Otolaryngology
Department of Otolaryngology
 and Facial Plastic Surgery
McGill University
Montreal, Quebec, Canada

Ravi N. Samy, MD
Assistant Professor of Otolaryngology
Department of Otolaryngology
University of Cincinnati/Cincinnati Children's Hospital
Cincinnati, Ohio

Barry M. Schaitkin, MD
Professor of Otolaryngology
Department of Otolaryngology
University of Pittsburgh School of Medicine
Pittsburgh, Pennsylvania

Richard L. Scher, MD, FACS
Associate Professor and Associate Chief
Department of Otolaryngology-Head and Neck Surgery
Duke University Health System
Durham, North Carolina

Samuel H. Selesnick, MD
Professor and Vice Chairman
Department of Otorhinolaryngology
Weill Medical College of Cornell University
New York, New York

Ashok R. Shaha, MD
Professor of Surgery
Department of Surgery–Head and Neck Surgery
Weill Medical College of Cornell University
Attending Surgeon
Head and Neck Service
Memorial Sloan-Kettering Cancer Center
New York, New York

Clough Shelton, MD
Professor of Otology, Neuro-otology,
 and Skull Base Surgery
Department of Otolaryngology–Head and Neck Surgery
Chief of Otolaryngology–Head and Neck Surgery
University of Utah School of Medicine
Salt Lake City, Utah

Larry Shemen, MD
Associate Clinical Professor of Otolaryngology
Department of Otolaryngology
Weill Medical College of Cornell University
Chief of Head and Neck Service
New York Hospital
New York, New York

James D. Sidman, MD
Associate Professor of Otolaryngology
Department of Otolaryngology
University of Minnesota
Childrens' Hospitals and Clinics of Minnesota
Minneapolis, Minnesota

Russell B. Smith, MD
Associate Professor of Otolaryngology–Head
 and Neck Surgery
Department of Otolaryngology–Head and Neck Surgery
Nebraska Medical Center
Omaha, Nebraska

Sarah A. Stackpole, MD
Clinical Assistant Professor of Otolaryngology
Department of Otolaryngology
Weill Medical College of Cornell University
New York, New York

Sherard A. Tatum III, MD
Associate Professor of Otolaryngology-Head
 and Neck Surgery
Department of Otolaryngology-Head and Neck Surgery
SUNY Upstate Medical University
Syracuse, New York

J. Regan Thomas, MD
Lederer Professor and Chairman of Otolaryngology–Head
 and Neck Surgery
Department of Otolaryngology–Head and Neck Surgery
University of Illinois at Chicago
Chicago, Illinois

Dean M. Toriumi, MD, FACS
Professor of Otolaryngology–Head and Neck Surgery
Division of Facial Plastic and Reconstructive Surgery
Department of Otolaryngology–Head and Neck Surgery
Director of Resident Research
University of Illinois
Chicago, Illinois

Jean Michel Triglia, MD
Professor of Otolaryngology
Department of Pediatric Otolaryngology–Head
  and Neck Surgery
University of Aix-Marseille
Hôpital de la Timone
Marseille, France

Harvey M. Tucker, MD, FACS
Professor of Otolaryngology–Head and Neck Surgery
Department of Otolaryngology–Head and Neck Surgery
Case Western Reserve School of Medicine
Cleveland, Ohio

Robert F. Ward, MD
Division Chief of Pediatric Otolaryngology
Weill Medical College of Cornell University
New York Presbyterian Hospital
New York, New York

Randal S. Weber, MD
Hubert and Olive Stringer Professor and Chair
  of Head and Neck Surgery
Department of Head and Neck Surgery
University of Texas M.D. Anderson Cancer Center
Houston, Texas

**William I. Wei, MS, FRCS, FRCSE, FACS,
FHKAM(ORL), FHKAM(Surg)**
Li Shu Pui Professor of Surgery
Chair in Otorhinolaryngology
Department of Surgery
The University of Hong Kong
Queen Mary Hospital
Hong Kong, China

Mark C. Witte, MD
Medical Staff
Department of Otolaryngology
Brainerd Medical Center
Brainerd, Minnesota

Peak Woo, MD
Professor of Otolaryngology
Department of Otolaryngology
Mount Sinai Medical Center
New York, New York

George C. Yang, MD
Private Practice
Millennium Facial Plastic Surgery
Lenox Hill Hospital
New York, New York

Michael T. Yen, MD
Associate Professor of Ophthalmology
Department of Ophthalmology
Baylor College of Medicine
Houston, Texas

**Anthony P. W. Yuen, MS, DLO, FRCSE,
  FACS, FHKAM(ORL)**
Professor of Surgery
Department of Surgery
The University of Hong Kong
Queen Mary Hospital
Hong Kong, China

Shane A. Zim, MD
Assistant Professor of Otolaryngology
Department of Otolaryngology–Head and Neck Surgery
Keck School of Medicine
University of Southern California
Los Angeles, California

I
General

Decision tree for hyperplastic lesions

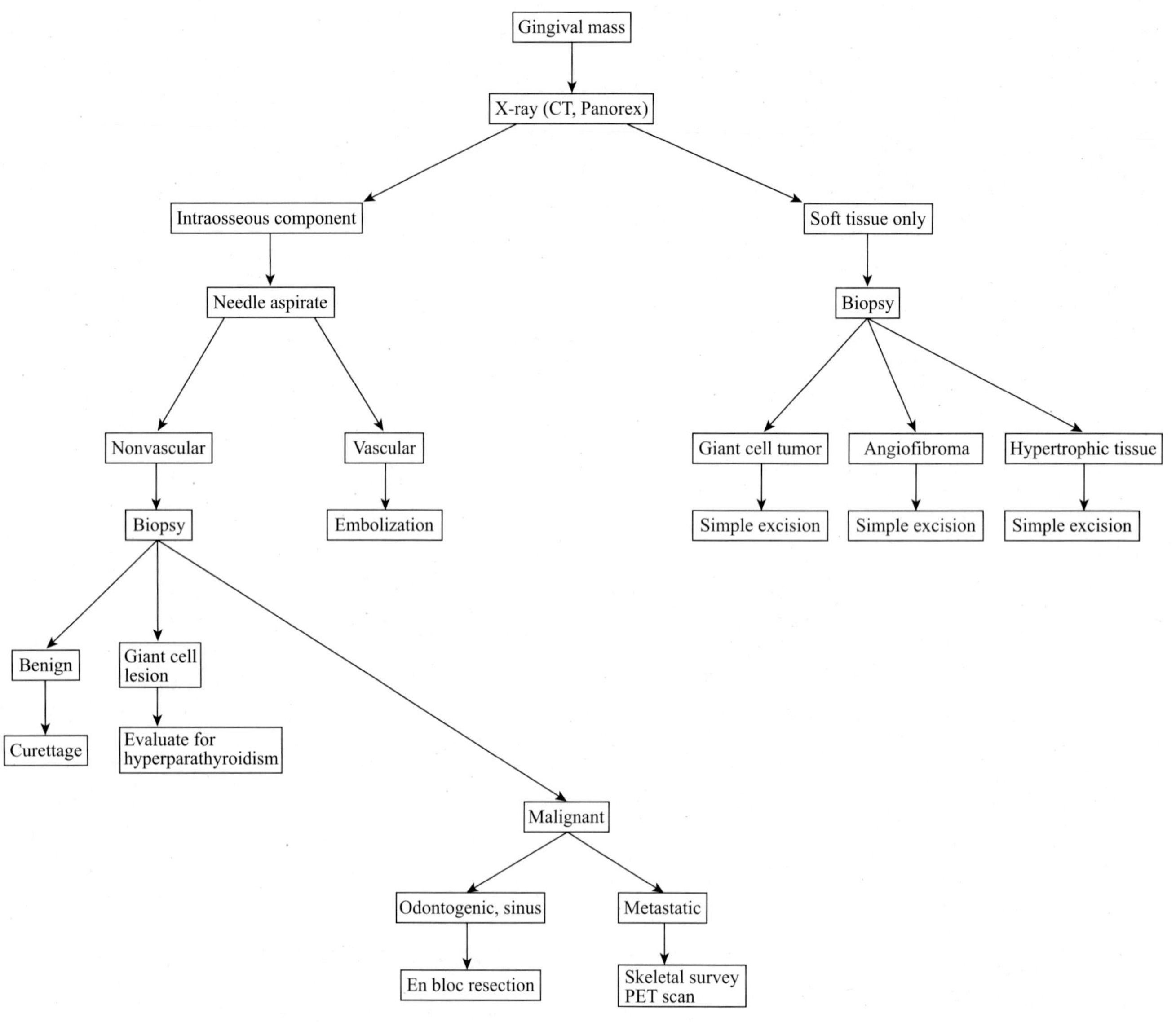

Management of Benign Oral Cavity Lesions

William Lawson

Oroantral Fistula

A permanent communication between the maxillary sinus and the oral cavity may result following the extraction of a maxillary bicuspid, or molar tooth. An attempt is often made at the time of the removal of the tooth to close a recognized perforation into the sinus by the dental surgeon, which may or may not be successful. Usually the communication goes unrecognized, and a permanent tract develops, with the patient presenting with a history of fluids draining through the nose while eating. One or several attempts at closure of the fistula ensue, which, again, may or may not be successful. The root cause of the fistula forming and persisting after an attempt has been made at repair is the presence of chronic maxillary sinus disease, which uses the tract for dependent drainage.

After a preliminary course of antral irrigations and antibiotic therapy, a computed tomography (CT) scan should be taken, which will generally reveal diffuse mucosal thickening, or total opacification of the maxillary sinus, often with adjacent disease in the ethmoid sinus. A foreign body from previous dental manipulation may also be identified in the sinus. It has been the author's experience that endoscopic sinus surgery directed at the middle meatus is insufficient to resolve the antral infection and permit sufficient removal of the irreversibly damaged mucosa necessary for the successful closure of the fistula.

The author favors an approach to the antrum through the canine fossa and the use of a buccal mucosa advancement flap to close the fistula (**Fig. 1.1**). The procedure consists of coring out the epithelium of the fistula tract with a no. 11 blade and curetting the granulation tissue present on

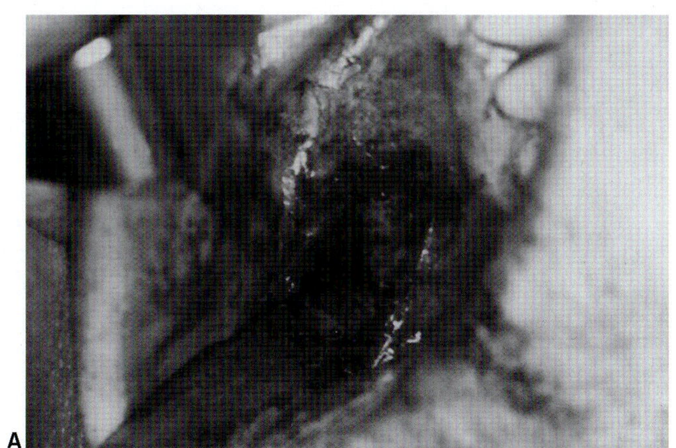
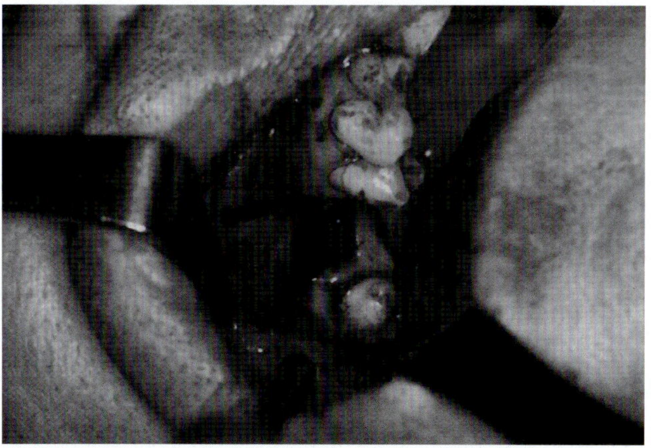
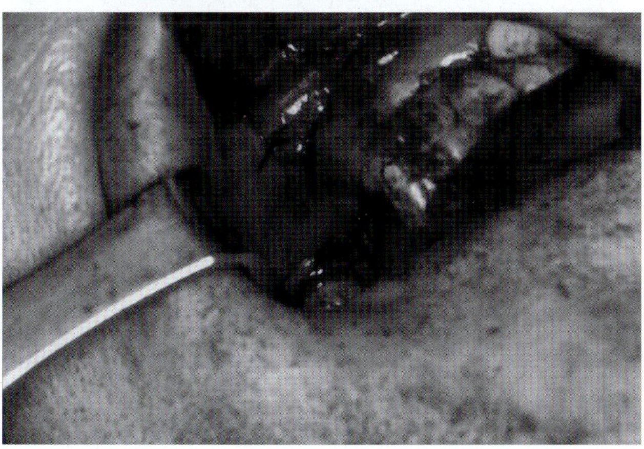

Fig. 1.1 (A–C) Repair of oroantral fistula.

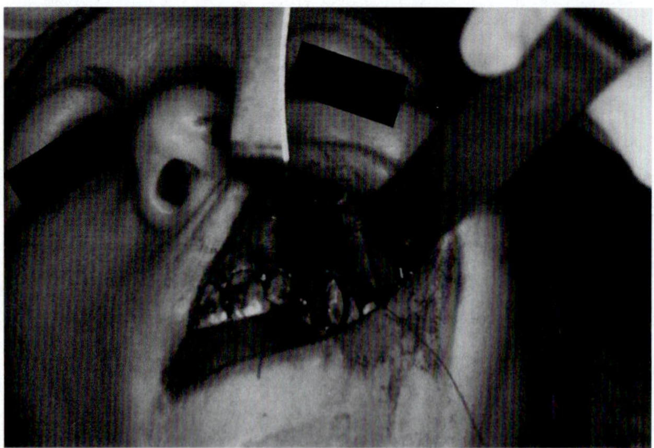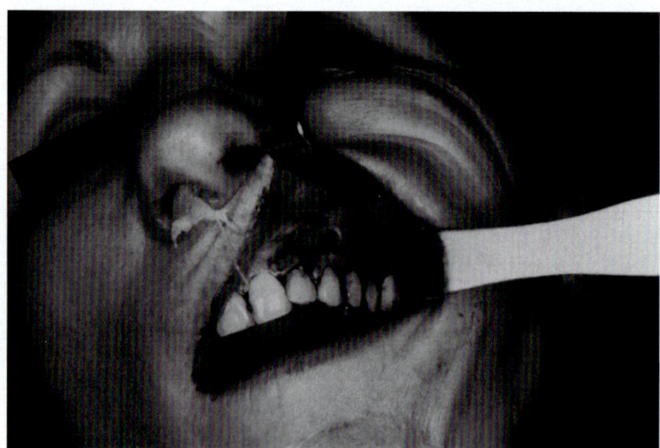

Fig. 1.2 (A, B) Excision of dentoalveolar lesion.

the adjacent bone. If one side of the fistula is not covered by bone, but by the root of an adjacent tooth, that tooth should be extracted; otherwise, complete epithelial closure over the defect will not be accomplished. Following this, two slightly divergent vertical incisions are made across the alveolus toward the cheek. A conventional transverse Caldwell-Luc incision would eliminate the ability to create this buccal advancement flap and should not be attempted. The flap to be elevated consists of mucoperiosteum and will not advance until the periosteum is incised on its undersurface with either a no. 15 blade or an iris scissors. The flap will then be freely mobile and is advanced and sutured to the palatal mucosal with interrupted 4–0 Vicryl sutures. Before the actual fistula closure is performed, another vertical incision is made along the long axis of the canine tooth, and the mucoperiosteum over the canine fossa is elevated. An opening into the antrum is made with a mallet and gouge and enlarged with a Kerrison-type punch forceps. This permits removal of the diseased mucosa directly and with endoscopic guidance. Another antrostomy is created in the inferior meatus, which facilitates cleansing of the sinus and will provide dependent drainage for the antrum. This incision is also closed with 4–0 Vicryl sutures. The key to oroantral fistula repair is removal of the diseased mucosa of the antrum, as a fistula does not develop following dental extraction when a healthy maxillary sinus is present.

Dentoalveolar Lesions

In patients with disease involving the dental alveolus, by extension downward from a benign maxillary sinus tumor, or inflammatory lesion, or by growth upward of a dental cyst or tumor into the antrum, complete exposure of the lesion and secure closure of the incision cannot be accomplished by the standard transverse Caldwell-Luc incision. Excision of the lesion will include removal of a portion of the alveolus and the lateral wall of the

antrum. An incision not supported by bone invites the postoperative formation of a fistula. If the extraction of a tooth is necessary, the opening in the alveolus cannot be closed primarily with such an incision. The use of a gingival flap obviates these difficulties (**Fig. 1.2**). This is created by incising the attached gingival with a no. 15 blade along the necks of the posterior maxillary teeth in the gingival sulcus. Posteriorly, the incision is carried over the maxillary tuberosity. Anteriorly, a vertical incision is made in the long axis of the canine tooth. Using a Freer elevator, the entire gingival and alveolar mucosa and the mucoperiosteum over the lateral wall of the maxillary sinus are elevated readily. The bone over the lesion is removed to expose its extent. The lateral wall of the antrum adjacent to it is also removed sufficiently to determine the degree of involvement of the sinus. The lesion is then removed, and the bone about it is curetted. The gingival flap is returned and fixed with interdental sutures of 4–0 Vicryl. If the removal of a single or multiple teeth has been necessary, relaxing incisions are made similar to those described in the previous section, and the buccal mucosa is advanced and sutured to the palatal soft tissues. If the antral mucosa is healthy, it is left undisturbed, and a small temporary antrostomy is made in the inferior meatus for dependent drainage. This approach provides wide access for removal of alveolar-antral lesions and permits the primary closure of the incisions about the resulting defect.

Hyperplastic Lesions

Giant Cell Granuloma

These lesions occur in the oral cavity on the gingiva and appear predominantly as broad-based reddish masses extending along the necks of several teeth. Occasionally, they are seen on the edentulous alveolus. They represent hyperplastic reparative growths composed of giant cells in a highly vascular stroma. Although histologically identical to the centrally occurring giant cell granuloma and tumor, they are self-limited and less destructive than their intraosseous counterparts and are not associated with hyperparathyroidism. These are completely benign soft tissue lesions, although they may cause minor bone erosion by compression. Treatment is by simple excision with a sickle knife (no. 12 blade), removing the marginal gingiva and the interdental papillae, with healing by secondary intention. With recurrent lesions, it may be necessary to extract the involved teeth, as the granuloma may be present in the periodontal membrane space. Clinically, it must be differentiated from the pregnancy tumor, which has an identical appearance and develops in response to elevated estrogen levels in gravid women. Many of these lesions spontaneously involute postpartum. However, surgery, which should be performed in the second trimester, may be indicated if the lesion persistently bleeds.

Palatal Papillary Hyperplasia

This inflammatory lesion develops on the hard palate of full denture wearers and presents as a large, but well-circumscribed, irregularly elevated papillary and nodular area (**Fig. 1.3**). The etiology is irritation by a poor-fitting denture, often exacerbated by secondary candidiasis. Should the lesion become friable and bleed, it can be removed by scalpel or electrocautery after preliminary treatment with an antifungal agent. The resection should not involve the periosteum of the hard palate, as its removal along with the lesion only results in prolonged healing. Prevention of recurrences is by the construction of a well-fitting new denture. The presence of a papillary

lesion on the hard palate of a nonedentulous person must be considered a neoplasm, and the patient should undergo incisional biopsy. The pathology will dictate the nature and extent of the subsequent treatment.

Epulis Fissuratum

This lesion develops at the periphery of a denture, with a fold of hypertrophic mucosa forming on one or on both sides of a denture flange (**Fig. 1.4**). The underlying edentulous alveolus is often atrophic, permitting motion of the denture and inciting the inflammatory mucosal response. Treatment is by excision of the excessive folds of mucosa with electrocautery after the infiltration of local anesthesia. The fabrication of a new full denture with a good soft tissue seal along the borders eliminates recurrence.

Hyperkeratotic Lesions

White Lesions

This is a global term that refers to areas in the oral cavity that appear white in color and are texturally rougher. Their appearance does not permit accurate assessment of the lesions with regard to the histologic changes that are present, which range from acanthosis, parakeratosis, and hyperkeratosis to dysplasia and invasive carcinoma. Most lesions have an identifiable irritative etiology, with genetically induced lesions being rare, and often having a cutaneous counterpart and a positive family history. The great majority of these lesions are benign; however, biopsy is essential to establish the correct diagnosis. Common sites of involvement are the floor of the mouth,

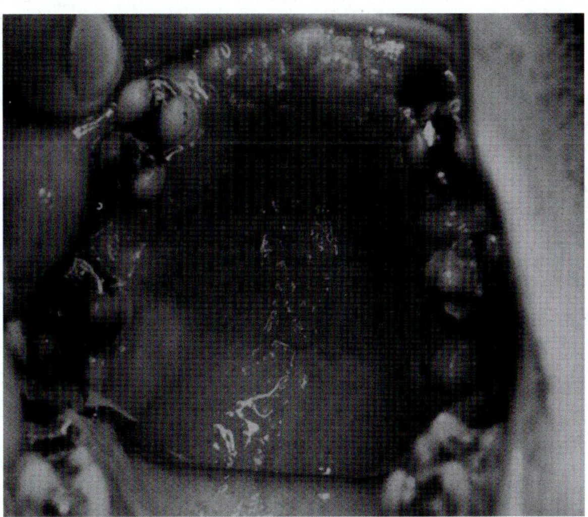

Fig. 1.3 Palatal papillary hyperplasia.

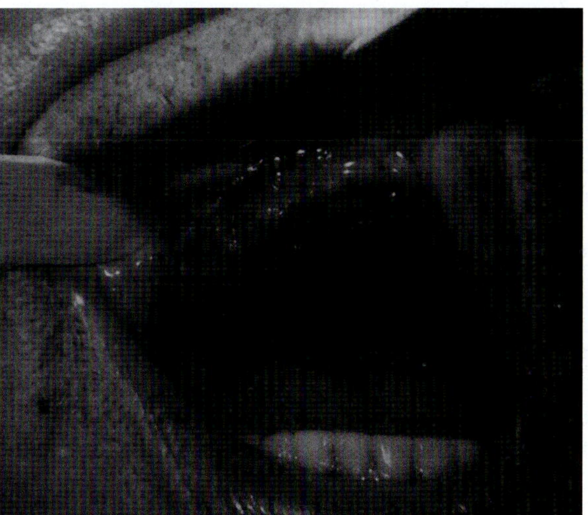

Fig. 1.4 Epulis fissuratum.

the ventral and lateral surfaces of the tongue, and the buccal mucosa. Small lesions are treated by excisional biopsy. Multiple whitish areas are often present, and removal by mucosal stripping would result in widespread scarring. Laser ablation is also discouraged because of postoperative pain, scarring, and tissue destruction, which do not permit histologic evaluation. Many patients who are prone to the development of these lesions experience recurrences despite the elimination of the irritative cause. Without the presence of necrosis, ulceration, and erythroplastic changes, the great majority of these lesions are benign. Accordingly, the author favors biopsy of each lesion with a small cup forceps after the application of topical anesthesia. The surface character and distribution of the lesions are mapped out at the time of the initial visit for comparison with the findings on subsequent visits. Wide excision would be prompted by the presence of marked atypia (pleomorphism, hyperchromatism), or dysplasia (disordered maturation) of the epithelium. If only hyperplastic changes in the epithelium are found, the patient should be observed at regular intervals. A change in the character of the surface epithelium of the lesion, such as ulceration, or the development of pain is an indication for rebiopsy. If the biopsy reveals malignant transformation, surgery appropriate to the management of carcinoma at the anatomical site and stage must be performed. In general, experience with the topical use of retinoids has been discouraging, with some patients applying them only forming new hyperplastic lesions and even carcinomas. The efficacy of the use of systemic retinoids must be weighed against their potential hepatic toxicity.

Lichen Planus

Lichen planus is a cell-mediated immunologic disorder of the oral mucosa and skin. It commonly appears on the buccal mucosa and tongue, but it may also involve the lips, gingiva, and floor of the mouth. These lesions are asymptomatic and commonly present with a reticular pattern of fine white lines (striae of Wickham). They may spontaneously regress and then recur. They are often biopsied for differentiation from other hyperkeratotic lesions. Histologically, they are characterized by hyperkeratosis, parakeratosis, elongation of the rete pegs, and necrosis and vascularization of the basal cell layer. The latter results in the formation of Civatte bodies (shrunken cells with pyknotic nuclei). Attempts at obliteration of these lesions by laser, cryotherapy, or excision fail because of recurrence. Similarly, regression induced by topical retinoids is short-lived, as the lesions reappear at the cessation of therapy. Consequently, treatment and removal of these lesions are discouraged.

There is an erosive, or bullous, form of lichen planus in which massive degeneration of the basal layer occurs, resulting in the separation of the epithelium from the submucosa. These lesions are painful, causing the patient to seek treatment. Healing may be achieved by the intralesion injection of triamcinolone, or low-dose oral steroid therapy (prednisone 20 mg). Biopsy and immunofluorescence studies are of value in differentiating these lesions from other bullous disorders.

Despite controversy that has raged for many years regarding the association of lichen planus with squamous cell carcinoma, long-term studies have shown the incidence (1.5%) is equal to that of leukoplakia and justifies its designation as a premalignant lesion. Consequently, patients with lichen planus should be routinely reexamined, and any change in the lesion should be biopsied for the presence of squamous cell carcinoma. The most common sites of transformation are the tongue, buccal mucosa, and alveolus.

Papillary Lesions

A spectrum of proliferative epithelial lesions occurs in the oral cavity and on the lips. Simple squamous papillomas generally have a narrow pedicle and often occur on the palate and tongue, the common sites of irritation. Simple excision is generally curative. The majority of oral cavity papillomas are produced by human papillomavirus, especially subtypes 6 and 11, and clinically are often broad based and multiple. Simple excision may result in a recurrence because of their viral etiology, and it is recommended that they be excised and the operative bed be electrocauterized, then left to heal by secondary intention. Particularly troublesome are the viral papillomas that are sexually transmitted and produce multiple, flat, wartlike lesions of the lip and oral cavity, termed condyloma acuminatum (**Fig. 1.5**). A variety of methods have been

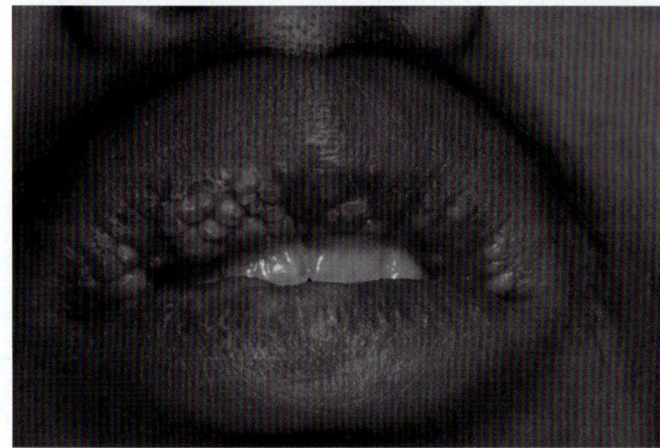

Fig. 1.5 Condyloma acuminatum.

employed for their removal, including carbon dioxide laser surgery, cryosurgery, and surgical excision, as well as chemical agents (e.g., podophyllin, 5-fluorouracil). The author has found electrocautery of individual lesions after the infiltration of a local anesthetic to the area to be highly curative and nondeforming. It is important to identify and treat the sexual partner to prevent recurrence and also to test the patient for any other sexually transmitted disease.

Vascular Lesions

Hemangiomas and Lymphangiomas

These lesions consist of simple endothelial lined spaces. Hemangiomas are subclassified into capillary and cavernous types, with the former containing capillary-sized vessels and the latter enlarged vascular lakes. Lymphangiomas are histologically similar but contain clear fluid (lymph). Hemangiomas can arise anywhere in the oral cavity, be simple or multiple, and may vary in size widely. Lymphangiomas show a predilection for the tongue and may be mixed with hemangiomatous elements. These lesions are present at birth and grow with the individual, although at highly different rates. Superficial hemangiomas at such sites as the lip, tongue, and buccal mucosa can be diagnosed by compressing the lesion with a glass slide and observing blanching. Bleeding upon biopsy can usually be controlled by pressure or suture ligatures, as these lesions are low-pressure systems. Preliminary biopsy is not necessary for small, superficial hemangiomas, with total excision performed. The presence of pulsations, or extensive soft tissue involvement, should alert the clinician to the occurrence of an arteriovenous malformation, which requires imaging studies to determine its extent and accordingly the management. Lesions arising on the mucosa over the jaws should undergo CT scanning to eliminate the possibility of an intraosseous component. These central lesions are capable of profuse hemorrhage, which may require radical management for control.

Treatment decision making involves consideration of the site, size, type, and growth history of the lesion to minimize operative morbidity. Small hemangiomas can be excised with primary repair of the defect. Larger lesions, especially those involving the tongue, may incur disabling consequences on attempting total removal, and alternative therapy, including intravascular embolization and the use of sclerosing solutions, should be considered.

Kaposi's Sarcoma

Kaposi's sarcoma is a multicentric tumor involving the skin and oral cavity as well as lymph nodes and multiple organs. It is the most common oral neoplasm in human immunodeficiency virus (HIV) seropositive individuals, and its presence is diagnostic of acquired immunodeficiency syndrome (AIDS). The lesions typically appear on the posterior hard palate, followed infrequently by the gingiva. They begin as multiple irregular red macules that eventually coalesce to form blue-purple nodules. These lesions are painless unless they ulcerate and become secondarily infected. The lesions do not blanch on compression and do not bleed on biopsy. Biopsy reveals spindle and endothelial cells surrounding small lumina interspersed with extravasated erythrocytes and hemosiderin deposits. Management is by the intralesional injection of vinblastine.

Cystic Lesions

Mucoceles and Ranulas

These cystlike lesions are the result of injury or obstruction of a minor salivary gland and accordingly are divided into two types. The extravasation type is produced by traumatic laceration of a duct, which permits pooling of mucus in the submucosa with the formation of granulation tissue and fibrin. This lesion is most commonly seen on the lower lip. The mucous retention type is less common and is produced by duct blockage, salivary obstruction, and cystlike dilatation of the duct. This lesion forms in the floor of the mouth from trauma to the submaxillary or sublingual gland ducts, and is termed a ranula. Although these lesions may fluctuate in size, or even appear to disappear, they tend to progressively enlarge from continued trauma to the exposed areas.

The mucocele, which commonly occurs on the lower lip, is treated by total excision. This is best done by making an elliptical incision over the top of the swelling at right angles to the long axis of the lip. Removing an ellipse of tissue eliminates redundant mucosa and makes perforation into the lesion during resection less likely. Following excision, a linear closure with absorbable or permanent sutures is performed. Removal of the mucocele in this fashion leaves no cosmetic deformity. If it is excised in the long axis of the lip, a noticeable depression will occur, so this method of removal should be avoided. The ranula is a more challenging lesion to remove, as it may grow greatly in size, with the larger lesions not only expanding in the submucosal tissues of the floor of the mouth but extending vertically through the mylohyoid muscle into the submandibular space, creating the so-called plunging ranula. Ranulas should be excised when they are small, as they tend to continue to grow and may involve both Wharton's duct and the lingual nerve, with injury to these structures possible when dissecting out the cyst sac. Marsupialization has been advocated for larger lesions, which tend to be adherent to the contiguous soft tissues in the floor of the mouth. This is accomplished by excising an ellipse of soft tissue over the height of the mass, which consists of the combined floor of mouth mucosa, and cyst lining and sewing the cut margins together circumferentially. In the author"s experience, this is often unsuccessful and only leads to further recurrence and expansion. Accordingly, an attempt should be made primarily to excise the ranula. This is done under general anesthesia with naso-endotracheal intubation, with the dissection performed using magnification to visualize the Wharton duct and the lingual nerve to prevent their injury. The incision is then closed primarily with absorbable 4–0 sutures. With recurrent and plunging ranulas, it may be necessary to excise the sublingual gland and its duct, which is often the main source of the pathology. Ranulas demonstrated on CT scan to have extension through the mylohyoid muscle into the submaxillary space may require a cutaneous incision to mobilize and remove the deep component of the lesion.

Granulomatous Lesions

Cheilitis Granulomatosis

This disorder is characterized by diffuse nontender enlargement of one or both lips (**Fig. 1.6**). The lip swelling is progressive and does not fluctuate in size, which differentiates it from angioneurotic edema of allergic origin. It is seen in association with facial paralysis and fissured tongue as part of the Melkersson-Rosenthal syndrome. It may appear as an isolated finding or accompany other oral or facial lesions, in patients with sarcoidosis, or inflamma-

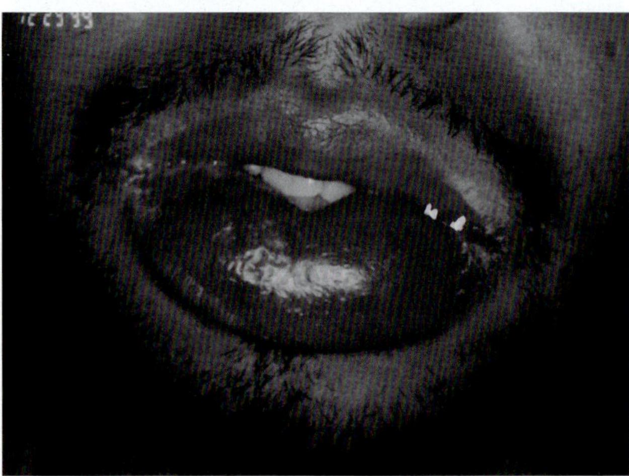

Fig. 1.6 Cheilitis granulomatosis.

tory bowel disease. Biopsy will reveal the presence of noncaseating granulomas containing giant cells, which are negative for the presence of microorganisms with specialized stains. The lip enlargement may progress to the point of extreme cosmetic deformity and functional impairment. Surgical excision requires transverse reduction in the entire lip, which is often followed by reenlargement by the continued activity of the inflammatory process. Accordingly, surgery should not be considered the primary method of management. Injection of triamcinolone directly into the lip produces reduction in its size, which persists for varying periods of time. The administration of clofazimine (100 mg daily for 6 months) has been found useful in steroid-resistant cases. Surgical incision should be considered only in refractory cases.

Suggested Reading

Chow JM, Skolnick EM. "Nonsquamous tumors of the oral cavity" in Nonsquamous Tumors of the Head and Neck I. Otolaryngologic Clinic of North America 1986;19(3):573–607.

Laskaris G. Color Atlas of Oral Diseases. 2nd ed. New York: Thieme Medical Publishers; 1994.

Lian TS. Benign tumors and tumor-like lesions of the oral cavity. In: Cummings CR et al, eds. Otolaryngology: Head and Neck Surgery. 4th ed. St. Louis: Mosby Elsevier; 2005: 1571–1577.

Decision tree for snoring treatment

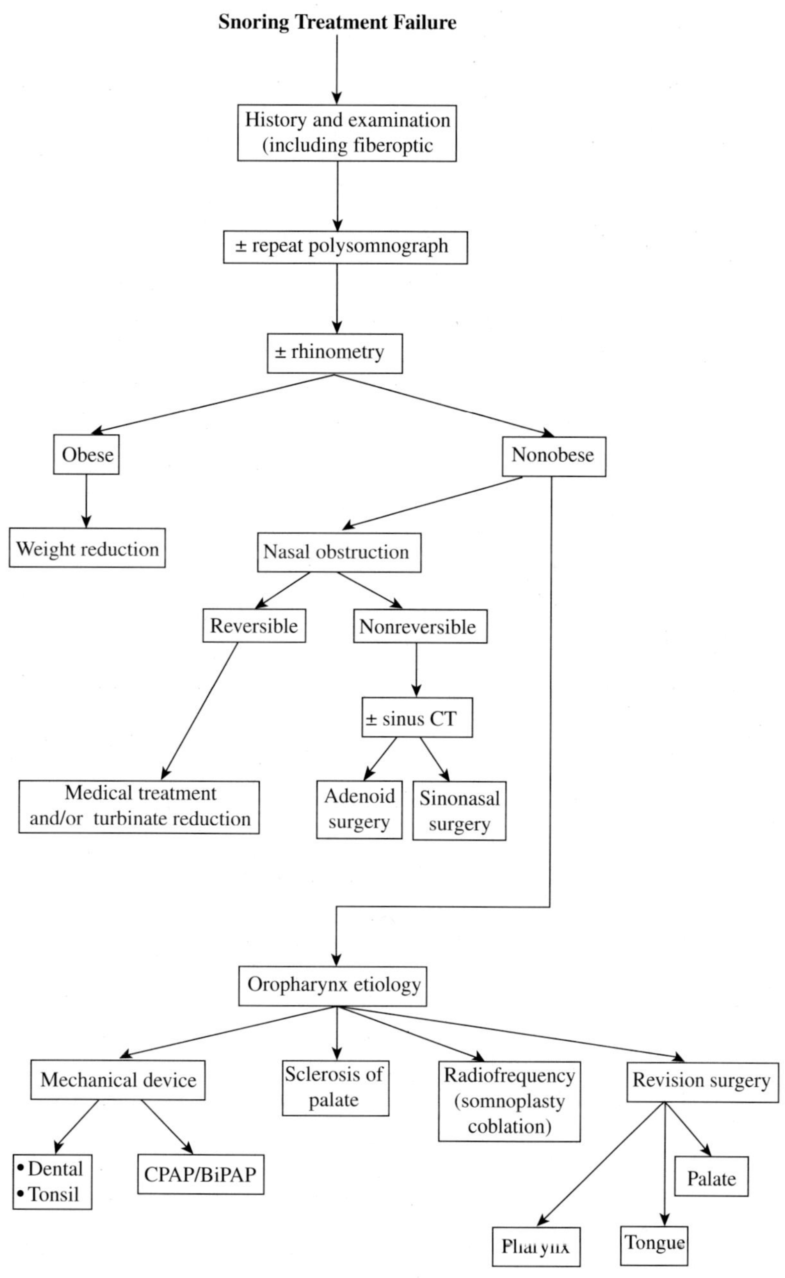

Decision tree for sleep apnea treatment

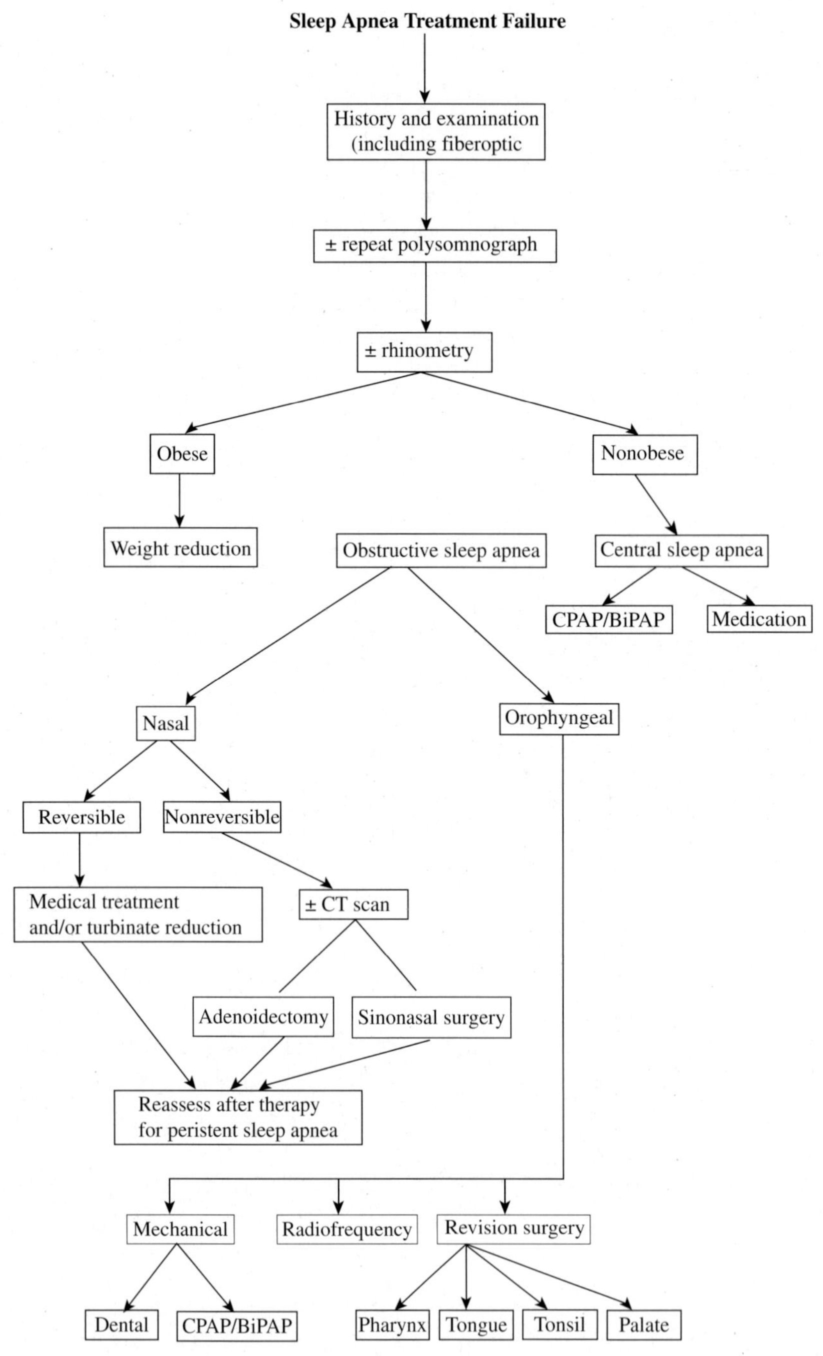

Revision Surgery for Snoring and Sleep Apnea

Larry Shemen

The evaluation and treatment for snoring and sleep apnea oftentime overlap. Both require a complete history and physical examination of the head and neck. Both require assessment with fiberoptic nasopharyngolaryngoscopy and polysomnography. Both may be treated with continuous positive airway pressure (CPAP), uvulopalatopharyngoplasty (UPPP), or tracheotomy. However, there is a great distinction between these two conditions. Snoring is largely of social concern, whereas sleep apnea has comorbidities that may be life threatening and warrants medical, if not surgical, treatment. The reasons why a given treatment may initially fail in treating either condition relate to errors in diagnosis, error in selection of treatment, or inadequate or improper treatment. Oftentimes, treatment of one site, such as the oropharynx, will improve but not eliminate the snoring or sleep apnea. However, if a second source of upper airways obstruction, such as the nasopharynx occluded with adenoid tissue, is identified and addressed at revision surgery, the snoring or sleep apnea may be further reduced or eliminated. Each of these issues will be addressed in the ensuing discussion.

A Clinical Evaluation

A detailed history relating to the upper airways is crucial in determining the diagnosis. One must inquire as to the presence or absence of snoring, alteration or cessation of breathing (sleep apnea), daytime somnolence, morning headaches, difficulty concentrating at work, and feeling tired or unrested upon awakening. The presence of nocturnal myoclonus, insomnia, narcolepsy (cataplexy, sleep paralysis, hypnogogic hallucinations), or short latency of sleep onset must be excluded. Nasal obstruction, congestion, allergies, and chronic sinusitis must be similarly questioned. The use of sedatives, sedating antihistamines, tranquilizers, and alcohol, especially prior to bedtime, must be questioned and if employed, must be eliminated. Any prior surgery of the upper aerodigestive tract, including rhinoplasty, tonsillectomy, or adenoidectomy, should be noted. A history of hypertension or arrhythmias should be questioned.

The general examination must include an evaluation of the general habitus of the patient, specifically regarding obesity. The nose must be examined to assess the septum and turbinates, rhinorrhea, and/or the presence of sinusitis. The nasal valve area should be assessed for collapse, particularly if the patient has undergone reduction rhinoplasty. The nasopharynx must be examined to rule out any adenoid enlargement, congenital obstruction, or tumors. The oral cavity and oropharynx must be assessed with specific attention to the size of the tongue, tonsils, uvula, and palate, and any redundancy or hypertrophy or tumors should be noted. The hypopharynx and larynx must be similarly evaluated to exclude any obstruction, such as lingual tonsil hypertrophy, obstructing vallecular cyst, or laryngeal tumor.

Nasopharyngolaryngoscopy is invaluable in analyzing the contributions to snoring or sleep apnea by the nasopharynx, soft palate, uvula, lateral pharyngeal walls, tonsils, lingual tonsils, or tongue. The Müeller maneuver consists of having the patient snore while the endoscope is in place and the anatomy can be viewed. The modified Müeller maneuver pertains to bending the endoscope forward to attempt to eliminate the palatal contribution to the obstruction. This technique is useful in predicting the outcome of UPPP.[1]

Laboratory Studies

Polysomnography is indispensable and mandatory in the assessment of patients with snoring and/or sleep apnea. The sleep laboratory must provide the apnea index and respiratory distress index. It is vital that the sleep laboratory provide results relating to the presence, frequency, loudness, and source of the snoring. The distinction between central, mixed, and obstructive sleep apnea must be made. Other conditions such as nocturnal myoclonus must be excluded. Prior to undergoing polysomnography, the patient must not take any sedatives, tranquilizers, alcohol, or sedating antihistamines for 48 hours, as these will corrupt the data.

Acoustic rhinometry may be used to assess the nasal resistance to airflow and the nasal volume. These tests are done before and after the instillation of a decongestant, thus permitting the distinction between reversible versus structural abnormalities causing the obstruction. Acoustic pharyngometry has been used to assess the resistance at the level of the palate and pharynx. Cephalometric and orthognathic measurements may be necessary if there is malocclusion or a small mandible and mandibular advancement is contemplated.

Once a patient fails a given modality of treatment, the assessment should include a nasal, nasopharyngeal, and oropharyngeal examination with the fiberoptic endoscope. Polysomnography, rhinometry, and pharyngometry may be repeated to evaluate if the patient has had any response to the prior treatment. If necessary, speech evaluation by a speech therapist should be conducted if there is any velopharyngeal incompetence or nasopharyngeal stenosis.

Medical Treatment

Allergic rhinitis or vasomotor rhinitis may cause significant airway obstruction, resulting in a negative nasopharyngeal pressure. This in turn promotes snoring, as the patient is forced to breathe transorally, and the elongated uvula is forced to vibrate. These conditions may be treated with the appropriate medicine, such as nasal steroids, systemic or topical antihistamines, and/or decongestants. Allergen avoidance and immunotherapy are also invaluable for the allergic patient. If all these measures fail to control rhinitis, turbinate injection may be indicated.

The mechanical treatment for snoring and sleep apnea is largely confined to CPAP and bilevel positive airway pressure (BiPAP). Both of these types of devices administer positive pressure so that the airway does not collapse and the obstruction is relieved. The amount of pressure applied is determined at polysomnography and may be titrated. Either of these devices may fail because of poor compliance or inability of the patient to wear the apparatus. For example, if the patient has a markedly S-shaped septal deviation, the positive pressure may cause significant discomfort, making the device intolerable. A mask that covers the nose and mouth may succeed in such cases. Other sources of failure are inadequate pressure, intolerable pressure, or excessive dryness. These settings are adjustable by the respiratory therapist. Other mechanical treatments include dental devices that are designed to thrust the jaw and tongue anteriorly and open the upper airway in this fashion. These devices may fail because of poor fitting or dental or periodontal disease, or if they cause temporomandibular joint dysfunction associated with pain.[2] Nasal devices are available that stent the nasal alae either internally or externally. These devices are useful only for nasal valvular collapse.

A more recent innovation in the nonsurgical treatment of snoring involves the injection of a sclerosing agent, such as sodium tetradechol sulfate (Sotradecol, Elkins-Sinn, Inc., Cherry Hill, NJ), commonly used for varicose veins, into the uvula and palate.[3] The goal of the injection is to cause contraction and superior retraction of the uvula. This treatment may fail if the uvula and inferior edge of the soft palate are not sufficiently retracted. Additional sclerosing agent may have to be injected. One should wait at least 1 month prior to reinjection, as the development of sclerosis and retraction may be prolonged. Long-term follow-up for this procedure is lacking.

Surgical Treatment

Surgical Treatment of the Nose for Snoring and Sleep Apnea

Septum

The deviated nasal septum is the most common nasal cause of upper airway resistance.[4] It may be corrected by submucous resection or nasoseptal reconstruction.[5]

Turbinates

Hypertrophied turbinates may be surgically reduced by one of several methods. A radiofrequency probe may be applied in either the unipolar or bipolar technique. The laser may alternatively be used to reduce the volume and reactiveness of the nasal mucosa. Coblation and somnoplasty are newer techniques that similarly reduce the turbinate volume. The turbinate bone and a portion of the mucosa may be reduced or laterally displaced (outfractured) in the operating room.

Revision Surgery of the Nose for Snoring and Sleep Apnea

It is not unusual for the septum to return to its deviated position even after successful initial surgery. The cartilage has memory and will return to its prior position unless the "spring" is broken. This can be accomplished either at the initial procedure or secondarily by either scoring or morselizing the cartilage. Silastic stents may be used to support the septum and ensure that it heals in a straight vertical position. Caution should be taken when doing revision septal surgery to avoid perforating the mucoperichondrium on both sides at the same location, as this will lead to a permanent perforation. This complication is more often encountered following revision septal surgery.

Revision turbinate reduction is, similarly, not an unusual procedure. Caution must be exercised during revision surgery not to overdo the reduction; otherwise, atrophic rhinitis will ensue. One must also be cautious when trimming the turbinates posteriorly to avoid injuring the sphenopalatine vessels and causing profuse intraoperative and postoperative epistaxis. Synechiae may develop between the septum and turbinates; these must be divided, as they can cause significant obstruction when debris is accumulated.

Surgical Treatment of the Nasopharynx for Relief of Upper Airway Obstruction

The most common nasopharyngeal cause of upper airway obstruction is adenoid hypertrophy. This can be treated with routine adenoidectomy. A newer innovation is the use of powered microshavers to remove the hypertrophied adenoid tissue. Complete or partial choanal atresia may cause upper airway obstruction. If membranous, this can be corrected with the laser with or without a stent. If bony, a palatal flap, drilling of the atretic plate, and stents may be necessary. There are several nasopharyngeal tumors that may cause upper airway obstruction. These must be biopsied and treated accordingly.

Revision Surgery of the Nasopharynx for Relief of Upper Airway Obstruction

Adenoid tissue may regrow, necessitating repeat adenoidectomy. Alternatively, adenoid tissue in the posterior choanae may have been missed during the initial surgery. Nasopharyngolaryngoscopy should therefore be routinely employed before any surgical procedure to relieve snoring/sleep apnea. The adenoid tissue in the posterior choanae may be removed using the nasal endoscopes and nasal forceps or the microdebrider (shaver). Choanal atresia may reform, secondary to scarring. As this usually consists of soft tissue, it can be removed using the laser.

Another problem encountered in revision nasopharyngeal surgery is the stenosed or scarred nasopharynx caused by aggressive initial adenoidectomy. Another etiologic factor for this condition may be when there is excessive resection of the soft palate that then becomes in contact with a de-epithelialized posterior nasopharyngeal wall and leads to scarification and stenosis. This may be corrected by using laser resection and steroid injections, posteriorly based pharyngeal mucosal flaps, free mucosal grafts,[6] Silastic stents, or prosthetic appliances.

Surgical Treatment of the Oropharynx for Relief of Upper Airway Obstruction

There are several surgical treatment options available for the relief of upper airway obstruction caused by the oropharyngeal tissues. The least invasive procedures involve applying a probe into the palate and uvula, which then causes volume reduction by cicatricial scarring. This may be performed with a radiofrequency unit with coated tips (sodium morrnuate; Ellman International, Inc., Hewlett, NY), somnoplasty (sodium tetradecylsulfate; Gyrus Medical, Maple Grove, MN), or coblation (ArthroCare Corp., Sunnyvale, CA).

The more invasive procedures involve resection of oropharyngeal tissues. Uvulectomy involves the removal of the uvula itself. Uvulopalatoplasty involves resection of the uvula and the redundant portion of the soft palate. In the technique espoused by Kamami, the uvula is reduced in size with the laser, and lateral trenches are made in the soft palate. This procedure could be repeated several times until the desired effect was accomplished.[7] An alternate approach is the partial resection of the soft palate and complete resection of the uvula in one stage. The more extensive procedure, favored when the tonsils are hypertrophied and contributing to the upper airway obstruction, is traditional UPPP with tonsillectomy.[8]

Revision Surgery of the Oropharynx for Relief of Upper Airway Obstruction

The overall success rate for laser-assisted uvulopalatoplasty (LAUP) in the treatment of snoring is 75 to 90%.[9] In the classic LAUP procedure, a "neo-uvula" is created, which can still vibrate and contribute to upper airway obstruction. The procedure was intended to be repeated several times, but one may opt, at revision, to convert to a full uvulopalatoplasty or traditional UPPP with tonsillectomy. The important factor is to limit the superior extension of the resection below the point of confluence of the muscles, so that velopharyngeal incompetence does not ensue.[10]

This problem may be encountered even when the entire uvula has been resected. In this case, an inadequate amount of soft palate was removed, and the goal of revision surgery is to remove additional palate while not causing velopharyngeal incompetence. Nasopharyngoscopy should be repeated prior to any further surgery, and the precise site of contact between the posterior palate and posterior pharyngeal wall should be noted. This site can be marked on the anterior palate with silver nitrate or with the laser itself. The resection can then be accurately and safely completed. The objective of the revision surgery is to resect the redundant palate while avoiding the junction of the levator palati, palatopharyngeus, and musculus uvulae (**Fig. 2.1**). Alternatively, if laser resection is unsuccessful, one may use one of the aforementioned techniques (injection, somnoplasty, coblation, etc.) to effect scarring of the palate and further retraction upward. The presence of adenoid tissue and the contribution of tonsillar tissue to obstruction should be noted and, if present, should be removed.

Scarring at the apex of the resection, on the posterior and lateral aspects, may narrow the vault of the remaining

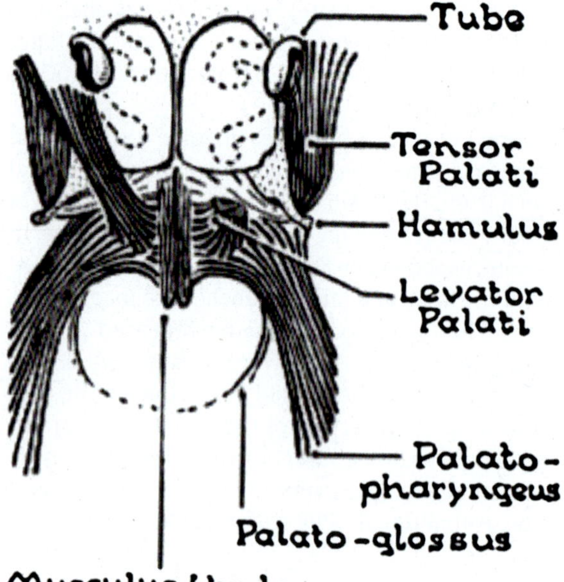

Fig. 2.1 The muscles of the soft palate—five on each side.

soft palate so that the opening into the nasopharynx is limited, and snoring resumes once again. Mucosal flaps may be necessary to enlarge the diameter of the nasopharynx. In the extreme case, which, fortunately, occurs rarely, consultation with a prosthodontist should be made, and a prosthesis with a stent should be worn, to maintain patency into the nasopharynx.

The opposite problem, namely, an overly patent oropharynx, may result in rhinolalia and regurgitation of fluids and/or solids into the nasopharynx and nose. This can be repaired with a superiorly based pharyngeal flap that is inset into the palate. Alternatively, the soft palate can be lengthened using cleft palate techniques.

Surgical Treatment of the Tongue for Snoring and Sleep Apnea

The oral or base of the tongue may be a major factor in snoring/sleep apnea. This can be seen on inspection or confirmed with cephalometric studies or acoustic pharyngometry. Causes of macroglossia should be ruled out. The large tongue will be retrodisplaced during sleep and will cause oropharyngeal obstruction.

The surgical correction for the enlarged tongue consists of measures that either suspend or reduce the volume of the tongue. The tongue may be resuspended by suturing it with a circumferential stitch through a drilled pivot point at the mandibular tubercle. Alternatively, the block of mandibular bone to which the genioglossus attaches (at the tubercle) may be retracted anteriorly. The volume of the tongue may be reduced with a wedge resection using the laser or radiofrequency. Somnoplasty or coblation may be considered, but no conclusive series has yet been reported at the time this chapter was written.

Revision Surgery of the Tongue and Tongue Base for Snoring and Sleep Apnea

The suture technique for tongue suspension may fail as the tissues become lax around the suture. Potentially, the wire suspension could be repeated, but an alternate technique would probably better suit the patient. Similarly, the genial tubercle suspension may weaken with time as the tissues become lax. The wedge resection of the base of the tongue may be repeated several times. Care, however, should be taken not to injure the lingual artery as one extends the incision laterally.

Mandibular and/or maxillary advancement procedures may be considered in the patient who has failed all the aforementioned techniques. Oral surgical and orthodontic consultations should be obtained.

Tracheal Surgery

Tracheotomy may be considered as the penultimate procedure when all other procedures have failed, or it may be the first procedure to consider in the obese, pickwickian patient in whom other procedures would be inadequate. The conventional tracheotomy tube or the Montgomery angled tube may be employed. Either tube will work satisfactorily, but patients must be monitored in a unit bed overnight and should have a suction machine at home and instruction with home care upon discharge.

References

1. Sher AE, Thorpy MJ, Spielman AJ, et al. Predictive value of Müller maneuver in selection of patients for UPPP. Laryngoscope 1985;95:1483–1487.
2. Miyazaki S. Prosthetic devices in the treatment of obstructive sleep apnea. Oper Tech Otolaryngol Head Neck Surg 1991;2:96–99.
3. Brietzke SE, Mair EA. Injection snoreplasty: how to treat snoring without all the pain and expense. Otolaryngol Head Neck Surg 2001;124:503–510.
4. Papsidero MJ. The role of nasal obstruction in obstructive sleep apnea syndrome. Ear Nose Throat J 1993;72:82–84.
5. Ellis PD, Harries ML, Ffowcs-Williams JE, et al. The relief of snoring by nasal surgery. Clin Otolaryngol 1992;17:525–527.
6. Chabolle F, Biacabe B, Sequert C, et al. Treatment of velopharyngeal stenosis after pharyngotomy for chronic snoring. Ann Otolaryngol Chir Cervicofac 1995;112(7):324–329.

7. Kamami YV. Outpatient treatment of sleep apnea syndrome with CO_2 laser: laser-assisted UPPP. J Otolaryngol 1994;23:395–398.

8. Davis JA, Fine ED, Maniglia AJ. Uvulopalatopharyngoplasty for obstructive sleep apnea in adults: clinical correlation with polysomnographic results. Ear Nose Throat J 1993;72:63–66.

9. Cheng DS, Weng JC, Yang PW, et al. Carbon dioxide laser surgery for snoring. Otolaryngol Head Neck Surg 1998;118:486–489.

10. Fairbanks DNF. Uvulopalatopharyngoplasty: strategies for success and safety. Ear Nose Throat J 1993;72:46–51.

Decision tree for vocal process granulomata

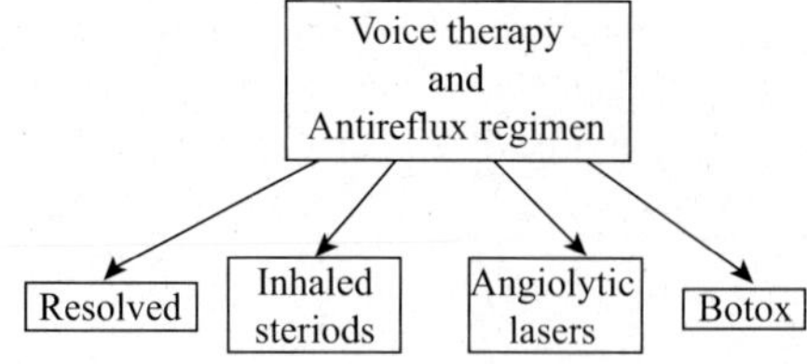

Decision tree for nodules and polyps

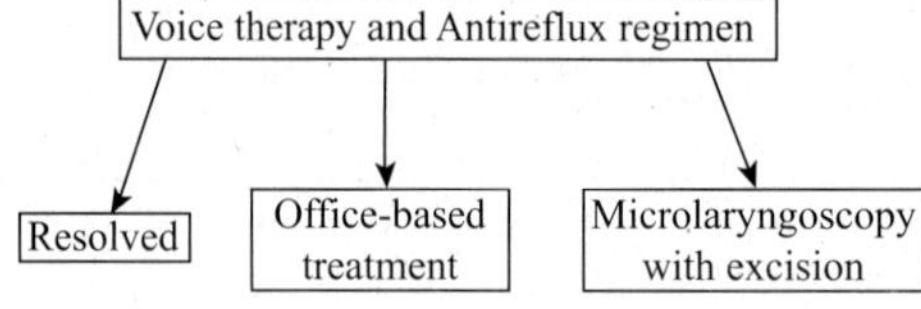

Recurrent Benign Glottic Lesions

Seth H. Dailey and *Marvin P. Fried*

Recurrence is either a real or an illusory phenomenon. A lesion may actually return after treatment, or it may simply not have been identified initially. The larynx has special properties that predispose it to benign recurrent lesions. First and foremost, adequate exposure to the larynx in an office setting has always been limited by lighting and by maneuverability of the examining instrument. Although mirror exam often provides a panoramic view with excellent color resolution, patient comfort limits the time available for evaluation. Furthermore, there is no permanent and reproducible record of the examination. Flexible fiberoptic examination allows for an extended examination and less interference with normal laryngeal biomechanics. However, the pixellated image produces worse resolution, and the color can be distorted. A permanent record is possible with this technology. Rigid stroboscopic examination with a rod-lens system permits excellent lighting, a digital recording medium, and the ability to examine subtle pathology at the glottal level. The increased cost, difficulty in interpreting the images, and controversy regarding the value of stroboscopy have influenced the availability of this tool. Nevertheless, it should be regarded as the method of choice in evaluating especially elusive or confusing laryngeal pathologies. Laryngeal lesions judged to be "recurrent" simply might not have been noticed or fully evaluated on primary inspection.

Second, some conditions are simply not common; as the saying goes, "The eye cannot see what the mind isn't prepared for." There is a background of considerable controversy and confusion regarding the etiology of such lesions as vocal process granulomata, glottal nodules and polyps, narrowing of the anterior larynx, and sulcus deformities.

With this background in mind, there are widely divergent strategies for treatment. When there are divergent strategies and lesions are uncommon, it is easy to see why a consensus viewpoint is a difficult goal and why lesions may not be treated optimally and may recur. Lastly, the presence of vocal trauma from overuse and the influence of laryngopharyngeal reflux disease may create an environment predisposing to recurrence.

Vocal Process Granuloma

Vocal process "contact ulcer" and vocal process granuloma (VPG) are most likely different manifestations of the same disease process. Although never definitely proven by serial biopsies and histologic examinations, a contact ulcer as described originally by Jackson in 1928, is a superficial erosion of the mucosa overlying the vocal process of the arytenoid cartilage.[1] This erosion turns into an aggregation of granulation tissue in the same place: a vocal process granuloma. It may occur unilaterally or bilaterally. An inciting event, whether iatrogenic (e.g., intubation) or spontaneous (e.g., vocal hyperfunction, violent cough) may cause the initial injury to the site. Aggravating factors are considered to be many, including chronic throat clearing, a low-pitched voice, a hard glottal attack, voice misuse in general, laryngopharyngeal reflux, smoking, and the chronic infection of the exposed cartilage. Therapies have thus been designed to address these aggravating factors. They include voice rest, voice therapy, medical management of allergy and sinus disease, medical management of laryngopharyngeal reflux, and botulinum toxin injection to reduce physical trauma on the arytenoids during adduction. A biopsy has been recommended to rule out malignancy. There is evidence to suggest that the disease may be from a perichondritis of the exposed arytenoid cartilage.

Clinical Evaluation

The clinical presentation of VPG can be a varied one. In his 40 years of clinical practice, Chevalier Jackson, who first described the entity in 1928, saw 127 cases.[1] He described it as a uni- or bilateral lesion that was best seen on abduction of the vocal folds. "Diffuse symptoms," as described by Ylitalo and Lindestad, are vocal fatigue, vocal discomfort, the need for excessive throat clearing, and the sensation of a foreign body in the throat.[2] Other common symptoms included hoarseness, uni- or bilateral throat pain, hemoptysis, dyspnea, and cough. This group of patients is often considered to be high-functioning professionally and to have a component of emotional stress responsible either for the initial damaging event or for its propagation. The vocal dysfunction can endanger the livelihoods of voice users. Additionally, the pain and general discomfort of an often-prolonged disease course, with the high likelihood of recurrence, can make this benign disease debilitating.

When lesions on the vocal process are noted early, they are called contact ulcers and are superficial erosions

Decision tree for anterior glottic webs

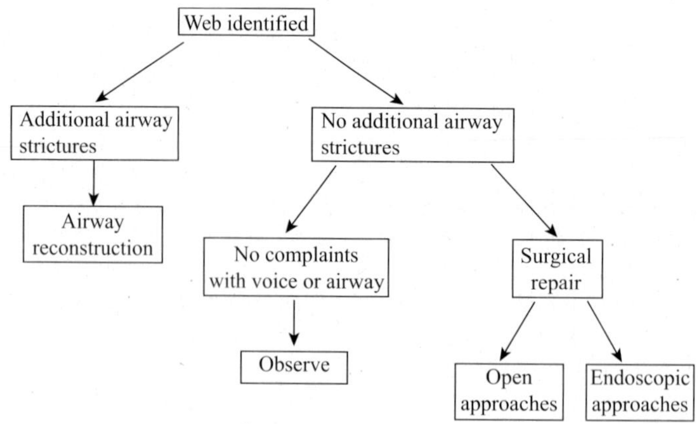

Decision tree for sulcus vocalis

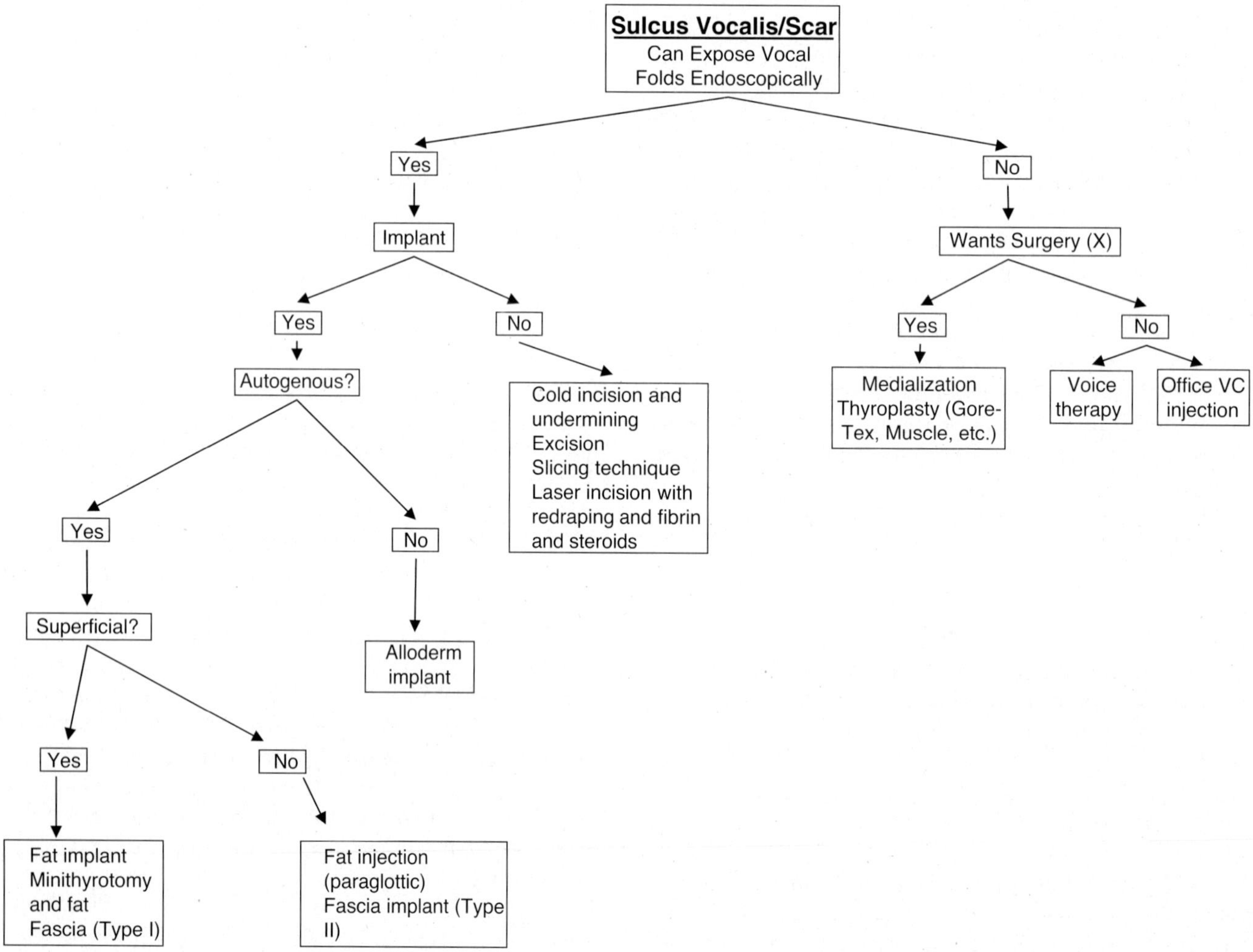

of the mucosa overlying the vocal process of the arytenoid. Even the original term *contact ulcer* speaks to its origin through physical trauma to the area. With time and aggravating factors, these contact ulcers may progress to VPG. Although there are no studies of serial histologic examinations of these ulcers as they progress, the clinical observation is that the originally superficial contact ulcers gradually enlarge as granulation tissue forms at the vocal process of the arytenoid cartilage and just superior to it. Ylitalo and Lindestad defined two different sites of the disease, one at the vocal process itself and the other posterosuperior to the vocal process.[2] They noted 25% and 75%, respectively. The development of reactive tissue at this site is presumed to be from the inflammatory cascade.

Etiology

Von Leden and Moore performed cinefluoroscopic examination of larynges during phonation of patients with VPG.[3] The laryngeal movements were assessed for the quality of motion of the arytenoids. These patients were noted to have a hard glottal attack and often what appeared to be significant force at the level of the arytenoids when using a low-pitched voice. Although no empiric data were derived from this study, the suggestion was made that a constant physical event was occurring at the level of the vocal process. Furthermore, the force involved might be responsible for the continued growth of the exuberant tissue at that site.

It has also been noted that men have the disorder more often than women. Hirano et al observed that the larynx achieves closure just above and posterior to the level of the true vocal folds, which implies that it is the arytenoids helping to achieve this closure.[4] The posterior glottic chink seen in women is a gap between the arytenoids during adduction. This gap may create a situation where the vocal processes simply do not make as much surface area contact as in men and may not be subject to the same irritating events. Additionally, women have higher pitched voices that do not require the adduction force of the arytenoids that von Leden and Moore described with low-pitched voices.[3]

Evidence to support the irritative etiology of this disease is also put forth by Ward et al, who described cinephotographic and cinefluoroscopic evidence that chronic throat clearing and repetitive coughing are violent and frequent events to the larynges of patients suffering from VPG.[5] The lead author invokes his own experience with laryngopharyngeal reflux (LPR) disease as a possible source for coughing and throat clearing. He claims that the constant irritation causes choking, violent coughing, laryngospasm, and overactive use of the larynx.

Fluoroscopic evidence of hiatal hernia with visualization of gastric contents into the larynx helped to confirm a source of inflammation. No prospective pH studies have been performed to date to compare data with his observations and techniques of evaluation. However, gastric acid as a possible cause of VPG was demonstrated by animal studies.

Delahunty and Cherry performed a study of application of gastric acid to the posterior vocal fold of two dogs.[6] Saliva was applied to the vocal fold of the control dog. After 29 applications, an appearance very similar to that of VPG developed, suggesting that the presence of gastric acid in the larynx may be responsible for VPG. There was no such appearance in the control dog. This is the only such study reported, and the significance of acid reflux has yet to be definitely proven either in its causality or in its perpetuation of the disease. The fact that the disease arises from chronic irritation is, however, difficult to ignore. Radiographic evaluation of the larynges of these patients suggests that the vocal processes themselves have been subjected to irritation.[7] Normal arytenoids are composed of hyaline cartilage in the body and elastic cartilage at the vocal process. Elastic cartilage does not normally calcify. Computed tomography (CT) scans of five patients with VPG showed calcification of the vocal processes of the arytenoids. This finding suggests that a chronic inflammatory process to that region had transformed it into an area capable of being calcified. In the diagnostic work-up and follow-up of patients with VPG, the use of a validated tool, such as the Voice Handicap Index (VHI), might provide longitudinal information regarding their presenting symptoms and improvement. Additionally, the routine use of esophageal probes to document LPR disease in scientific studies might validate the suspected role reflux plays in this entity. As the supposition of chronic irritation is an attractive and justifiable one, however, therapies should be directed toward the possible inciting agents.

Treatment

Jackson himself recommended absolute voice rest as the mainstay of primary therapy for these patients, under the assumption that vocal use or misuse perpetuates the disease.[1] Voice therapy has been explored as the primary therapy for VPG with mixed results. Ylitalo and Lindestad retrospectively reviewed 123 patients with VPG.[2] Twenty-nine out of 120 patients not cured by surgery used only voice rest as their therapy. The remaining 91 were patients who recurred after surgery or who chose voice therapy as their only treatment. At 6 months, the cure rates for these three groups of patients were 24%, 23%, and 29%. These results changed to 31%, 35%, and 51% at

12 months and 34%, 50%, and 58% at 18 months after voice therapy. This suggests that either voice therapy may take a long time to help heal the ulcer or simply that time will cure most of these lesions. Additionally, the recovery time was twice as long for patients who had undergone surgery as for patients who had not had surgery. It should be noted that the recurrence rate after surgery was 92% and that this was a retrospective study.

Peacher documented the progress of 70 patients with VPG to voice therapy and arrived at similar conclusions.[8] She found that with enough time (follow-up from 1 to 12 years), 65 of 70 patients healed completely and did not recur. Also, the patients who received surgical intervention of at least one operation took 6.5 months to heal compared with 2.5 months for those who had no operations. Peacher also observed the healing rate was the same for patients who received concentrated voice therapy versus those whose appointments were more spread out. Also, the more operations a patient underwent, the longer was the healing time. No antireflux therapy was administered.

Antireflux therapy has been supported as a mainstay for the treatment of VPG, but no studies have prospectively shown its efficacy. Although Delahunty and Cherry's dog study is suggestive, the role of LPR in the propagation of VPG remains to be seen.[6]

Botulinum toxin A (Botox) injection has been introduced with favorable initial results. Botox has been used in the thyroarytenoid muscle and lateral cricoarytenoid muscle to control the hyperdynamic state of the larynges.[9] Six patients were included in the study by Nasri et al, and all were cured of the VPG, with three patients having follow-up of less than 1 year. The treatment with Botox amounts to chemical voice therapy. Botox stops the hyperadduction of the arytenoids and decreases the force with which the vocal processes collide. It may be useful for refractory cases, as it is not without risks, which include a breathy voice, dysphagia, and reaction to the drug itself.

Topical inhalant steroid therapy with budesonide has been used for the treatment of VPG.[10] In a prospective study, 20 patients were given the topical inhalant 4 times a day (two puffs of 50 mcg), and a control group of 14 patients received voice rest, antacids, "anti-inflammatory agents," and oral corticosteroids. In the treatment group, the VPG disappeared completely in 19 of 20 patients (95%) at 1 year. In the control group, 6 of 14 patients (42.8%) were free of granuloma at 1 year. Microlaryngeal surgery was performed on the eight failures in this group, resulting in six successes out of eight in this subgroup. The only side effect was oral monoliasis in two patients who received the steroid inhalant. A success rate of 95% is indeed impressive and represents the highest reported rate.

Radiotherapy has been used for treatment failures with some success. Obvious disadvantages include induction of malignancy and exclusion of radiation therapy should the patient develop an upper aerodigestive tract cancer in the future. A typical radiation course would be a total of 12 Gy in four daily fractions using 6 MV photons centered on the larynx.[11] Radiation has been used to treat other inflammatory conditions, such as keloid scarring, heterotrophic bone formation, and conjunctival pterygia. These conditions are similar to VPG in that they are benign inflammatory processes that result in tissue proliferation. The suggestion of the authors is to first surgically debride the area and then radiate. Clearly, this approach is not suggested for all cases, but it can be considered in treatment failures.

A less invasive and repeatable intervention is now possible with office-based laser therapy. The 585 nm pulsed dye laser was designed to target vascular lesions of neonatal skin. It was initially applied to papillomatosis of the larynx under microlaryngoscopic conditions, as the fibrovascular cores of each frond are prime targets. The flexible fiber has been adapted to pass through the working channel of flexible transnasal endoscopes, allowing for application of the laser to laryngeal lesions with only topical anesthesia.[12] In a preliminary experience with this laser in 10 patients with VPG, Clyne et al showed complete resolution of VPG in 5 cases and partial response in 3 cases, with no change in 2.[13] Although the technology is sound, this approach should be viewed as adjunctive to voice therapy because control of vocal hyperfunction and reflux is likely to produce the most reliable long-term results.

Initial inciting events may be difficult to prevent, but aggravating factors may be addressed. The pathophysiology is still unclear, and no histologic studies have been performed to prove the development of VPG from contact ulcer. It should be noted that repeated resection either with the laser or with a "cold" technique does not eradicate the disease, and surgery as a sole therapy should be avoided. No randomized controlled trial of different treatments such as antireflux therapy with and without voice therapy has been undertaken because of the uncommon nature of the disease and the need for a multi-institutional trial. It may be true that no therapy would produce the same results as those practiced to date. However, considering the years of experience and the evidence that repetitive trauma and irritation cause VPG, and that antireflux management, voice therapy, inhaled steroids, Botox, and 585 nm pulsed dye laser have shown some efficacy, clinical trials to optimize care can be of significant value.

Nodules and Polyps

Etiology

Benign lesions of the glottis include cysts, nodules, and polyps (**Figs. 3.1, 3.2**). (Because keratin cysts are derived from epithelial rests and do not recur once excised, nodules

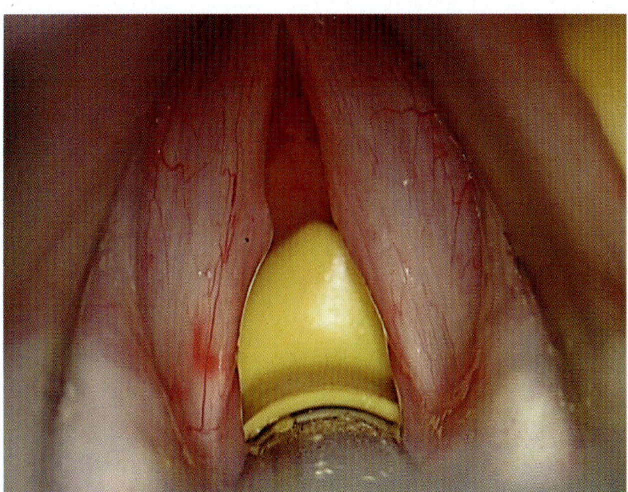

Fig. 3.1 Patient with bilateral vocal cord nodules that appear at the midmusculomembranous vocal cord.

and polyps are more central to the discussion of recurrent lesions. Nodules and polyps are believed to appear in the hyperkinetic larynx where microtraumatic events to the vocal folds do not heal within the extracellular matrix of the lamina propria. Furthermore, the dysfunctional state that the nodules and polyps create only exacerbates the hyperkinetic habits of these patients. In an effort to compensate for the dysfunctional voice, greater effort is exerted, and the condition worsens. Many authors have noted anecdotally an association between hyperkinetic voice use and nodules and polyps.[14–16] Few hard data exist, however, even from an epidemiological standpoint, to justify this association. More recent examinations of histologic sections, however, point to microtrauma of the vocal folds as the central culprit, confirming the suspicion

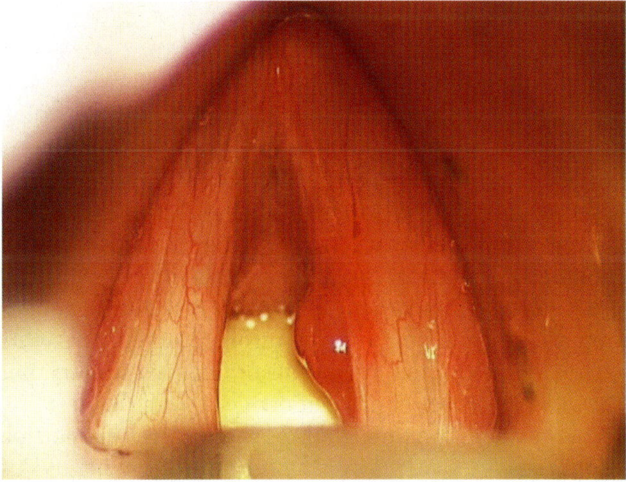

Fig. 3.2 Patient with a large right vocal cord polyp, which causes a very breathy voice and chaotic vibration.

that overactivity may be at the root of these benign growths.[17]

G. E. Arnold observed that nodules and polyps were more common in patients who used their voices extensively.[18] Moreover, he described predisposing, precipitating, and aggravating causes. Predisposing causes included an athletic body type, a "personality structure" that was "vociferous and aggressive," and often included a misshapen larynx. Arnold made the comparison of glottic polyps to nasal polyps, where hyperplastic nasal mucosa was noted in athletic patients and ozena was noted in "asthenic" individuals. This observation was anecdotal and did not necessarily imply causality. Laryngeal changes that Arnold cited were asymmetry, a poorly elevated or infantile epiglottis, crossing arytenoids upon adduction, and a larynx that is generally constricted and hard to inspect, a situation now termed hyperfunction. Extralaryngeal musculature is often employed in this type of patient for voice production. Precipitating factors include medical conditions such as allergy, thyroid imbalance, hormonal imbalance, especially in women, and "emotional maladjustment." Aggravating factors included injudicious voice use, particularly in the context of tobacco and alcohol use. Arnold notes that a single event of acute vocal trauma producing hoarseness will persist as chronic laryngitis if voice rest and proper vocal hygiene are not observed. Other studies have attempted to address the validity of these claims.

In 1981, Baker et al performed a retrospective review of 10 patients with hoarseness after surgical excision of benign glottic lesions.[19] Detailed histories of each patient were obtained and compared for predisposing factors for their recurrent hoarseness. Only cumulative medical history was significant by univariate analysis. Points were assigned for each medical condition affecting the upper aerodigestive tract and added together for a "cumulative medical history" value. Of note, behavior after surgery and behavioral history were not significant. This study is limited by a lack of stroboscopic exam (not widely available in 1981) and histologic analysis of the lesions themselves and by a small patient population. It is, however, a reasoned approach to examine recurrent lesions. Baker et al suggested that the medical problems of these patients should be addressed more aggressively and that the issue of voice rest and even retraining postoperatively are called into question. Modern histologic studies, however, are highly suggestive of a traumatic etiology for these lesions, which implies that judicious voice use is paramount in avoiding these lesions or preventing recurrence.[17]

Gray and associates performed an immunohistochemical examination of archived benign laryngeal lesions to determine the amount of fibronectin present in the superficial layer of lamina propria of the vocal folds.[17] Fibronectin is present normally in the vocal folds, but it is seen to increase in the context of injury. Gray et al also tested for the presence of collagen type IV, which is normally present in the basement membrane zone (BMZ) and whose disruption can be used to detect injury. Thirty-three specimens were examined and revealed two basic patterns of injury. For polyps, there was minimal if any damage to the BMZ and little additional fibronectin deposition. For nodules, distinct damage to the BMZ was noted along with an increased deposition of fibronectin. Using electron microscopy, Dikkers et al also noted disruption of the basement membrane with disorganized architecture in patients with benign phonotraumatic lesions.[20] The same group also performed histologic studies showing thickening of the basement membrane in polyps, Reinke edema, and nodules.[21] These findings are highly suggestive of a traumatic etiology for most if not all benign subepithelial pathology.

Treatment

These microscopic changes bear on recurrence in two different ways. First, the damage occurring in the superficial lamina propria (SLP) and BMZ may be reversible, and the voice may return to normal. However, if the damage does not heal, then despite voice therapy the lesions may persist and produce the "chronic laryngitis" that Arnold described.[18] Second, the overzealous voice use that may have produced these lesions initially, if not modified, will place the patient at risk for recurrent nodules. Modification of voice use is best managed by voice therapy to "unlearn" the habits of hyperfunction. Voice therapy seems most useful in two situations: in patients with a recent diagnosis of nodules that may still heal without surgery and in patients who are about to undergo surgery for the nodules. Voice therapy is a mainstay of treatment for vocal fold nodules, with surgery reserved for refractory cases.

Further epidemiological and microscopic study of vocal fold nodules and polyps is needed to better define the nature of the lesions. Current evidence seems to support a microtraumatic etiology for nodules. Polyps are best managed with phonosurgical resection with or without angiolytic lasers under general anesthesia for maximum control. Voice results have been favorable using this technique.[22–24] Recurrence of these lesions is linked to overzealous voice use and probably to poor vocal hygiene. Management with voice therapy, along with cessation of smoking and alcohol and control of LPR disease, is the mainstay of therapy, with surgery reserved for refractory cases.

Anterior Laryngeal Narrowing

Anterior glottic webs (AGWs) have always proven a difficult problem to correct (**Fig. 3.3**). Because these lesions narrow the rima glottidis and tether the vocal folds,

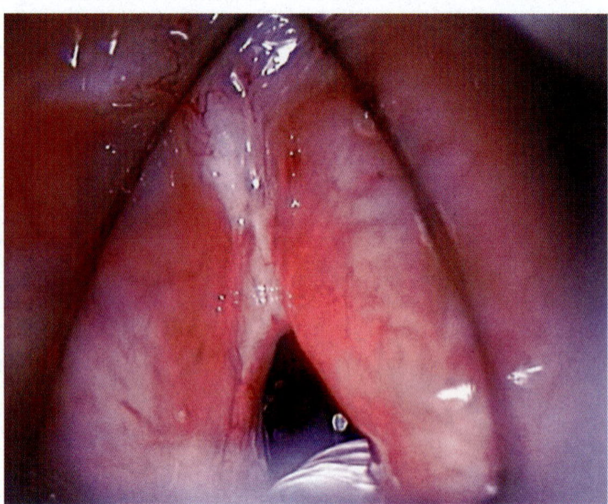

Fig. 3.3 Microlaryngoscopic view of a long iatrogenic vocal fold web. This patient underwent multiple procedures for papillomatosis of the glottis.

patients complain of an inadequate airway and poor voice quality. Although historically due to infection, AGWs are now most commonly iatrogenic. Until recently, assessment has been only clinical. The advent of formal voice evaluation and more advanced endoscopic equipment has made these evaluations more accurate and uniform. No single approach has proven definitive because of the relative rarity of clinically significant anterior webs and the difficulty in achieving treatment success.

Etiology

In the 1900s, infectious sources such as diphtheria, tuberculosis, and syphilis were the most common cause of glottic stenosis of all varieties, including anterior stenosis.[25] Because these infections are now less common and because of the relative frequency of endotracheal intubation and laryngeal procedures, iatrogenesis is now the most important source of anterior glottic stenosis.[26] Congenital glottic webs, although overall quite rare, still constitute a significant proportion of this disorder. Most studies report about a 40% incidence.[26] Presentation is somewhat uniform. Specifically, patients have exercise-induced dyspnea with or without biphasic stridor and dysphonia. These voice irregularities would probably include a decrease in range, a decrease in volume, an increase in pitch, and an increase in air loss during phonation. AGWs are not a self-limiting problem; patients either live with their symptoms or undergo surgery, but they do not get better on their own.

In the adult, the rima glottidis is the narrowest portion of the airway.[27] Therefore, any further narrowing of this area will exert a maximum effect on airflow, producing symptoms of dyspnea in the patient and often stridor. The stridor is biphasic, as this is a fixed airway lesion. The voice quality is disturbed in several ways. The normal voice range is modulated by the ability of the vocal folds to undergo changes in tension and length.[28] With an anterior stenosis, the vocal folds are tethered such that tension and length cannot be easily changed. Volume is also altered. Increased volume is generated by a subglottal pressure being transmitted through an efficient glottis.[26] Glottic efficiency is permitted by symmetry of the mucosal wave with a limited space between the vocal folds. With a web, the vibratory surface of the vocal folds is limited, and an effective mucosal wave is diminished. Overall, pitch is increased because the vibratory length of the membranous vocal fold is decreased. The effect is the same as shortening the string of a violin, for example. Glottal air leak is probably produced by a midcord bowing with adduction, producing a wide opening for air escape. Additionally, the web itself may prevent proper rotation of the arytenoids, altering overall efficiency.[26] The goals in treatment are an adequate airway first and a serviceable voice second.

Clinical Evaluation

The evaluation of an anterior glottic web requires a full history, a view of the anatomical obstruction, a voice evaluation, and an evaluation of airway function. A full history must investigate trauma, infections, and iatrogenesis. Complete visualization of the lesion is essential in decision making. The rod-lens system, fiberoptic endoscopes, and stroboscopy all facilitate this visualization. If the web extends posteriorly beyond the vocal processes of the arytenoids, then a posterior glottic repair is required. The repair can be accomplished either concomitantly with the anterior stenosis or as a staged procedure. Also, if the thickness of the web in the superior-inferior dimension is too great for an endoscopic repair, an open approach is required. Voice evaluation can include stroboscopy, sonograms/voice spectrography, and measurements of fundamental frequency, voice range profile, and voice duration. Although currently not included as a standard procedure, flow-volume loop or pulmonary function tests should be included.

Treatment

AGWs are treated surgically. Options are endoscopic, open, or a combination of the two. Iglauer was the first to make sense of the anatomic dilemma of AGW repair.[29] Namely, exposed tissues must be separated, or else the edges will heal from their adjoining apex outward. In 1924, Haslinger was the first to attempt the endoscopic treatment of AGWs.[30] He endoscopically placed a silver plate between the true vocal folds and tied it externally to the skin with metal wires. Poe and Seager, Alonzo et al, Lynch and LeJeune, Frazer, and Pennington all elaborated on Haslinger's attempt.[25,30–34] The improvements included different methods to pass the wires from outside to inside the larynx. Dedo introduced Teflon as his keel of choice and cut the keel to conform to the shape of the anterior commissure.[35] Specifically, the edge abutting the endolarynx had an angle of ~120 degrees. Dedo extolled the advantages of the endoscopic approach, noting that it is easier on the patient, a normal voice is achieved, and there is a decrease in cost, operating room time, and hospital days. One disadvantage is erosion of the anterior neck skin. When the keel is tied to the neck skin with wires, swallowing produces differential movement of the wires, and the keel and the wires erode the skin. An endoscopic advance was put forth by McGuirt et al, who introduced the concept of turning the web into a microflap.[26] In this manner, it is possible to cover one vocal fold and to let the other epithelialize separately. This technique requires no tracheotomy or exogenous materials, but it often requires "touch-up" procedures. McGuirt et al reported a good voice outcome in five out of six patients.

Open techniques date from 1950, when McNaught inserted a tantalum keel through a limited thyrotomy to separate the vocal folds from one another.[36] The fixation of the keel to the thyroid cartilage eliminated the differential movement of the larynx and the neck skin with swallowing. This approach, however, required an external incision to place the keel and a second to remove it. Since then, modifications have included the use of a plastic sheet by Knight and the use of a silicone "umbrella" keel by Montgomery and Gamble.[37,38] Montgomery and Gamble noted that silicone induces less granulation to form at the surgical site than metal and that the keel should not be left in place for more than 3 weeks because of excess granulation.

Isshiki et al in 1991 promoted the use of the open approach with a soft silicone stent to hold in place a mucosal graft taken from the oral cavity.[39] This approach required two procedures, one to place the stent and another to remove it. Tracheotomy is required in both Montgomery and Gamble's and Isshiki et al's techniques, a distinct disadvantage when compared with the endoscopic approaches.

Hsaio reported a combined endoscopic and external approach in which a video microlaryngoscope is used to place a very thin silver sheet through an incomplete midline thyrotomy.[40] The silver sheet is fixed to the thyroid cartilage and removed during a second procedure. A tracheotomy is not required. The return to silver sheeting, which had been seen as promoting granulation formation, is unusual. Indeed, one of the two patients reported required removal of granulation during the second procedure.

Each patient had only a 2 to 3 mm anterior web after treatment. The voice measurements of maximum phonation time, intensity range, and pitch range all improved significantly in both patients.

Novel approaches have been attempted with success more recently. Using novel flap elevation and suture technique, Schweinfurth and Akst have reported successful single-stage endoscopic repair of a anterior webs.[41,42] In 2004 Unal reported a single case of congenital web repair with lysis and topical mitomycin C application.[43] These techniques will likely take hold in the field, as they offer significantly less morbidity to the patient with equal success.

The treatment of AGWs remains difficult. There is the temptation to lyse the web and to expect a patent airway and functional voice. However, the proximity of the two raw surfaces allows the vocal folds to fuse back together. The dilemma is thus evident. What is the most effective and least traumatic way to separate the two raw surfaces? The endoscopic approach is less invasive, does not always necessitate a tracheotomy, and is more cosmetically favorable. Montgomery and Gamble"s results lend credence to its effectiveness.[38] The open approach, although more invasive, offers a logical option to the endoscopic route and may be more appropriate for larger lesions in the anteroposterior dimension. Formal voice evaluation and pulmonary studies might help to standardize future reports.

This lesion presents special challenges for the physician to prevent recurrence. First and foremost, the physician must establish concordance between the expectations of the surgeon and those of the patient. If there are reasonable expectations, then neither the surgeon nor the patient will desire return trips to the operating room to improve a less than perfect airway and/or voice. Misdiagnosis can cause recurrence if the etiology and extent of injury are not accurate or if there is an untreated evolving process. Furthermore, the extent of the pathology should dictate the repair. The more extensive web will require an external approach.

Sulcus Vocalis

Sulcus deformities may be seen as a recurrent benign laryngeal lesion, as they are prone to misdiagnosis and inappropriate treatment. Vocal scar and sulcus vocalis are part of a continum of abnormal lamina propria fibroplasia. *Sulcus vocalis* is a term meaning "furrow" or "indentation"; it has been used to describe glottic lesions that possess this appearance. It is a lesion that generally produces a breathy voice with a strained quality, requiring increased vocal effort and producing a decrease in range. Functional studies such as those by Hirano et al have helped to better characterize this disease entity.[44] Sulcus deformities may affect one or both vocal folds. It is unclear whether they are congenital or acquired or both. Clinically, they are suspected by

history and indirect laryngoscopy, but they are often missed on initial exam and require diligence for proper identification and categorization. Once identified, there are multiple treatment options available. Voice therapy has been regarded as an essential adjunctive measure because many of these patients attempt to decrease the glottal incompetence by using supraglottal speech—trying to use their false vocal folds as the resonating site in their vocal tract. Clearly, this compensatory behavior must be addressed for a good outcome. Other options include the injection of collagen, Teflon, and steroids. Also, undermining of the lesion with or without its excision has been described.[45] A "slicing" technique is also available, as is medialization thyroplasty. Even with these techniques available, results are not always excellent.

Classification

Often used in the context of entities with a spindle-shaped appearance, sulcus vocalis has more recently been categorized according to its different morphologies. Ford et al described three types of sulcus deformities.[46] Type 1 is a "physiologic sulcus" that may be apparent on examination but produces little if any voice alteration and is essentially an incidental finding. Of note, these sulci do not alter the normal mucosal wave when examined with videostroboscopy and produce no focal stiffness to the vocal fold. Type 2 is the sulcus vergeture, as described by Bouchayer et al.[47] It is a furrow along the medial surface of the true vocal fold created by an attachment of the epithelium of the vocal fold directly to the underlying vocal ligament; in type 2 sulcus, the SLP does not separate the epithelium from the vocal ligament as it does normally. Type 3 sulcus is designated as sulcus vocalis. Morphologically, it is a focal indentation of the epithelium onto the vocal ligament; here also the SLP does not intervene. It is possible that sulcus deformities are derived from epithelial cysts that may have ruptured. Ford et al reports finding the coexistence of cysts with sulci in 9 out of 20 patients in their series.[46] Bouchayer et al also observed epidermoid cysts together with mucosal bridges and glottic sulci in 23 out of 157 patients.[47] Histologically, these lesions often have prominent fibrosis and vasculature.[4] Because sulci were identified in 48% of the whole mount sections with laryngeal cancer, it is thought that cancer may play a causative role, or at least suggests that sulci may be acquired lesions.

Clinical Evaluation

Patients with sulcus deformities generally present with a history of increased vocal fatigue, a breathy and strained voice, significant air loss, and sometimes odynophonia. Ages range from 5 to 59, 10 to 68, and 24 to 79 in different series.[44,46,47] Presentation therefore can be in both pediatric and adult populations. Bouchayer et al note several characteristics of this population of patients, including (1) lowering of the average pitch of the voice in women and elevation in men; (2) monotone speech; (3) a weak voice; (4) husky, breathy, and strained qualities; (5) pitch breaks and diplophonia; and (6) frequent glottal attacks.[48] Hirano et al described many functional characteristics of this group.[46] Specifically, the majority of patients had a breathy voice. Stroboscopy revealed a small vibratory amplitude, a small mucosal wave, and incomplete glottic closure. The maximum phonation time, fundamental frequency range, and sound pressure level were all decreased. Airflow during phonation was increased. The pitch perturbation quotient, amplitude perturbation quotient, and normalized noise energy were increased. Abnormal test results were more common and more marked for bilateral lesions than for unilateral lesions. Of note, 95 of 126 patients had bilateral lesions. From a diagnostic standpoint, sulci are generally seen as a member of the "spindle-shaped" glottis category. Spindle-shaped lesions include, but are not limited to vocal fold paralysis, thyroarytenoid atrophy, and presbylaryngis. Therefore, in patients with spindle-shaped glottic lesions, sulci should always be considered.

Etiology

There is conflicting evidence as to when these lesions arise. As noted above, the age range is wide. Bouchayer et al argued for a congenital origin of these lesions based on the presentation of 55% of their patients during childhood.[47] Also, cysts were often associated with the sulci, suggesting a copresentation. The researchers further noted that the lesions did not recur with adequate excision and that there may be a familial pattern. Their theory is an embryological maldevelopment of the fourth and sixth branchial arches, which may have yielded ruptured or unruptured epidermoid cysts of the true vocal folds.[47] Arnold argues a congenital basis for sulci based on studies of comparative anatomy.[48]

The arguments for sulci as acquired lesions date from Van Caneghem's observation that they appear secondary to infectious causes, including tuberculosis.[49] Sulci are also seen to appear in adults. Evidence for an acquired pathogenesis is found in a review of whole mount laryngeal specimens; 48% of the specimens with laryngeal cancer were found to have sulci.[50]

Treatment

The treatment options for sulcus deformities are many, but all focus on the basic principle of trying to restore glottic sufficiency. Again, sulci are a cause of spindle-shaped deformity, so the treatment goal is to decrease the glottic gap, thereby increasing glottal efficiency and improving the vocal quality. Local injections have been used to fill the local gaps of the sulci. These include steroids,[50] bioimplants,[51,52] and Teflon.[53] Medialization thyroplasty also has been used to restore the glottal gap.[54] A more direct approach has been directed at the actual anatomical lesion, including laser or microdissection of the sulcus deformity.[46] The tethering effect of the sulcus has been addressed with techniques that undermine the tethered area and redrape the mucosa directly or with vertical "slicing" incisions.[55] Ford et al describe a graded approach to the sulcus deformity.[46] For type 1, or "physiologic," sulcus patients, treatment is directed by the degree of the deformity and also its cause. If the sulcus deformity is secondary to a paralyzed true vocal fold or atrophy, then a medialization procedure is suggested. For type 1 patients, Ford et al warn against direct intervention on the true vocal folds, as their anatomical structure is intact; their cover-body relationship has not been interrupted. However, for type 2 and 3 patients, the SLP is not fully interposed between the vocal ligament and the overlying epithelium, and the cover-body relationship is disturbed. Type 2 and 3 patients are thus good candidates for surgical intervention on the focal defects themselves. In Ford et al's series of 20 sulcus patients, the majority benefited from intervention.[46] In Bouchayer et al's series of 157 cases, which included epidermoid cysts, sulci, and mucosal bridges, the researchers judged that only 15 out of 157 cases had "very good" voice results, indicating that even in the best of hands, the treatment of sulci is still difficult.[47] Fat and fascia implantation into the superficial vocal fold via endoscopic approaches have also been reported with favorable results.[57,58] It may be that tissue engineering techniques with injectable bioactive gels may represent the best long-term pathway for treatment of this refractory problem.[59]

Sulci present difficulty for the clinician in terms of both proper diagnosis and treatment. Their elusive qualities may delay a diagnosis until focused stroboscopic and direct microlaryngoscopic exam reveal their influence. They may thus be seen as "recurrent" because of this difficulty in diagnosis or because of the necessity for secondary procedures. It is for these reasons that return to a normal voice is rare, and both patient and physician should be prepared for this reality.

Conclusion

The discussion here has been limited to several distinct entities. However, the themes of difficult evaluation, lack of consensus, and rarity of presentation can be extrapolated to other intralaryngeal and extralaryngeal paradigms. To improve treatment for these entities, different paths can be pursued. Less expensive, more available evaluation techniques with less qualitative and more quantitative information would be helpful in standardizing evaluation. Although stroboscopy is a powerful tool, it is certainly not available to all, nor should it be. Alternative tools for evaluation may become available with technological advances.

Greater clarity will be gained regarding these and other lesions by using the power of prospective randomized trials. With large numbers of patients, the limits of anecdotal experience and varied treatments can be overcome, resulting in better outcomes for the patient and greater clarity for the physician and the specialty.

References

1. Jackson C. Contact ulcer of the larynx. Ann Otol Rhinol Laryngol 1928;37:227–230.
2. Ylitalo R, Lindestad P. A retrospective study of contact granuloma. Laryngoscope 1999;109:433–436.
3. Von Leden H, Moore P. Contact ulcer of the larynx: experimental observations. Arch Otolaryngol 1960;72:746–752.
4. Hirano M, Kiyokawa K, Kurita S, et al. Posterior glottis: morphologic study in excised human larynges. Ann Otol Rhinol Laryngol 1986;95:576–581.
5. Ward PH, Zwitman D, Hanson D, et al. Contact ulcers and granulomas of the larynx: new insights into their etiology as a basis for more rational treatment. Otolaryngol Head Neck Surg 1980;88:262–269.
6. Delahunty JE, Cherry J. Experimentally produced vocal cord granulomas. Laryngoscope 1968;78:1941–1947.
7. McFerran DJ, Abdullah V, Gallimore AP, et al. Vocal process granulomata. J Laryngol Otol 1994;108:216–220.
8. Peacher GM. Vocal therapy for contact ulcer of the larynx: a follow-up of 70 patients. Laryngoscope 1961;71:37–47.
9. Nasri S, Sercarz JA, McAlpin T, et al. Treatment of vocal fold granuloma using botulinum toxin type A. Laryngoscope 1995;105:585–588.
10. Roh HJ, Goh E, Chon K, et al. Topical inhalant steroid (budesonide, Pulmicort™ nasal) therapy in intubation granuloma. J Laryngol Otol 1999;113:427–432.
11. Mitchell G, Pearson CR, Henk JM, et al. Excision and low-dose radiotherapy for refractory laryngeal granuloma. J Laryngol Otol 1998;112:491–493.
12. Zeitels SM, Franco RA, Dailey SH, et al. Office-based treatment of glottal dysplasia and papillomatosis with the 585-nm pulsed dye laser and local anesthesia. Ann Otol Rhinol Laryngol 2004;113(4):265–276.
13. Clyne SB, Halum SL, Koufman JA. Pulsed dye laser treatment of laryngeal granulomas. Ann Otol Rhinol Laryngol 2005;114(3):198–201.
14. Ash JE, Schwartz L. The laryngeal (vocal cord) node. Trans Am Acad Ophthalmol Otolaryngol 1943–44;48:323–332.
15. Jackson CL. Vocal Nodules. Trans Am Laryngol 1941; 63: 185–193.
16. Zerffi WAC. Vocal nodules and crossed arytenoids. Laryngoscope 1935;45:532–534.
17. Gray SD, Hammond E, Hanson DF. Benign pathologic responses of the larynx. Ann Otol Rhinol Laryngol 1995; 104:13–18.
18. Arnold GE. Vocal nodules and polyps: laryngeal tissue reaction to habitual hyperkinetic dysphonia. J Speech Hear Disord 1962;27:205–217.
19. Baker BM, Fox SM, Baker CD, et al. Persistent hoarseness after surgical removal of vocal cord lesions. Arch Otolaryngol 1981;107:148–151.
20. Dikkers FG, Hulstaert CE, Oosterbaan JA, et al. Ultrastructural changes of the basement membrane zone in benign lesions of the vocal folds. Acta Otolaryngol 1993;113(1):98–101.
21. Dikkers FG, Nikkels PG. Benign lesions of the vocal folds: histopathology and phonotrauma. Ann Otol Rhinol Laryngol 1995;104(9 Pt 1):698–703.
22. Hirano S, Yamashita M, Kitamura M, Takagita S. Photocoagulation of microvascular and hemorrhagic lesions of the vocal fold with the KTP laser. Ann Otol Rhinol Laryngol 2006;115:253–259.
23. Johns MM, Garrett CG, Hwang J, Ossoff RH, Courey MS. Quality-of-life outcomes following laryngeal endoscopic surgery for non-neoplastic vocal fold lesions. Ann Otol Rhinol Laryngol 2004;113(8):597–601.
24. Ivey C et al. Office pulsed dye laser treatment for benign laryngeal vascular polyps: a preliminary study. Ann Otol Rhinol Laryngol 2008;117:353–358.
25. Frazer JP. Treatment of thin laryngeal webs with suspended metallic plates. Trans Am Acad Ophthalmol Otolaryngol 1968;72:581–587.
26. McGuirt WF, Salmon J, Blalock D. Normal speech for patients with laryngeal webs: an achievable goal. Laryngoscope 1984;94:1176–1180.
27. Titze IR. Fluid flow in respiratory airways. In Titze IR, ed. Principles of Voice Production. Englewood Cliffs, NJ: Prentice Hall; 1993.
28. Titze IR. Voice classification and life-span changes. In Titze IR, ed. Principles of Voice Production. Englewood Cliffs, NJ: Prentice Hall; 1993.
29. Iglauer S. A new procedure for the treatment of web in the larynx. Arch Otolaryngol 1935;22:597–602.
30. Haslinger F. Ein Fall von Membranbildung im Larynx. Eine neue Methode zu ihrer Behebung. Monatsschr. F. Ohrenheilk v. Ann Otol Rhinol Laryngol 1924;58:174.
31. Poe DL, Seager PS. Congenital laryngeal web: its eradication. Arch Otolaryngol 1948;47:46–48.
32. Alonso JM, Alonso Regles JE. Treatment of membranes and synechiae of the anterior part of the glottis. Arch Otolaryngol 1957;65:111–115.
33. Lynch MG, LeJeune FE. Laryngeal stenosis. Laryngoscope 1960;70:315–317.
34. Pennington CL. The treatment of anterior glottic webs: a re-evaluation of Haslinger's technique. Laryngoscope 1968;78:728–741.

35. Dedo HH. Endoscopic Teflon keel for anterior glottic web. Ann Otol Rhinol Laryngol 1979;88:467–473.
36. McNaught RC. Surgical correction of anterior web of the larynx. Laryngoscope 1950;60:264–272.
37. Knight JS. Laryngeal stenosis: method of surgical correction. Laryngoscope 1964;74:564–574.
38. Montgomery WW, Gamble JE. Anterior glottic stenosis: experimental and clinical management. Arch Otolaryngol 1970;92:560–567.
39. Isshiki N, Nose K, Taira T, Kojima H. Surgical treatment of laryngeal web with mucosa graft. Ann Otol Rhinol Laryngol 1991;100:95–100.
40. Hsiao TY. Combined endolaryngeal and external approaches for iatrogenic glottic web. Laryngoscope 1999;109(8):1347–1350.
41. Schweinfurth J. Single-stage, stentless endoscopic repair of anterior glottic webs. Laryngoscope 2002; 112(5): 933–935.
42. Akst LM, Broadhurst MS, Burns JA, Zeitels SM. Microflap laryngoplasty for treating an anterior-commissure web with papillomatosis. Laryngoscope 2007;117:1496–499.
43. Unal M. The successful management of congenital laryngeal web with endoscopic lysis and topical mitomycin-C. Int J Pediatr Otorhinolaryngol 2004;68(2):231–235.
44. Hirano M, Tanaka S, Yoshida T, Hibi S. Sulcus vocalis: functional aspects. Ann Otol Rhinol Laryngol 1990;99: 679–683.
45. Remacle M, Lawson G, Deglos JC, Evrard I, Jamart J. Microsurgery of sulcus vergeture with carbon dioxide laser and injectable collagen. Ann Otol Rhinol Laryngol 2000;109:141–148.
46. Ford CN, Inagi K, Khidr A, et al. Sulcus vocalis: a rational analytical approach to diagnosis and management. Ann Otol Rhinol Laryngol 1996;105:189–200.
47. Bouchayer M, Cornut G, Loire R, et al. Epidermoid cysts, sulci, and mucosal bridges of the true vocal cord: a report of 157 cases. Laryngoscope 1985;95:1087–1094.
48. Arnold GE. Dysplasia dysphonia: minor anomalies of the vocal cords causing persistent hoarseness. Laryngoscope 1958;68:142–158.
49. Van Caneghem D. L'étiologie de la corde vocale á sillon. Ann Maladies Oreille Larynx Nez Pharynx 1928;47: 121–130.
50. Nakayama M, Ford CN, Brandenburg JH, et al. Sulcus vocalis in laryngeal cancer: a histopathologic study. Laryngoscope 1994;104:16–24.
51. Bouchayer M, Cornut G. Microsurgery for benign lesions of the vocal folds. Ear Nose Throat J 1988;67:446–466.
52. Ford CN, Bless DM. Selected problems treated by vocal fold injection of collagen. Am J Otolaryngol 1993;14:257–261.
53. Ford CN, Bless DM, Loftus JM. Role of injectable collagen in the treatment of glottic insufficiency: a study of 119 patients. Ann Otol Rhinol Laryngol 1992;101:237–247.
54. Lee ST, Niimi S. Vocal fold sulcus. J Laryngol Otol 1990; 104:876–878.
55. Ford CN, Bless DM, Prehn RB. Thyroplasty as primary and adjunctive treatment of glottic insufficiency. J Voice 1992;6:277–285.
56. Pontes P, Behlau M. Treatment of sulcus vocalis: auditory perceptual and acoustic analysis of the slicing mucosa surgical technique. J Voice 1993;7:365–376.
57. Neuenschwander MC, Sataloff RT, Abaza MM, Hawkshaw MJ, Reiter D, Spiegel JR. Management of vocal fold scar with autologous fat implantation: perceptual results. J Voice 2001;15:295–304.
58. Tsunoda K, Kondou K, Kaga K, Niimi S, Baer T, Nishiyama K, Hirose H. Autologous transplantation of fascia into the vocal fold: long-term result of type-1 transplantation and the future. Laryngoscope 2005;115(12 Pt 2 Suppl 108):1–10.
59. Duflo S, Thibeault SL, Li W, et al. Vocal fold tissue repair in vivo using a synthetic extracellular matrix. Tissue Eng 2006;12(8):2171–2180.

Decision tree for preoperative evaluation

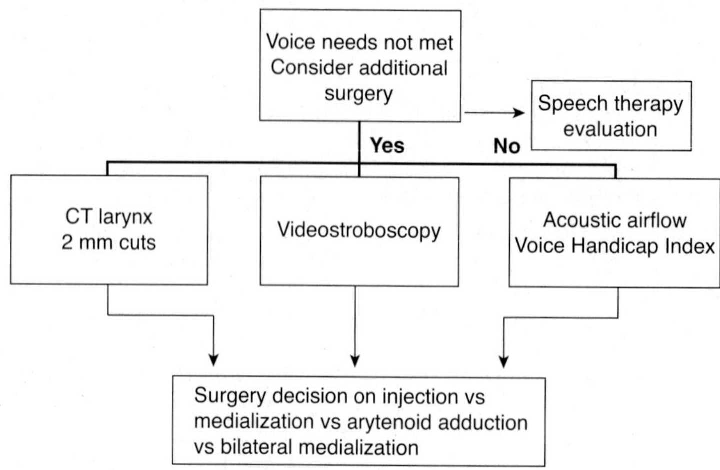

Decision tree for revision medialization laryngoplasty

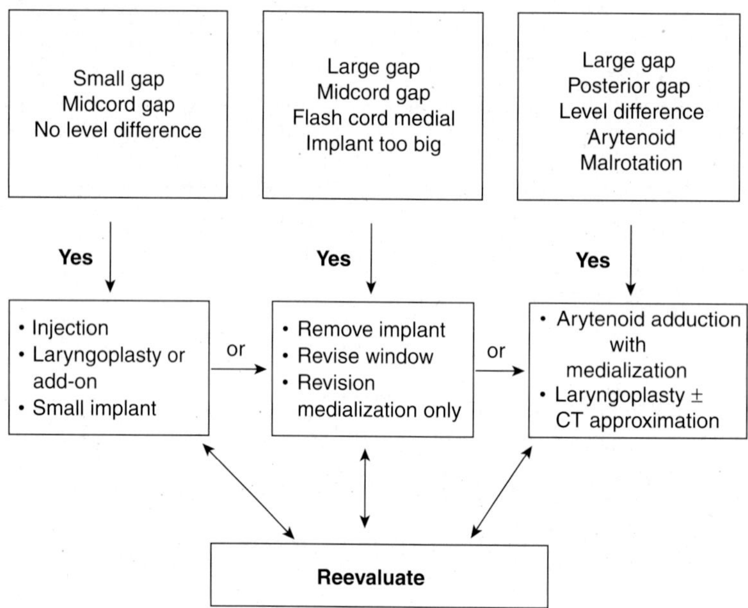

Revision Medialization Laryngoplasty

Peak Woo

The concept of medialization laryngoplasty has been with us since the turn of the last century. Payr in 1915 first described medialization laryngoplasty using an anterior pedicled U-flap on the thyroid cartilage.[1] Seiffert and Meurman described the implantation of a rib cartilage into the paraglottic space to medialize the vocal folds.[2,3] However, the laryngeal framework fell into disfavor because of airway compromise, postoperative infections, and the introduction of injection laryngoplasty. In 1911, Brünnings successfully reported the use of intracordal paraffin injections to medialize vocal folds in glottic insufficiency.[4] This method fell into disrepute because patients developed complications such as paraffinomas and distal spread of paraffin. Arnold, in 1962, described the use of Teflon (polytetrafluoroethylene), which is still used today but is gradually diminishing in popularity because of the numerous complications associated with its use.[5–7] Other materials, such as collagen and autologous fat, have come to the forefront and are popularly used today.[8,9] It was not until 1974, when Isshiki et al described a systematic approach to surgery of the vocal skeleton to change the tension and mass of the vocal fold, enabling many surgeons to similarly achieve good results, did laryngeal framework surgery become popular.[10] They described four different types of laryngeal framework surgery for different clinical conditions. Type 1 thyroplasty (medialization laryngoplasty) is the most popular method of laryngeal framework surgery because it addresses the most common clinical disorder of glottic incompetence caused by vocal fold paralysis.[11]

Indications and Contraindications

Medialization laryngoplasty reduces glottic incompetence and helps prevent aspiration. Glottic incompetence may arise from

1. Paralysis of the vagus nerve
2. Vocal fold atrophy (e.g., presbyphonia)
3. Sulcus vocalis

When the vagus nerve is damaged, the vocal fold may assume one of three positions: median, paramedian, or lateral.

In patients with a unilateral vocal fold paralysis with the vocal fold in the paramedian or lateral position, the uninvolved side often compensates for a glottic gap by coming across to meet the paralyzed side, thereby resulting in a good or satisfactory voice. However, there are instances when this compensatory mechanism is insufficient and will result in a patient who is dysphonic and breathy. Often the patient then acquires undesirable compensatory measures, such as excessive laryngeal squeezing or laryngeal muscle tension, resulting in a strained, effortful voice. At this point, the patient often presents to the clinic requesting professional help. Medialization laryngoplasty aims to restore vocal strength, loudness, sustainability, and projection.

In high vagal lesions, there may be paresthesia or hypoesthesia of the supraglottis, resulting in laryngeal penetration and aspiration. Medialization thyroplasty has been shown to help reduce aspiration in these patients.

Treatment

Medialization laryngoplasty can be divided into

1. Injection laryngoplasty
2. Laryngeal framework surgery
   a. Vocal fold medialization
   b. Arytenoid adduction
   c. Cricothyroid approximation

Nonsurgical Treatment

Injection laryngoplasty improves the voice quality by injecting a material into the vocal fold. Materials may be injected medially into the superficial lamina propria (e.g., vocal fold scarring) or laterally in the vocal ligament or vocalis muscle. Superficial injection techniques aim to re-create the superficial layer of the vocal fold in an attempt to re-create the mucosal wave. Lateral or deep injections attempt to augment the vocal fold by adding bulk and improving glottic closure. This lateral injection is most useful in treating vocal fold paresis, paralysis, and vocal fold atrophy.

Materials

Over the last 2 decades, many different materials have been tried and tested. The choice of material depends on

Decision tree for evaluation of failed medialization laryngoplasty

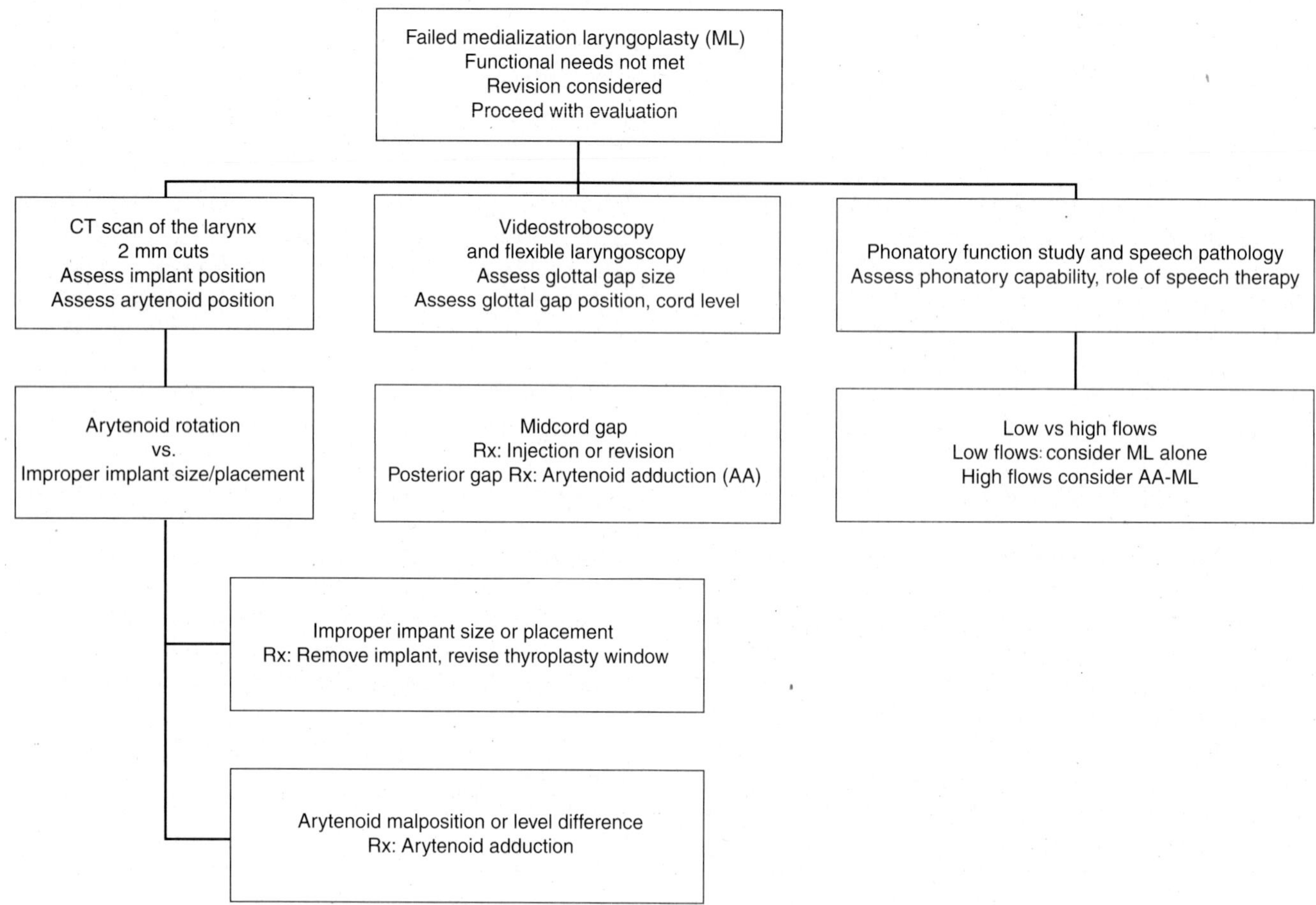

patient factors, safety profile of the material, resorption characteristics, and the surgeon's experience with the material. Fat, micronized dermis, collagen, Gelfoam, and hydroxylapatite are some of the materials being used today.[8,9,12,13]

- Teflon: Teflon is a polymer of polytetrafluoroethylene. After injection into the paraglottic space, an acute inflammatory reaction ensues that later becomes chronic and encapsulates the polymer. Although good results are achieved immediately, the long-term results are more difficult to predict and may deteriorate over time. Another problem associated with Teflon use is migration superficially within the vocal fold, eroding the overlying mucosa and leading to granuloma formation. This affects the mucosal wave adversely and causes stiffness. Local spread to lymph nodes and the thyroid gland has been described.[7] The current indication for Teflon injection is for patients with vocal fold paresis or paralysis with terminal disease and short life expectation.
- Gelfoam: Gelfoam, which is supplied as a powder and mixed with a buffered saline solution to form a paste, is used for vocal fold injection. Because it lasts only 6 to 8 weeks, it is ideal for temporary treatment for vocal fold paralysis when recovery is expected. It can also be used repeatedly in the first few months before recovery when vocal fold function is essential.
- Fat: Autologous fat is readily harvested and available. It does not give a foreign body reaction and is well tolerated. There are different methods of harvesting fat. Some surgeons prefer harvesting abdominal fat with a liposuction machine, whereas others prefer careful dissection with minimal trauma to maintain integrity of the lipocytes. The harvested fat is processed and loaded into a Brünings syringe for injection. The author washes the fat in Ringer's lactate solution followed by Depo-Medrole steroid solution before loading it into a syringe. Other authors prefer centrifuging the fat to remove impurities. Approximately 30 to 50% of injected material will reabsorb within the first month; hence it is advisable to overcorrect when performing lipoinjection. Fat is injected lateral to the vocal folds in vocal fold paralysis.
- Collagen: The use of collagen was popularized by Ford et al in the human larynx.[8] Safety issues with bovine collagen, such as hypersensitivity reactions, have led to the introduction of autologous human collagen for injection laryngoplasty. Although collagen is absorbed by the body, the amount and rate of it are less than those of fat.
- Other materials: Materials such as autologous fascia harvested from the fascia lata have been reported with good success in a small series.[14] The rate of resorption is low, and the free grafts survive as living tissue.

Micronized dermis is an off-the-shelf product that is reconstituted by the surgeon and is well tolerated. The material does not require hypersensitivity testing and may be given as an office procedure, as there is no donor morbidity. Absorption is still high, and overinjection by 50% is necessary.[12]

Advantages and Disadvantages

The advantages of injection laryngoplasty are as follows:

1. It is easily performed.
2. It is quick and effective.
3. It is convenient, for both the patient and the surgeon, if performed using indirect laryngoscopy transorally under local anesthesia or transcutaneously as an office procedure.

There are also several disadvantages:

1. The anatomy of the vocal fold and arytenoid cartilage is altered in paralysis. The arytenoid is tilted anteriorly and rotated laterally. There is a vertical phase difference between the two vocal folds. Injection laryngoplasty does not address these issues.
2. The diffusion pattern of the substances injected follows the path of least resistance and may not adequately augment the areas intended.
3. Although the substances are biologically inert and are generally well accepted by the body, hypersensitive and inflammatory reactions can occur, resulting in granuloma formation and vocal fold scarring.
4. These substances may interfere with the mass, volume, and pliability of the vocal fold.
5. These procedures are irreversible and difficult to correct.
6. Several repeated procedures may be required because of absorption.
7. If performed under general anesthesia, voice monitoring is not possible. If performed under local anesthesia, the procedure may be technically demanding, as patient cooperation is required.

Surgical Treatment

Isshiki et al described four types of laryngeal framework surgery.[15] Type 1 thyroplasty medializes the vocal fold by insinuating an implant between the thyroid cartilage and the thyroarytenoid muscle, thus medializing the vocal fold. This is the most popular thyroplasty procedure, and it addresses the glottic insufficiency resulting from vocal fold paresis or paralysis. It may be supplemented with arytenoid adduction when there is a large posterior glottic gap that cannot be corrected by medialization alone.[16] Type 2 thyroplasty lateralizes a segment of the thyroid cartilage, thus lateralizing the vocal fold. It increases the glottic chink, resulting in a breathy voice. It was first proposed as an alternate treatment for adductor spasmodic dysphonia. Type 3 thyroplasty shortens the anteroposterior distance, resulting in a lax vocal fold and pitch lowering. It is used in the treatment of therapy-resistant mutational dysphonia and vocal fold atrophy. Type 4 thyroplasty increases the anteroposterior dimensions of the thyroid ala, thus thinning out the vocal folds with consequent increase in pitch. This is appropriate for patients undergoing gender reassignment or those with cricothyroid muscle paralysis.

Medialization laryngoplasty can be unilateral or bilateral. Bilateral medialization is indicated for patients with presbylaryngis, unilateral paralysis with contralateral vocal fold bowing/atrophy, bilateral vocal fold paresis, and recalcitrant abductor spasmodic dysphonia.

In addition, two other procedures can be performed with medialization laryngoplasty: arytenoid adduction or arytenoidopexy cricothyroid approximation and subluxation.

The classical arytenoid adduction procedure described by Isshiki et al achieves rotation of the arytenoid by suture placed through the muscular process.[15] The suture is directed anteriorly through the thyroid lamina, thus mimicking the lateral cricoarytenoid muscle and the thyroarytenoid muscles. The arytenoidopexy technique described by Zeitels simulates the agonist-antagonist adductor function of the other intrinsic muscles (lateral thyroarytenoid, interarytenoid, posterior cricoarytenoid) as well.[17] Zeitels showed it to be more effective than the classic arytenoid adduction in closing interarytenoid gaps through cadaveric studies.

Cricothyroid approximation mimics the function of the cricothyroid muscle in lengthening the vocal folds. In vocal fold paralysis, there may be anterior tilting of the arytenoids cartilage, leading to a vertical phase height difference. The denervated vocal fold also undergoes atrophy and becomes flaccid. Some surgeons will perform routine manual cricothyroid approximation intraoperatively to see if correcting the vocal fold tension will further improve the voice.

Criocothyroid subluxation was described by Zeitels to complement his arytenoidopexy technique because of the disruption to the cricothyroid joint during the procedure.[17] This caused the thyroid lamina to be retrodisplaced with relation to the cricoid, resulting in a foreshortened vocal fold. Zeitels also found that cricothyroid subluxation improved the aerodynamic efficiency of the glottal valve, leading to better acoustic maximal-range capabilities.

Complications of medialization laryngoplasty have been reviewed by Tucker and by Rosen.[18,19] These include immediate and delayed complications. Immediate complications include airway edema, stridor, and bleeding. Delayed complications include poor voice outcome, implant extrusion, dysphagia, and airway obstruction. The

impact of physician experience, selection of the implant, and medialization laryngoplasty versus medialization with arytenoid adduction all have an impact on outcome.

For the patient with poor voice or airway outcome after prior medialization laryngoplasty, revision surgery may be necessary. Revision surgery may be accomplished by simple injection laryngoplasty to major revision, such as revision medialization with arytenoid adduction.[20] Careful assessment and analysis should reveal the deficit that needs further correction in these patients. After a complete analysis, revision surgery based on surgery designed to correct the deficit will often offer an improvement in the functional capacity of the patient.

Preoperative Evaluation

History

A general systemic and comprehensive voice evaluation is performed. A detailed history into the symptoms and duration of disability is taken. The specific vocal needs and outcome expectations are discussed, and treatment is recommended.

Examination

An extensive evaluation, including a thorough examination of the head, neck, and chest region, is performed to exclude an obvious cause of the vocal fold paralysis. Computed tomography (CT) scans assist in evaluating the entire course of the vagus nerve. In the patient with prior surgery, a CT scan of the larynx done without contrast at 2 mm intervals is recommended. The CT scan serves the following functions: (1) it delineates the position of the implant and the site of medialization, (2) it will show the position of the arytenoid cartilage on the paralyzed side relative to the normal side, (3) it will show whether there is adequate soft tissue coverage of the implant and will show an impending extrusion, (4) it will demonstrate the position of the previous thyroplasty window, and (5) it will demonstrate the level differences between the vocal folds.

A neurological examination of the cranial nerves is performed. In particular, soft palatal movement and gag reflex are evaluated. In some patients, additional procedures such as unilateral palatoplasty may be necessary to reduce hypernasality.

Stroboscopic examination is crucial to identify the glottic configuration. Because there is no fixed glottic configuration in vocal fold paralysis, the vocal fold can assume one of three configurations:

1. Midmembranous gap
2. Bilateral midmembranous vocal fold defects
3. Midvocal fold and posterior glottal gap

Patients with a midmembranous gap are ideal candidates for revision surgery by medialization thyroplasty alone because they have small midmembranous vocal fold gaps. When there is no rotation of the arytenoid cartilage posteriorly, the results by medialization alone will be good. On phonatory testing, patients with a midcord gap will typically have phonation times of 5 to 10 s, phonatory airflow between 200 and 300 cm^3/s, with moderate voice quality. Perceptually, the voice sounds breathy with restricted pitch and loudness range. Improvement with the manual compression test is a useful guide to success with medialization thyroplasty alone. In patients with a midcord gap, medialization compression testing on the affected thyroid cartilage improves the voice quality and loudness. When there is arytenoid malrotation associated with a large posterior glottal gap, the voice improvement is negligible with medial compression testing.

Patients with bilateral midmembranous vocal fold defects have bilateral bowing with or without vocal fold paralysis. They will have a greater degree of breathiness and airflow, as well as decreased laryngeal resistance. Several authors have shown the benefits of bilateral medialization in these patients.[21] The current indications for bilateral medialization are unilateral paralysis with contralateral bowing, bilateral defects of the vocal folds secondary to aging, atrophy, bowing, and scarring.

The most dysphonic patients are those with combined midvocal fold and posterior glottal gaps. These patients also frequently have problems with dysphagia and aspiration. Although often seen in high vagal paralysis, they may also occur in patients with recurrent nerve paralysis. This anatomical defect arises from anterior tilting of the arytenoid cartilage with foreshortening of the vocal folds. Phonation time is usually < 5 s, and the phonatory airflow is usually > 300 cm^3/s.

These patients are ideal candidates for combined medialization thyroplasty and arytenoid adduction procedures.

Phonatory Function Analysis

This has been well studied by numerous authors. Acoustic analyses and aerodynamic analyses should be routinely performed to (1) obtain quantitative data on the physiologic abnormality, (2) help analyze the functional deficits to be revised, and (3) document the change due to revision surgery.

Acoustic analysis includes pitch perturbation (jitter), amplitude perturbation (shimmer), and signal-to-voice ratio. This is performed with a sustained vowel /i/ at habitual loudness and pitch.

Aerodynamic analyses include mean flow rate, maximum phonation time, and S/Z ratio. (The S/Z ratio measures the sustained production of the sounds /s/ and /z/.)

In many patients, there is a compensatory hyperkinetic supralaryngeal constriction. The role of the speech therapist is to identify this compensatory laryngeal behavior before surgery and to teach the patient to "unload" to assess the underlying glottal condition.

The Voice Handicap Index (VHI) is a validated outcomes instrument that can be used to survey the voice handicap of the patient with residual voice disorder.[22] It has also been used to document pre- and postoperative voice improvement.

Postoperative Evaluation

Postoperatively, aerodynamic measurements and acoustic analysis are repeated at ~3 months after surgery. Netterville et al[23] note that the initial voice improvement acquired intraoperatively may decrease and become raspy because of intraoperative edema. The voice quality continues to improve for up to 1 year after surgery. It is because of this cycle of events that the postoperative measurements are performed after about 3 months. The surgeon and the patient should be aware of this so as to avoid unnecessary anxiety and disappointment in the initial postoperative month.

Several authors have studied the impact of medialization laryngoplasty on acoustic and phonatory function.[24,25] In these studies, there is consistently a significant improvement in pitch range, phonation time, S/Z ratio, signal-to-noise ratio, and pitch and amplitude perturbation. Aerodynamic measures such as air pressure, average airflow, and laryngeal resistance were also improved. Some studies showed positive change in the fundamental frequency, whereas others did not. Gray et al[26] found that despite an overall satisfaction with surgery (92%), most patients did not feel their voice was completely better. Most of the difficulty occurred at work, with 27% needing a change in employment. Although perceptual qualities in pitch, intonation, and loudness did improve, strain, breathiness, hoarseness, harshness, and unsteadiness did not.

From these studies, we are able to counsel our patients preoperatively and give them a realistic expectation of their postoperative voice. Additional studies are necessary to demonstrate the added value of laryngeal reinnervation procedures.

Implant Materials and Sizing

Various implant materials are used to medialize the vocal fold. They include

1. Silastic blocks
2. Gore-Tex strips

3. Prefabricated blocks and implant systems
4. Hydron gel implants
5. Hydroxylapatite implants
6. Titanium implants

Since Isshiki et al first described their technique in 1974, some criticism has been leveled against it. Many surgeons find the procedure of carving the implant laborious and time consuming. Because each implant is individually handcrafted, several implants may have to be tried and tested before an optimal voice result is found. Numerous commercial implant systems with prefabricated implants have been designed with this in mind. Examples of these are the Montgomery Thyroplasty System (Boston Medical Products, Westborough, Massachusetts) and the Netterville Thyroplasty Set (Medtronic Xomed, Jacksonville, Florida).[27,28] Both sets come with a measuring device and surgical instruments. The measuring device helps to predetermine the correct implant size and may reduce the need for revisions. The Montgomery system comes with an elegantly designed precarved Silastic implant, which helps stabilize it in place while reducing the total time of surgery. The cost of convenience, however, should be considered. Other systems have been described and are available commercially. They include titanium vocal fold medializing and hydroxylapatite laryngeal implants.[29,30]

Gore-Tex (expanded polytetrafluoroethylene) has a good track record in vascular surgery and is used in cosmetic surgery too. It does not seem to incite as strong an inflammatory response as Teflon and is therefore more easily removed, should revision surgery be necessary. The meshlike structure of Gore-Tex allows tissue in growth and cell attachment. McCulloch reported on using this material instead of solid implants in medialization.[31] Because Gore-Tex is soft and pliable, its insertion, placement, and intraoperative adjustment are easier. Intraoperative time is reduced because there is no need to customize an implant. The thyroid cartilage window is smaller, and the risk of fracturing the inferior strut of thyroid cartilage is less.

Contraindications

Although medialization laryngoplasty is generally safe, it should be avoided when

1. There is a bleeding disorder if the patient was previously on an anticoagulant (the patient should be told to stop taking the anticoagulant or to replace the anticoagulant medication before surgery)
2. A vertical hemilaryngectomy has been previously performed if the absence of the thyroid cartilage as a

lateral buttress prevents adequate medialization from the implant against the scarred neoglottis
3. Previous laryngeal irradiation has been performed if the vocal fold is stiff and scarred and will not yield easily to medialization from the implant

Although medialization procedures are generally performed under local anesthesia, some patients suffer from extreme anxiety. In these cases, general anesthesia may be preferable.

Complications

Medialization laryngoplasty and arytenoid adduction have become a popular and successful treatment of vocal fold paralysis. As more surgeons perform these operations, the number of complications will also rise.

Complications associated with the procedure include

1. Airway obstruction
2. Hematoma formation and vocal fold hemorrhage
3. Implant migration and extrusion
4. Failure to improve voice
   a. Improper implant position
   b. Incorrect patient selection
5. Allergic reaction to implant
6. Local wound infection

Airway obstruction after medialization procedures is uncommon. It ranges from 0% (Cotter et al[32]) to 1% (Montgomery and Montgomary[27]) to 10% (Tucker[33]). Airway compromise is more likely to occur in patients who have had arytenoid adduction because of the resultant mucosal edema and hematoma. Medical measures such as oxygenation with an oxygen mask, nebulizing with racemic epinephrine, intravenous steroids, and use of mixed helium and oxygen (80%/20%) should be attempted first. If these fail, intubation or a tracheotomy is performed. Most patients requiring a tracheotomy did so within the first 18 hours. The median time to development of significant postoperative stridor was 9 hours, and the average time was 16.3 hours. Postoperative edema and postoperative hematoma, overzealous medialization in the anterior commissure, and overrotation of the arytenoid cartilage are possible causes of airway obstruction. Overnight hospitalization is therefore recommended for medialization laryngoplasty, especially when arytenoid adduction is performed. Another predisposing factor that may contribute to airway compromise is the presence of underlying neuromuscular disease.

The rate of wound hematoma ranges from ~10 to 24% of patients.[32,33] Although usually mild and limited to the vocal folds, hematoma can involve the paraglottic space, necessitating a tracheotomy. This can occur anytime between the first 24 hours to the fifth postoperative day. Some patients underwent wound exploration, whereas others were managed conservatively. In cases of delayed hemorrhage, there was an association with sudden transient increased intracranial pressure (lifting, straining), and the majority of cases involved people > 50 years old. Cases managed conservatively usually regress after about 3 weeks of observation.

The incidence of implant extrusion ranges from 0 to 8%. This occurred anytime between the fifth postoperative day to 15 months postoperatively.[33] This is possibly due to a breach in the inner perichondrium during surgery or due to an implant that is too large. Even after the removal of the implant, the voice improvement may persist. Some implants are coughed up, whereas others are removed endoscopically or externally through the previous incision site.

Failure to improve voice after medialization surgery is usually related to the inability to close the glottic gap adequately. The problem commonly lies in the posterior gap, where a secondary combined arytenoid adduction is required. Other problems, such as the size of the implant, implant migration, and subsequent vocal fold atrophy, also contribute to failure to close the glottal gap.

The implants used are generally regarded as biocompatible. Allergy to a silicone implant has been reported in one patient.[34] She presented with urticaria, pruritus, and erythema over pressure points on her body that resolved after the implant was removed. Foreign body reactions to Silastic have also been encountered but are rare.

A national survey by Rosen, which represented 14,621 cases of medialization laryngoplasty, showed that complications were higher in surgeons who had performed fewer than 10 such cases in their career and had fewer than two medialization laryngoplasties in the past year.[19] He concluded that there was a learning curve involved and that a certain familiarity with the procedure was required to minimize postoperative complications.

Revision Surgery

Timing

Medialization laryngoplasty has the advantage of reversibility, which the other injectable materials do not have.

Despite the best of intentions, voice failures do occur. These patients continue to have dysphonia, dysphagia, and dyspnea after medialization surgery, necessitating a revision laryngoplasty.

The rate of revision laryngoplasty ranges from 5.4 to 16.0%. In Woo et al's study, the median time interval between primary and revision surgery was 15.7 months (0.5–132 months).[20]

As in primary surgery, it is preferable to perform revision surgery under local anesthesia. There will be instances when general anesthesia is required, such as potential airway compromise or if the patient is intolerant of another local anesthetic procedure.

Causes of Failure of Primary Surgery

Failures of primary surgery may be classified as early or late.

Early Failures

Early failures are patients whose voice quality continued to be poor at 4 to 6 weeks postsurgery. Causes of early failure include

- Inappropriate patient selection and procedure
- Problem with implant size, position, and shape
- Implant migration or extrusion
- Contralateral vocal fold atrophy/bowing
- Hyperkinetic compensatory voice

The most common reason for failure is the persistence of a large posterior glottic gap. When performing stroboscopic assessment for first-time medialization laryngoplasty patients, the surgeon should look for the presence of anterior tilting of the arytenoid cartilage on the paralyzed side, vertical height difference between the two sides, and the failure to improve voice on the manual compression test. These indicate that arytenoid adduction may be necessary.

The presence of a midmembranous gap postoperatively may be due to undercorrection or the presence of contralateral vocal fold atrophy. To correct this, one should estimate the size of the gap. If it is small, fine-tuning with injection laryngoplasty is sufficient. However, if it is large, bilateral medialization is recommended.

The intention of medialization laryngoplasty is to medialize the true vocal folds. Only the membranous vocal folds can be easily pushed to the midline by a solid surgical implant. The superior extent of the vocal folds lies just below the midpoint between the thyroid notch and the inferior thyroid cartilage in the midline. A common mistake is to place the prosthesis too high. Such action will result in false cord medialization. The resultant voice will be rough and strained. Koufman and Isaacson point out that there are some patients with a large inferior thyroid notch that could distort the perceived level of the vocal fold.[35] They recommend that the bottom of the thyroid cartilage should be palpated separately from the inferior notch and the measurement taken as if the inferior notch did not exist.

There is always the temptation to place a big implant in the mistaken belief that this will result in a better voice result. Big implants may give rise to a foreign body sensation in the neck, have a higher tendency to migrate, and impinge on the vocal process of the arytenoid cartilage. Although this may aid in partially reducing the posterior glottic gap, no implant can fully address this issue. It is far better to consider adding an arytenoid adduction procedure here. Furthermore, a big implant may hinder the amount of arytenoid rotation achievable with an adduction procedure.

An extruding implant should be removed. This can be done endoscopically or externally through the previous incision site. If the implant has breached the endolarynx, antibiotics should be given and the surrounding strap muscles swung in to provide cover. When the airway has been entered, the treatment is the removal of the foreign body. The placement of a new implant should be deferred until a later date.

The presence of contralateral bowing should always be sought on stroboscopy, especially in older patients. The voice may continue to be poor after unilateral medialization and arytenoid adduction. A contralateral medialization procedure will often improve the voice.

A strained, raspy, hyperkinetic voice secondary to muscle tension dysphonia present preoperatively may persist into the postoperative period. A speech therapist will need to teach the patient to unload this compensatory mechanism to achieve a better quality voice.

Late Failures

Late failures are patients who have had an initially good result but experienced deterioration of voice quality because of subsequent atrophy of the vocal folds. This happens when concomitant medialization is performed to prevent aspiration after skull base surgery (high vagal lesion). With time, however, the vocal fold continues to atrophy, leaving a large glottic chink, which results in the voice deterioration. Therefore, delaying medialization laryngoplasty for 6 months, while waiting for atrophy to complete itself, is recommended. If there are issues with aspiration, then an injection laryngoplasty with fat, Gelfoam, or collagen is preferable. If the patient is to have an open procedure, he or she should be advised of the possible need for future revision if the voice is not satisfactory.

Preoperative and Postoperative Evaluation

Preoperative evaluation before revision surgery comprises

- Videostroboscopy
- CT scans (fine cuts) of the larynx
- Phonatory voice analysis

Videostroboscopy is performed to identify the errors that occurred during the first operation. This includes

- Evaluating the status of the glottic aperture and configuration
- Assessing arytenoid rotation and anterior tilt
- Performing implant extrusion
- Determining the presence of undesired hyperfunctional compensatory mechanisms

CT scans of the larynx (2 mm cuts) are useful in assessing the relationship of the implant to the vocal folds and the arytenoid cartilages. Magnetic resonance imaging also has been used to assess implant size and position.[36]

Pre- and postoperative phonatory voice analysis allows both surgeon and patient to quantify any improvement to the voice. In Woo et al's study, only improvement in airflow reached statistical significance.[20] There was no significant change in phonation time, fundamental frequency, jitter, shimmer, or noise-to-harmonic ratio. **Figure 4.1** comprises four CT scans showing the various implant malpositions that may result in failure. **Figure 4.2** is a videostroboscopic photograph showing a left arytenoid malposition.

Surgical Decisions

Should the Initial Implant Be Removed?

Silastic is the most commonly used implant today. Although it is inert and biocompatible, it does cause a surrounding inflammatory reaction, resulting in a fibrous capsule formation. In the majority of cases, the amount of scarring is not excessive and will allow another implant to be inserted. However, it may be necessary to incise into the scar tissue to achieve adequate medialization. If the implant is too large, or if there is severe capsule formation, the revision may be simply the removal of the implant, while leaving the fibrous capsule to remain and medialize the vocal fold. There is more difficulty revising patients who have had previous medialization with hydroxylapatite implants because the implant becomes well incorporated with the surrounding tissue. There are no reports regarding local tissue reaction to Gore-Tex, but anecdotal experiences have shown that Gore-Tex can be placed improperly, with formation of irregular edges causing poor voice.

In general, unless surgery is performed only on the contralateral side (bilateral medialization), the original implant should be removed and a new one inserted. Sometimes the desired voice can be achieved just with the addition of new shims or with just arytenoid medialization on the ipsilateral side. **Figure 4.3** shows a very small implant placed in a mobile vocal fold. After the

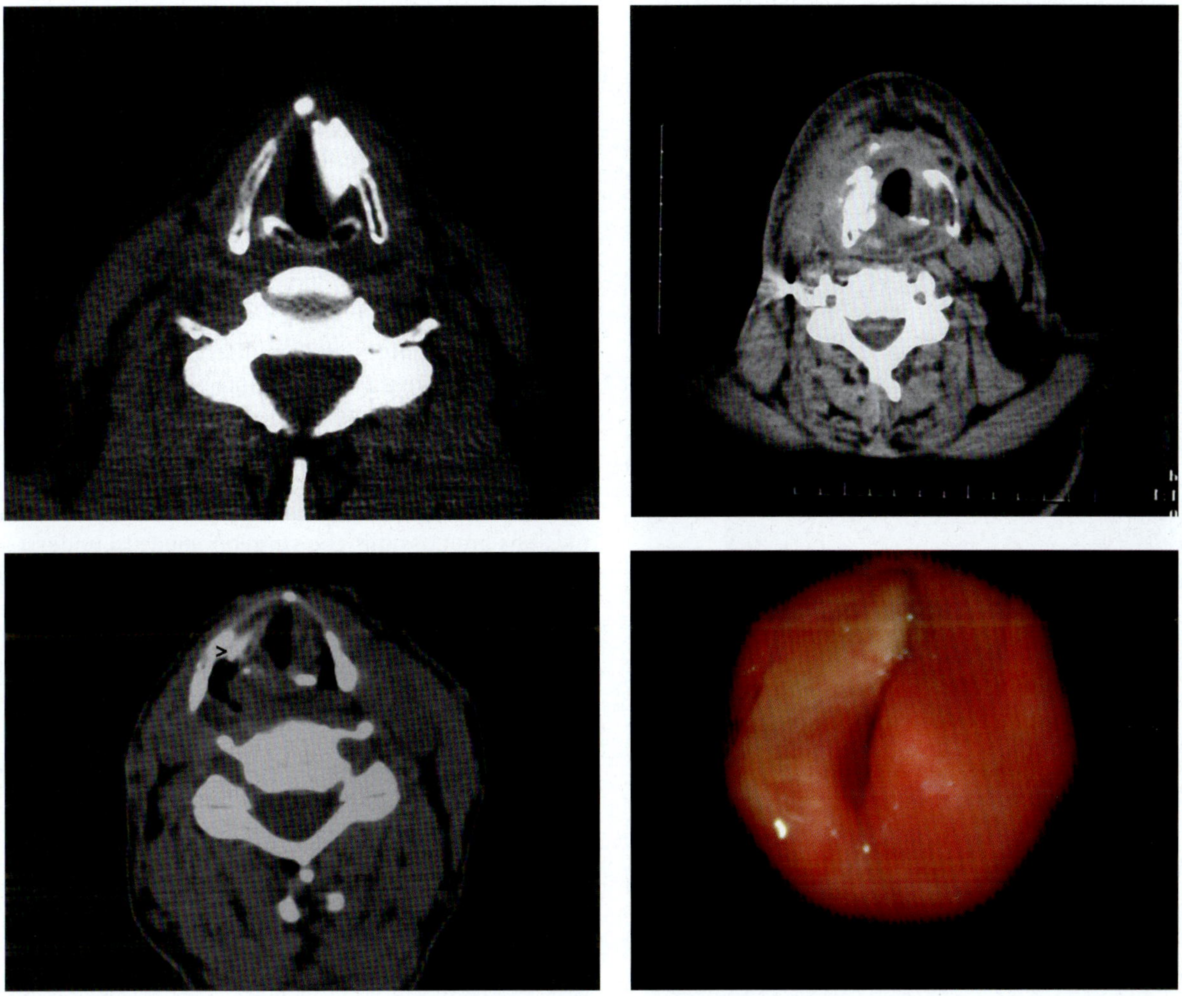

Fig. 4.1 CT scans of the larynx showing poor implant placement. **(A)** The Silastic implant with a large capsule around it, which was suggestive of a foreign body reaction. **(B)** CT scan showing a high implant. The figure shows the thyroid cartilage window and implant to be above the level of the vocal cords; also seen is the superior aspect of the arytenoid. **(C)** CT scan showing inadequate medialization. The image shows the implant to be low and small (not medializing the vocal cord) and a large posterior glottic gap due to the arytenoid malposition (*arrow*, rotated arytenoid). **(D)** Malposition of the implant. The CT scan shows two implants. The anterior implant is just deep to the mucosa.

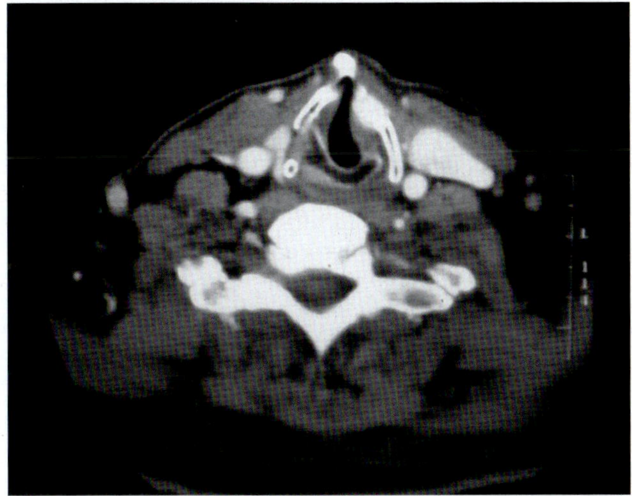

Fig. 4.2 Videostroboscopic view of the larynx demonstrating large posterior glottic gap and left arytenoid malrotation.

implant was removed, the voice returned to normal. In all likelihood, the small implant was not necessary, and the mobility of the vocal fold continued to cause inflammatory response against the foreign body.

Should Arytenoid Adduction Be Performed?

In general, arytenoid adduction should be performed whenever there is a significant posterior glottal gap that cannot be closed by a medialization alone.

Should Cricothyroid Approximation Be Performed?

If the patient has vocal fold flaccidity on preoperative stroboscopy, or if the voice quality remains low pitched

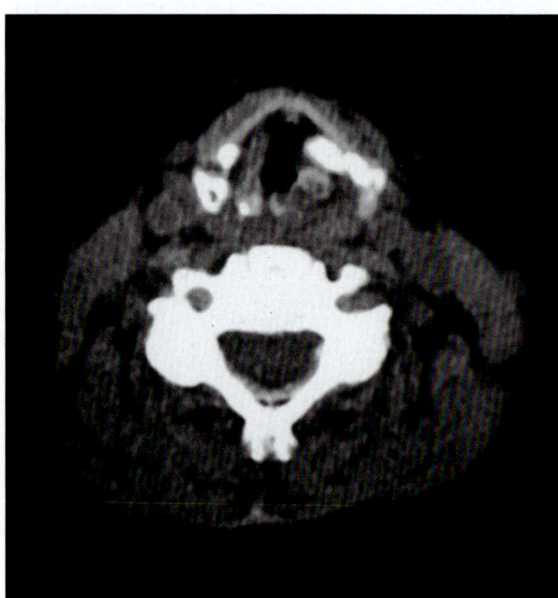

Fig. 4.3 A very small Gore-Tex implant placed in a mobile vocal fold. The patient experienced dysphonia until it was removed.

and weak after medialization, one can perform a manual cricothyroid approximation to see if the voice quality improves before proceeding with cricothyroid approximation during the surgery.

Is There a Role for Augmentation Injection Laryngoplasty after Failed Medialization Laryngoplasty?

There is a role for augmentation injection laryngoplasty. Although unsuitable for large defects, it is ideal for small gaps and "fine-tuning" of the voice.

Conclusion

Over the last century, many different techniques have evolved in the treatment of glottic insufficiency. Most recently, the technique of medialization laryngoplasty with a combination of arytenoid adduction has become popular because of its effectiveness and consistently good results. Although these operations are reversible and revisions are possible, the surgeon needs to understand the causes for failure and address all the issues in the first attempt at surgery.

The patient should be evaluated comprehensively with videostroboscopy, CT scanning, and phonatory function measurements and counseled preoperatively on the expectations of surgery.

In the event of failure to improve voice, the surgeon should reevaluate the reasons for this and be aware of the surgical options available before attempting to correct the situation.

References

1. Payr E. Plastik am Schildknorpel zur Behebung Folgen einsetiger Stimmbandlähmung. Dtsch Med Wochenschr 1915;43:1265–1270.
2. Seiffert A. Operative Wiederherstellung des Glottisschlusses bei einsteiger Recurrenslähmung und stimmddefekten. Arch Ohr Nas Kehlkheilk 1942;152:366–368.
3. Meurman Y. Mediofixation der Stimmalippe bei ihrer vollstandigen Lahmung. Arch Ohr Nas Kehlkheilk 1944;154:296–304.
4. Brünings W. Uber eine neue behandlungsmethode der rekurrenslähmung. Verh Veh Laryngol 1911;18:93–151.
5. Arnold GE. Vocal rehabilitation of paralytic dysphonia: 8. Phoniatric methods of vocal compensation. Arch Otolaryngol 1962;76:76–83.
6. Rubin HJ. Pitfalls in treatment of dysphonias by intracordal injection of synthetics. Laryngoscope 1965;75:1381–1397.
7. Lewy RB. Teflon injection of vocal cord: complications, errors, precautions. Ann Otol Rhinol Laryngol 1983;92:473–474.
8. Ford CN, Gilcrist K, Bartell T. Persistence of injectable collagen in the human larynx: a histopathological study. Laryngoscope 1987;97:724–727.
9. Brandenburg JH, Unger J, Koschkee D. Vocal cord injection with autogenous fat: a long-term magnetic resonance imaging evaluation. Laryngoscope 1996;106(2 Pt 1):174–180.
10. Isshiki N, Morita H, Okamura H, et al. Thyroplasty as a new phonosurgical technique. Acta Otolaryngol 1974;78(5–6):451–457.
11. Isshiki N, Okamura H, Ishikawa T. Thyroplasty type I (lateral compression) for dysphonia due to vocal cord paralysis or atrophy. Acta Otolaryngol 1975;80(5–6):465–473.
12. Pearl AW, Woo P, Ostrowski R, et al. A preliminary report on micronized AlloDerm injection laryngoplasty. Laryngoscope 2002;112(6):990–996.
13. Lee B, Woo P. Use of injectable hydroxy apatite in the secondary setting to restore glottic competence after partial laryngectomy with arytenoidectomy. Ann Otol Rhinol Laryngol 2004;113:618–622.
14. Rihkanen H. Vocal fold augmentation by injection of autologous fascia. Laryngoscope 1998;108(1):51–54.
15. Isshiki N, Morita H, Okamura H, et al. Experimental and clinical study of thyroplasty as a new type of phonosurgery. In: Loebell E, ed. XVIth International Congress of Logopedics and Phoniatrics. Basel: Karger; 1976:213–216.
16. Noordzij JP, Perrault D, Woo P. Biomechanics of combined arytenoid adduction and medialization laryngoplasty in an ex vivo canine model. Otolaryngol Head Neck Surg 1998;119(6):634–642.
17. Zeitels SM. New procedures for paralytic dysphonia: adduction arytenopexy, Gor-Tex medialization laryngoplasty,

and cricothyroid subluxation. Otolaryngol Clin North Am 2000;33(4):841–854.

18. Tucker HM. Anterior commissure laryngoplasty for adjustment of vocal fold tension. Ann Otol Rhinol Laryngol 1985;94(6 Pt 1):547–549.

19. Rosen CA. Complications of phonosurgery: results of a national survey. Laryngoscope 1998;108:1697–1703.

20. Woo P, Pearl AW, Hsiung MW, et al. Failed medialization laryngoplasty: management by revision surgery. Otolaryngol Head Neck Surg 2001;124(4):615–621.

21. Postma GN, Blalock PD, Koufman JA. Bilateral medialization laryngoplasty. Laryngoscope 1998;108(10):1429–1434.

22. Benninger MS, Ahuja AS, Gardner G, et al. Assessing outcomes for dysphonic patients. J Voice 1998;12(4):540–550.

23. Netterville JL, Jackson CG, Civantos F. Thyroplasty in the functional rehabilitation of neurotologic skull base surgery patients. Am J Otol 1993;14(5):460–464.

24. Lu FL, Casiano RR, Lundy DS, et al. Longitudinal evaluation of vocal function after thyroplasty type I in the treatment of unilateral vocal paralysis. Laryngoscope 1996;106(5 Pt 1):573–577.

25. Omori K, Kacker A, Slavit D, et al. Quantitative criteria for predicting thyroplasty type I outcome. Laryngoscope 1996;106(6):689–693.

26. Gray SD, Barkmeier J, Jones D, et al. Vocal evaluation of thyroplastic surgery in the treatment of unilateral vocal fold paralysis. Laryngoscope 1992;102(4):415–421.

27. Montgomery WW, Montgomery SK. Montgomery thyroplasty implant system. Ann Otol Rhinol Laryngol Suppl 1997;170:1–16.

28. Netterville JL, Stone RE, Luken ES, et al. Silastic medialization and arytenoid adduction: the Vanderbilt experience. Ann Otol Rhinol Laryngol 1993;102:413–424.

29. Friedrich G. External vocal fold medialization: surgical experiences and modifications. Laryngorhinootologie 1998;77(1):7–17.

30. Cummings CW, Purcell LL, Flint PW. Hydroxylapatite laryngeal implants for medialization: preliminary report. Ann Otol Rhinol Laryngol 1993;102(11):843–851.

31. McCulloch TM, Hoffman H. Medialization laryngoplasty with expanded polytetrafluoroethylene: surgical technique and preliminary results. Ann Otol Rhinol Laryngol 1998;107(5):427–432.

32. Cotter CS, Avidano MA, Crary MA, et al. Laryngeal complications after type 1 thyroplasty. Otolaryngol Head Neck Surg 1995;113(6):671–673.

33. Tucker HM. Complications after surgical management of the paralyzed larynx. Laryngoscope 1983;93(3):295–298

34. Hunsaker DH, Martin PJ. Allergic reaction to solid silicone implant in medial thyroplasty. Otolaryngol Head Neck Surg 1995;113(6):782–784.

35. Koufman JA, Isaacson G. Laryngoplastic phonosurgery. Otolaryngol Clin North Am 1991;24(5):1151–1177.

36. Ford CN, Unger JM, Zundel RS, et al. Magnetic resonance imaging (MRI) assessment of vocal fold medialization surgery. Laryngoscope 1995;105(5 Pt 1):498–504.

Decision tree for secondary reconstruction of post-traumatic mandibular deformities

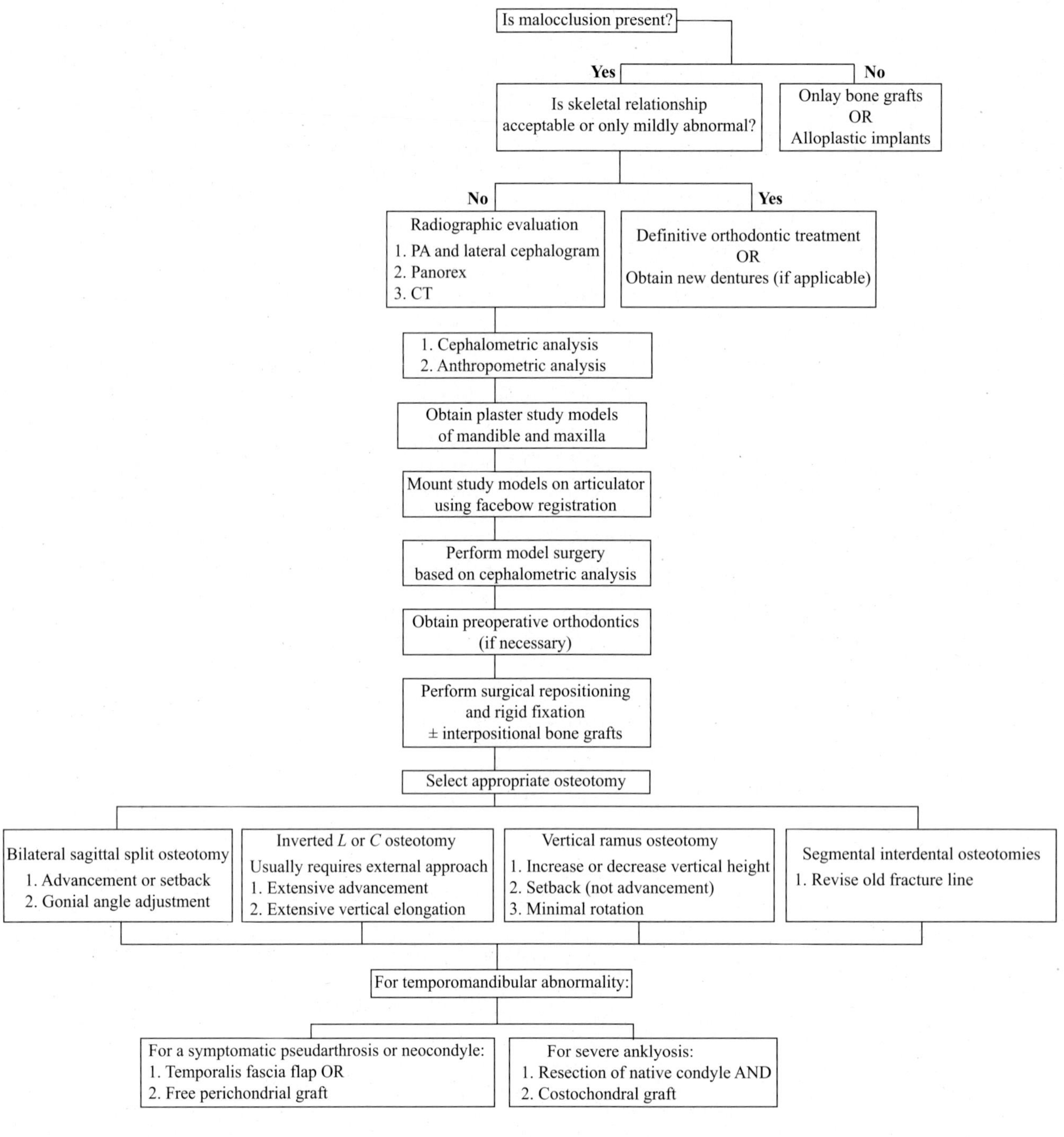

5 **Mandibular Facial Fractures**

Shane A. Zim, Sherard A. Tatum III, and Robert M. Kellman

Post-traumatic facial deformities pose some of the most challenging problems confronting the reconstructive surgeon. The main objectives in the initial repair of facial fractures are restoration of function and reestablishment of the preinjury appearance. Even in the best of hands, acute management of maxillofacial trauma may be less than optimal. Delay in initial management due to associated life-threatening injuries, failure to recognize the magnitude of injury, unsuccessful exposure and reduction, and operative complications may all contribute to secondary cosmetic deformity and dysfunction. Such deformities may cause pain and impair mastication, vision, speech, and hearing. The cosmetic abnormality may lead to deleterious emotional and social sequelae.[1] Secondary reconstructive procedures for correction of persistent post-traumatic maxillofacial deformities can provide excellent outcomes when used appropriately, and improvement in any preexisting, preinjury deformities may even be possible. However, adequate repair of the initial injuries in a timely fashion is still the optimal management.

This chapter focuses on secondary reconstruction of post-traumatic mandibular deformities, and the following chapter focuses on secondary reconstruction of post-traumatic maxillary deformities. Many of the basic principles remain the same regardless of the site of injury. Minor deformities not affecting occlusion can occasionally be adequately camouflaged with onlay bone grafts or alloplastic implants. However, severe deformities and those causing malocclusion are usually not adequately corrected with simple bone grafts and implants. In these cases, restoration of normal anatomical position of facial bones typically involves complete exposure, osteotomies with repositioning of displaced bone, rigid internal fixation, and bone grafts to fill gaps left by the movements.[2] Multiple staged operations are frequently necessary to correct complex deformities involving multiple facial bones.[3]

Occlusion and Classification of Malocclusion

An understanding of normal occlusion and classification of malocclusion is critical in the management of post-traumatic deformities, especially those involving the mandible. Simply stated, occlusion is the relationship of the maxillary teeth to the mandibular teeth. Accurate evaluation of occlusion requires evaluation in the sagittal, transverse, and vertical dimensions.

Molars usually have four cusps, with grooves between these cusps (**Fig. 5.1**). The cusps adjacent to the tongue are the lingual or palatal cusps, and those adjacent to the cheek are the buccal cusps. Those cusps located anterior on the molar toward the dental midline (the space between the central incisors) are referred to as mesial, and those located posterior on the molar away from the dental midline are distal. This dental terminology, in which the molars are distal and the incisors are mesial, should not be confused with other terminology that uses the vertical center of the body as midline in which the molars are proximal and the incisors are distal. The term *intercuspation* refers to the fitting together of opposing molar cusps and grooves. The posterior maxillary teeth are normally shifted one-half tooth width distal (or posterior) to the corresponding mandibular teeth because the maxillary central incisors are approximately one-half tooth wider than the mandibular central incisors. This shifting prevents the cusps from striking end on end, allowing for normal intercuspation.

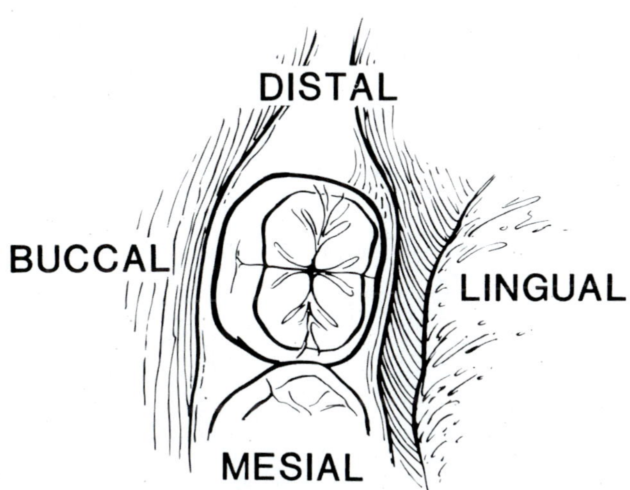

Fig. 5.1 Dental terminology. *Mesial* means toward the dental midline (the space between the central incisors). *Distal* means away from the dental midline. *Buccal* is adjacent to the cheek. *Lingual* is adjacent to the tongue. (From Donald PJ. The Surgical Management of Structural Facial Disharmony: A Self-Instructional Package. Washington, DC: American Academy of Otolaryngology–Head and Neck Surgery; 1985:12. Reprinted with permission.)

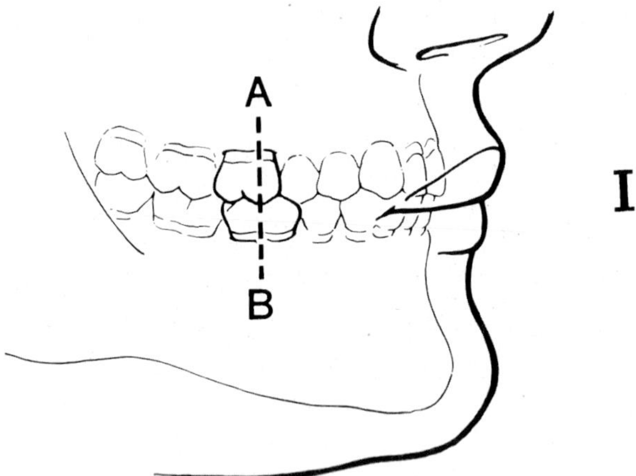

Fig. 5.2 Angle's classification of occlusion. Class I normal or centric occlusion. (From Donald PJ. The Surgical Management of Structural Facial Disharmony: A Self-Instructional Package. Washington, DC: American Academy of Otolaryngology–Head and Neck Surgery; 1985:13,14, 15. Reprinted with permission.)

In the sagittal plane, molar relationships are described independent of anterior dentition relationships. The Angle classification system refers only to the anteroposterior (mesial-distal) relationship of the maxillary first molar with the mandibular first molar. In Angle class I occlusion, which is considered normal or centric occlusion, the mesial buccal cusp of the first maxillary molar intercuspates with the buccal groove of the first mandibular molar (**Fig. 5.2**). In Angle class II malocclusion, the mesial buccal cusp of the first maxillary molar is mesial (anterior) to the buccal groove of the first mandibular molar. In Angle class III malocclusion, the mesial buccal cusp of the first maxillary molar is distal (posterior) to the buccal groove of the first mandibular molar. A posterior open bite occurs when there is no intercuspation at all and a vertical space exists between the mandibular and maxillary molars.

Relationships of the anterior teeth are described independently of molar relationships. The term *overjet* refers to the horizontal relationship of the maxillary incisors to the mandibular incisors. Normal overjet occurs when the maxillary incisors are 2 to 4 mm anterior to the mandibular incisors. Inadequate overjet, also termed *anterior crossbite,* is present when the maxillary incisors are posterior to the mandibular incisors, and excessive overjet is present when the maxillary incisors are > 4 mm anterior to the mandibular incisors. The term *overbite* refers to the vertical relationship of the maxillary incisors to the mandibular incisors. Normal overbite occurs when the incisal edges of the maxillary incisors overlap the incisal edges of the mandibular incisors by 2 to 4 mm. Excessive overbite, also called deep bite, is present when there is > 4 mm of vertical overlap between the mandibular and maxillary incisors. An anterior open bite exists when there is no overlap and a vertical space exists between the mandibular and maxillary incisors (**Fig. 5.3**).

Transverse relationships refer to the side-to-side positioning of the posterior dentition. Because the maxillary arch is wider than the mandibular arch (due to the greater width of the maxillary central incisors compared with the mandibular central incisors), the maxillary dentition normally overlaps the mandibular dentition in the transverse plane. The maxillary incisors and cuspids are normally anterior (labial) to the mandibular incisors and cuspids. The lingual cusps of the maxillary bicuspids and molars normally fit in the grooves between the lingual and buccal cusps of the mandibular bicuspids and molars,

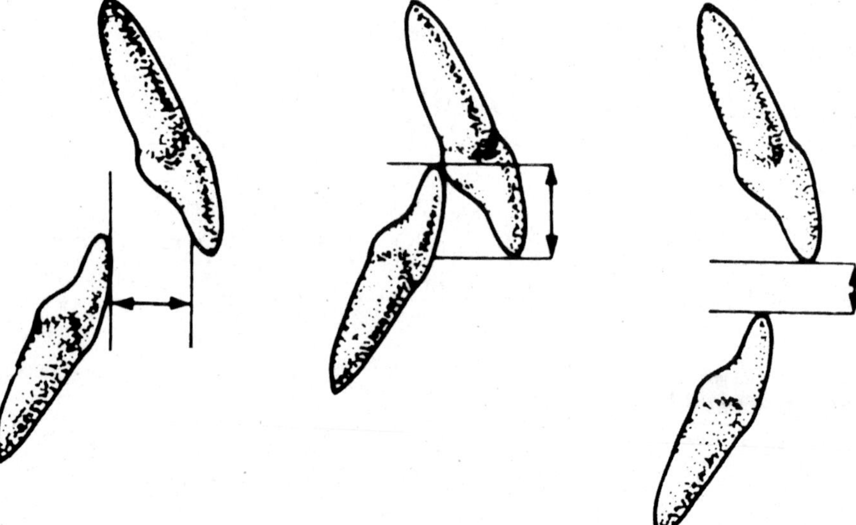

A–C

Fig. 5.3 Incisor relationships. **(A)** Overjet. **(B)** Overbite. **(C)** Open bite. (From Bailey LJ, Simmons KE, Warren DW. Orthodontic problems in children. In: Bluestone CD, Stool SE, Kenna MA, eds. Pediatric Otolaryngology. Vol 2. Philadelphia: WB Saunders; 1996:1030. Reprinted with permission.)

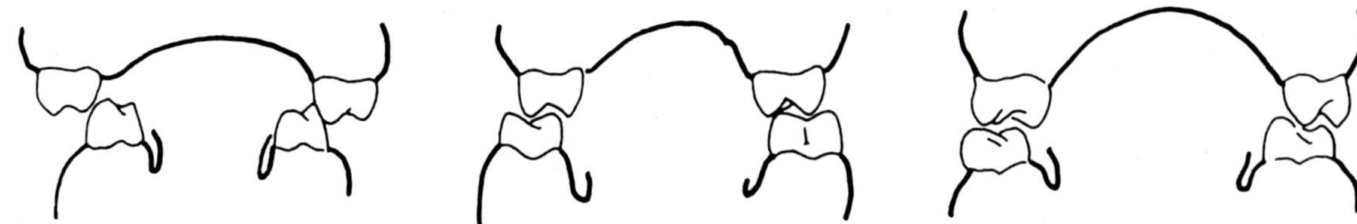

A–C

Fig. 5.4 Transverse dental relationships. **(A)** Bilateral buccal crossbite. **(B)** Bilateral lingual crossbite. **(C)** Unilateral lingual crossbite (*left*) and normal relationship (*right*). (From Powell N, Humphreys B. Considerations and components of the aesthetic face. In: Powell N, Humphreys B, eds.: Proportions of the Aesthetic Face. New York: Thieme-Stratton; 1984:11. Reprinted with permission.)

whereas the buccal cusps of the mandibular bicuspids and molars normally fit in the grooves between the lingual and buccal cusps of the maxillary bicuspids and molars. A lingual crossbite is present when the maxillary buccal cusps either fit end to end with or are lingual (medial) to the mandibular buccal cusps. When the maxillary lingual cusps are buccal (lateral) to the mandibular buccal cusps, a buccal crossbite exists (**Fig. 5.4**).

Another important occlusal concept to be aware of is the curve of Spee, which represents a gentle superior curvature in the occlusal plane from posterior to anterior (**Fig. 5.2**). Abnormalities in this curvature can result in vertical malocclusion. For example, an anterior open bite exists when the maxillary curve of Spee is greater than the mandibular curve of Spee, whereas a posterior open bite occurs when the mandible has a greater curve of Spee than the maxilla. The anterior plane of occlusion may be abnormal as well. For example, an asymmetric mandibular or maxillary arch can result in an obliquely oriented bite (**Fig. 5.5**). Finally, the abnormal position of one or two teeth is not always a reflection of an underlying bony abnormality. The term *version* refers to a single tooth in crossbite with surrounding teeth that are in a normal relationship. The abnormally positioned tooth is labeled by the direction in which it is displaced, such as in lingual, palatal, or buccal version.

A patient with a post-traumatic deformity may have had a preinjury malocclusion. Although often difficult to delineate, the preinjury malocclusion can sometimes be determined from flat surfaces on the teeth caused by occlusal contact, termed wear facets. Radiographs and intraoperative visualization may also aid in evaluating preinjury relationships. However, as the secondary post-traumatic deformity ages, new wear facets form and skeletal deformities remodel, making it even more difficult to determine the preinjury state. In some instances it may be possible and desirable to correct preinjury malocclusion, which must be planned in conjunction with correction of the post-traumatic deformity.

Once the concepts of occlusion have been grasped, it is important to understand that any combination of these occlusal relationships can occur in the post-traumatic deformity as a result of malunion or nonunion. Maxillary and mandibular position can be excessive, deficient, or simply malaligned in the sagittal, transverse, and/or vertical dimension. These deformities must be thoroughly analyzed and characterized to determine the appropriate means of correcting the post-traumatic deformity.

Pretreatment Assessment

Successful management of post-traumatic facial deformities begins with a comprehensive pretreatment assessment followed by a well-organized treatment plan, which may include orthodontics and multiple staged procedures. Diagnosis begins with a history of the mechanism of injury, any previous attempted repairs, and any subsequent complications. Insight into the condition of the tissues involved in the deformity is important because fibrosis of surrounding soft tissue from scar contraction limits skeletal movements and the success of bone grafts.[2] During physical

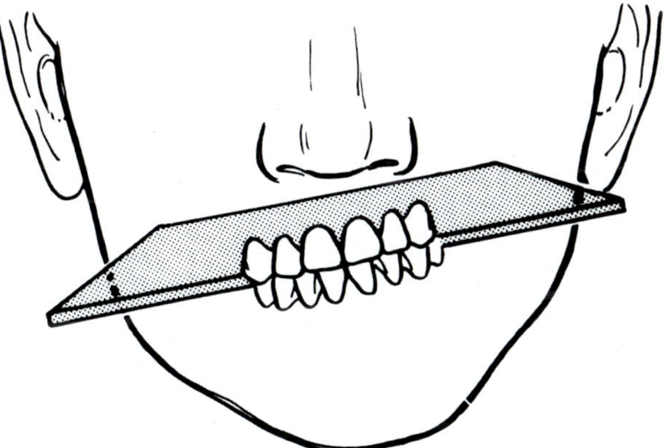

Fig. 5.5 Obliquely oriented bite. (From Donald PJ. The Surgical Management of Structural Facial Disharmony: A Self-Instructional Package. Washington, DC: American Academy of Otolaryngology–Head and Neck Surgery; 1985:17. Reprinted with permission.)

examination, skeletal abnormalities and classification of occlusion are evaluated. In particular, temporomandibular joint function should be documented, including interincisal opening distance, translation of the joint, and crepitus or pain in the joint. Any cranial nerve or vision dysfunction should also be documented.[1] Anthropometric measurements should be obtained to provide quantitative analysis of specific facial structures and their relationships with each other.[4] Pre- and postinjury photographs are helpful both as a baseline record and in treatment planning.

Radiographic studies provide the definitive analysis of skeletal abnormalities. A panoramic radiograph provides excellent information about the craniofacial skeleton. Lateral cephalograms are crucial in assessing skeletal and occlusal relationships, and anteroposterior cephalograms are required for any asymmetry. There are multiple cephalometric analysis systems described in the literature, each with its own strengths and weaknesses (**Fig. 5.6**).[5] The surgeon must choose a system with which he or she is comfortable and become very familiar with its particular normative data as well as its strengths and weaknesses. Some of the typical cephalometric angular measurements are listed in **Table 5.1**. When correlated with anthropometric measurements, cephalometric measurements allow determination of which dimensions are normal versus abnormal. Pencil tracings on acetate paper then provide for precise planning of surgical movements. Alternatively, the cephalometric analysis and surgical planning can be done on a computer. High-resolution axial and coronal computed tomography (CT) scans, especially those with three-dimensional reconstruction, provide invaluable information on the entire craniomaxillofacial skeleton. CT scans provide visualization of fragments, evaluation of degree of bony

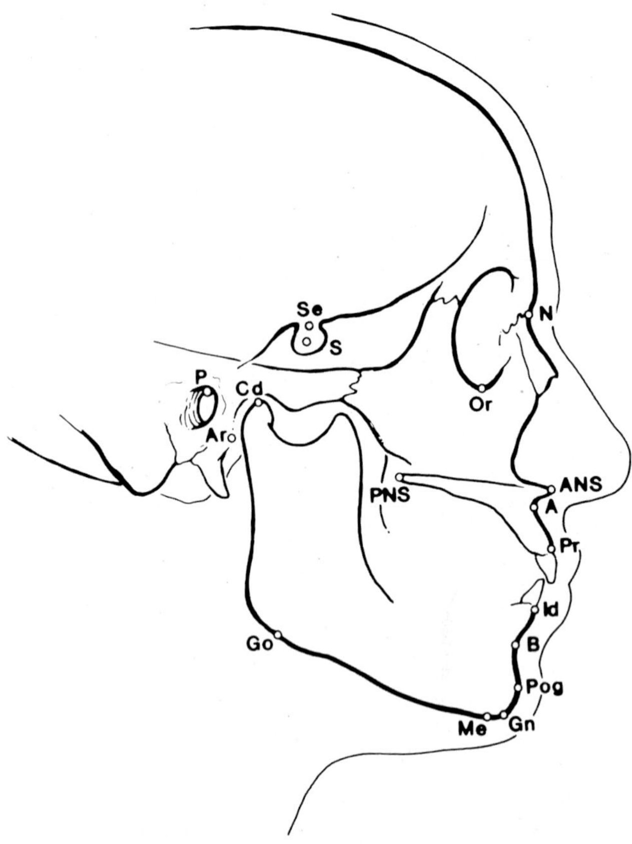

Fig. 5.6 Common skeletal landmarks used in cephalometric analysis. A, subspinale; ANS, anterior nasal spine; Ar, articulare; B, supramentale; Cd, condylion; Gn, gnathion; Go, gonion; Id, infradentale; Me, menton; N, nasion: OR, orbitale; P, porion; PNS, posterior nasal spine; Pog, pogonion; Pr, prosthion; S, sella; Se, sellaturcica. (From Sykes JM, Donald PJ. Orthognathic surgery. In: Papel ID, Nachlas NE, eds. Facial Plastic and Reconstructive Surgery. St. Louis: Mosby Year Book; 1992:237. Reprinted with permission.)

Table 5.1 Typical Cephalometric Angle Measurements

Points of the Angle	Definition	Mean Value
N-S-Ar	Saddle angle	123 ± 5 degrees
S-Ar-Go	Articular angle	143 ± 6 degrees
Ar-Go-Me	Gonial angle	128 ± 7 degrees
Ar-Go-N	Upper gonial angle (GOI)	52 to 55 degrees
N-Go-Me	Lower gonial angle (GOI)	70 to 75 degrees
SNA	Anteroposterior position of maxilla	82 degrees
SNB	Anteroposterior position of mandible	80 degrees
ANB	Difference between SNA and SNB	2 degrees
SN-MP	Angle between SN and mandibular plane	35 degrees
Pal-MP	Angle between palatal and mandibular plane	25 degrees
O-P intersecting	Frankfort mandibular plane angle	20 to 29 degrees

A, subspinale; Ar, articulare; B, supramentale; Go, gonion; Me, menton; MP, mandibular plane; N, nasion; O, orbitale; P, porion; Pal, palatal plane; S, sella.

Source: From Rakowski T. An Atlas and Manual of Cephalometry Radiography. Philadelphia: Lea and Febiger; 1982. Adapted with permission.

displacement and bony defects, and definition of soft tissue disruption.[1] Holographic projection of three-dimensional reconstructions enhances the depiction of the abnormality. Furthermore, software is being developed that will permit simulated surgery on three-dimensional images with prediction of soft tissue results. Finally, intraoperative CT and image-guided navigation systems offer the promise of more precise skeletal movements.[6]

Articulator-mounted dental study models are essential for planning surgical correction of malocclusion.[7] Using alginate or acrylic rubber, dental impressions of the maxillary and mandibular teeth are taken, followed by construction of plaster study models of the dentition made from these impressions. A face bow registration is then taken, and the information obtained is used to place the maxillary study model in the same position relative to the articulator joints that the patient's maxillary dentition has relative to the temporomandibular joints. Once the maxillary study model is mounted, a wax bite registration is taken from the patient to show the current relationship between the maxillary and mandibular teeth. This bite registration is placed on the maxillary study model, then the mandibular study model is placed into the underside of the bite registration and mounted in this position on the articulator (**Fig. 5.7**). The patient's current occlusion is now accurately represented on the articulator-mounted model. Subsequently, the plaster bases of the study models are marked with a millimeter scale parallel and perpendicular to the occlusal plane. One or both of the plaster bases are cut, simulating osteotomies. Based on the cephalometric tracings, the occlusal relationship is normalized and the plaster bases refixed. The amount of movement required is determined from the marked scale on the plaster bases. Alternatively, articulators with adjustable bases are available to allow the model movements to be done without plaster cuts. Occlusal splints for intraoperative use can be created from the normalized articulated study models if desired. This detailed presurgical preparation can reveal subtle asymmetries in the skeletal movements necessary to achieve normal occlusion.

Treatment

Nonsurgical Treatment

Orthodontics

It is important to decide whether to manage post-traumatic malocclusion surgically or nonsurgically. Correction of very minor malocclusions such as premature contact of a single set of cusps may consist of grinding the contacting teeth to provide better intercuspation.[8] Minor skeletal abnormalities can sometimes be fixed by obtaining new dentures. If a greater degree of malocclusion is present with either acceptable skeletal relationships or a minor skeletal abnormality, orthodontics may be adequate management. More severe skeletal abnormalities and malocclusion require surgical movement, with or without preoperative orthodontics. It should be understood that orthodontic movements intended to compensate for skeletal abnormalities without surgery are quite different from orthodontic movements planned in combination with surgery. Therefore, the decision for surgery should be made prior to any orthodontic treatment. Finally, additional orthodontic treatment may be required even after skeletal surgery is completed to fine-tune occlusion.

Surgical Treatment

Incisions and Approaches

Essentially, the entire mandible can be exposed intraorally through an inferior gingivobuccal sulcus incision or extensions thereof superiorly along the mandibular ramus, though extraoral incisions may be necessary for wider and freer manipulation in some areas (e.g., the condylar region) (**Fig. 5.8**). If free bone grafting of the mandible is intended, extraoral incisions will more likely provide a successful result by avoiding contamination of the graft with oral flora. Standard Risdon or submental incisions

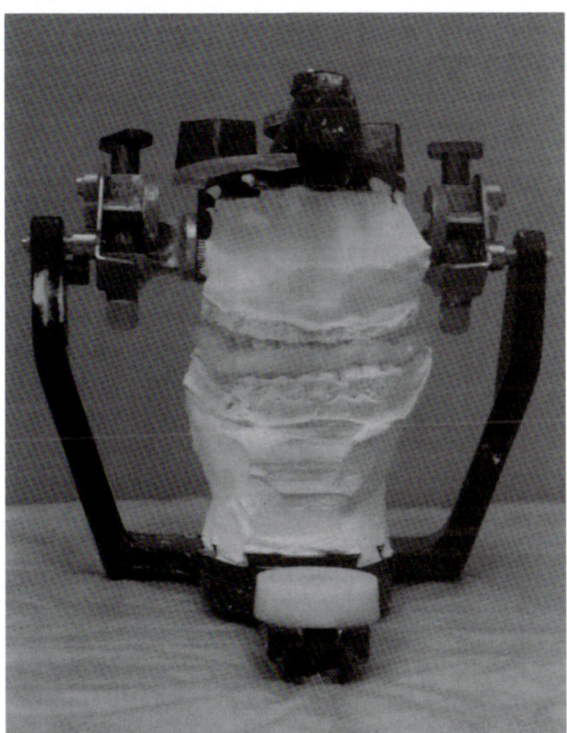

Fig. 5.7 Plaster dental models mounted on an articulator, with bite registration in place.

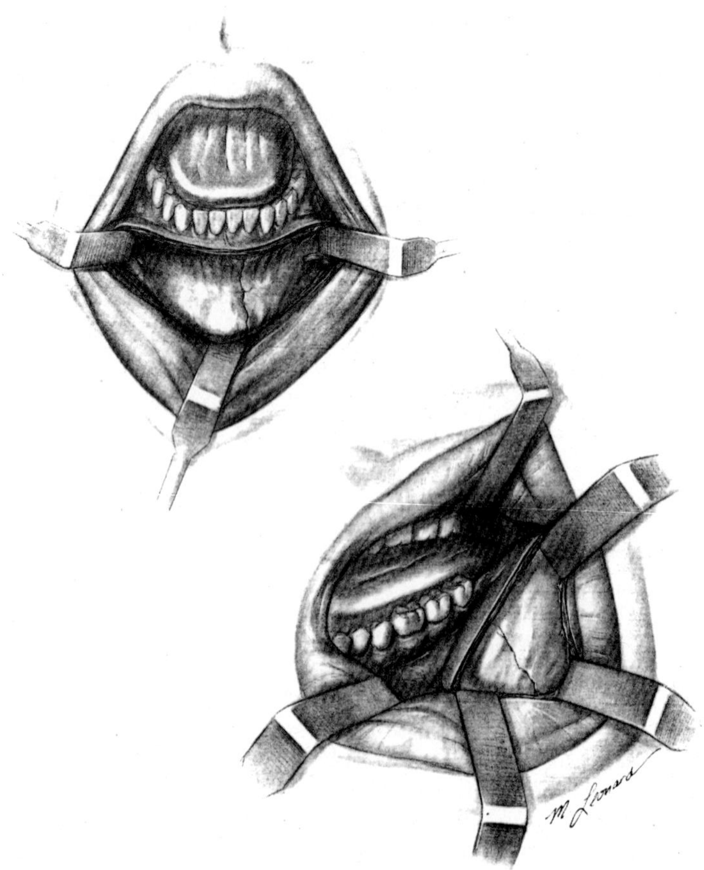

A

B

Fig. **5.8** Inferior gingivobuccal sulcus incisions for mandible exposure. **(A)** Exposure of anterior mandible. **(B)** Exposure of posterior mandible. (From Kellman RM, Marentette LJ. Surgical approaches. In: Kellman RM, Marentette LJ, eds. Atlas of Craniomaxillofacial Fixation. New York: Raven Press; 1995:73,79. Reprinted with permission.)

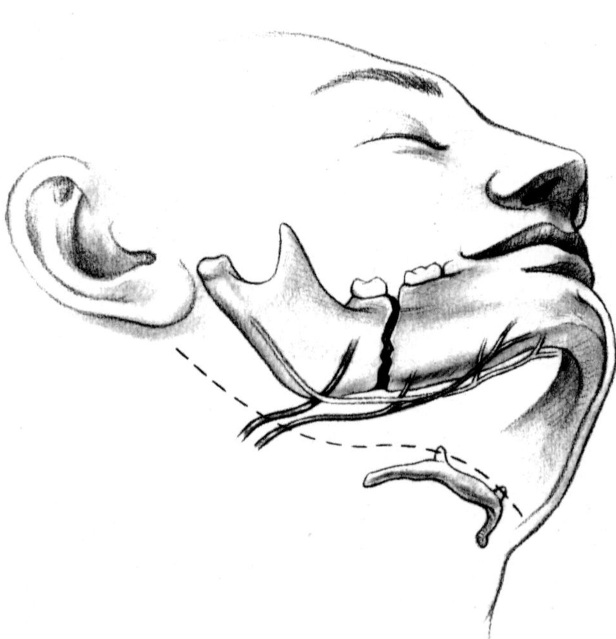

Fig. **5.9** External approach for mandible exposure. Extraoral incision. (From Kellman RM, Marentette LJ. Surgical approaches. In: Kellman RM, Marentette LJ, eds. Atlas of Craniomaxillofacial Fixation. New York: Raven Press; 1995:83,84. Reprinted with permission.)

provide adequate extraoral access when required (**Fig. 5.9**). Some surgeons advocate transoral approaches for mandibular bone grafting, so it may be acceptable for small grafts in otherwise healthy patients.

If an intraoral approach is selected, the oral cavity is prepared with povidone and/or hydrogen peroxide solution. After the mucosa is injected with a vasoconstricting agent, the incision is made with a scalpel or with electrocautery. It is important to leave enough tissue on the gingival side to facilitate closure but not leave too much tissue to interfere with visualization of the mandibular cortex. The incision is carried down through periosteum, followed by elevation of periosteum down to the inferior border of the mandible to clearly expose the areas of interest. The mental nerve, which usually exits its foramen between the canine tooth and the first bicuspid, must be identified and preserved to avoid sensory disturbance in the lower lip. Elevation of the periosteum on the lingual cortex of the upper ramus is required if sagittal split osteotomies are planned. In this case, the mandibular nerve must be identified and protected as it enters the mandibular foramen at the lingula. Before closing the inferior gingivobuccal sulcus incisions, the mentalis muscle should be resuspended either from residual muscle or from small drill holes in the anterior cortex of the mandible to prevent "witch's chin" or mentalis ptosis. Incisions are closed in a watertight fashion to reduce the chance of wound dehiscence and subsequent infection of osteotomy sites or fixation hardware. Two-layer closure where possible is beneficial.

If an extraoral approach is chosen, the skin is prepared with a povidone solution. The proposed incision site is injected with a vasoconstricting agent. An incision is made through the skin and subcutaneous tissue in a natural skin crease approximately one finger breadth below the inferior border of the mandible to decrease the amount of skin retraction required. If exposure of the high ramus and condyle is required, the incision can be curved superiorly toward the back of the ear. Dissection proceeds inferiorly in a plane superficial to the platysma for 1 to 2 cm. The platysma is then incised, and the dissection proceeds superiorly toward the mandible in a plane deep to the platysma. The marginal mandibular branch of the facial nerve should be identified and preserved as it courses immediately deep to the platysma. Alternatively, the dissection may be taken deeper through the cervical fascia to the level of the submandibular gland until the capsule of the gland is identified. The dissection then continues in a subfascial plane superiorly toward the mandible, deep to the marginal mandibular branch of the facial nerve. However, the nerve is not identified in this latter approach. Once it has been exposed, the periosteum of the inferior border of the mandible is incised. Attachments of the masseter muscle are also incised, followed by elevation of the periosteum to adequately expose the areas of interest. The incision is closed in layers, and a drain is usually placed because dead space may be created during the dissection.

Osteotomies

Mandibular osteotomies can be designed to allow a variety of movements. If anterior horizontal mandibular advancement is required, sagittal split ramus osteotomy is typically performed. During this osteotomy, the lingual and buccal cortices of the ramus, angle, and occasionally posterior body of the mandible are divided while preserving the inferior alveolar nerve (**Fig. 5.10**).[9] The gonial angle of the mandible can theoretically be altered after sagittal split osteotomy by rotating the mandible clockwise or counterclockwise (from a right lateral perspective), although the permanence of this maneuver is debated.[10] The bone segments are rigidly fixed with plates and screws or with three fixation screws placed through the overlapping cortical segments. Lag screws and compression plates are avoided to protect the inferior alveolar nerve from compression and to protect the temporomandibular joint from torsion. Alternatively, inverted L- or C-shaped full-thickness, bicortical ramus osteotomies with interposition bone grafts are used when the horizontal advancement necessary is too extensive for sagittal split osteotomy or when significant vertical elongation of the ramus is required (**Fig. 5.11**).

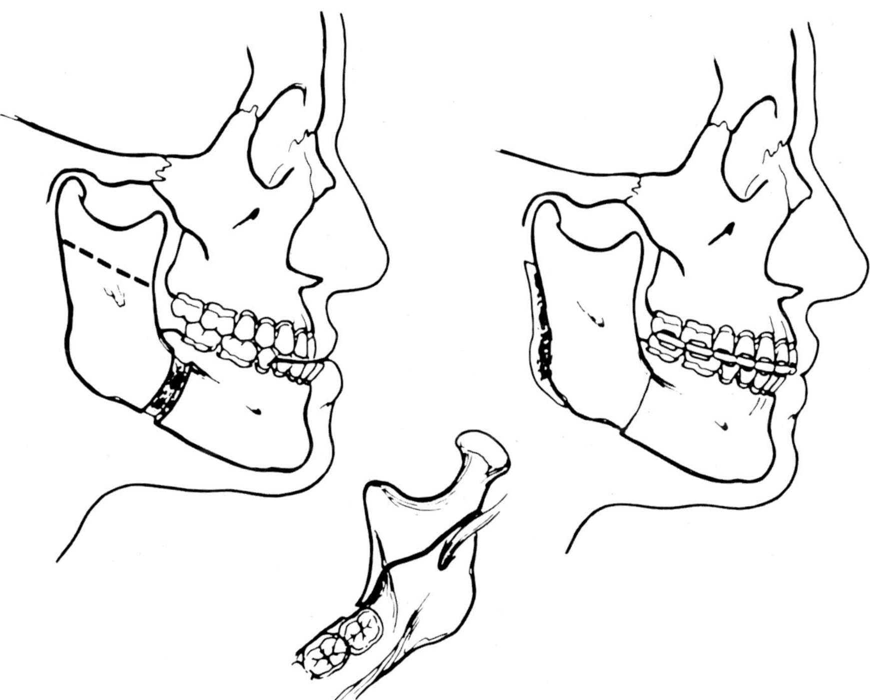

Fig. 5.10 Sagittal split osteotomy of the mandibular ramus allowing advancement or recession of the mandible as well as rotation of the gonial angle. Bone cuts consist of a horizontal osteotomy of the lingual cortex superior to the lingula, a vertical osteotomy of the buccal cortex near the second molar, and an osteotomy along the oblique line connecting the first two. (From Sykes JM, Donald PJ. Orthognathic surgery. In: Papel ID, Nachlas NE, eds. Facial Plastic and Reconstructive Surgery. St. Louis: Mosby Year Book; 1992:243. Reprinted with permission.)

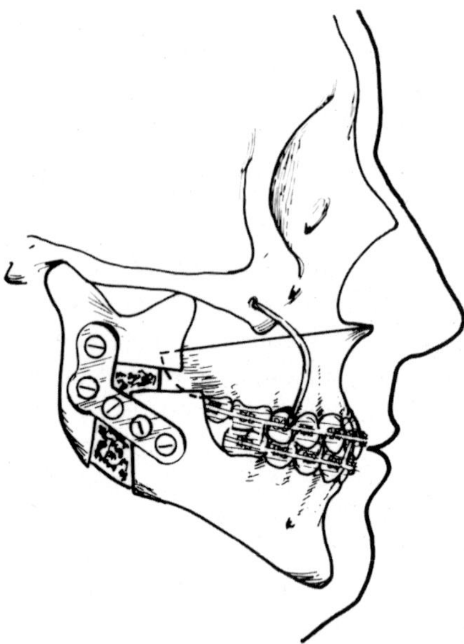

Fig. 5.11 L-shaped bicortical osteotomy of the mandibular ramus, allowing extensive horizontal or vertical advancement. Completed osteotomy with interposition bone graft and rigid fixation plate. (From Carlotti AE, Schendel SA. Surgical management of short mandibular ramus deformities. In: Bell WH, ed. Modern Practice in Orthognathic and Reconstructive Surgery. Vol 3. Philadelphia: WB Saunders; 1992:2017. Reprinted with permission.)

Vertical or vertical oblique ramus osteotomies allow increase or reduction of vertical ramus height, posterior horizontal setback (but not anterior horizontal advancement), and some minimal rotation (**Fig. 5.12**). These full-thickness, bicortical osteotomies extend from just anterior to the condylar neck down through the posterior border of the mandibular angle, running behind the mandibular foramen. When asymmetric

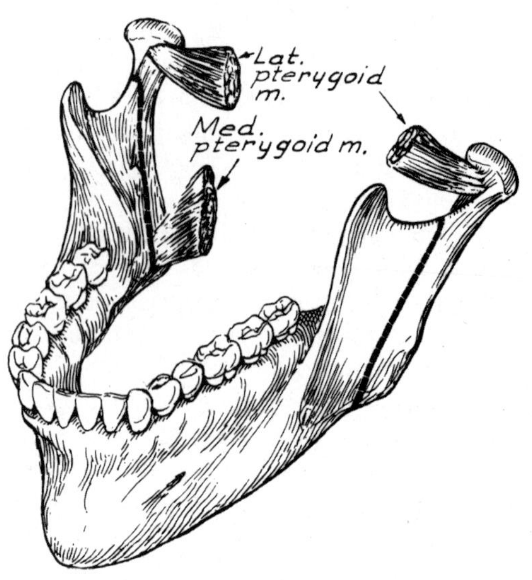

Fig. 5.12 Vertical mandibular ramus osteotomies. Design of osteotomy running posterior to the mandibular foramen. (From McCarthy JG, Kawamoto H, Grayson BH, et al. Surgery of the jaws. In: McCarthy JG, ed. Plastic Surgery. Vol 2. Philadelphia: WB Saunders; 1990:1239. Reprinted with permission.)

movements are required, vertical ramus osteotomies are preferred because less torsion is placed on the temporomandibular joints. These osteotomies usually do not require fixation when performed for mandibular setback. Moreover, the bone overlap is in a "favorable" position so that the surrounding muscle forces provide for excellent healing after 4 to 6 weeks of mandibulomaxillary fixation. When used to alter vertical ramus height, rigid fixation with plates and screws is more likely to be necessary (**Fig. 5.13**).

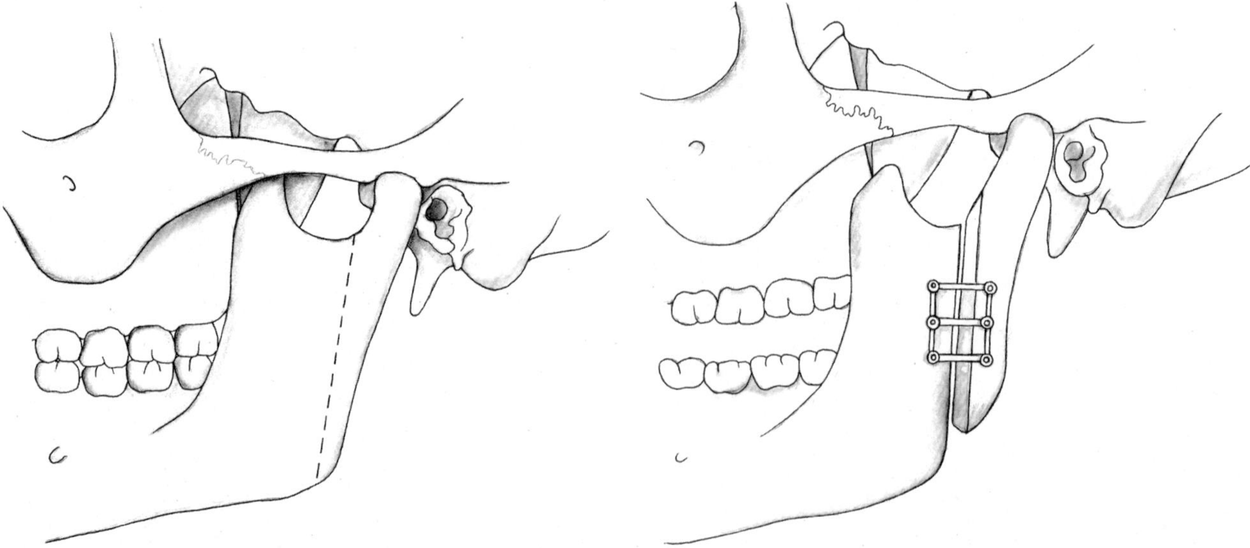

Fig. 5.13 A rigid fixation plate used to stabilize a vertically repositioned bony segment after vertical mandibular ramus osteotomy.

Segmental interdental osteotomies through previous fracture lines are often needed to revise mandibular fractures (**Fig. 5.14**). The inferior alveolar nerve should be drilled out and transposed to protect it from being transected while performing these osteotomies. Due to bony remodeling after the original trauma, the edges of the osteotomies may require contouring to ensure proper fit.

Sliding genioplasty through a subapical osteotomy of the menton provides three-dimensional chin movement independent of the remainder of the mandible (**Fig. 5.15**). An alternative to ramus osteotomies in the correction of an anterior open bite associated with bilateral subcondylar fractures involves posterior maxillary impaction using a Le Fort I osteotomy combined with a sliding genioplasty to camouflage mandibular recession. This approach may provide superior resistance to the strong relapsing forces

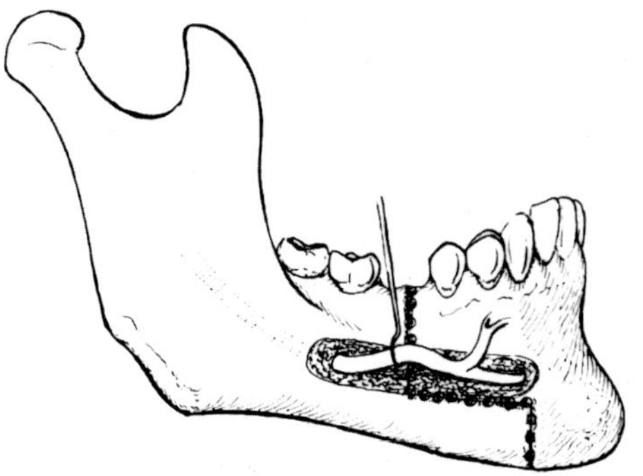

Fig. 5.14 Segmental interdental mandibular osteotomies. Inferior alveolar nerve drill-out allowing interdental osteotomies. (From McCarthy JG, Kawamoto H, Grayson BH, et al. Surgery of the jaws. In: McCarthy JG, ed. Plastic Surgery. Vol 2. Philadelphia: WB Saunders; 1990:1267. Reprinted with permission.)

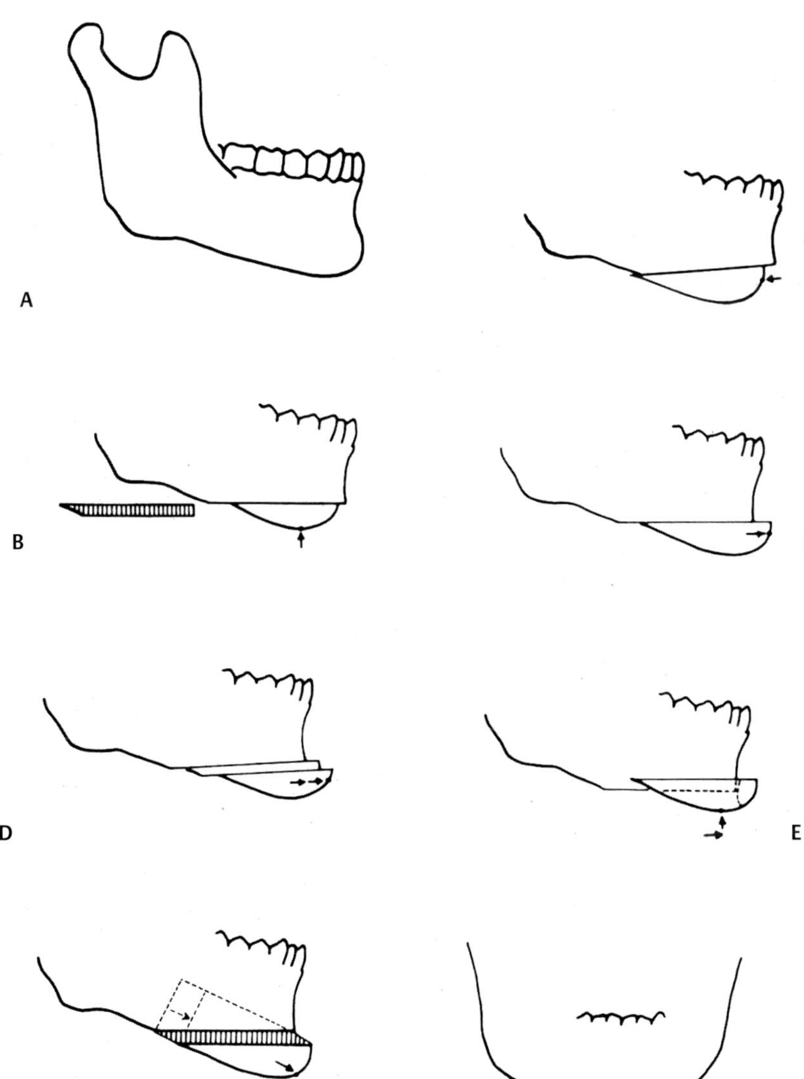

Fig. 5.15 Sliding genioplasty allowing three-dimensional chin movement to correct a variety of deformities. **(A)** Posterior slide. **(B)** Vertical reduction. **(C)** Anterior advancement. **(D)** Two-tiered anterior advancement. **(E)** Jump. **(F)** Anterior advancement with augmentation. **(G)** Transverse slide. (From McCarthy JG, Kawamoto H, Grayson BH, et al. Surgery of the jaws. In: McCarthy JG, ed. Plastic Surgery. Vol 2. Philadelphia: WB Saunders; 1990:1313. Reprinted with permission.)

caused by the muscles of mastication.[7] However, the loss of facial height must be carefully considered before choosing this alternative approach.

The temporomandibular joint must be carefully evaluated in post-traumatic deformities of the mandible. A functioning, asymptomatic pseudarthrosis or neocondyle should be left undisturbed. Vertical deficiency may be best managed with a vertical oblique ramus osteotomy to reestablish appropriate ramus height (**Fig. 5.13**). If the pseudarthrosis or neocondyle is symptomatic or poorly functioning, then the temporomandibular joint should be reconstructed. The joint must be opened, and an attempt to locate the meniscus should be performed. An inferiorly based temporalis fascia flap or free perichondrial graft is transposed to line the joint. It may also be wrapped around the native condylar remnant (**Fig. 5.16**). Severe ankylosis with complete obliteration of the joint necessitates resection of the native condyle and reconstruction with a costocartilage graft (**Fig. 5.17**). Alloplastic prosthetic temporomandibular joints are controversial and are not recommended until biomechanical problems with them are worked out.[7,11,12]

Case Study

A 20-year-old woman involved in a motor vehicle accident sustained multiple facial fractures, including a comminuted left mandibular body fracture and bilateral subcondylar fractures. All fractures except the left subcondylar fracture were repaired primarily by open reduction and internal fixation (**Fig. 5.18A**). Several months later, she returned with secondary deformities, including nonunion of the left mandibular body fracture and left vertical mandibular ramus deficiency due to loss of the condylar fragment with subsequent premature contact of the posterior teeth. She underwent revision surgery consisting of débridement of the left mandibular body nonunion with an iliac crest cancellous bone graft to fill the resulting gap and placement of a mandibular reconstruction plate, followed by a left vertical oblique mandibular ramus osteotomy with miniplate fixation to restore ramus height (**Fig. 5.18B**).

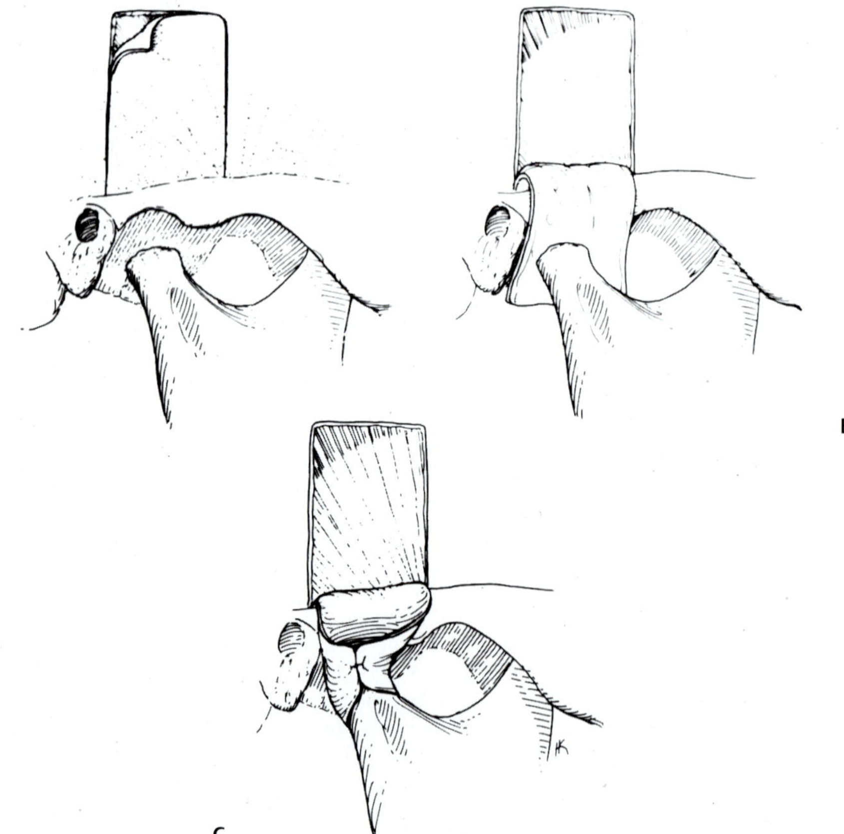

Fig. 5.16 Reconstruction of a poorly functioning temporomandibular joint. **(A)** Elevation of the temporalis fascia flap. **(B)** Transposition of the temporalis flap into the joint. **(C)** The temporalis flap wrapped around the condyle. (From Kawamoto HK. Correction of established traumatic deformities of the facial skeleton using craniofacial principles. In: Schultz RC, ed. Facial Injuries. Chicago: Year Book Medical Publishers; 1988:629. Reprinted with permission.)

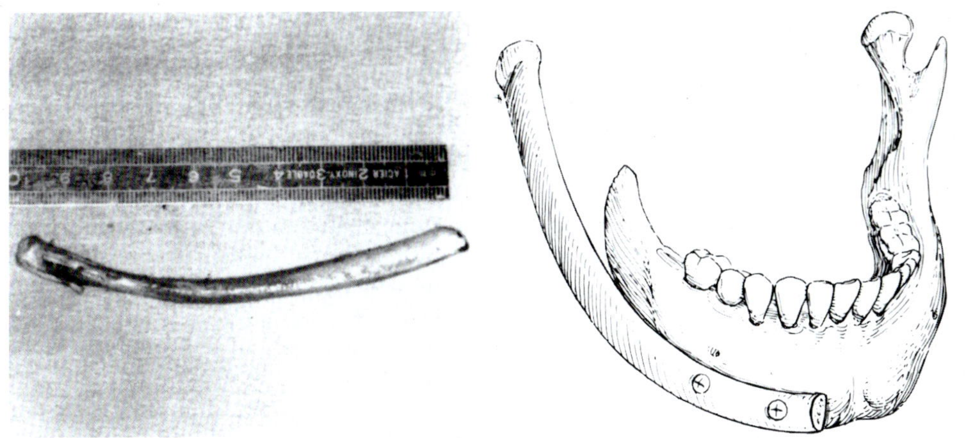

A

B

Fig. 5.17 Reconstruction of the temporomandibular joint after resection for severe ankylosis. **(A)** A costochondral graft harvested with a cartilage cap as the neocondyle. **(B)** Lag screw fixation of a graft to the mandible. (From Kawamoto HK. Correction of established traumatic deformities of the facial skeleton using craniofacial principles. In: Schultz RC, ed. Facial Injuries. Chicago: Year Book Medical Publishers; 1988:630. Reprinted with permission.)

Complications

Complications that can occur as a result of the initial trauma can also occur as a result of revision surgery.[13] Incision-related complications include bleeding, infection, and wound dehiscence leading to infected osteotomy sites or hardware. The mandibular nerve is at risk for stretching, avulsion, or transection resulting in numbness of the mandibular teeth and lower lip. Injury to the neurovascular supply to the tooth roots leads to nonviability of the teeth.

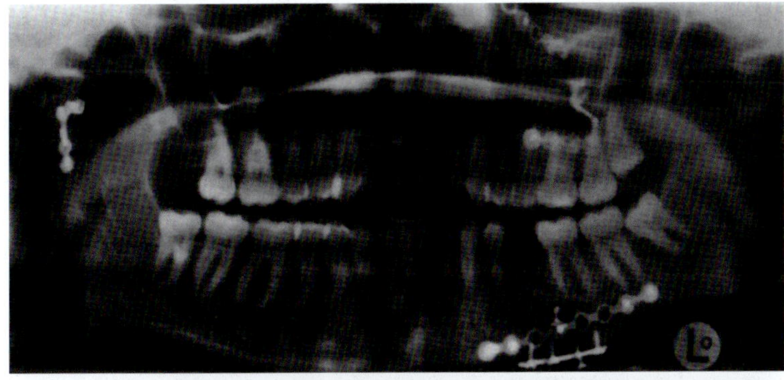

A

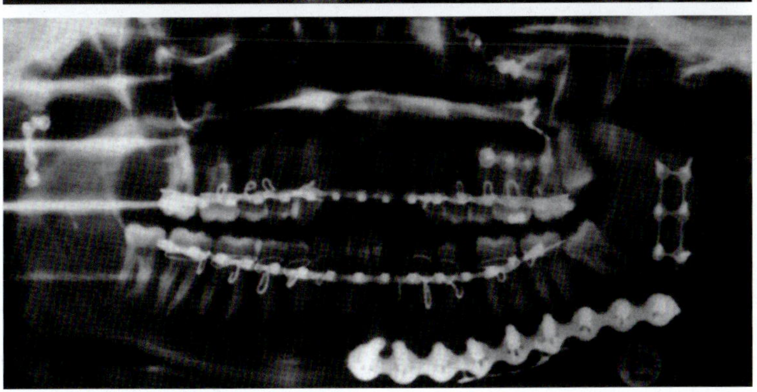

B

Fig. 5.18 Case study. **(A)** Panorex following primary repair illustrating nonunion of the left mandibular body and loss of left vertical ramus height. **(B)** Panorex following revision surgery illustrating bony continuity of the left mandibular body after an iliac crest cancellous bone graft and placement of a reconstruction plate, as well as restoration of left vertical ramus height after a vertical oblique ramus osteotomy and placement of a miniplate for rigid fixation. (From Tatum SA. Correction of post-traumatic maxillofacial deformities involving occlusion. Facial Plastic Surgery Clinics of North America 1998;6:535–556. Reprinted with permission.)

Osteotomy-specific complications include nonunion, malunion, bony relapse, and ankylosis of the temporomandibular joint. Care must be taken to ensure proper placement of the condyles in the glenoid fossae to avoid improper positioning of the mandible and subsequent malocclusion. Propensity for skeletal relapse increases proportionately with the extent of bony repositioning. Because skeletal relapse can occur up to several years postoperatively, patients should be followed with serial cephalograms for a minimum of 2 years after surgery.

Conclusion

Post-traumatic mandibular deformities can be corrected using craniomaxillofacial principles to provide improved facial aesthetics and mastication. Careful evaluation of the deformity, including a detailed analysis of occlusion, coupled with a well-thought-out treatment plan, allow for a very precise correction of occlusion. Well-hidden incisions, wide exposure, appropriate osteotomies with subsequent repositioning of bone, rigid internal fixation, and bone grafting as indicated all contribute to an acceptable reconstructive result.

References

1. Hardesty RA , Coffey JA. Secondary craniomaxillofacial deformities: current principles of management. Clin Plast Surg 1992;19:275–300.
2. Gruss JS. Craniofacial osteotomies and rigid fixation in the correction of post-traumatic craniofacial deformities. Scand J Plast Reconstr Surg Hand Surg Suppl 1995;27:83–95.
3. Cohen SR, Kawamoto HK. Analysis and results of treatment of established posttraumatic facial deformities. Plast Reconstr Surg 1992;90:574–584.
4. Posnick JC, Farkas LG. Anthropometric surface measurements in the analysis of craniomaxillofacial deformities: normal values and growth trends. In: Posnick JC, ed. Craniofacial and Maxillofacial Surgery in Children and Young Adults. Philadelphia: WB Saunders; 2000:55–79.
5. Grayson BH. Cephalometric analysis for the surgeon. Clin Plast Surg 1989;16:633–644.
6. Stanley RB. Use of intraoperative computed tomography during repair of orbitozygomatic fractures. Arch Facial Plast Surg 1999;1:19–24.
7. Kawamoto HK. Correction of established traumatic deformities of the facial skeleton using craniofacial principles. In: Schultz RC, ed. Facial Injuries. Chicago: Yearbook Medical Publishers; 1998:601–630.
8. Zachariades N, Mezitis M, Michelis A. Posttraumatic osteotomies of the jaws. Int J Oral Maxillofac Surg 1993;22:328–331.
9. Bloomquist DS. Mandibular body sagittal osteotomy in the correction of malunited mandibular fractures. J Maxillofac Surg 1982;10:18–23.
10. Tatum SA. Correction of post-traumatic maxillofacial deformities involving occlusion. Facial Plast Surg Clin North Am 1998;6:535–556.
11. Rubens BC, Steolinga PJW, Weaver TJ, Bludorp PA. Management of malunited mandibular condylar fractures. Int J Oral Maxillofac Surg 1990;19:22–28.
12. Patel A, Maisel R. Condylar prostheses in head and neck cancer reconstruction. Arch Otolaryngol Head Neck Surg 2001;127:842–846.
13. Mathog RH, Rosenburg Z. Complications in the treatment of facial fractures. Otolaryngol Clin North Am 1976;9:533–552.

Decision tree for secondary reconstruction of post-traumatic maxillary deformities

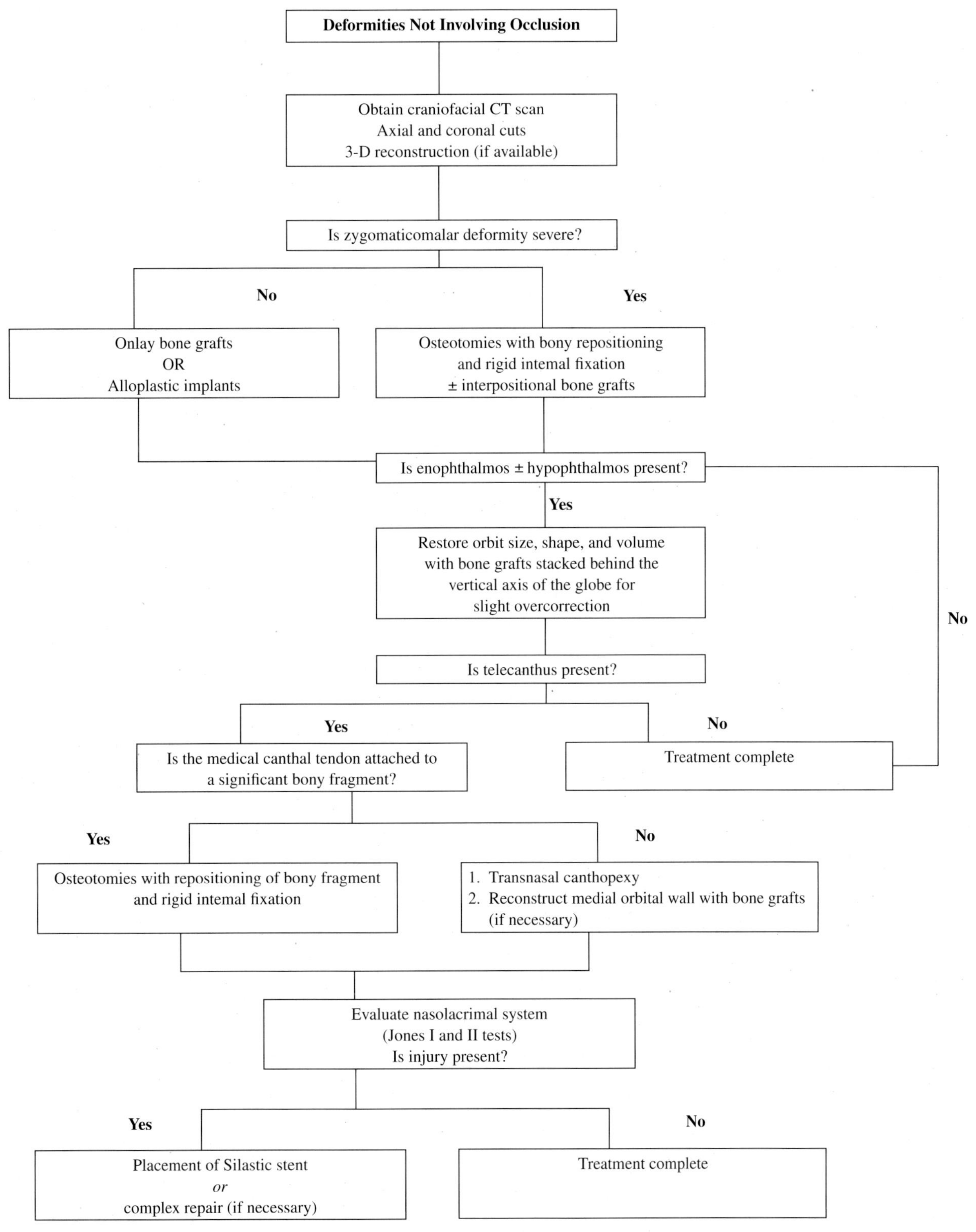

Decision tree for secondary reconstruction of post-traumatic maxillary deformities

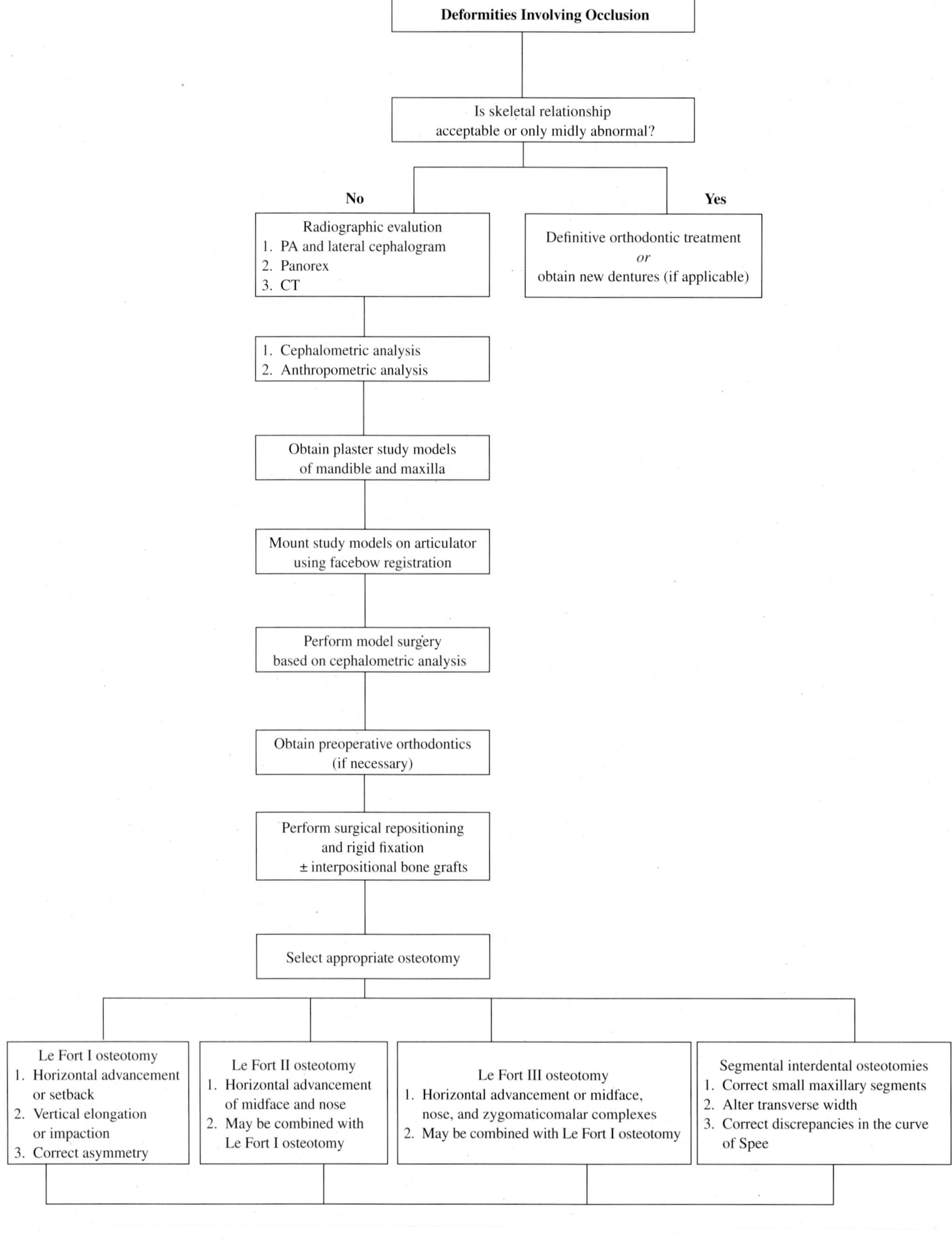

6 Maxillary Facial Fractures

Shane A. Zim, Robert M. Kellman, and Sherard A. Tatum III

This chapter, which focuses on secondary reconstruction of post-traumatic maxillary deformities, is a continuation of the preceding chapter, which discusses management of post-traumatic mandibular abnormalities. Common post-traumatic deformities of the midface include enophthalmos, vertical ocular dystopia, malar flattening, telecanthus, collapse of the naso-orbito-ethmoid area, and malocclusion.[1] The guiding principles for successful management of post-traumatic abnormalities remain the same regardless of the site of injury, whether it is the mandible or maxilla. These principles include a comprehensive pretreatment analysis followed by a well-organized treatment plan, which may entail multiple staged procedures.[2] Craniomaxillofacial techniques for reconstruction of such deformities consist of complete exposure, osteotomies with repositioning of displaced bone, rigid internal fixation, and bone grafts to fill gaps left by the movements.[1] For a detailed discussion of occlusion, pretreatment assessment, and orthodontics, the reader is referred to the previous chapter on mandibular fractures. The remainder of this chapter will focus on analysis, incisions, and osteotomies for deformities of the maxilla and the naso-orbito-zygomatic region.

Incisions

Essentially, the entire midface can be exposed through three incisions: a maxillary vestibular (gingivobuccal sulcus) incision, either a transconjunctival incision or a subciliary incision, and a coronal incision (**Fig. 6.1**). The maxillary vestibular (gingivobuccal sulcus) incision can be extended from tuberosity to tuberosity to expose the maxilla up to the orbital rim.[1]

To perform the maxillary vestibular incision, the oral cavity is prepared with povidone and/or hydrogen peroxide solution. The mucosa at the proposed incision site is injected with a vasoconstricting agent. It is important to leave enough tissue on the gingival side to facilitate closure, but not too much tissue to interfere with visualization of the maxilla. The incision is carried down through the periosteum, followed by elevation of the periosteum superiorly to the inferior orbital rims. The infraorbital nerve must be identified and preserved to avoid sensory disturbance in the cheeks. If a Le Fort I osteotomy is to be done, a less extensive incision should be made to preserve additional blood supply to the osteotomized palate and upper teeth. When higher osteotomies are required, more superior exposure can be achieved by converting the maxillary vestibular incision into a midfacial degloving approach through nasal circumvestibular and intercartilaginous incisions.[3] In this fashion, the upper lip can be retracted up to the glabella. A watertight closure is important to reduce the risk of wound dehiscence and subsequent infection of osteotomy sites or fixation hardware. If tension is present, the mucosa is closed with a simple interrupted absorbable suture; otherwise, a simple running stitch is usually adequate. When extensive repositioning of the maxilla has been performed, a V → Y closure of the labial mucosa reduces the tendency for lip shortening. Further, a cinching suture should be placed from ala to ala either through or beneath the nasal base to prevent splaying out of the alar base by the advanced maxilla.

The malar eminence, inferior orbital rim, and orbital floor can be exposed through a transconjunctival or subciliary incision. A transconjunctival incision with or without lateral cantholysis is preferable to a subciliary incision in most cases to decrease the risk of ectropion and avoid a visible scar. A corneal shield may be beneficial. After skin preparation, the proposed incision should be injected with a vasoconstricting agent. A lateral canthotomy incision is made 5 to 10 mm out into the facial skin and down through the lateral canthal tendon, separating its upper and lower components. Fine scissors are then used to perform the inferior cantholysis by separating the lower half of the lateral canthal tendon from the lateral orbital rim. The incision is then extended through the conjunctiva 3 to 5 mm inferior to the tarsal plate, followed by dissection down to the infraorbital rim. The importance of maintaining a preseptal plane of dissection is debated. The periosteum on the facial side of the infraorbital rim is incised, with care taken to preserve the infraorbital nerve. A subperiosteal dissection is performed to expose the orbital floor, the lateral orbital wall, the medial orbital wall, and the frontozygomatic suture as needed. The conjunctiva may be closed with a fast-absorbing buried knot suture. A permanent or slow-absorbing suture is required to resuspend the lateral canthal tendon.

Limited exposure to the superior and superolateral orbit can be achieved through a lateral brow or a superior lid crease incision. If cranial bone grafts are to be obtained, however, a coronal incision provides superior

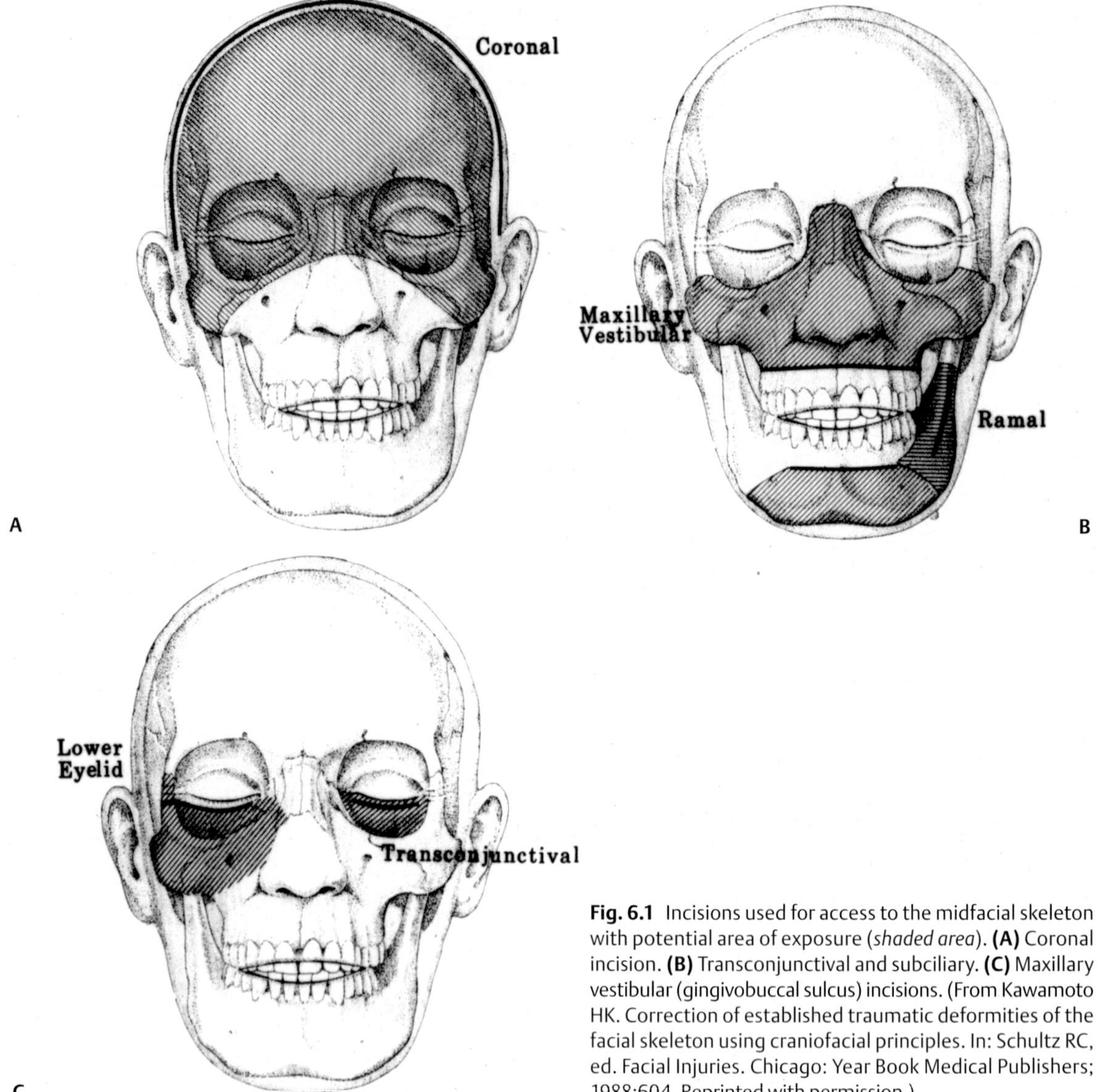

Fig. 6.1 Incisions used for access to the midfacial skeleton with potential area of exposure (*shaded area*). **(A)** Coronal incision. **(B)** Transconjunctival and subciliary. **(C)** Maxillary vestibular (gingivobuccal sulcus) incisions. (From Kawamoto HK. Correction of established traumatic deformities of the facial skeleton using craniofacial principles. In: Schultz RC, ed. Facial Injuries. Chicago: Year Book Medical Publishers; 1988:604. Reprinted with permission.)

periorbital exposure.[4] A wavy line coronal incision is recommended over a straight coronal incision to reduce the visibility of the scar. After skin preparation with or without scalp shaving, the proposed incision should be injected with a vasoconstricting agent. An incision is made down through the periosteum in the midline and extended laterally until the superior temporal line is identified on both sides. The coronal flap is elevated anteriorly in the subperiosteal plane medial to the superior temporal lines. Lateral to the superior temporal lines, care must be taken to elevate the flap deep to the temporoparietal fascia to prevent injury to the frontal branch of the facial nerve. If exposure of the zygomatic arch is necessary, the superficial layer of the deep temporal fascia is incised just inferior to the temporal line of fusion to expose the temporal fat pad. Dissection is then continued down to the zygomatic arch, with care taken to avoid disruption of the temporal fat pad. The periosteum is incised along the superior portion of the arch and then carefully dissected off the arch laterally. Frequently, the supraorbital neurovascular bundle exits through a foramen, which must be converted to a groove with a small osteotome to free the bundle. During closure, the superficial layer of the deep temporal fascia should be reapproximated. Drains are often used, although suction drains may not be optimal when dural repairs or sinus leaks are present. Certain key areas of the soft tissue, including the medial and lateral canthal tendons, the anterior aspect of the temporalis muscle, and the periosteum over the malar eminence, should be resuspended to the skeleton prior to closure. Closure of the scalp consists of a meticulous galeal repair with medium- to long-term absorbable sutures followed by reapproximation of the skin with sutures or staples. A subcuticular closure is recommended in small children.

Deformities Involving Occlusion

Pretreatment Evaluation

A maxillary fracture can be malunited in any position but is most often displaced posteriorly and inferiorly along an inclined plane at the skull base, which results in premature contact of the molars, an anterior open bite deformity, and an inferiorly displaced chin. This abnormality gives the appearance of an elongated face with a deceiving prognathic appearance due to an undisturbed mandible.[5] As part of the physical examination, the middle third of the face should be evaluated for nonunion by grasping the anterior alveolar ridge while stabilizing the skull and applying force in the anteroposterior direction to determine if there is movement. Principles of management are similar to those of elective orthognathic surgery, and the reader is referred to the previous chapter on mandible fractures for an in-depth discussion of occlusion, orthodontics, and pretreatment assessment, including radiographic evaluation. One additional important aspect of the maxilla to understand is the buttress concept.[6] The skeletal framework of the midface consists of relatively thick segments of bone acting as a major structural support system that transmits the powerful forces of mastication to the skull base (**Fig. 6.2**). The intervening thin sheets of bone have a separating rather than a structural role. These buttresses, which give three-dimensional (3-D) strength to the facial skeleton and prevent soft tissue collapse, are typically the areas where rigid fixation and bone grafts are placed.[7]

Surgical Treatment

Standard midfacial osteotomies resemble the classic Le Fort fracture patterns. However, rather than cutting through the pterygoid plates, as is usually the case with

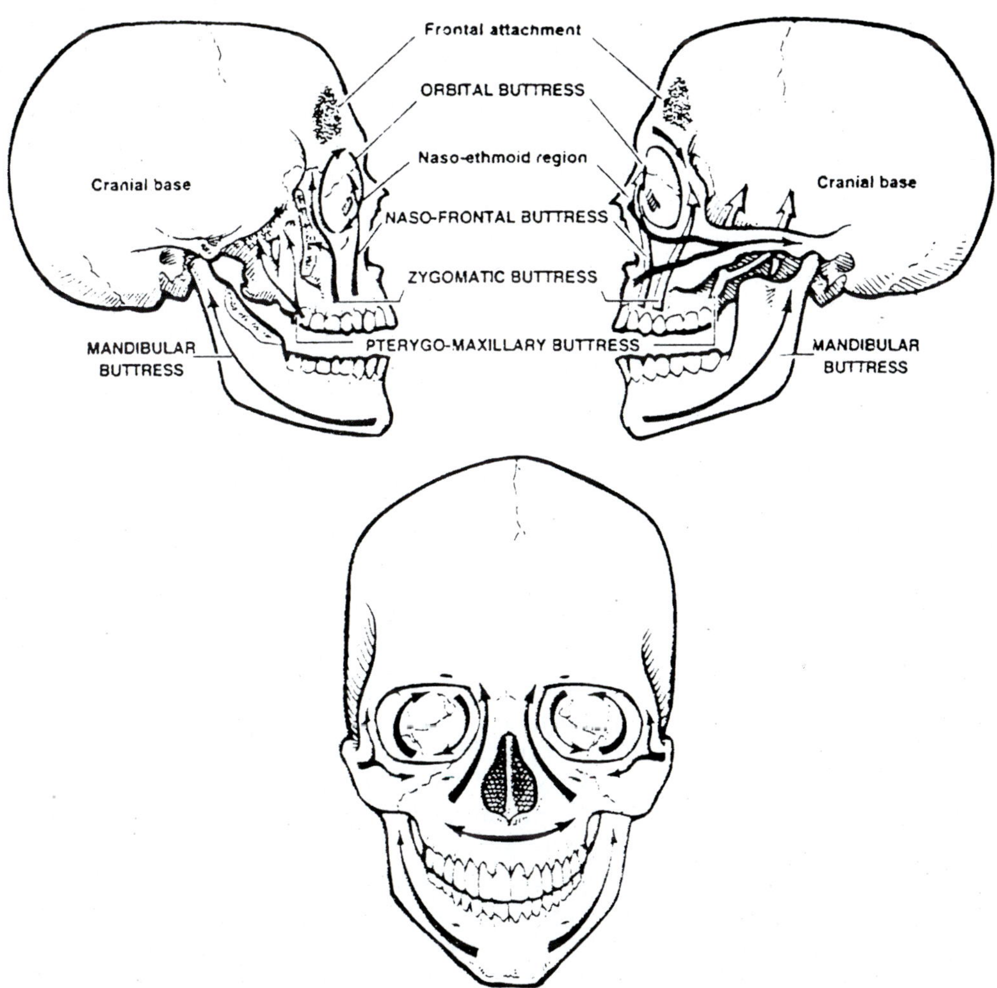

Fig. 6.2 Horizontal and vertical buttresses of the facial skeleton. (From Hardesty RA, Coffey A. Secondary craniomaxillofacial deformities: current principles of management. Clin Plast Surg 1992;19:275–300, as adapted from Manson PW, Hoopes JE, Su CT. Structural pillars of the skeleton: an approach to the management of Le Fort fractures. Plast Reconstr Surg 1980;66:54–61. Reprinted with permission.)

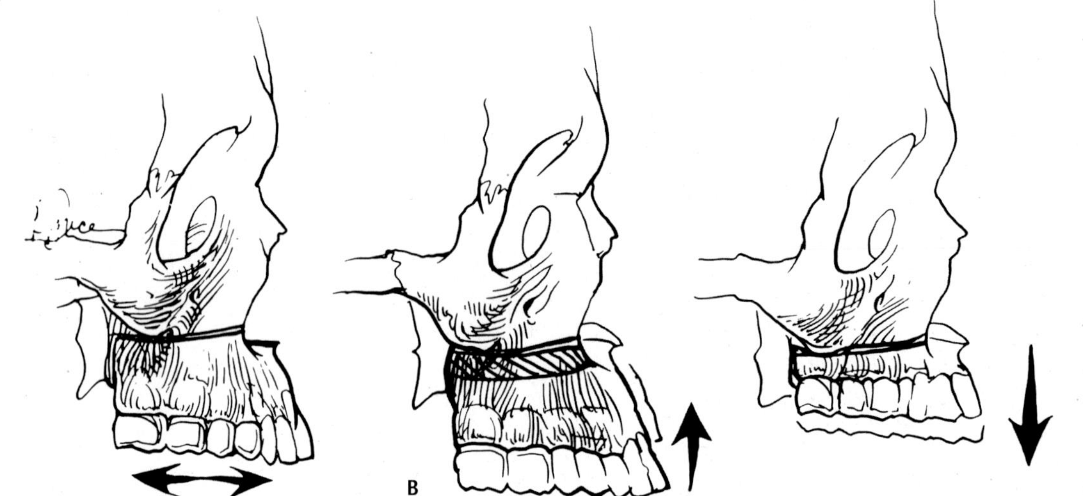

Fig. 6.3 The versatile Le Fort I osteotomy, which allows a variety of maxillary movements. **(A)** Maxillary recession or advancement. **(B)** Vertical impaction. **(C)** Vertical elongation. (From McCarthy JG, Kawamoto H, Grayson BH, et al. Surgery of the jaws. In: McCarthy JG, ed. Plastic Surgery. Vol 2. Philadelphia: WB Saunders; 1990:1369. Reprinted with permission.)

Le Fort fractures, the pterygomaxillary fissure is osteotomized instead.[8] The classic Le Fort I osteotomy cuts parallel to the occlusal plane just above the floor of the nose and the floor of the maxillary sinus. Considered the workhorse of maxillary occlusal surgery, the versatile Le Fort I osteotomy can be altered or angulated in a variety of ways, allowing the maxilla to be moved in any direction in space (**Fig. 6.3**). The addition or removal of bone from the osteotomized maxilla provides vertical height increase or vertical impaction, respectively. Using the Le Fort I osteotomy, posterior or anterior horizontal advancement of the maxilla can be accomplished. Rotating or shifting the osteotomized maxilla to one side can be used to correct asymmetry, and the occlusal plane can be leveled by the appropriate asymmetric vertical changes. By angling the Le Fort I osteotomy downward and forward, simultaneous maxillary advancement and vertical height increase can be achieved. The bone cut can be angled upward from medial to lateral, passing either just beneath the infraorbital nerve or through the orbit out into the zygomaticomalar complex. This slight modification increases the midfacial fullness in the inframalar area by advancing that area with the maxillary dentition. Interdental osteotomies may be necessary to correct small maxillary segments or individual teeth in crossbite, to alter the transverse width of the dental arch, or to fix discrepancies in the curve of Spee (**Fig. 6.4**). If the palate has been split to increase the transverse width of the maxilla, a plate across the palate osteotomy and an occlusal splint are especially useful to help prevent transverse relapse, which is particularly prone to occur in this area.[9]

The standard Le Fort II osteotomy is primarily used to provide anterior horizontal advancement of the midface and nose. The standard Le Fort III osteotomy advances the zygomaticomalar complex in addition to the midface and nose (**Fig. 6.5**).[10] Alternatives to the standard zygomatic arch osteotomy in the coronal plane allow bony continuity after repositioning, thereby reducing the need for bone grafts (**Fig. 6.6**). However, Le Fort II and III osteotomies permit very limited vertical or asymmetric movement compared with the Le Fort I osteotomy. When the degree of midface movement necessary does not correlate with the degree of movement necessary to correct the occlusion, a Le Fort I osteotomy can be combined with a Le Fort III osteotomy to achieve the desired result. Finally, the surgeon must realize that standard Le Fort osteotomies may not always be adequate for correction of post-traumatic deformities of the maxilla. To optimize reconstruction, creativity must frequently be employed to design custom osteotomies that mimic the original fracture line.[11,12]

When bony repositioning > 4 or 5 mm is performed, corticocancellous bone grafts harvested from the ilium or calvarium should be used to fill the gaps between bone segments and to help reduce the tendency for relapse. In general, all osteotomies should be rigidly fixed with titanium plates and screws in the 1 to 2 mm range to stabilize the bony segments in their newly acquired positions and to help prevent relapse. Moreover, mandibulo-maxillary fixation can often be discontinued immediately postoperatively if all bony segments are rigidly fixed and the occlusal result is satisfactory.

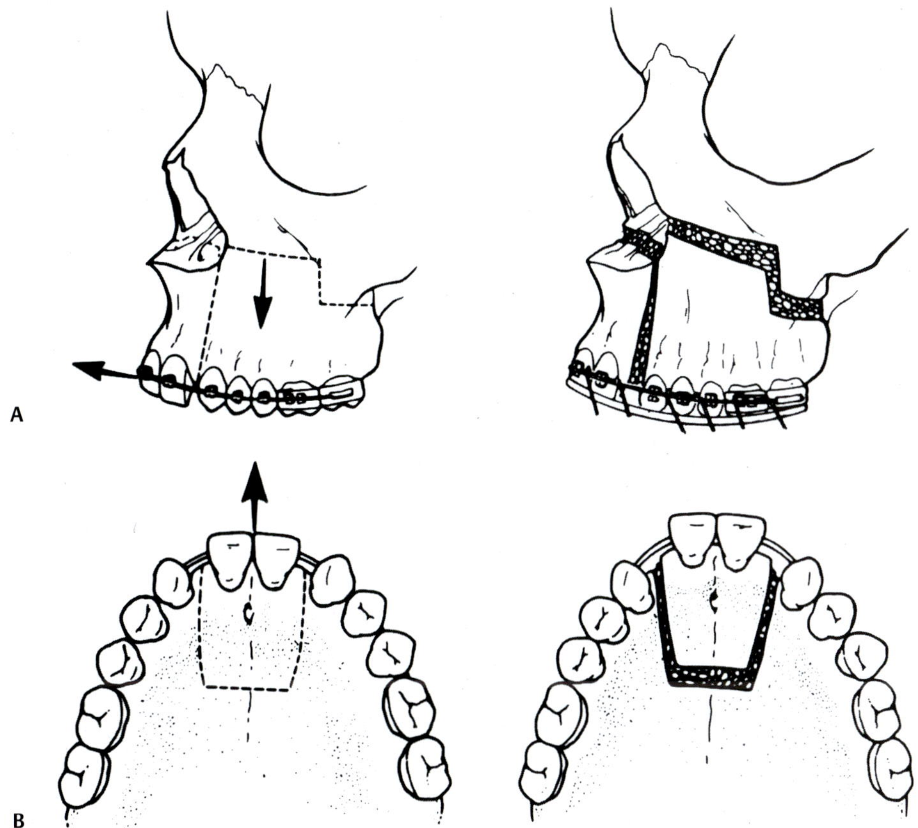

Fig. 6.4 Two-piece Le Fort I osteotomy with interdental osteotomies. **(A)** Design of osteotomies. **(B)** Completion of osteotomies, allowing independent movement of the anterior and posterior segments with interposition bone grafts. (From Bell WH, Darab D, You Z. Maxillary and midface deformity, I: Individualizing the osteotomy design for the Le Fort 1 downfracture. In: Bell WH, ed. Modern Practice in Orthognathic and Reconstructive Surgery. Vol 3. Philadelphia: WB Saunders; 1992:2220. Reprinted with permission.)

Deformities Not Involving Occlusion

Pretreatment Evaluation

Characteristic deformities resulting from post-traumatic orbitozygomatic injuries include a decreased anteroposterior projection of the zygomaticomalar complex, increased facial width due to collapse of the zygomatic arch, and rotation of the zygomatic body.[1] Secondary sequelae can produce enophthalmos due to increased orbital volume, diplopia, vertical orbital dystopia, and decreased sensation in the cheek from injury to the infraorbital nerve. The deformities associated with post-traumatic nasoethmoid injuries are telecanthus, loss of dorsal nasal height, and an increase in nasal width. Impaction of the central face in the area of the nasal root with lateral displacement of the medial orbital walls is responsible for these abnormalities.

Analysis begins with a thorough ophthalmologic evaluation, including documentation of visual acuity, visual fields, and extraocular movements, as well as inspection of the retina. A formal ophthalmologic consultation is indicated if any abnormality is identified. Specific attention should be given to the status of the lacrimal drainage system, the integrity of the medial and lateral canthal tendons, and the position and protection of the globes. Important orbital surface measurements that should be obtained include intercanthal distance, bony interorbital distance, palpebral fissure height and width, interpupillary distance, and vertical pupil position (**Fig. 6.7**).[13] Through a system of prisms and mirrors, the Hertel exophthalmometer is used to determine the anteroposterior distance between the anterior corneal surface and the orbital rim. A difference between the injured side and the normal side > 3 mm is usually clinically and surgically significant. The validity of measurements obtained with the exophthalmometer is uncertain if there has been damage to the orbital rim, because the bony reference point may have been altered. In this case, an alternative method to obtain globe position is by paraxial longitudinal orbital computed tomography (CT) scan reformatted images.[13] Evaluation for vertical dystopia involves comparing the pupillary plane of one eye with the other eye. A difference of > 3 mm represents a significant vertical dystopia. Although the uninjured side provides reference measurements in unilateral injuries, normative data tables must be used in bilateral injuries.[14] Generally, the interpupillary distance is approximately equal to the distance from the nasion to the vermillion-cutaneous junction of the upper lip. The normal intercanthal

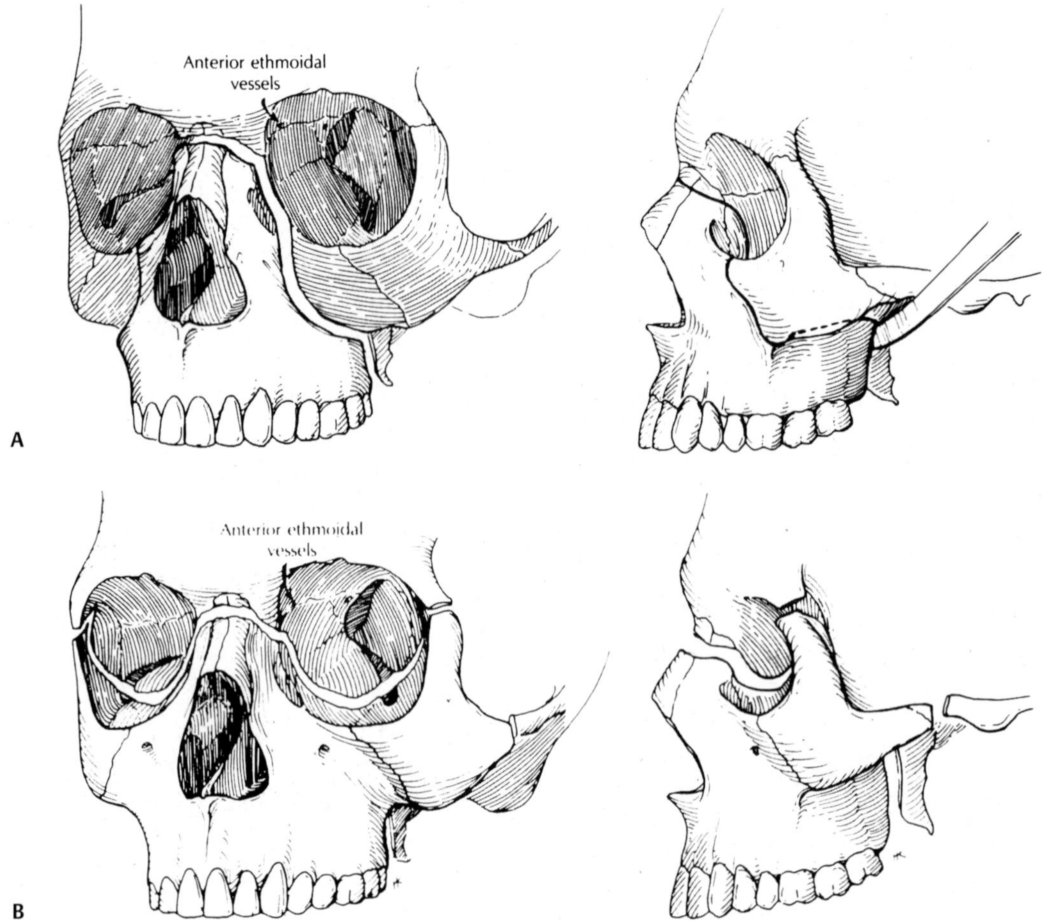

Fig. 6.5 Le Fort II and III osteotomies. **(A)** Le Fort II osteotomy, allowing nasomaxillary advancement. **(B)** Le Fort III osteotomy, allowing advancement of the entire maxilla. (From Ferraro J. Mandible: aesthetic changes with advancement and setbacks. In: Ousterhout DK, ed. Aesthetic Contouring of the Craniofacial Skeleton. Boston: Little, Brown; 1991:497,499. Reprinted with permission.)

distance should roughly equal the palpebral fissure width and half the interpupillary distance, usually between 30 and 35 mm in the adult.

Particular attention should be paid to the evaluation of telecanthus, which is especially difficult to repair secondarily. Telecanthus is most commonly caused by fracture and subsequent lateral migration of the bony fragment on which the medial canthal tendon is inserted, or rarely by complete avulsion of the tendon from its insertion on the lacrimal crests. Due to the tension exerted by the unchecked orbicularis oculi muscle, the intercanthal distance is increased, the palpebral fissure width is decreased, and the medial canthal region is rounded rather than elliptical. With time, the medial canthal region settles in a position that is generally lateral, inferior, and anterior to its normal position. In the acute situation and during the initial healing period, attachment of the tendon can be determined by performing the eyelid traction (or bowstring) test, in which the upper eyelid is pulled laterally while the medial canthal tendon is palpated. The tendon will not tighten with traction if it is detached. However, over time, the development of scar formation can make this test misleading.

The bony orbit is essentially a pyramid-shaped structure, with the optic foramen forming the apex (**Fig. 6.8**). It is crucial to understand that the medial orbital floor and the medial orbital wall have a convex shape behind the vertical axis of the globe in the middle third of the orbit (**Fig. 6.9**). The bulge resulting from this convexity is critical in maintaining the proper position of the globe, because loss of the convexity produces increased orbital volume and subsequent enophthalmos with frequently accompanying hypophthalmos. Failure to address the loss of convexity when repairing post-traumatic orbital injuries will result in persistent enophthalmos and hypophthalmos.[1] It is also important to remember that the optic foramen is located in the superomedial

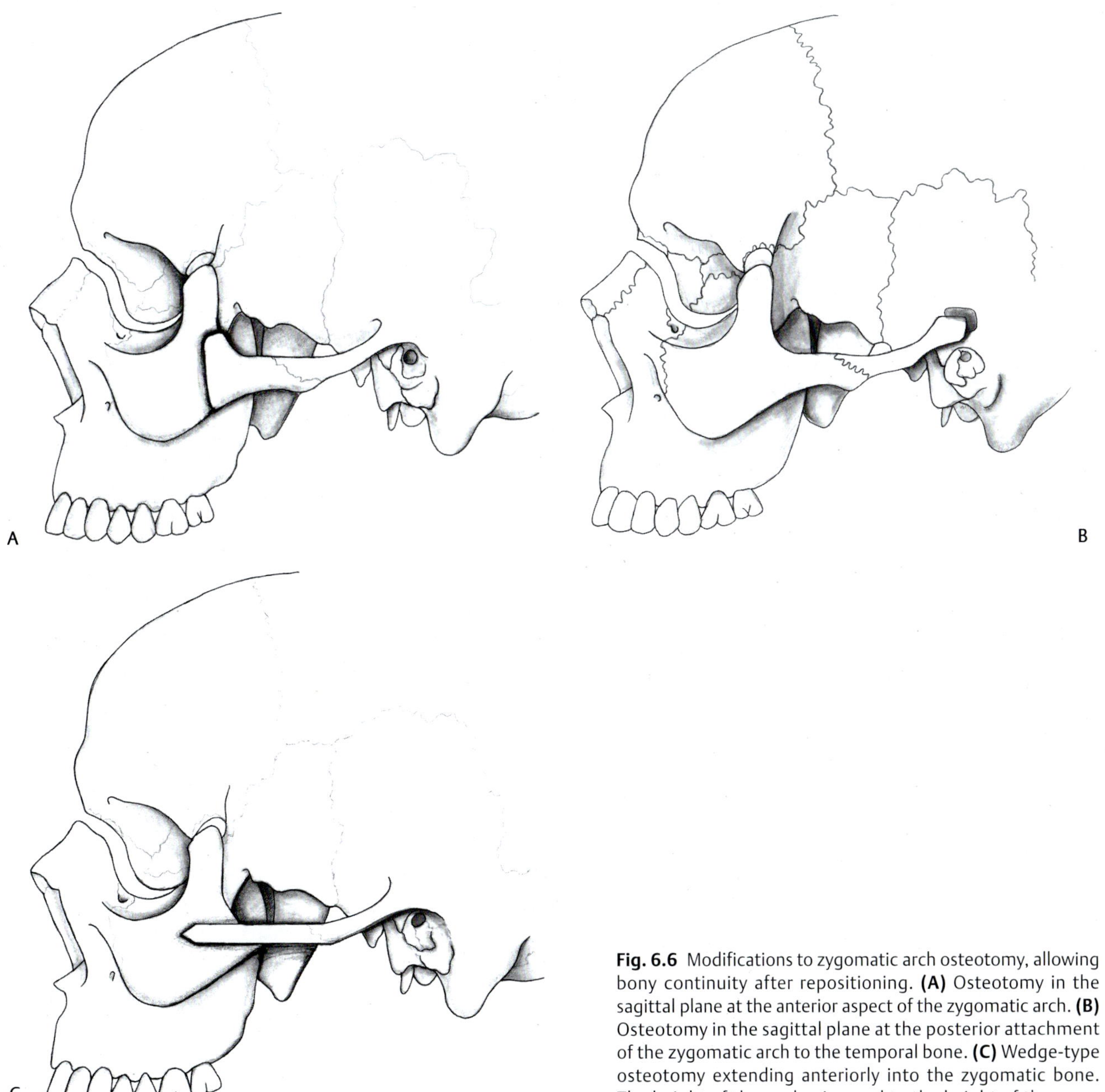

Fig. 6.6 Modifications to zygomatic arch osteotomy, allowing bony continuity after repositioning. **(A)** Osteotomy in the sagittal plane at the anterior aspect of the zygomatic arch. **(B)** Osteotomy in the sagittal plane at the posterior attachment of the zygomatic arch to the temporal bone. **(C)** Wedge-type osteotomy extending anteriorly into the zygomatic bone. The height of the wedge is equal to the height of the zygomatic arch.

aspect of the orbit ~40 to 45 mm posterior to the inferior orbital rim (**Fig. 6.10**). The definitive study of skeletal anatomy of the naso-orbito-zygomatic region is provided by axial and coronal CT with thin sections through the orbit. CT not only delineates skeletal deficiencies and malpositioning but also allows quantitative orbital measurements. Finally, 3-D reformatting of CT scans provides a detailed, high-quality image of the naso-orbito-zygomatico complex.[15] Three-dimensional reconstructions are best developed from 1.5 mm cuts (either axial or coronal).[16]

Surgical Treatment

Because post-traumatic enophthalmos is a result of increased bony orbital volume relative to soft tissue orbital volume, treatment is aimed at restoring the size and shape of the bony orbit and/or compensating for a bony volume discrepancy. For fractures confined to the orbital floor and/or medial orbital wall, access is usually adequately gained through a transconjunctival incision. Subperiosteal dissection is performed to identify and expose the entire defect, including the posterior edge. If present,

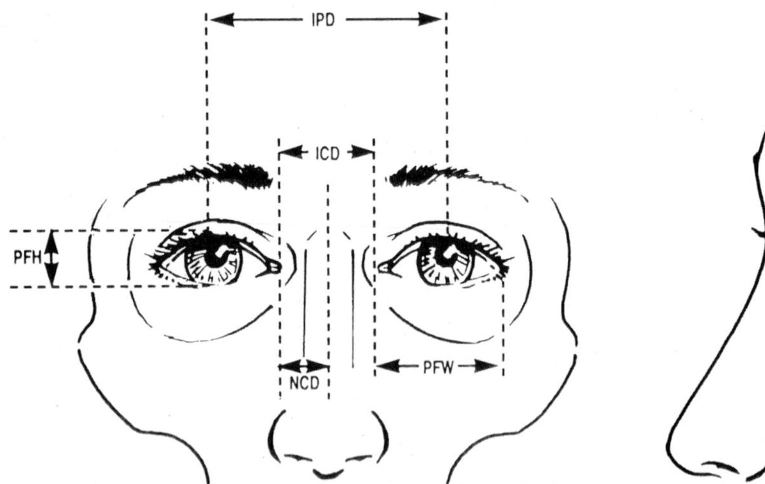

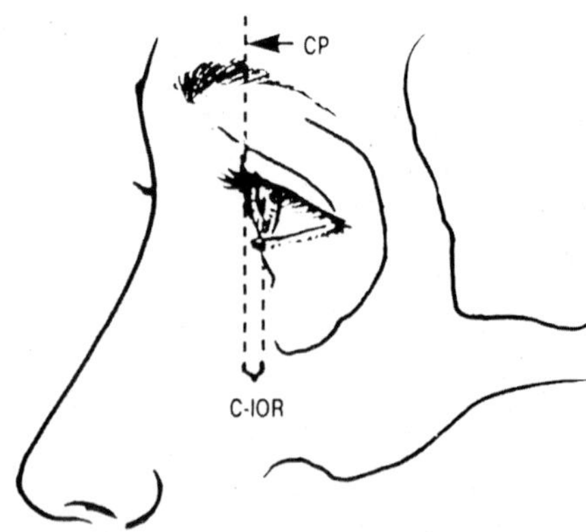

Fig. 6.7 Orbital surface measurements. C-IOR, cornea–inferior orbital rim distance; CP, corneal plane; ICD, intercanthal distance; IPD, interpupillary distance; NCD, nasocanthal distance; PFH, palpebral fissure height; PFW, palpebral fissure width. (From Hardesty RA, Coffey A. Secondary craniomaxillofacial deformities: current principles of management. Clin Plast Surg 1992;19:275–300, as adapted from Marsh JL. Blepharocanthal deformities in patients following craniofacial surgery. Plast Reconstr Surg 1978;61:842–853. Reprinted with permission.)

herniated tissue is subsequently returned to the orbit. For large, posterior defects and with difficulty delivering herniated tissue, an inferior orbitotomy provides exceptional exposure of the orbital floor (**Fig. 6.11**).[17] The defect is then covered with a split calvarial bone graft. Orbital volume is corrected by placing further bone grafts behind the vertical axis of the globe to thrust the globe forward, with emphasis on restoring the inferomedial convexity to achieve slight overcorrection of the enophthalmos. When the inferior periorbital tissue is fibrosed, it may need to be incised several times to release it and allow the orbital contents to come forward as the bone grafts are placed.

Mild post-traumatic zygomatic deformities due to bony depression that do not include enophthalmos can occasionally be managed with onlay grafts fixed with lag screws. However, severely displaced zygomatic deformities with enophthalmos are best managed with osteotomies that re-create the fracture and subsequent repositioning of the displaced bony segments into their normal position. Interposition bone grafts are used to fill gaps. Of paramount importance is adequate exposure of the entire orbit, which is usually achieved through a coronal incision combined with a transconjunctival incision. Additional exposure to the zygomaticomaxillary buttress is obtained via an intraoral maxillary vestibular incision. Following incisions, subperiosteal dissection is performed in the orbit to identify all bony defects and facilitate adequate freedom of movement. To improve exposure, the lateral canthal tendon may be stripped from its insertion into Whitnall's tubercle and later resuspended. Using a saw and/or an osteotome, orbitozygomatic osteotomies are performed at the frontozygomatic suture, extended down the lateral orbital wall, through the inferior orbital rim and lateral maxillary buttress, and through the zygomatic arch (**Fig. 6.12**).[1] Malunited fracture lines, if present at other locations, are osteotomized

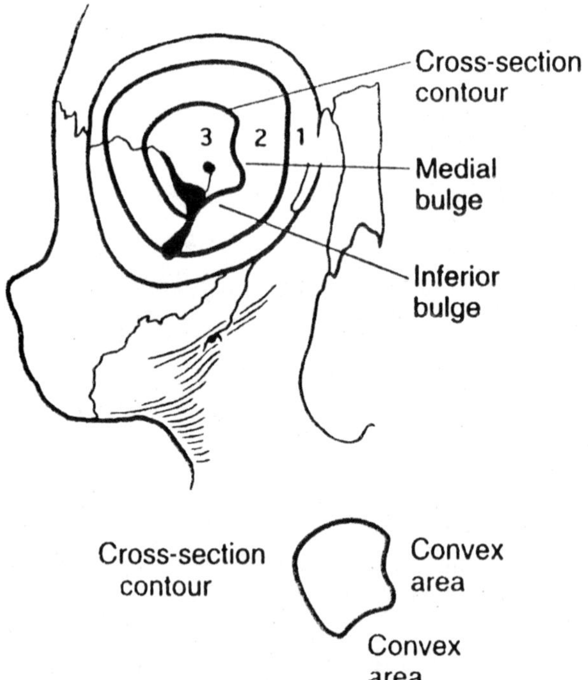

Fig. 6.8 Bony orbit. Note the convex shape of the medial orbital floor and medial orbital wall in the middle third of the orbit. (From Gruss JS. Craniofacial osteotomies and rigid fixation in the correction of post-traumatic craniofacial deformities. Scand J Plast Reconstr Hand Surg Suppl 1995;27:83–95. Reprinted with permission.)

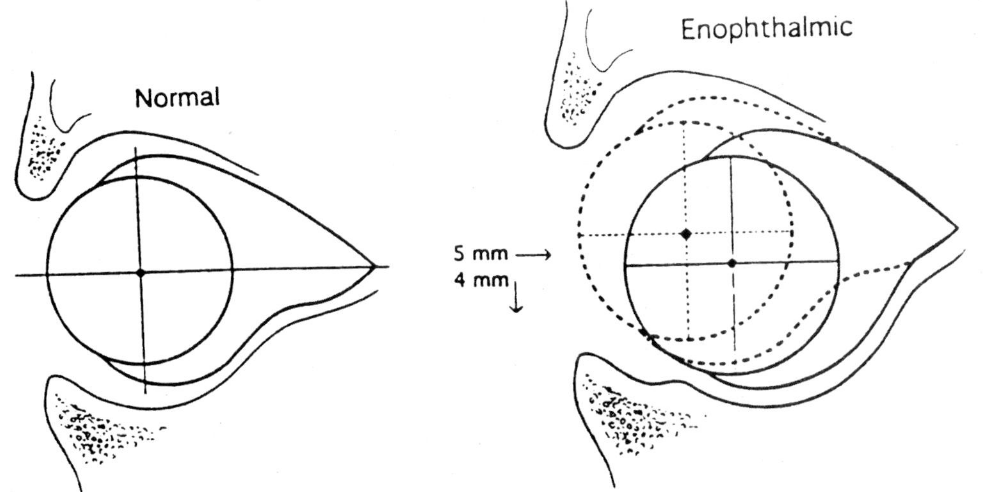

Fig. 6.9 Sagittal view of the bony orbit. **(A)** The convex bulge lies posterior to the vertical axis of the globe. **(B)** Loss of the convex bulge increases orbital volume, resulting in enophthalmos and hypopthalmos.

(From Gruss JS. Craniofacial osteotomies and rigid fixation in the correction of post-traumatic craniofacial deformities. Scand J Plast Reconstr Hand Surg Suppl 1995;27:83–95. Reprinted with permission.)

as well. The entire zygomaticomalar complex, which should be completely mobile, is then returned to its normal anatomical location. During repositioning, the zygomatic arch often becomes outwardly bowed and commonly requires an additional osteotomy to ensure its proper configuration (**Fig. 6.13**). It is important to appreciate that the normal anatomical shape of the zygomatic arch is a slope, rather than a gentle curve (a common misunderstanding).[1] Split calvarial bone grafts are used to fill in any gaps, and the zygomaticomalar complex is rigidly fixed with plates and screws at the frontozygomatic suture, lateral maxillary buttress, inferior orbit rim, and zygomatic arch. Bone graft is also stacked in layers behind the vertical axis of the globe to allow for slight overcorrection of enophthalmos if present.

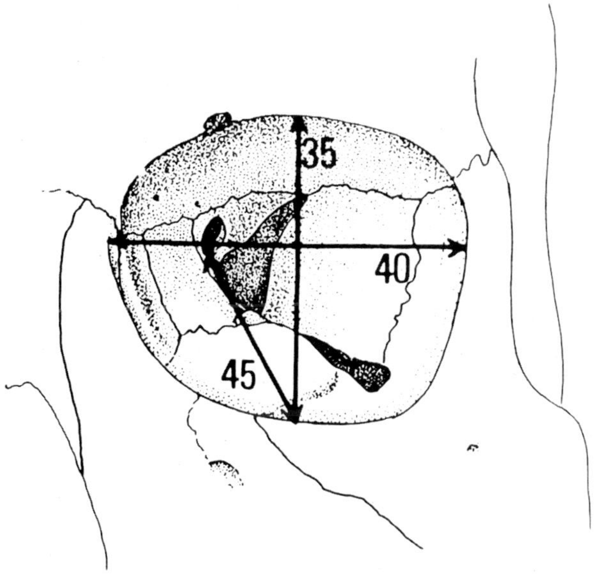

Exposure for repair of traumatic telecanthus is accomplished through a coronal incision. Because the medial canthal tendon often remains attached to a significant bony fragment of the medial orbital wall, management may consist of osteotomies to mobilize the canthus-bearing bony segment, followed by rigid fixation with plates and screws after repositioning into proper alignment. If the canthal tendon has been avulsed from its bony attachment, or if the bone fragment is too small for rigid fixation, a transnasal canthopexy is performed (**Fig. 6.14**).[18] A wire or heavy permanent suture through the medial canthal tendon is passed through the nasoethmoid complex behind the lacrimal fossa and tied around a screw placed in the supratrochlear region of the contralateral orbit to pull the tendon posteriorly, medially, and superiorly. Excessive overcorrection is almost impossible, particularly when a long delay has resulted in horizontal reduction of the intracanthal distance. Occasionally, the medial orbital wall must be reconstructed with bone grafts. In this situation, the canthal wire/suture is passed through a hole drilled in the graft where the lacrimal fossa would normally be. Although a split calvarial bone graft cantilevered from the frontal bone may be used to restore dorsal nasal height, it should not be used to increase nasal length. Nasal lengthening requires techniques of rhinoplasty, a discussion of which is beyond the scope of this chapter. Lacrimal drainage system dysfunction is surprisingly infrequent after naso-orbito-ethmoid fractures. If such an injury is suspected, Jones I and II tests should be

Fig. 6.10 Average orbital measurements (in millimeters). The optic foramen is located ~45 mm behind the inferior orbital rim. (From Habal MB, Aryian S, eds. Facial Fractures. Toronto: BC Decker; 1989:156. Reprinted with permission.)

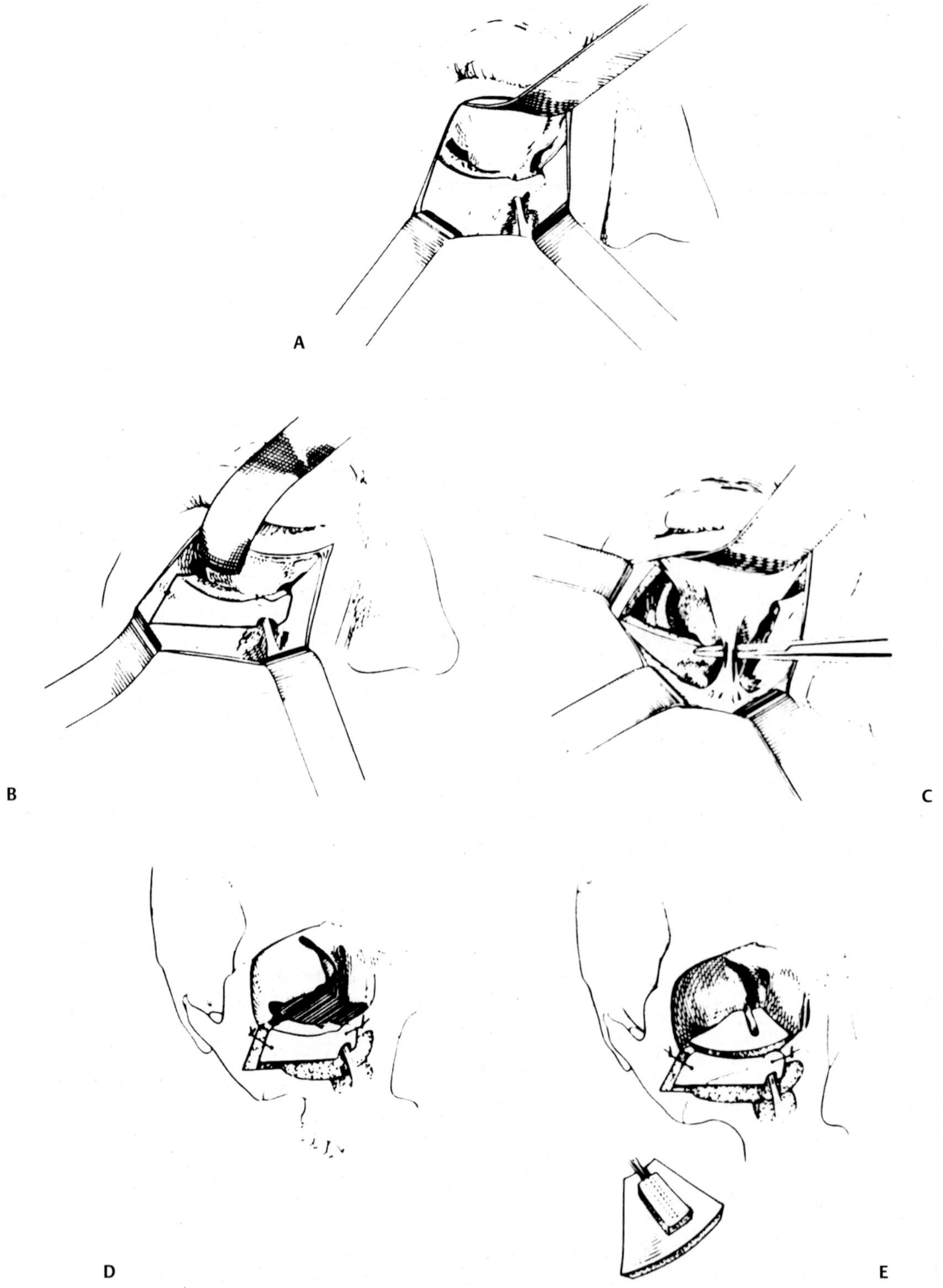

Fig. 6.11 Inferior orbitotomy allowing access to large, posterior orbital floor defects. **(A)** Inferior orbital rim exposure. **(B)** Design of osteotomy. **(C)** Exposure of the orbital floor and reduction of herniated tissue after removal of the rim. **(D)** Replacement of the orbital rim. **(E)** Placement of a bone graft to cover the orbital floor defect. (From Tessier P. Inferior orbitotomy—a new approach to the orbital floor. Clin Plast Surg 1982;9:569. Reprinted with permission.)

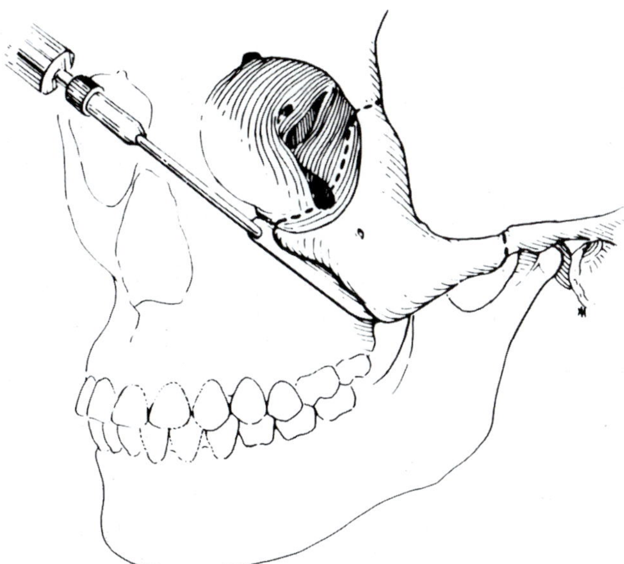

Fig. 6.12 Orbitozygomatic osteotomies re-creating zygomatic complex fracture, allowing repositioning into its normal anatomical location. (From Kawamoto HK. Late posttraumatic enophthalmos: a correctable deformity? Plast Reconstr Surg 1982;69:423–430. Reprinted with permission.)

performed. If indicated, a Silastic stent (Crawford or Guibor tube) may be inserted through the canaliculi and removed in 4 to 6 weeks. Rarely, a complex repair of the lacrimal drainage system is required.

Case Studies

Case 1

A 36-year-old man involved in a motor vehicle accident sustained multiple facial fractures, including a severely displaced right zygomaticomaxillary complex fracture (**Fig. 6.15**). Due to the severity of his injuries, which included aortic dissection, celiac vessel injury, and right carotid artery thrombosis, he was unable to undergo primary repair of the facial fractures. Fourteen months later, the patient returned with secondary deformities, including significant right malar retrusion, enophthalmos, and hypophthalmos. He underwent revision surgery consisting of right orbitozygomatic osteotomies at the old fracture sites, followed by repositioning and rigid fixation of the zygomaticomaxillary complex. Split calvarial bone grafts were used to fill in the resulting gaps at the lateral maxillary buttress, frontozygomatic suture, zygomatic arch, lateral orbital wall, and orbital floor. Split calvarial bone grafts were also stacked in layers behind the vertical equator of the globe to correct enophthalmos and hypophthalmos (**Fig. 6.16**).

Case 2

A 34-year-old man involved in a motor vehicle accident sustained multiple Le Fort fractures that were not repaired primarily. He subsequently returned with posttraumatic maxillary retrusion, resulting in a significant cosmetic deformity and an Angle class III malocclusion. He underwent a Le Fort III osteotomy with advancement and a Le Fort I osteotomy with asymmetric advancement of the maxilla to restore his appearance and occlusion. Rigid fixation was used at all osteotomy sites (**Fig. 6.17**).

Complications

Complications that can occur as a result of the initial trauma can also occur as a result of revision surgery.[19] Incision-related complications include bleeding, infection, and dehiscence leading to infected osteotomy sites or hardware. The supraorbital nerve, the infraorbital nerve,

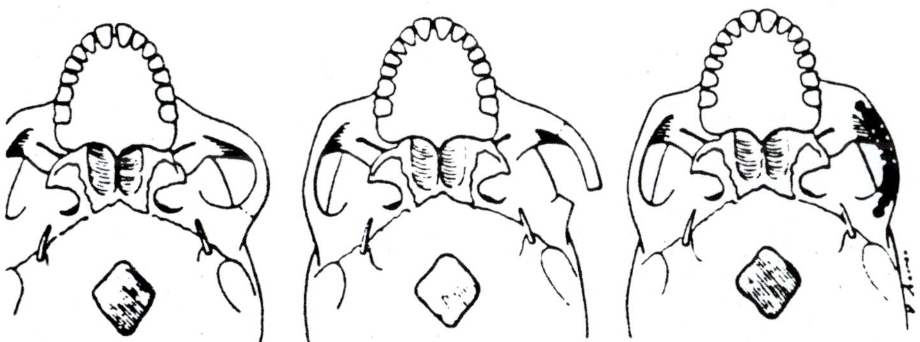

Fig. 6.13 An additional zygomatic arch osteotomy is often required to correct outward bowing of the arch that commonly occurs after zygomatic complex osteotomy and repositioning. The remaining defects in the posterior arch are bridged with a bone graft and a mini- or microplate. (From Gruss JS. Craniofacial osteotomies and rigid fixation in the correction of post-traumatic craniofacial deformities. Scand J Plast Reconstr Hand Surg Suppl 1995;27:83–95. Reprinted with permission.)

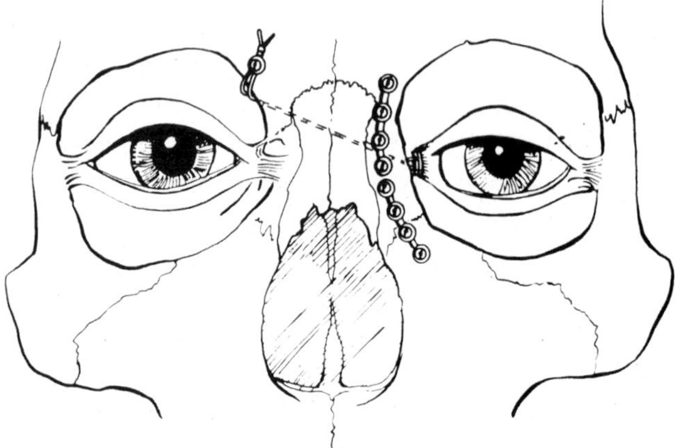

Fig. 6.14 Repair of traumatic telecanthus via transnasal canthopexy to secure avulsed medial canthal tendon and microplates for rigid fixation of bony fragments. (From Stanley RB. Maxillofacial trauma. In: Cummings CW, Fredrickson JM, Harker LA, et al, eds. Otolaryngology—Head and Neck Surgery. Vol 1. St. Louis: Mosby Year Book; 1998:476. Reprinted with permission.)

and the frontal branch of the facial nerve are at risk for stretching, avulsion, or transaction, resulting in numbness of the scalp, numbness of the cheek, and weakness of the forehead, respectively. Osteotomy-specific complications include nonunion, malunion, malocclusion, and skeletal relapse. Damage to the palatine vessels in combination with a wide maxillary vestibular incision can lead to ischemic loss of the entire palate and maxillary arch. Nonviable teeth result from interruption of the neurovascular supply to the tooth roots. Periorbital osteotomies risk damage to the globe, optic nerve, extraocular muscles, and lacrimal drainage system. Persistent telecanthus, enophthalmos, and vertical orbital dystopia are usually due to suboptimal reconstruction. Transient exophthalmos and diplopia are expected and usually resolve within a few months. If diplopia persists beyond 6 months, extraocular muscle surgery may be necessary.

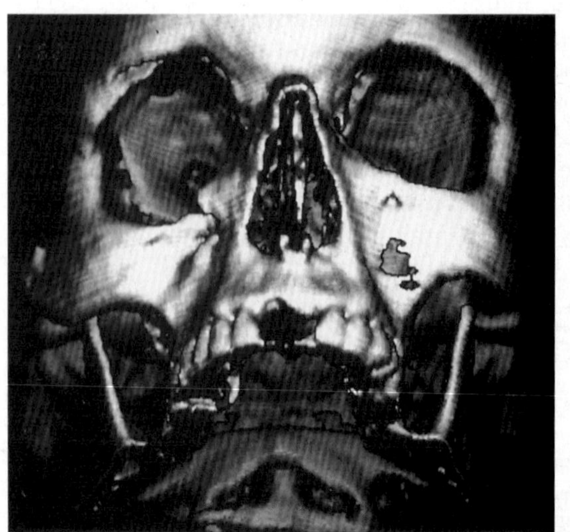

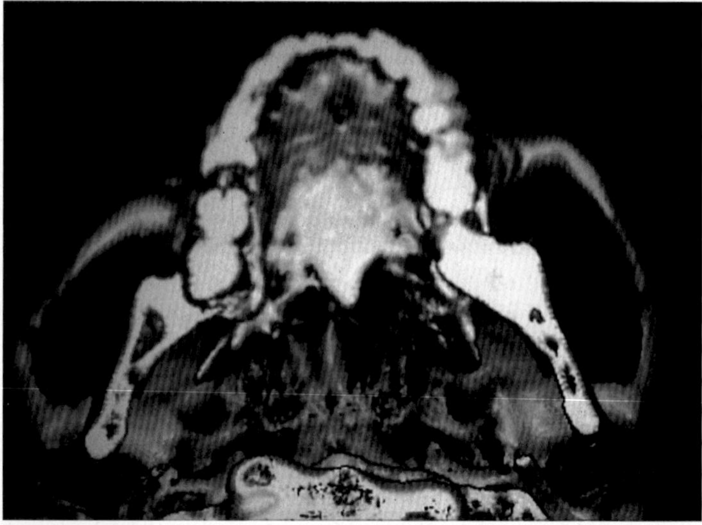

Fig. 6.15 Preoperative CT images illustrating right zygomaticomaxillary deformity. **(A)** Anteroposterior 3-D reconstructed CT image. **(B)** Axial 3-D reconstructed CT image. **(C)** Axial CT image.

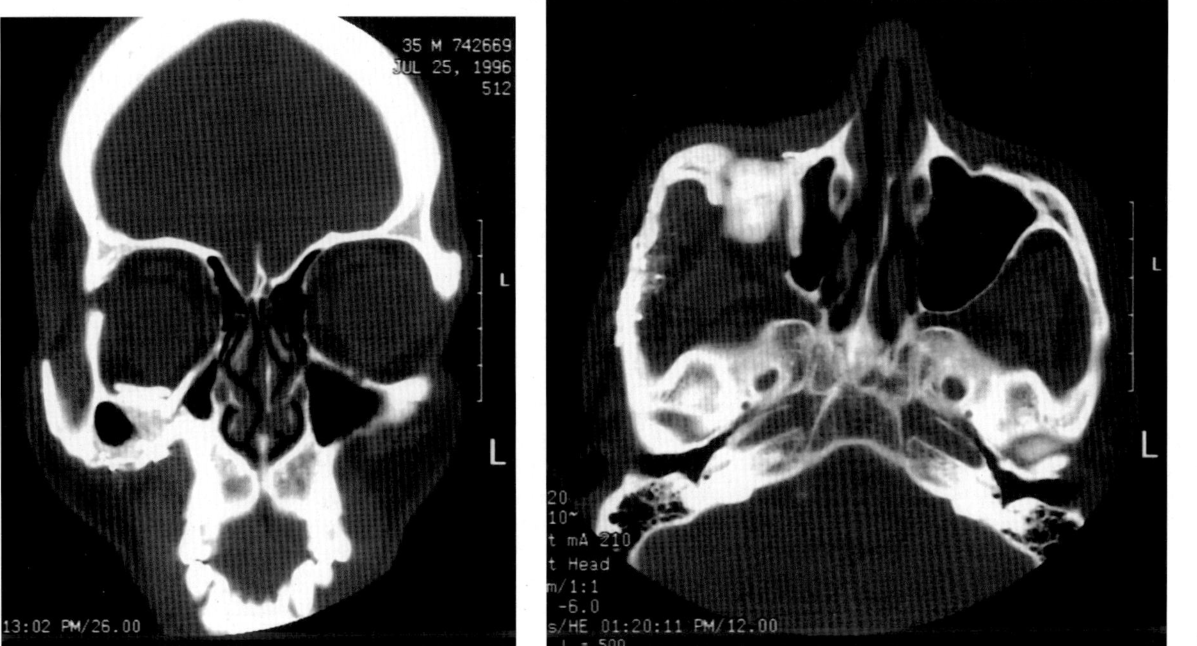

Fig. 6.16 Postoperative CT images illustrating bony repositioning with miniplate rigid fixation of right zygomaticomaxillary complex, along with orbital reconstruction with split calvarial bone grafts. **(A)** Coronal CT image. **(B)** Axial CT image.

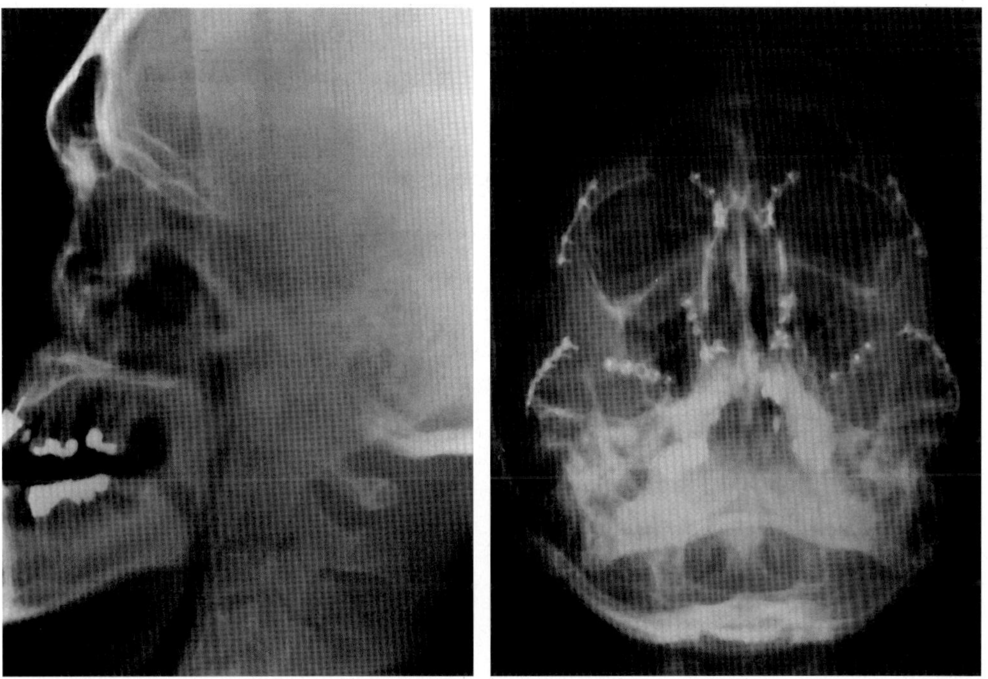

Fig. 6.17 (A) Preoperative lateral cephalogram demonstrating maxillary retrusion. **(B)** Postoperative radiograph illustrating improved maxillary position with rigid fixation at osteotomy sites. (From Tatum SA. Correction of post-traumatic maxillofacial deformities involving occlusion. Facial Plast Surg Clin North Am 1998;6:535–556. Reprinted with permission.)

Conclusion

Post-traumatic midface deformities are difficult to correct and are best reconstructed in the acute phase. However, secondary repair of these injuries can be satisfactorily accomplished using craniomaxillofacial principles. Thorough evaluation of the deformity, including a detailed analysis of occlusion and of orbital relationships, coupled with a well-designed treatment plan, allows for improvement in facial aesthetics, malocclusion, and enophthalmos. Well-hidden incisions, wide exposure, appropriate osteotomies with subsequent repositioning of bone, rigid internal fixation, and bone grafting when indicated all contribute to an acceptable reconstructive result. Finally, resuspension of all affected soft tissues is critical for achieving the desired result.

References

1. Gruss JS. Craniofacial osteotomies and rigid fixation in the correction of post-traumatic craniofacial deformities. Scand J Plast Reconstr Surg Hand Surg Suppl 1995;27: 83–95.
2. Cohen SR, Kawamoto HK. Analysis and results of treatment of established posttraumatic facial deformities. Plast Reconstr Surg 1992;90:574–584.
3. Casson PR, Bonanno PC, Converse KM. The midfacial degloving procedure. Plast Reconstr Surg 1974;53:102–103.
4. Wolfe SA. Treatment of post-traumatic orbital deformities. Clin Plast Surg 1988;15:225–238.
5. Hardesty RA, Marsh JL. Malunion and non-union of facial fractures. In: Habal MB, Aryian S, eds. Facial Fractures. Toronto: BC Decker; 1989:195–229.
6. Mathog RH, ed. Atlas of Craniofacial Trauma. Philadelphia: WB Saunders; 1992.
7. Tatum SA. Concepts in midface reconstruction. Otolaryngol Clin North Am 1997;30:563–592.
8. Rabuzzi DD. Revision surgery of malaligned midfacial fractures. Otolaryngol Clin North Am 1974;7:107–117.
9. Merville LC, Derome T, de Saint-Jorre G. Fronto-orbitonasal dislocations: secondary treatment of sequelae. J Maxillofac Surg 1983;11:71–82.
10. Tessier P. Complications of facial trauma: principles of later reconstruction. Ann Plast Surg 1986;17:411–420.
11. Furnas WD. Transverse maxillary osteotomy for malunion of maxillary fractures. Plast Reconstr Surg 1968;42: 378–383.
12. Khosla VM, Berk LH. Unilateral oblique osteotomy for correction of open bite after multiple facial fractures. J Oral Surg 1971;29:821–824.
13. Hardesty RA, Coffey JA. Secondary craniomaxillofacial deformities: current principles of management. Clin Plast Surg 1992;19:275–300.
14. Marsh JL. Blepharocanthal deformities in patients following craniofacial surgery. Plast Reconstr Surg 1978;61:842–853.
15. DeMarino DP, Steiner E, Poster R, et al. Three dimensional computed tomography in maxillofacial trauma. Arch Otolaryngol Head Neck Surg 1986;112:146–150.
16. Levy RA, Rosenbaum AE, Kellman RM, et al. Assessing whether the plane of section on CT affects accuracy in demonstrating facial fractures in 3-D reconstruction using the dried skull. AJNR Am J Neuroradiol 1991;12:861–866.
17. Tessier P. Inferior orbitotomy: a new approach to the orbital floor. Clin Plast Surg 1982;9:569–575.
18. Whitaker LA, Yaremchuck MJ. Secondary reconstruction of posttraumatic orbital deformities. Ann Plast Surg 1990;25:440–449.
19. Mathog RH, Rosenburg Z. Complications in the treatment of facial fractures. Otolaryngol Clin North Am 1976;9:533–552.

II

Otology

Decision tree for revision tympanoplasty/ossiculoplasty

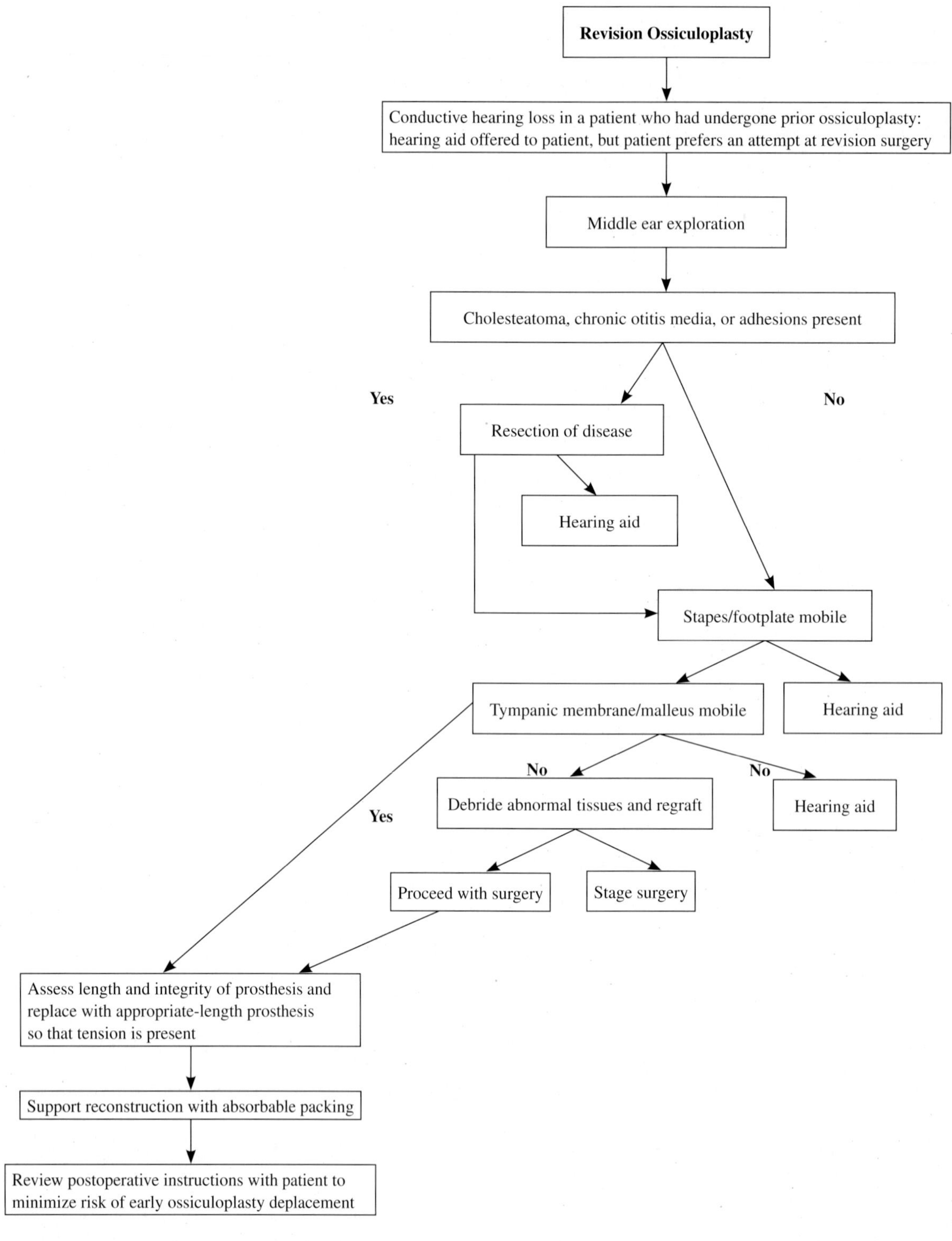

Tympanoplasty/Ossiculoplasty

Robert A. Goldenberg

The fact that revision surgery results from failed primary surgery is obvious; however, the reasons for that failure and how to address them often are not. This chapter identifies the causes for failure of primary surgery, review the indications for revision surgery, discuss the increased risks of revision surgery, and offer suggestions to reduce the chances of another failure at reoperation. This chapter also discusses principles of revision tympanoplasty and ossiculoplasty separately even though the two are often performed at the same time as well as in staged procedures.

Failure in tympanoplasty and ossiculoplasty is due to one of two reasons. The first reason relates to the art of surgery and includes patient selection, preoperative judgment, perioperative management, and intraoperative surgical technique. Increased skill, knowledge, and experience of the surgeon result in less chance for error in judgment and/or execution; the surgeon must keep abreast of new technology, maintain a competent skill level, and consider referral to a more experienced or specialized surgeon if the case requires it. The second reason for failure is the disease process itself. The overwhelming majority of cases of tympanoplasty and ossiculoplasty involve ears damaged by chronic otitis media. The operation occurs in a pathologic continuum that may or may not be altered permanently by surgical intervention. It is critical to remember this fact when counseling a patient preoperatively and when assessing postoperative results.

As well as the otologic disease process, there are many nonotologic factors that can influence surgical outcome. Systematic diseases such as tuberculosis, diabetes, immunodeficiency syndromes, and craniofacial anomalies are but a few. Of major significance is respiratory disease, particularly that of an allergic or infectious nature. Smoking can be a significant cause for failure in some cases. Other factors, such as unhealthy diet, poor nutrition, poor health in general, noncompliance with medical treatment, and lifestyle choices, such as swimming and scuba diving, may also increase the chance for unsatisfactory results.

It is important to evaluate a patient preoperatively with regard to the specific objectives of surgery. The often-stated objectives of chronic ear surgery are elimination of disease, creation of a dry, functional ear, and maintenance of or improvement in hearing. In most cases, the objectives are prioritized in the order presented. In other words, it is difficult to obtain a dry ear or improve hearing for any length of time if otologic disease is still present. Although these objectives are important in primary cases, they are critical in performing revision surgery. This chapter will address only tympanoplasty and ossiculoplasty; mastoidectomy is discussed in the following chapter.

Most importantly, before considering whether revision surgery is indicated, whether the objectives of surgery can be met, or what revision procedure should be recommended, the surgeon must answer one simple question: Why did the previous surgery fail?

Causes of Failure of Primary Surgery

Tympanoplasty

Tympanoplasty failure can be classified as one of the following condition: reperforation, graft lateralization, or atelectasis. Of course, any or all can occur together. The success rate for tympanoplasty is considered quite high; it is usually reported as upwards of 90% in simple myringoplasty, although the failure rate is somewhat higher when associated with mastoid surgery, severe infections, or congenital anomalies.[1,2] There may be a higher failure rate in children, although this is not universally agreed upon.[3,4] Merchant et al stated that chronic otitis media with granulation tissue is much harder to control than chronic otitis media with cholesteatoma.[5]

The causes of reperforation may occur early or late. Early causes of reperforation are most often due to faulty technique; late causes of failure are usually due to infection or graft shrinkage.[6] There are many reasons that could be attributed to faulty technique. Poorly constructed surgical incisions may have resulted in inadequate exposure of the tympanic membrane and surrounding structures, thus limiting visibility during the procedure. The graft may have been made too small, not allowing for shrinkage as the graft dries or heals. The recipient bed of the tympanic membrane remnant may have been prepared improperly by not creating a large enough surface for the graft to adhere to the recipient bed. In a large or total perforation with little or no anterior remnant, the graft may have been inserted improperly onto the bony external auditory canal, again, creating inadequate adherence. The graft may also have been placed improperly, allowing an edge to pull away from the supporting tympanic membrane remnant.

It may not have been anchored sufficiently with packing or the various techniques to interpose the graft between skin and bone of the external canal. Faulty technical factors are almost infinite and, in reality, may not be readily identifiable in the postoperative analysis.

Late causes of reperforation often relate to infection or graft atrophy. A preoperative infection may have been unrecognized and doomed the procedure to failure before it was even started. There may have been a postoperative hemorrhage or collection of fluid that caused the graft to pull away from supporting structures or reperforate. The graft itself may atrophy over time due to an infectious or autorejection process.

Persistent middle ear disease is undeniably the most common factor underlying a late graft reperforation. Residual cholesteatoma, persistent mucosal disease, and disease in the mastoid cell system are major contributing factors. The common denominator for all middle ear disease is ultimately eustachian tube dysfunction; this fact is so basic that it seems almost trite to discuss it, yet it is necessary to emphasize this reason. Many of the failures of chronic ear surgery in general, and tympanoplasty in particular, relate to the inability to adequately solve this difficult physiological problem at the present time. Long-term follow-up in tympanoplasty surgery is important to monitor this complication, which may be asymptomatic in the early stage.

Failure may also occur with graft lateralization. This most often occurs with the overlay technique of tympanic membrane grafting and is an inherent complication of the technique itself. Because the graft has been placed lateral to the tympanic membrane remnant, it can become displaced outwardly due to improper placement, hemorrhage, serous fluid collection, inadequate packing, or Valsalva effect in the immediate postoperative period. If lateralization occurs in the anterior portion of the tympanic membrane, these conditions can be the result of the anterior angle. Blunting in this area may also be caused by an iatrogenic cholesteatoma that results from incomplete removal of all squamous epithelium from the lateral surface of the anulus or tympanic membrane prior to placement of the graft.

Lateralization of the graft can also occur when using an underlay technique or some modification thereof. The graft can slip from the tympanic membrane bed or not adhere to the malleus handle. Lateralization of the graft from the malleus long process may occur in the "over-under" technique, where the graft is placed "under" the anterior remnant but "over" the malleus handle. Graft lateralization creates insufficient conduction of sound through the transformer mechanism of the middle ear and can be quite difficult to reconstruct satisfactorily at a subsequent operation.

Although lateral grafting techniques are excellent methods for tympanoplasty and are used widely by many surgeons, the technique itself causes this complication, and usually not the disease process. Paying meticulous attention to the details of graft placement, replacing the canal skin and/or flaps meticulously without any squamous epithelium turned under, and using firm packing material are technical ways to avoid this problem. By no means should these overlay techniques be abandoned, but avoidance of this inherent complication is obviously the best solution.

The third way in which a tympanoplasty can fail is by postoperative atelectasis. This may be technical, caused by using too thin a graft, not reinforcing the graft with other materials, such as cartilage, using a thicker graft, or not ventilating the ear at the primary surgery. It is often an error in judgment not to stage the surgery. Thick Silastic sheeting can maintain the middle ear space while the tympanoplasty heals, to reduce the incidence of this complication.

Although technical factors may play a role, the most common cause of postoperative atelectasis is the disease process, specifically, eustachian tube dysfunction. As mentioned previously, this is the underlying etiology of almost all chronic ear disease and is, unfortunately, without adequate solution at the present time. Atelectasis may also be due to weakening of the tympanic membrane from recurring infections, recurrent disease of the mastoid cell system, or the development of a monomeric tympanic membrane during the healing process. As with reperforation, long-term follow-up is critical to monitor the progression of atelectasis. It may be possible to reduce its incidence by ventilation of the middle ear in the postoperative period.

Postoperative myringitis is another condition that should be considered to be a graft failure. Hearing may be satisfactory and the middle ear protected; however, the patient may complain of pain, fullness, or otorrhea. In actuality, this is a granular reaction of the lateral surface of the tympanic membrane graft. It can have an angry red or a velvety pink appearance. The etiology is uncertain, although an autoimmune response, reaction to topical agents used intraoperatively (including packing material), or a postoperative infection may be factors. If topical antibiotics, débridement, or silver nitrate cautery is not successful, revision tympanoplasty with excision of the diseased area may be necessary.

Ossiculoplasty

Ossiculoplasty may fail for one of three basic reasons: a problem with the prosthesis, postoperative adhesions, and recurrent disease.

The first cause of failure, a problem with the prosthesis, may be immediate or delayed. Immediate failure is most likely due to technical factors. The prosthesis may have been measured inappropriately; too long a prosthesis may lead to slippage or dislocation into the vestibule, and too short may lead to inadequate sound conduction. The ossicular remnant (malleus or stapes superstructure) to which the prosthesis is attached may erode. There may be an unrecognized fixation of the stapes footplate.[7] Delayed failure can also be due to slippage of the prosthesis within the middle ear space.[8] This can be from inadequate contact with supporting ossicles, scar tissue, adhesions, or tympanosclerosis. Extrusion of the prosthesis can occur with any implant and can result from a foreign body reaction to autograft, homograft, or synthetic biomaterial. Prosthesis extrusion can result from the disease process as well and may be due to collapse and adherence of the tympanic membrane/graft around the prosthesis and not actually due to the ossiculoplasty itself.[8] Although this should be considered an extrusion, it relates more to otopathology than to the technical aspects of ossiculoplasty. The incidence of extrusion of a synthetic prosthesis may be reduced by using a cartilage interface between the prosthesis and the tympanic membrane graft.

Unrelated, nonotologic events can cause the prosthesis to become displaced after proper insertion. These include postoperative head injury, trauma, and sports-related injuries (soccer, scuba diving, wrestling, etc.), as well as a simple sneeze or other Valsalva episodes, which are sometimes unavoidable.

It is also possible to have a malfunction of the prosthesis by reabsorption. This is rather uncommon with most biomaterials, except with cartilage used to reconstruct the ossicular chain.[9]

Determination of which technical factor caused the failure in ossiculoplasty may be difficult or impossible; an accurate operative note or personal knowledge if the revision is accomplished by the initial surgeon is desirable. The patient's history, however, will be helpful in identifying whether the lack of hearing improvement was immediate or delayed.

A second cause of failure in ossiculoplasty is from postoperative adhesions in the middle ear. As with any epithelial surface in a cavity, the method of handling middle ear mucosa can create adhesions postoperatively. Bone dust, glove powder, or packing material itself can create a foreign body reaction that causes adhesions. Manipulation of the mucosa can create raw surface areas that will adhere to the graft material or opposing epithelium. The disease process itself, either recurrent or primary, can promote granulation tissue formation.[5] Inadequate removal of diseased mucosa can create excessive scar tissue. Each of the conditions may promote adhesion formation. Modification in surgical technique can reduce the incidence of adhesions, but the underlying disease process will often create a situation where adhesions arise.

Ossiculoplasty may also fail because of recurrent disease. A recurrent or residual cholesteatoma can displace a prosthesis or simply render it nonfunctional. The persistence of granulation tissue, reperforation of the tympanic membrane, or persisting otorrhea can cause a failure in ossiculoplasty. Atelectasis and nonaeration of the middle ear affect the transformer mechanism of the middle ear, although the ossiculoplasty itself may be intact. All of these conditions can also cause the prosthesis to become immobilized or to migrate or extrude.

The causes of failure of tympanoplasty and ossiculoplasty have been considered separately, but obviously, many of the factors that affect one can affect the other. It is important to recognize the causes of failure when considering the indications for revision surgery.

Indications for Revision Surgery

General

The indications for revision surgery relate to the objectives of surgery. The basic objectives for revision surgery are identical to those for primary surgery: eliminating residual disease, obtaining a dry, functional ear, and improving or maintaining hearing. It is just as critical at revision surgery (perhaps even more so) to consider the specific objectives of both the surgeon and the patient. Does the patient only want a dry ear at the expense of hearing improvement? Does the surgeon note residual or recurrent disease that must be addressed to prevent complications? Does the patient want to hear better, even if it means never swimming again? Answering these questions accurately is important in counseling the patient preoperatively and improves the chances of satisfactory surgical outcome. With these thoughts in mind, we will consider for each of the two procedures the indications for revision surgery and will try to identify noncorrectable causes of failure and, specifically, when not to reoperate.

Tympanoplasty

The indications for revision tympanoplasty are persisting otorrhea, hearing loss, reperforation, graft lateralization, atelectasis, and residual and/or recurrent disease. These factors must be considered with respect to the objectives just discussed to allow appropriate patient selection preoperatively.

There are several noncorrectable causes of failure that may preclude revision tympanoplasty. Eustachian tube dysfunction is the underlying factor behind many surgical failures and may be irreversible. Other coexisting conditions discussed in the overview may or may not be correctable.

For example, if a heavy smoker cannot stop, a decision not to perform revision surgery may be appropriate. Persisting mucosal disease may not be reversible if associated with severe respiratory illness. In some of these cases, preservation of a perforation may actually be desirable to ventilate the middle ear. Conversely, otorrhea caused by external contamination from an open perforation may be readily corrected by closure of the perforation.

A decision not to reoperate is appropriate when several conditions exist. Severe eustachian tube dysfunction that requires middle ear ventilation is a contraindication to revision tympanoplasty for reperforation. Multiple, unsuccessful procedures previously for the same indication would appear to be a relative contraindication to revision surgery. Although it is always tempting to use a new technique (as well as a new surgeon), each attempt at revision surgery lowers the chance of success for the next procedure should another failure occur. Often it is difficult to decide when to give up, but at some point it is appropriate. If there is no progressive disease present, or persistent otorrhea can be controlled with medication, not advising revision surgery may be the best option. Guidelines in making this type of decision should relate to the specific objectives of surgery and should be individualized to each case.

Ossiculoplasty

The indication for revision ossiculoplasty is persisting or recurrent conductive hearing loss. Revision ossiculoplasty may result in hearing improvement alone or hearing improvement with the use of a hearing aid. Each case must be assessed individually, and recommendations should be based on a judgment of the hearing level that can be realistically obtained. The less cochlear reserve, the less opportunity for successful revision ossiculoplasty.

There are several noncorrectable causes that will lead to failure in revision ossiculoplasty. Persistent atelectasis of the tympanic membrane creates a dysfunctional, conductive mechanism despite a technically satisfactory ossiculoplasty. Lack of vibratory surface area and improper contact between the prosthesis and an atelectatic tympanic membrane are significant factors in not achieving improvement in hearing. Although eustachian tube dysfunction is the underlying cause behind many problems in the middle ear, tissue factors such as scarring of the epithelial surface, tympanosclerosis, a thickened tympanic membrane graft, and loss of support structures for the graft may lead to failures in revision surgery. Adhesions or tympanosclerosis in the middle ear and tympanosclerosis of the oval or round windows are conditions that also may preclude correction.

A decision not to reoperate is appropriate if one (or more) of several conditions exist. Severe atelectasis or collapse of the tympanic membrane, as demonstrated by previous tympanoplasty failure, would be a contraindication to revision ossiculoplasty. Ossiculoplasty is only one factor in reconstruction of the sound transformer mechanism of the middle ear; a tympanic membrane properly positioned to provide an aerated middle ear space and to create an efficient area ratio is just as important. If this can be accomplished with a ventilation tube, ossiculoplasty may be advisable. Multiple previous procedures may predict failure with revision ossiculoplasty. De la Cruz et al described certain unique conditions that preclude revision surgery.[10] Congenital anomalies, unilateral hearing loss, and other associated factors are examples. Another is a dehiscent facial nerve overlying the oval window niche that made insertion of a prosthesis impossible at the first procedure.

Certain congenital anomalies of the middle ear, such as an absent oval or round window, are probably contraindications to surgery, although techniques have been described to address these problems.[11] Although individual experts and otologists have reported success in performing these unique and challenging operations, positive results are usually not the norm.[10]

Having discussed the indications for revision surgery, there are several increased risks that should be considered in revision surgery.

Increased Risks of Revision Surgery

Most of the risks for revision surgery are the same as those for primary surgery. Postoperative hemorrhage, infection, otalgia, and transient vertigo are most common. Postoperative hearing loss, transient or permanent injury to the facial nerve, and vestibular problems resulting in vertigo are infrequent, but possible, complications of middle ear surgery. There are several additional complications for revision surgery.

There is increased likelihood of the previously described complications to occur. All of the above-mentioned complications of primary surgery can occur, but because normal anatomical landmarks have been altered by scar tissue, adhesions, or surgical resection, there is an increased opportunity for surgical misadventure. This does not mean that revision surgery cannot be accomplished safely; it simply means that these risks should be fully considered and explained. Additionally, there may be a slightly greater chance of hearing loss in revision tympanoplasty.

Probably the greatest risk in revision surgery is the risk of another revision. The risk of failure increases with each progressive operation even in the most skilled surgical hands. Chronic ear disease is very much like dental disease where routine periodic examinations, dental fillings, root canal surgery, and crown and bridge work may be required repeatedly over time to prevent full mouth extraction and dentures. If this analogy is valid, revision procedures should be considered to be part of routine maintenance. This must be fully explained to the patient preoperatively, particularly when multiple procedures have already occurred. Patient dissatisfaction should be considered a complication and must always be addressed; it often results from unrealistic expectations and insufficient communication between patient and surgeon. This will be addressed further in the next section.

Having considered the reasons for failure as well as the indications and risks for revision surgery, surgical techniques that will increase the chance of a successful revision procedure will be discussed.

Revision Surgery or Revision Surgical Treatment

General Surgical Considerations to Reduce the Chance of Another Failure

Earlier in the chapter, it was suggested that before deciding whether to perform revision surgery at all, one simple question should be asked: Why did the previous surgery fail? Answering this question accurately will increase the likelihood of a successful outcome. Failure in tympanoplasty/ossiculoplasty is most often from one of two reasons: surgical technique or the disease process. The preceding discussion suggested methods to address the disease process; this section will address the art of surgery.

Surgical success is determined by three basic factors: the skill of the surgeon, the selection of the technique and the patient, and the level of care in the preoperative period. The chance of success in revision surgery will be increased by addressing each of these factors and asking the same question: Why did the previous procedure fail?

The skill of the surgeon is one of the most significant factors in determining surgical results, be it primary or revision. In a revision tympanoplasty/ossiculoplasty, it is incumbent upon the surgeon to evaluate his or her own individual skill level and consider referral to a more experienced or subspecialized otologic surgeon. This is not meant to imply that all cases of revision surgery should be referred; it is simply offered as one method to increase the chance for a good result.

Preoperative Evaluation

The patient history should obtain information about the procedure and coexisting pathological conditions. If the primary surgery was performed by the same surgeon who is revisiting the case, the history may not be important except as a reminder. If the surgery was performed elsewhere, obtaining information from the patient or direct communication with the initial surgeon can be most helpful. A history of disease conditions, particularly coexisting systemic disease, is necessary. Addressing such problems preoperatively may make the difference between success and failure. Determination of whether or not the failure in tympanoplasty/ossiculoplasty was immediate or delayed may allow the surgeon to determine why the previous procedure failed.

Microscopic examination of the ear is an important part of the preoperative evaluation. Assessment of the condition of the tympanic membrane, middle ear mucosa, location of the perforation, and presence of the ossicles is also important. Tympanometry or pneumatic otoscopy can aid in assessing the mobility of the tympanic membrane, a critical component of the hearing mechanism. Despite the fact that there are no totally adequate tests of eustachian tube function, a general assessment of the eustachian tube, by any means, is still desirable, even if controversial.[12] Examination of the auricular area will reveal previous surgical scars, general tissue health, and the size of the external canal. A complete otolaryngological examination may discover a coexisting disease that would have an impact on the surgical outcome. Other ancillary tests, such as medical imaging of the temporal bone, sinuses, or related structures, may be helpful.[13,14] Evaluation of the respiratory mucosa, particularly as it relates to chronic infections and/or allergic manifestations, also may be helpful. Direct visualization of the eustachian tube opening by nasopharyngoscopy may demonstrate tubal pathology. Endoscopic examination of the middle ear and mastoid, as well as other endoscopic techniques, has been introduced and should become more popular in the future.[15–17]

The patient should undergo audiometric evaluation to assess the air–bone gap and cochlear reserve. This is absolutely required for ossiculoplasty, but it is also important with tympanoplasty. Assessment of the air–bone gap is necessary to decide whether or not to perform an ossiculoplasty at all. Word discrimination testing in quiet and noise is essential for accurate preoperative counseling. Cochlear reserve will be helpful in assessing whether or not amplification will be required even with a complete closure of the air–bone gap (**Fig. 7.1**).

Several preoperative findings are usually positive predictors of success. The presence of a dry perforation without otorrhea or a central perforation (vs a marginal one) and the presence of the malleus (particularly in ossicular reconstruction) are generally associated with good surgical outcomes. Several preoperative factors that are predictive of unsatisfactory results are allergic tubotympanitis (as confirmed by history or nasopharyngoscopy), an anterosuperior perforation (particularly when marginal), and persistence of mucosal disease in the middle ear.

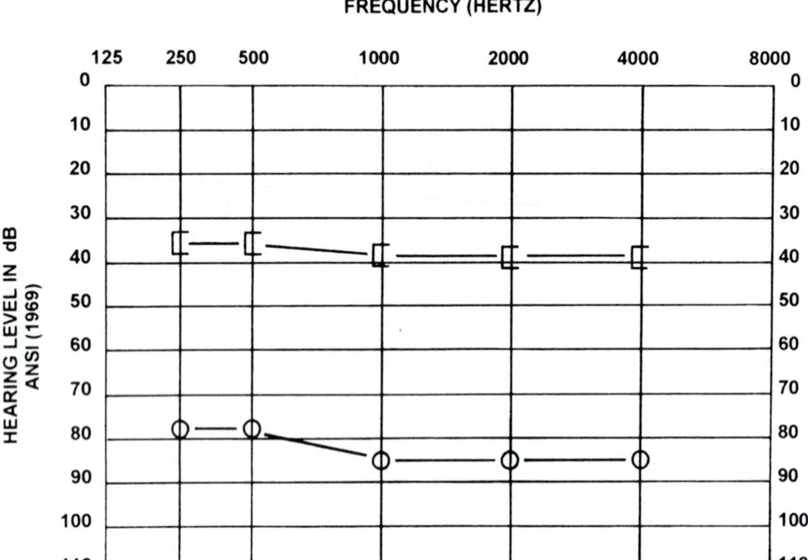

Fig. 7.1 Audiogram demonstrating a significant air–bone gap and adequate cochlear reserve.

Patient selection and counseling are a critical part of the preoperative evaluation. Appropriate selection of the surgical candidate is probably the single most important factor in obtaining successful surgical results. Preoperative counseling is based on realistic expectations of the surgeon and the patient; it will reduce the potential for dissatisfaction that is inherently higher with revision surgery.

Having completed the preoperative evaluation, specific technical factors will now be discussed for both tympanoplasty and ossiculoplasty.

Tympanoplasty

Results of revision surgery, although inherently having a lesser chance of success, can still be quite successful. Veldman and Braunius in 1998 reported the results of revision surgery as follows: a dry ear 90% of the time, reperforation 10%, otorrhea 10%, and recurrent cholesteatoma 5%.[18]

One basic principle that may be helpful in performing successful revision surgery is to simply use a different approach or technique from that used previously. With respect to approach, a different incision could be used for exposure. If the initial procedure had been performed transcanal, the revision procedure could be through a postauricular incision. If the initial graft was an overlay, an underlay technique could be used.

Preservation of the anterior anulus will allow for accurate graft placement with either an overlay or underlay technique; maintaining this structure can make the difference between success and failure in cases of superior-anterior perforations. In creating canal skin flaps, wide exposure is important for proper visualization of the graft recipient bed. There should be a wide meatus, the external canal should be enlarged, and there should be a broad lateral exposure to allow for good visualization. It is important to avoid turning skin under when replacing the flap, particularly when scar tissue has altered the normal contours. Turned under skin creates iatrogenic cholesteatoma pearl formation; for this reason, an underlay technique may be preferable in revision cases. The margins of the perforations should be excised and the recipient bed stripped of mucosa or epithelium to allow for a large surface area to adhere to the graft. However, as much tympanic membrane remnant as possible should be preserved.

Removal of an area of diseased tympanic membrane can be effective in improving the chance for a successful revision. An area of granulation tissue, atelectasis, or certainly graft cholesteatoma should be sharply excised, leaving as much normal tissue behind as possible. Whether or not to remove tympanosclerosis is controversial. The tympanosclerotic plaque may indicate an area of vasulature compromise and lessen the opportunity for a successful graft take; removing a large area of tympanosclerosis will often create a total perforation with limited anterior margin, thus creating a difficult technical problem. A helpful technique is to sharply elevate a portion of the outer squamous layer from the plaque before removing it, thereby ensuring a greater recipient bed for an underlay graft.

Instrumentation can be quite useful in more difficult revision cases. Use of the laser may allow for more delicate tissue handling. The laser is particularly helpful in removing tympanosclerosis of the middle ear, particularly around the oval or round window. The use of a nerve monitor can be helpful in identifying the facial nerve in revision cases.[19] The use of new and sharp burs for the surgical drill, adequate hemostatic material, and suction irrigation are a few examples of standard techniques that should be mastered for successful revision cases.

The pathological condition of the middle ear must be corrected. Diseased mucosa should be meticulously removed. Bone chips, adhesions, tympanosclerosis, and other foreign material should be removed, when appropriate, to allow for maximal aeration of the middle ear space.

There are several techniques for handling the graft in revision surgery. The choice of graft material itself may be limited. Multiple revision tympanoplasties may leave no obvious remaining temporalis fascia. If temporalis fascia is desirable, revision surgery may create the need for an extended middle fossa–type incision on the lateral skull to allow for harvesting of temporalis fascia superiorly; except for troublesome bleeding, temporalis fascia should almost always be obtainable. The use of totally different tissue as graft material should be considered. Perkins and Bui described the use of formaldehyde-formed fascia grafts as an effective method of closing large perforations, particularly in cases of revision surgery.[20] Wehrs recommended a homograft tympanoplasty technique in revision cases.[21] Heerman has used cartilage for a graft material.[22,23] This technique may be useful, particularly in cases where the graft failure was partially due to atelectasis or collapse of the previous graft. Perichondrium, vein, pericranium (medial to the temporalis muscle), homograft dura, and fascia lata have been used for tympanic membrane grafts as well.

The most critical step in tympanoplasty is proper placement and stabilization of the graft (**Fig. 7.2**). Whether employing the overlay or underlay technique, it is often helpful in revision surgery to use a graft that has been dried sufficiently and trimmed precisely to specific proportions. The use of a large, dried graft with a sharp, neat anterior edge will allow for exact placement anteriorly, whether lateral or medial to the anterior anulus, as well as an ample overlap of graft and tympanic membrane recipient area. The same principle can be applied when a "window shade" technique is used and the anterior margin of the graft is inserted between a remnant of the anterior canal skin and the bony external auditory canal. Meticulous placement of the leading edge of the graft under direct visualization can often be the difference between success and failure in tympanoplasty surgery, be it primary or revision.

The use of packing in the middle and external auditory canal is not universally accepted. The use of packing can stabilize the graft during the immediate postoperative period, but packing should not be relied on for long-term stability. Accurate placement of the graft circumferentially, as well as medially or laterally to the long process of the malleus, is a useful technique in creating a stable reconstructive situation without the need for packing. There is some debate whether or not absorbable middle ear

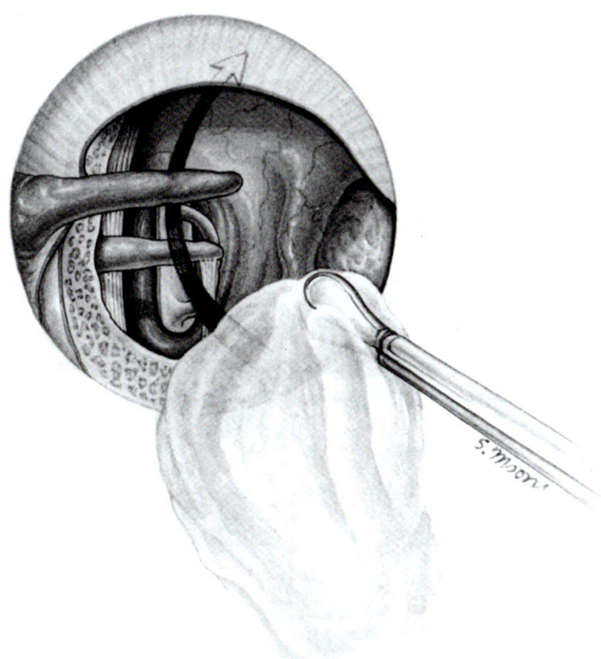

Fig. 7.2 Meticulous placement of the anterior (leading) edge of the tympanic membrane graft.

packing can cause tissue reaction. If such a reaction had been suspected in the previous operation, it should certainly not be used in a subsequent procedure.

The use of a ventilation tube in the tympanic membrane postoperatively is often successful in maintaining aeration of the middle ear, thus preventing atelectasis. Ventilation tube insertion is often difficult intraoperatively; therefore, the patient must be followed closely if atelectasis is suspected. The use of a ventilation tube in a tympanic membrane graft as early as 3 to 4 weeks postoperatively may avert a surgical failure. Certainly, the use of a ventilation tube in the longer-term postoperative period can help to avoid further collapse of an otherwise successful tympanic membrane graft. Dornhoffer and Kartush both described techniques of using cartilage blocks as a method of preserving the middle ear space and preventing atelectasis.[24,25]

Ossiculoplasty

Selection of the prosthesis in revision ossiculoplasty should be accomplished with great care and forethought. Simply using a different prosthesis may increase the chance for a successful result. Therefore, the surgeon should have the ability to use several of the different synthetic prostheses commercially available as well as autograft or homograft bone or cartilage. Schuring observed that no one prosthesis solves all problems.[26] The choice of

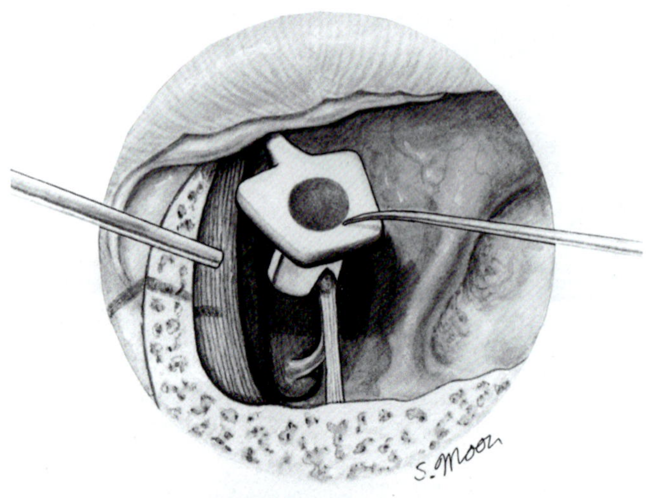

Fig. 7.3 Hydroxyplastic middle ear implant for hearing reconstruction (author's design).

material, technique, and prosthesis may have to be made intraoperatively (**Fig. 7.3**).

In some cases, the prosthesis may have slipped or migrated from the proper position. If this is observed intraoperatively, it is tempting to simply reposition the same prosthesis. This temptation should be avoided; whatever caused the prosthesis to slip the first time may indeed cause slippage again. It is more prudent to remove the old prosthesis and reinsert a new one. The remaining ossicles should be palpated for ankylosis of an existing ossicle or an undetected fibrous union ossicle that looks like a sound conducting assembly but is not.

The use of a laser in revision ossiculoplasty may be helpful. In cases of tympanosclerosis involving the oval window, use of the laser for delicate removal of the tympanosclerosis plaque is far safer than mechanical removal or drilling techniques; preservation of cochlear function and avoidance of injury to the vestibule can be more readily accomplished. The use of a laser may also be helpful in removing disease from remaining ossicles or dissecting the prosthesis from the oval window or vestibule without excessive trauma.

The principle of staging ossicular reconstruction is just as important in revision surgery as it is in primary surgery. It may be even more so due to the existence of severe mucosal disease. One of several biomaterials available, such as Silastic or Epifilm, should be used to prevent adhesions between the tympanic membrane graft and the medial aspect of the middle ear, as well as to create an adequate tympanum for subsequent ossiculoplasty. Although the desire to avoid a second procedure is laudable, staging is a technique that can ultimately lead to an increased chance of successful hearing reconstruction, particularly in revision cases.[27–29]

With ossiculoplasty, postoperative follow-up is essential to ensure good long-term results. Should the tympanic membrane begin to retract, a ventilation tube may prevent or reduce the amount of postoperative atelectasis that may develop. Should middle ear fluid collect, the resulting conductive hearing loss can be corrected. Subsequent migration or extrusion of the prosthesis can often be noted through periodic examination. This obviously is most important in cases of chronic disease, as opposed to trauma or congenital fixation of the ossicular chain.[30]

Basic Principles of Middle Ear Reconstruction

There are five basic principles of middle ear reconstruction that apply to revision ossiculoplasty as well as primary surgery. In revision cases, it is important to adhere to these basic concepts to achieve maximal hearing improvement.

The first principle is aeration of the middle ear. To have an efficient transformer mechanism of the middle ear, a true tympanum with efficient vibration of the tympanic membrane must be created. Staging, the use of ventilation tubes, and patient selection are critical factors in maintaining a well-aerated tympanum.

A perpendicular columella for optimal conduction of vibratory energy from the tympanic membrane to the oval window is the second principle (**Fig. 7.4**). In chronic ear surgery, reconstruction of the lever action of the ossicular chain is difficult and often impractical; unlike stapes surgery, it is of minimal importance in hearing improvement. A maximal area ratio of the tympanic membrane to

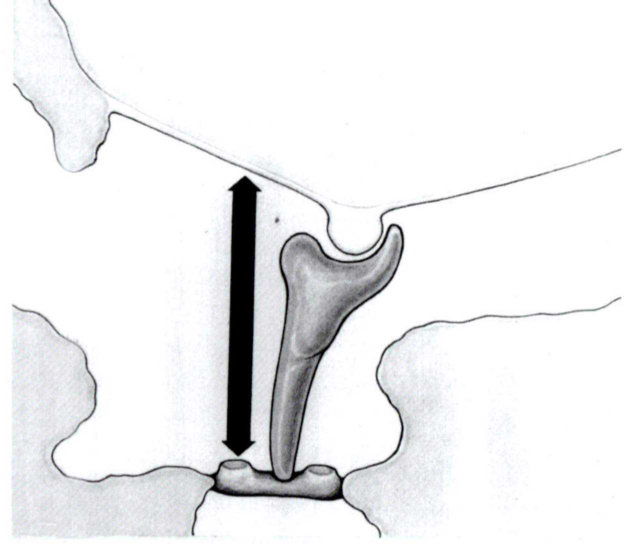

Fig. 7.4 Perpendicular columella for optimal conduction of energy in the transformer mechanism of the middle ear.

the oval window, along with a perpendicular columella to connect the two, will achieve the most satisfactory reconstruction of the sound transformer mechanism.

Preservation of the malleus handle is the third principle. Whenever possible, preservation of this structure will allow for accurate graft placement and the creation of a conical tympanic membrane. This reconstruction increases the stability of the prosthesis and prevents lateralization of the tympanic membrane graft. Preservation of the malleus handle creates a more efficient ossicular reconstruction and results in improved hearing.[31]

The fourth principle, sound protection of the round window, maintains the phase differential between the oval and round windows and enhances the efficiency of the transformer mechanism of the middle ear. Every attempt should be made to protect the round window even if a prosthesis cannot be used for ossicular reconstruction.

A snug fit of the prosthesis is essential for maximal conductivity of sound. This fifth principle is often accomplished better by "feel versus fit." In other words, although accurate and precise measurements should be attempted, it is more important to fit the prosthesis by feel between the tympanic membrane/malleus handle and the stapes superstructure/footplate. This must be accomplished without undue pressure to avoid dislocation of the prosthesis into the vestibule, but with firm enough pressure that the maximal conductivity of sound can be created and maintained.

Conclusion

Revision tympanoplasty/ossiculoplasty is required because of a previous failure due to either technical or disease factors. Revision surgery is indicated to correct the initial problem (or possibly a new or coexisting one). Although there are several indications for tympanoplasty and ossiculoplasty, this discussion has focused on the most common and difficult indication: chronic otitis media. The same principles apply to other indications, such as congenital anomalies, trauma, and miscellaneous etiologies.

As with any surgery, it is important to have realistic expectations from the patient and surgeon alike. The patient must be able to prioritize what is most important (e.g., sacrificing hearing results for a dry, safe ear). The surgeon must be able to prioritize the objectives of surgery (e.g., improving hearing at the expense of swimming). Communication between the surgeon and patient, as well education of the patient regarding his or her particular condition, is essential to achieving satisfaction. Despite the many advancements of tympanoplasty/ossiculoplasty over the past 50 years, these procedures are often associated with failures and complications secondary to conditions beyond the surgeon's control. Long-term follow-up is critical because, despite the many successes that can be achieved at the present time, today's success may be tomorrow's failure.

With all these disclaimers, the overwhelming majority of patients who undergo revision surgery should still be able to achieve primary objectives of eliminating disease, obtaining a dry, functional ear, and maintaining or improving hearing.

Acknowledgments The author would like to thank Shelley Dukate for her tireless efforts in preparing this chapter, and give credit to the outstanding artwork prepared by Stephen J. Moon, M.S.

References

1. Vartiainen E. The results of chronic ear surgery in training programme. Clin Otolaryngol 1998;23:177–180.
2. Albu S, Babighian G, Trabalzini F. Prognostic factors in tympanoplasty. Am J Otol 1998;19:136–140.
3. Stangerup SE, Drozdziewicz D, Tos M, Trabalzini F. Surgery for acquired cholesteatoma in children: long-term results and recurrence of cholesteatoma. J Laryngol Otol 1998;112:742–749.
4. Tos M, Lau T. Stability of tympanoplasty in children. Otolaryngol Clin North Am 1989;22:15–28.
5. Merchant SN, Wang P, Jang CH, et al. Efficacy of tympanomastoid surgery for control of infection in active chronic otitis media. Laryngoscope 1997;107:872–877.
6. Attallah MS. Revision tympanoplasty: surgical findings and results in Riyadh. ORL J Otorhinolaryngol Relat Spec 1996;58:36–38.
7. Wehrs RE. Incus interposition and ossiculoplasty with hydroxyapatite prostheses. Otolaryngol Clin North Am 1994;27:677–688.
8. Goldenberg RA, Driver M. Long-term results with hydroxylapatite middle ear implants. Otolaryngol Head Neck Surg 2000;122:635–642.
9. Chole RA. Ossiculoplasty with presculpted banked cartilage. Otolaryngol Clin North Am 1994;27:717–726.
10. De la Cruz A, Doyle KJ. Ossiculoplasty in congenital hearing loss. Otolaryngol Clin North Am 1994;27:799–811.
11. Sterkers JM. Congenital absence of the oval window. Laryngoscope 1991;101:220.
12. Kumazawa T, Iwano T, Ushiro K, et al. Tubotympanoplasty. Acta Otolaryngol Suppl 1993;500:14–17.
13. Campbell JP, Pillsbury HC III. The use of computerized tomographic imaging in revision mastoid surgery for chronic otitis media. Am J Otol 1990;11:387–394.
14. Blevins NH, Carter BL. Routine preoperative imaging in chronic ear surgery. Am J Otol 1998;19:527–535.
15. Bottrill ID, Poe DS. Endoscope-assisted ear surgery. Am J Otol 1995;16:158–163.

16. Youssef TF, Poe DS. Endoscope-assisted second-staged tympanomastoidectomy. Laryngoscope 1997;107:1341–1344.
17. Rosenberg SI. Endoscopic otologic surgery. Otolaryngol Clin North Am 1996;29:291–300.
18. Veldman JE, Braunius WW. Revision surgery for chronic otitis media: a learning experience. Report on 389 cases with a long-term follow-up. Ann Otol Rhinol Laryngol 1998;107:486–491.
19. Beck DL, Benecke JE Jr. Intraoperative facial nerve monitoring: technical aspects. Otolaryngol Head Neck Surg 1990;102:270–272.
20. Perkins R, Bui HT. Tympanic membrane reconstruction using formaldehyde-formed autogenous temporalis fascia. Otolaryngol Head Neck Surg 1996;114:366–379.
21. Wehrs RE. Ossicular reconstruction in ears with cholesteatoma. Otolaryngol Clin North Am 1989;22:1003–1013.
22. Heermann J. Auricular cartilage palisade. Clin Otolaryngol Allied Sci 1978;3:443–446.
23. Heerman J. Autograft tragal and conchal palisade cartilage and perichondrium in tympanomastoid reconstruction. Ear Nose Throat J 1992;71:344–349.
24. Dornhoffer JL. Surgical modification of the difficult mastoid cavity. Otolaryngol Head Neck Surg 1999;120:361–367.
25. Kartush JM. Ossicular chain reconstruction. Otolaryngol Clin North Am 1994;27:689–715.
26. Schuring AG. Ossiculoplasty with semi-biologic and composite prostheses. Otolaryngol Clin N Am 1994;747–757.
27. Hirsch BE, Kamerer DB, Boshi S. Single-stage management of cholesteatoma. Otolaryngol Head Neck Surg 1992;106:351–354.
28. Schuring AG, Lippy WH, Rizer FM, Schuring LT. Staging for cholestetoma in the child, adolescent, and adult. Ann Otol Rhinol Laryngol 1990;99:256–260.
29. Dodson EE, Hashiaki GT, Hobgood TC, Lambert PR. Intact canal wall mastoidectomy with tympanoplasty for cholesteatoma in children. Laryngoscope 1998;108:977–983.
30. Rosenfeld RM, Moura RL, Bluestone CD. Predictors of residual-recurrent cholesteatoma in children. Arch Otolaryngol Head Neck Surg 1992;118:384–391.
31. Fisch U, Schmid S. Total reconstruction of the ossicular chain. Otolaryngol Clin North Am 1994;27:785–797.

Revision Surgery for Cholesteatoma or Chronic Otitis Media

Simon C. Parisier and Jose N. Fayad

The primary goal of surgery for cholesteatoma is complete eradication of the disease process. Additionally, the surgeon seeks to preserve or restore hearing and to provide the patient with a trouble-free dry ear.[1,2] Revision surgery presents the otologic surgeon with special problems.[3,4] Landmarks frequently have been distorted by the disease process as well as by the prior surgery. Also, patients who have recidivistic disease tend to have the most severe form of chronic ear disease, with poor eustachian tube function and failure of middle ear ventilation. This chapter reviews the experience gained in the diagnosis and treatment of recidivistic cholesteatoma in 162 ears. Highlights of the surgical technique will be discussed. Results in adults and children with respect to production of safe, dry ear, along with hearing results and rates of recidivism, will be reviewed.

Causes of Failure of Primary Surgery

The causes of failure in surgery for cholesteatoma may be incomplete resection of the disease (residual disease) and poor surgical technique, but the cause may also be a severe form of chronic ear disease with poor eustachian tube function or the failure of middle ear ventilation (recurrent disease). In our hands, the rate of recidivism (whether recurrent or residual disease) is 11% in the pediatric population and 14% in the adult population. These numbers vary greatly between different centers and different surgeons with varied approaches to the treatment of chronic otitis media with cholesteatoma.

Revision Surgery

Surgical Technique for Residual Cholesteatoma

The following are the highlights of our surgical technique in treating recidivistic cholesteatomatous disease. In patients who have had a skillfully performed canal wall down operation, a residual cholesteatoma may present as a localized "pearl" in the mastoid and can be marsupialized in the office. The area is anesthetized either with a 50% topical phenol solution or by use of local anesthetic infiltration. The lateral wall of the cyst is excised, and the keratin accumulation is aspirated. The epidermal base is preserved, and, having been unroofed, it will form a stable skin lining. Residual disease localized within the middle ear cleft will usually require only a tympanotomy for removal, but if the disease has extended into the sinus tympani, its removal will be more difficult. To expose this area, the bone anterior and lateral to the vertical portion of the facial nerve must be removed. Exposure of this area may be facilitated by performing a canal wall down mastoidectomy. An alternative is to perform an extended hypotympanotomy via a canal wall intact mastoidectomy, preserving the posterior canal wall. This procedure will increase exposure of the sinus tympani, but not to the degree obtained in a canal wall down approach.

Isolated residual disease within the mastoid cavity following an intact canal wall procedure occurs relatively infrequently. In such cases, performing a revision mastoidectomy will allow for its complete removal. The mastoid cortex may have regenerated, especially in children. If the mastoid has adequate aeration after the initial procedure, the surgeon may find an otherwise air-filled, mucosa-lined cavity, and the disease can be removed and the canal wall preserved. However, when residual keratinizing epithelium invades air cells, it may insidiously grow extensively within the temporal bone. Its removal will require meticulous exenteration of the remaining "accessible cells," a process that can be time consuming and technically demanding. Even in large, cellular mastoids, sacrificing of the posterior canal wall may be required to obtain the necessary exposure to permit the complete removal of existing disease when the pathology is found to be clinically more aggressive, as in massive cholesteatoma regrowth.

Recurrent Cholesteatoma

Recurrent disease is a frequent problem in intact canal wall cholesteatoma surgery.[5] Recurrent disease occurs when the underlying eustachian tube function is inadequate to equalize pressures within the middle ear mastoid complex. It must be recognized that removal of middle ear

Decision tree for cholesteatoma

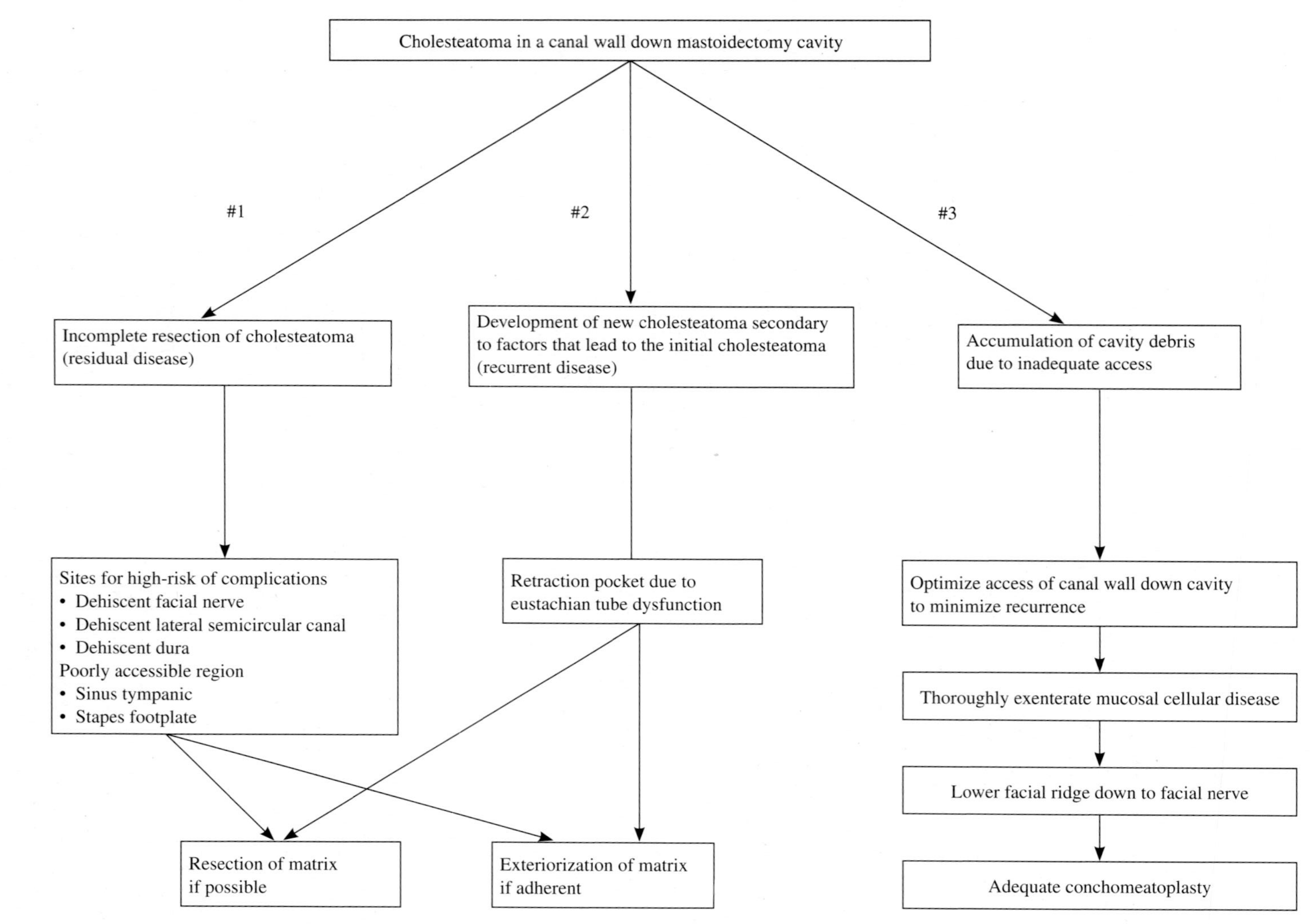

or mastoid disease will not affect disorders intrinsic to the eustachian tube. Regretfully, otologists are not able to predictably evaluate or to improve the physiologic function of the eustachian tube, even though nasal, nasopharvngeal, and sinus disease may have been successfully treated. Effective eustachian tube surgery or treatment that improves tube function has not yet been developed. Thus, following canal wall up surgery, recurrent cholesteatomas may develop.

Prevention of the recurrence of cholesteatoma may be possible by inserting middle ear ventilating tubes or by meticulous reconstruction of canal wall defects. In canal wall up surgery, Silastic sheeting is often placed from the middle ear through the facial and epitympanic recesses into the mastoid cavity to restore aeration to these areas. However, this does not consistently succeed in providing the desired middle ear–mastoid aeration. Recurrent disease removal can still occur in spite of these maneuvers due to persistent eustachian tube dysfunction. When confronted with such a recurrence, the surgeon must avoid the development of yet another recurrent cholesteatoma in the future by using a canal wall down, open technique.

Marsupializing the mastoid into the ear canal eliminates it as an air-containing cavity and precludes the need for ventilation. A canal wall down procedure provides an unobstructed exposure of the middle ear, anterior epitympanic-zygomatic area and may facilitate eradication of disease from the sinus tympani. When a patient with a cholesteatoma develops a labyrinthine fistula or a significant intracranial complication in an ear having had a canal wall up procedure, it is essential to convert it to a canal wall down mastoidectomy.

Often, a patient with localized erosion from an attic cholesteatoma, or with a prior limited atticotomy, will present with an epitympanic retraction despite a well-aerated middle ear. In such ears, the loss of underlying bony support may have led to a collapse of the overlying keratinizing epithelium. If canal skin collapses onto the floor of the epitympanum, it may block mastoid aeration. The attic defect progressively retracts behind the posterior canal wall into the antrum, producing a recurrent cholesteatoma. One may suggest that removal of the retraction and reconstruction of the lateral epitympanic wall with a cartilage graft could eliminate the problem. However, if there is poor eustachian tube function, over time recurrent disease may still develop in some of these reconstructed ears.

Indications for Revision Surgery

Revision surgery is indicated in the treatment of recidivistic disease whether due to recurrent or residual cholesteatoma.

Table 8.1 Summary of the Senior Author's Experience in the Surgical Treatment of Cholesteatoma and Recidivism

	Initial Operation	Revision	Total Operations by Author
Adult	172	109	281
Pediatric	184	53	237
Total	356	162	518

The clinical data from the senior author's experience with 518 ears operated upon for cholesteatoma were reviewed. Three hundred fifty-six were primary cases, 172 (48%) adults and 184 (52%) children.

Recidivistic cholesteatoma accounted for 162 (31%) of the total cases (**Table 8.1**). Fifty-three (10% of total patients) were children, and 109 (21% of total patients) were adults. Half of the adult cholesteatomas occurred in males, whereas in children males accounted for 65% of patients. Right and left ears were affected equally. The mean age for the adults was 42.6 ± 15 years and for children was 8.6 ± 4.7 years.

The patients with cholesteatoma regrowth in this series can be subdivided into two groups (**Table 8.2**). The first is composed of 120 ears initially operated elsewhere and referred to the senior author for treatment of recidivistic disease. The second is composed of 42 cases of cholesteatomatous regrowth in ears previously operated on by the senior author. These were analyzed separately. Many of the patients in this latter group were asymptomatic, the regrowth being discovered during the course of office follow-up examinations.

The following parameters were analyzed: presenting signs and symptoms of recidivism, interval of time between initial surgery and diagnosis of recidivism, types and incidence of complications in the recidivism group, and results of revision surgery.

Presenting Symptoms

The regrowth of a cholesteatoma produced symptoms similar to those produced by the original disease (**Table 8.3**). Drainage and hearing loss were the most commonly

Table 8.2 Summary of the Nature of the Recidivism in the Senior Author's Revision Cholesteatoma Cases

	Revisions Referred to Author	Author's Recidivism	Total
Adult	86 (53%)	23 (14%)	109 (67%)
Pediatric	34 (22%)	19 (11%)	53 (33%)
Total	120 (75%)	42 (25%)	162 (100%)

Note: % reflects the percentage of all recidivistic cholesteatomas undergoing surgery by the senior author.

Table 8.3 Clinical Presentation of the Patients with Recidivistic Cholesteatoma Who Were Referred to the Senior Author for Revision Surgery

Clinical Presentation	Adult (n = 86)	Pediatric (n = 34)	Total (n = 120)
Hearing loss	81 (94.2%)	30 (88.2%)	111 (92.5%)
Otorrhea	77 (89.5%)	32 (94.1%)	109 (90.8%)
Retraction pocket	42 (48.8%)	12 (35.3%)	54 (37.5%)
Vertigo*	36 (41.9%)	2 (5.9%)	38 (31.7%)
Tinnitus	21 (24.4%)	2 (5.9%)	23 (19.2%)
Middle ear mass	10 (11.6%)	7 (20.6%)	17 (14.2%)
Facial weakness	7 (8.1%)	0	7 (5.8%)

* Includes both patients with vertigo and those with a positive fistula test.

observed symptoms. Usually, there was a recurrence of foul-smelling otorrhea in a previously dry ear and a deterioration in hearing. Otalgia occurred quite frequently in children (41%) and was less common (19%) in adults. Episodes of vertigo were commonly reported by adults (42%) but rarely in children. Eight percent of adults with cholesteatoma regrowth presented with a facial nerve paralysis, whereas no children in this series suffered this disfigurement.

Otologic Findings

Regrowth of cholesteatoma occurred regardless of the type of initial procedure performed (**Table 8.4**). Patients having had a closed, canal wall up technique developed both residual or recurrent cholesteatoma and cholesteatoma of unknown origin (**Table 8.5**). In these ears, residual middle ear cholesteatoma presented as a whitish mass displacing the overlying tympanic membrane or as a collection of keratin debris seen through a drum defect. Residual growths occurred less frequently in the mastoid than in the middle ear. However, if a closed technique was used for the initial excision, residual mastoid cholesteatoma would silently grow without being detected until it became infected or caused a complication. Alternatively, recurrent cholesteatomas in

Table 8.5 Type of Cholesteatoma Regrowth in Patients Who Were Referred to the Senior Author with Recidivistic Cholesteatoma

Types of Cholesteatoma Regrowth	Adult (n = 86)	Pediatric (n = 34)	Total (n = 120)
Recurrent	30 (34.9%)	11 (32.4%)	41 (34.2%)
Residual	43 (50%)	19 (55.9%)	62 (51.7%)
Unknown Origin	13 (15.1%)	4 (11.8%)	17 (14.2%)

Table 8.4 Prior Surgeries Performed on Patients Who Were Referred to the Senior Author for Revision Cholesteatoma Surgery

Prior Surgeries	Adult (n = 86)	Pediatric (n = 34)
Tympanotomy	11 (12.8%)	5 (14.7%)
Canal wall up mastoidectomy	42 (48.8%)	12 (35.3%)
Canal wall down mastoidectomy	22 (25.6%)	11 (32.4%)
Atticotomy	11 (12.8%)	6 (9.4%)

ears having had canal wall up procedures presented as retraction pockets filled with keratin. These retractions often extended superiorly into the attic, posteriorly toward the antrum, or deep into the sinus tympani. Frequently, pyogenic-like granulation and foul-smelling otorrhea were present.

Patients having had a properly performed canal wall down procedure in which the mastoid recess had been marsupialized into the ear canal developed residual but not recurrent cholesteatoma. Retained keratinizing epithelium presented as a whitish mass either in the marsupialized mastoid or displacing or eroding the grafted tympanic membrane. If infected, foul-smelling otorrhea and granulation tissue were present.

Surgical Procedures Performed for Recidivism

Each ear was individually assessed to attempt to determine the type of recidivism, why the initial operation failed, and which operative procedure would permanently eliminate the disease process (**Table 8.6**). Most adults who presented with cholesteatomatous regrowth having had an initial closed technique were treated with canal wall down mastoidectomies (87.2%). However, in children with recidivism, it was elected to preserve the posterior canal wall (closed technique) in 26.5%. In children

Table 8.6 Type of Surgery Performed as Revision for Recidivistic Cholesteatoma in Patients Referred to the Senior Author

Type of Surgery Performed	Adult (n = 86)	Pediatric (n = 34)
Canal wall down mastoidectomy	75 (87.2%)	21 (61.8%)
Canal wall up mastoidectomy	4 (4.47%)	9 (26.5%)
Excision/marsupialization	4 (4.7%)	0
Tympanotomy	3 (3.35%)	4 (11.8%)

Table 8.7 Intraoperative Findings at Revision Surgery for Recidivistic Cholesteatoma in Patients Referred to the Senior Author with Recidivism

Intraoperative Findings at Revision Surgery	Adult ($n = 86$)	Pediatric ($n = 34$)
Facial dehiscence	32 (37.2%)	6 (17.6%)
Semicircular canal fistula	15 (17.4%)	0
Intracranial extension	8 (9.3%)	0
Petrous extension	5 (5.8%)	1 (2.9%)

who originally had tvmpanotomy-type procedures for congenital cholesteatoma, it was possible to excise small residual cholesteatomas in 11.8% by repeating the same middle ear approach. Thus, 38% of children with recidivistic cholesteatoma were treated with closed techniques.

Intraoperative Findings

Semicircular canal fistulas were present in 17.4% of adults, though none occurred in children (**Table 8.7**). It must be noted that some patients with fistulas did not complain of vertigo, while conversely, many who had labyrinthine symptoms did not have fistulas. The facial nerve was observed to be dehiscent in 37.2% of adults, but only 8% presented with a facial paralysis. In children, even though the facial nerve was observed to lack some portion of its bony covering in 17.6%, this exposure did not result in any facial paralysis either preoperatively or postoperatively. Petrous apex involvement occurred in 5.8% of adults and in only one child (2.9%). Intracranial extension occurred in 9.3% of adults but fortunately in none of the children.

Results

Following revision surgery, 10 (11.6%) adults and 9 (26.4%) children experienced persistent or frequently recurrent otorrhea (i.e., requiring more than four visits a year). A perforation was observed in no adults and in seven children. Following canal wall up (closed) surgery, otorrhea occurred in no adults and in seven children. In canal wall down (open) surgery, drainage postoperatively was a slightly greater problem, occurring in 10 adults and 9 children.

In adults and children, the hearing results were analyzed by comparing the changes between pre- and postoperative air conduction pure tone averages (AC-PTAs), air–bone gaps (ABGs), discrimination scores (DSs), bone conduction pure tone averages (BC-PTAs), and bone conduction at 4 kHz. A repeated measures analysis of variance (RMANOVA) was used to assess statistical significance.

In adults, the average preoperative AC-PTA was 48 ± 17 dB, postoperative 47 ± 19 dB. ABGs were preoperative 34 ± 13, postoperative 30 ± 11 dB. Bone conduction at 4 kHz was preoperative 26 ± 15 dB, postoperative 26 ± 17 dB. DS was preoperative 93% ± 7%, postoperative 90% ± 15%, the only statistically significant change ($p > .004$); all other comparisons were unchanged. This observation should be interpreted in relation to the unchanged BC-PTA and BC at 4 kHz.

In children, a statistically significant improvement was noted when comparing AC-PTA pre- (51 ± 16 dB) and postoperatively (44 ± 21 dB), $p = .01$, and ABG pre- (43 ± 13 dB) and postoperatively (35 ± 15 dB), $p = .01$. However, bone conduction rates at 4 kHz pre- and postoperatively (pre- 19 ± 17dB, post- 20 ± 19 dB, $p = .01$) were statistically different, though the BC-PTA and DS remained unchanged.

Recidivism in Primary and Revision Cholesteatoma Surgery

One hundred and twenty of these patients (86 adults and 34 children) presented with recidivistic disease after having their primary excision performed elsewhere. The rate of recidivism in these two groups was analyzed using a Kaplan-Meier surgical analysis.

Kaplan-Meier analysis, frequently used in evaluating surgical survival in cancer studies, seeks to correlate the incidence of an adverse event (e.g., patient death or recurrence of disease) in subjects who have been followed for an identical length of time, thereby arriving at a rate of occurrence of this event. The adverse event in our study is the recidivism of the cholesteatoma. Usually, in an analysis of this type, the median time to the adverse event would be determined. However, the number of patients who developed recidivism in our study was too small to allow the median to be estimated. Therefore, the data were summarized as the 10-year recidivism rates (± standard error).

Eighty-six adults presented to the senior author with recidivistic disease, and 3 developed further regrowth of cholesteatoma. The rate of recidivism was calculated as 6% ± 4% at 5 years and 6% ± 4% at 10 years. Thirty-four children presented to the author with recidivistic disease, and 5 developed further regrowth of cholesteatoma. The rate was calculated as 21% ± 10% at 5 years and 34% ± 10% at 10 years.

These results were compared with those obtained following the first surgery for primary or secondary acquired cholesteatomas. In adults, the group operated for recidivistic disease had a smaller rate of regrowth than those operated upon for acquired cholesteatomas. The

Table 8.8 Recidivistic Cholesteatoma in Those Patients Whose Initial Excision Was Performed by the Senior Author

Type of Recidivistic Cholesteatoma	Adult	Pediatric	Total
Recurrent	4	6	10
Residual	19	13	32
Total	23	19	42

opposite was true in children: those who presented with acquired disease and who had their initial surgery performed by the author had a smaller rate of regrowth than those who presented with recidivistic disease and required revision surgery. In neither the adult nor the pediatric groups were the differences statistically significant.

Revision Cholesteatoma Surgery in Patients Whose Primary Excision was Performed by the Author

As mentioned in the last section, the senior author has operated on 476 ears for the primary excision of cholesteatoma (**Table 8.1**) using a tympanotomy, a (closed) canal wall up mastoidectomy, or an (open) canal wall down mastoidectomy. These patients were treated with a single individualized definitive operation rather than relying on a staged approach in which a planned second procedure is performed to verify that the ear is free of disease or to complete the removal of cholesteatoma.

To detect recidivistic disease in these ears, the author examined the ears over time using an operating microscope and sequential audiometric studies. In selected cases, CT scans were obtained and occasionally these too were repeated sequentially. Of these patients who were operated on by the senior author, 42 patients (23 adults and 19 children) developed recidivistic cholesteatoma (**Table 8.8**). These consisted of 10 recurrences (4 adults and 6 children) and 32 residuals (19 adults, and 13 children). The types of surgery required to eradicate the regrowth were individualized (**Table 8.9**). Simple marsupialization for residual disease, generally performed as an office procedure, was used in some children (31%) and many adults (74%). In this carefully monitored group of patients, cholesteatoma regrowth was detected when the disease became evident on clinical examination rather than by performing staged re-explorations. There was little progressive destruction observed. In one child and one adult, both of whom had normal symmetrical facial movement, the fallopian canal that had been intact at the first operation was found to have become eroded at the revision procedure. Progressive ossicular erosion was observed in one adult in whom the stapes arch became eroded and in two children (the long process of the incus was eroded in one, and the stapes arch was eroded in the other). Following the revision surgery on this selected group of patients, hearing was analyzed by assessing the ability to achieve a postoperative speech reception threshold (SRT) of 30 dB (**Table 8.10**). The SRT went from worse to better than 30 dB in seven adults and in one child. In nine adults and nine children, it remained worse than 30 dB postoperatively. In two children the hearing deteriorated postoperatively, the SRT falling from better than 30 dB both pre- and postoperatively in seven adults and seven children. In summary, after these revisions for recidivism, 14 adults had an SRT better than 30 dB, and 9 adults had an SRT worse than 30 dB. In children, after revision surgery, the SRT was better than 30 dB in 8 and was worse than 30 dB in 11. None of these cases developed a neurosensory hearing loss.

Table 8.9 Types of Revision Surgery Performed on Patients with Recidivistic Cholesteatoma Whose Initial Excision Was Performed by the Senior Author

Type of Revision Surgery Performed	Pediatric Residual (*n* = 13)	Pediatric Recurrent (*n* = 6)	Adult Residual (*n* = 19)	Adult Recurrent (*n* = 4)
Canal wall down mastoidectomy	3 (23%)	6 (100%)	2 (11%)	2 (50%)
Canal wall up mastoidectomy	1 (8%)	0	2 (11%)	0
Tympanotomy	5 (38%)	0	1 (5%)	0
Excision/ marsupialization	4 (31%)	0	14 (74%)	2 (50%)

Table 8.10 Hearing Results following Revision Surgery Performed on Patients with Recidivistic Cholesteatoma Whose Initial Excision was Performed by the Senior Author

Hearing Results following Revision Surgery	Adult (*n* = 23)	Pediatric (*n* = 19)
Hearing unchanged, SRT > 30 dB	9	9
Hearing unchanged, SRT > 30 dB	7	7
Hearing improved*	7	1
Hearing worsened*	0	2

* Improved hearing was that which began with a speech reception threshold (SRT) better than 30 dB and was less than 30 dB after the operation. The converse is true for worsening.

Lowering the Risk of a Second Failure

Revision cholesteatoma surgery can be very challenging even for the most experienced otologic surgeon. When dissecting cholesteatoma in the areas of the semicircular canals, cochlea, or footplate, the possibility of a fistula should be kept in mind to prevent sensorineural hearing loss, anacusis, and postoperative vertigo.

Perfect knowledge of the anatomy and location of the facial nerve is required to avoid injuring the nerve, which can be dehiscent and exposed under surrounding infected, bleeding mucosa and granulation tissue. Facial nerve monitoring in these cases can be very helpful to identify and protect the nerve from injury. But facial nerve monitoring cannot be a substitute to mastering the anatomy, such as identification of the nerve using fixed landmarks as the tensor tympani muscle, the digastric groove, and the oval and round windows.

In other cases, the possibility of brain tissue protruding into the mastoid cavity due to a meningoencephalocele should be kept in mind in the presence of soft tissue in the mastoid. A cerebrospinal fluid otorrhea can be induced if the anatomy is obscured by granulation tissue or the dura is exposed and invaded by aggressive cholesteatoma. Exposed major vessels, such as the internal carotid artery and sigmoid sinus, will be seen in certain cases, and care should be taken to avoid injury to those vessels. Only knowledge of the tridimensional anatomy of the temporal bone and rigorous surgical technique will ensure total removal of the disease and avoidance of complications.

In the body of the text, we outlined our strategy in dealing with recidivistic disease and explained our microdissection techniques and our approach to avoid a second failure. Although we do not routinely use the laser in cholesteatoma surgery, the argon or CO_2 laser can be used to vaporize tissue in the area of the footplate or the superstructure. Using the laser will minimize manipulation of the inner ear and is an effective tool in ablating disease in the areas of the windows.

When it comes to reconstruction, our preference is using cartilage harvested from the concha and the inferior part of the cartilaginous external auditory canal while performing the meatoplasty. Attic bony defects are reconstructed with cartilage to avoid recurrent retraction pockets due to poor eustachian tube function. Mastoid obliteration when indicated is achieved using bone pate when available and musculoperiosteal flaps.

Conclusion

Revision cholesteatoma surgery represents a true challenge to the otologic surgeon. The goals of cholesteatoma surgery, whether primary or revision, are the complete eradication of disease, the preservation or restoration of hearing, and the creation of a dry, safe ear. It would seem that these goals are best achieved at the initial surgical intervention. Revision will be needed in cases of recidivism (residual or recurrent cholesteatoma), persistent otorrhea due to chronic mucosal disease, canal stenosis, or conductive hearing loss. Revision surgery can be complicated by the absence or alteration of important temporal bone landmarks, either by the persistent disease or the prior surgery. Careful evaluation must include an objective assessment of the reasons for failure in the first operation and a detailed computed tomography scan.

The key to successful revision cholesteatoma surgery is the early identification of the facial nerve. This can be accomplished by its identification in a location where the anatomy is often unchanged at the time of revision, such as the stylomastoid foramen or the cochleariform process. A canalplasty and meatoplasty will often be needed at the time of revision. All remaining diseased mucosa and unexenterated air cells must be removed. The conductive hearing mechanism can usually be reconstructed at the time of the revision surgery.

The choice of revision procedure used depends on the reasons for and type of failure in the original operation. Poorly performed open mastoidectomies may need revision due to problematic cavities in the absence of recidivistic disease. Removal of residual cholesteatoma may require a mere marsupialization of the lesion or may require massive revision. Recurrent cholesteatoma will often require that an intact canal mastoidectomy be converted into an open cavity.

The results of revision surgery are not as good in children as in adults. This is related to a variety of factors. In many children with cholesteatoma, the mastoid air cell system is well developed, which technically makes the complete eradication of disease more difficult. Most adults have sclerotic mastoids that serve to localize the process and facilitate its removal. Endogenous growth factors present in children may stimulate cholesteatomatous proliferation, making recidivism a greater problem in this population.[6] Also, the increased frequency of upper respiratory infections in the pediatric age group may affect the middle ear, resulting in a greater incidence of graft perforations, postoperative otorrhea, and recurrent cholesteatoma.

Attentive long-term office observation following surgery for cholesteatoma is an effective way of detecting recidivism. Residual and recurrent growths detected in this manner produced little, if any, additional erosion. These cholesteatomas could readily be excised with good results.

References

1. Parisier SC. Management of cholesteatoma. Otolaryngol Clin North Am 1989;22:927–940.
2. Parisier SC, Weiss MH, Edelstein DR. Treatment of cholesteatoma. Otolaryngol Head Neck Surg 1991;5:107–141.
3. Sheehy JL. Recurrent and residual cholesteatoma surgery. Clin Otolaryngol 1978;3:393–403.
4. Sheehy JL. Brackmann De, Graham MD. Cholesteatoma surgery: residual and recurrent disease. A review of 1024 cases. Ann Otol Rhinol Laryngol 1977;86:451–462.
5. Glasscock ME, Miller GW. Intact canal wall tympanoplasty in management of cholesteatoma. Laryngoscope 1976;86:1639–1657.
6. Edelstein DR, Parisier SC, Ajuha GS, et al. Cholesteatoma in the pediatric age group. Ann Otol Rhinol Laryngol 1988;97:23–29.

Revision Stapedectomy and Stapedotomy

Samuel H. Selesnick, George C. Yang, and Mukesh Prasad

Since the reintroduction of stapes surgery in the 1950s, surgeons have come to realize that improved methods for revision stapes surgery must be developed. Revision stapes surgery is not unusual. Some studies estimate that up to 25% of stapes surgeries will require revision.[1] Although the literature on revision stapes surgery can be difficult to interpret due to the large variations in patient selection criteria, outcome measures, and operative techniques, some generalizations can be made to help today's otologic surgeon best treat the revision surgical candidate.[2]

Because primary otosclerosis is less common now than only a few decades ago, current trends reveal an increased percentage of revision stapes procedures in the overall number of surgeries for otosclerosis.[3] Although the exact cause of this decrease in otosclerosis is unknown, many postulates have been offered. Increasing evidence correlates the etiology of otosclerosis to the measles virus, so that the near universal vaccination of children against measles in developed countries may have resulted in the decreased incidence of new cases of otosclerosis noted today.[4,5] Further, the addition of fluorides to drinking water may have played a role in the recent fall in incidence.[6,7] Finally, because there are fewer primary stapes surgeries being performed, young surgeons have less experience in performing stapes surgery. This may translate into a higher failure rate in primary surgeries, which adds to the increase in the number of revision stapes procedures seen today.[8,9]

The central issues in revision stapedectomy are the decreased potential for the repair of the conductive component and the increased potential risk of inner ear damage when compared with primary stapes surgery. Outcomes depend on the pathology encountered at revision surgery, as well as the management of the oval window. Technological advances, including the use of the laser, have proved to be important tools in improving hearing results and in decreasing the morbidity of performing both primary and revision stapes procedures.

Historical Overview

The goal of stapes surgery is to circumvent the inefficient sound transmission of an ossicular chain immobilized by otosclerosis. A group of surgeons from the 19th century, Kessel, Boucheron, Miot, Faraci, and Passow, pioneered procedures intended to mobilize or remove a fixed stapes.[5] However, due to the lack of adequate illumination, magnification, and sterile technique, as well as a lack of understanding of the need for oval window and stapes reconstruction, these surgeries often ended in inner ear injury and infection. In 1938, Julius Lempert introduced a one-stage fenestration technique for otosclerosis, bypassing surgery on the stapes.[10] He used an endaural approach and a dental drill to create a labyrinthine fenestra, which became the standard for otosclerosis at the time. This procedure was challenged in 1952, when Samuel Rosen reintroduced stapes mobilization for otosclerosis.[9] Finally, in 1956, it was John J. Shea's technique of total stapedectomy that replaced both Lempert's fenestration procedure and Rosen's mobilization operation and ultimately became the dominant procedure performed throughout the world for otosclerosis. Shea's technique involved the removal of the entire stapes, followed by grafting of the oval window with a vein graft. An artificial stapes made of polytetrafluoroethylene (Teflon) was placed on the vein graft in the oval window and attached to the incus.[11] Variations have been made in Shea's procedure in three major areas: the design of the prosthesis, the nature of the oval window seal, and the small fenestration technique.

Technological improvements in biocompatible materials, operating microscopes, intraoperative monitoring, and laser tissue vaporization raised stapes surgery to a higher level.

Meta-analysis of the Literature

A series of Medline literature searches spanning the time period from 1969 to 2001 was performed. The list of search words included *otosclerosis, stapes surgery, reoperation, stapedectomy, stapedotomy,* and *revision.* A review of the bibliographies of the studies that were found through this search process was also conducted. The criteria for inclusion in this meta-analysis were studies of a defined group of patients that required revision stapes surgery whose outcomes were measured and whose etiologies for failure of the primary stapes surgery were recorded. Studies selected contained data that could be extracted and pooled with those from other studies. No duplication of patient populations between studies was permitted. Sixteen studies met the selection criteria.[2,3,7,12–24] Their data can be seen in **Table 9.1.** Each study

Decision tree for revision stapes surgery

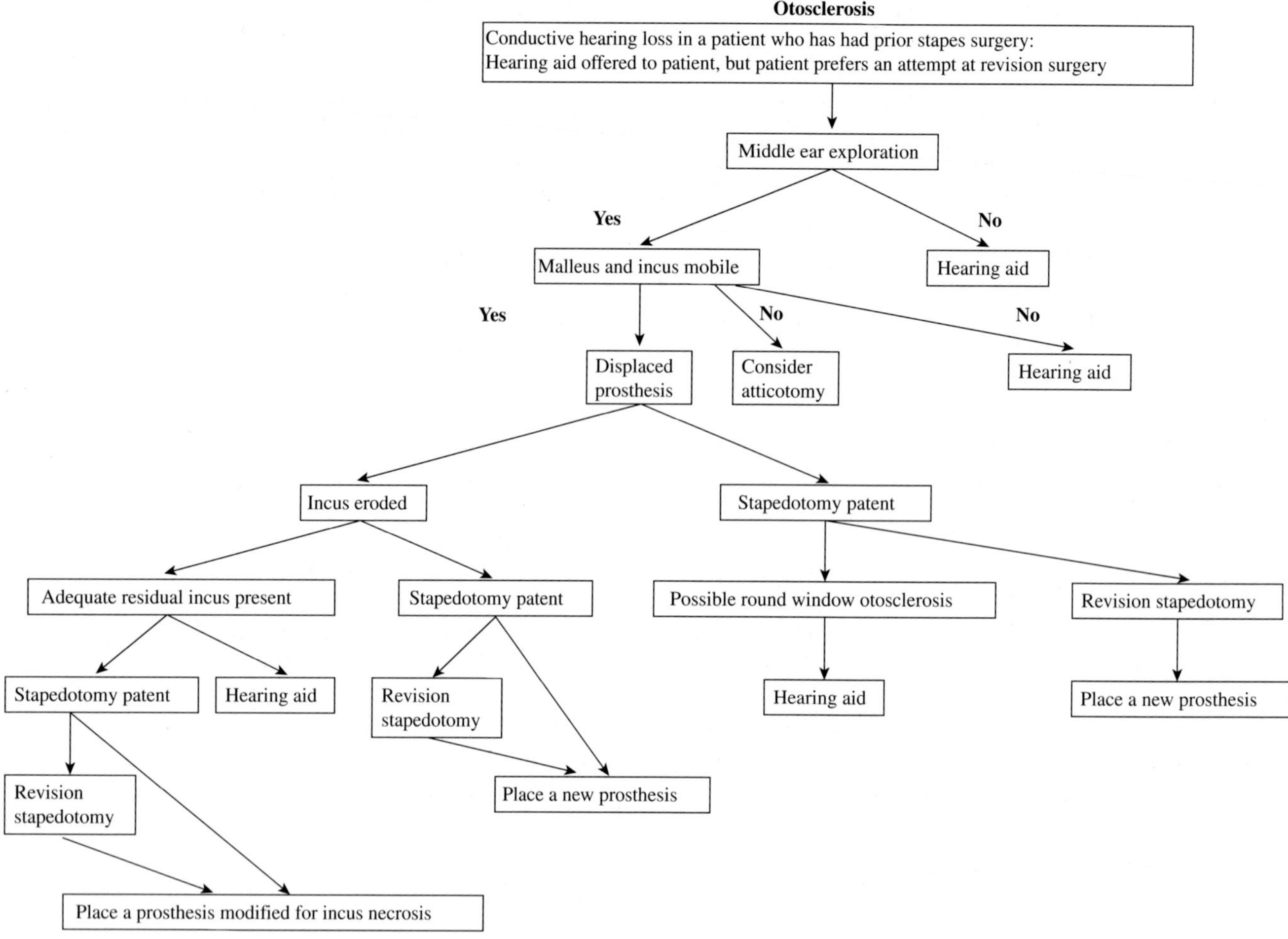

Table 9.1   Causes of Failure and Their Incidence for Revision after Stapes Surgery

	Feldman and Schuknecht, 1970 (12)	Lippy et al, 1980 (16)	Crabtree et al, 1980 (17)	Sheehy et al, 1981 (7)	Pearman and Dawes, 1982 (18)	Derlacki, 1985 (19)	Glasscock et al, 1987 (20)	Bhardwaj and Kacker, 1988 (21)	Farrior and Sutherland, 1991 (3)	McGee et al, 1993 (22)	Langman and Lindeman, 1993 (15)	Han et al, 1997 (23)	Somers et al, 1997 (2)	Lesinski, 1997 (14)	Hammerschlag et al, 1998 (24)	De la Cruz and Fayad, 2000 (13)	Totals	Percentage of Total Findings
Patient Number	154	63	35	258	74	217	79	120	102	185	66	74	226	200	250	356	2459	–
Prosthesis Dislocation	22	3	16	120	31	178	24	37	44	16	16	43	22	148	61	188	969	34.0%
Loose Prosthesis	18	5	5	0	3	0	0	8	0	17	16	7	37	2	2	19	139	4.9%
Short Prosthesis	5	5	0	31	4	0	6	8	0	4	0	3	6	12	35	42	161	5.6%
Long Prosthesis	5	1	0	0	0	0	2	14	0	0	0	1	9	0	2	13	47	1.6%
Prosthesis Related	50	14	21	151	38	178	32	67	44	37	32	54	74	162	100	262	1316	46.1%
Incus Necrosis	15	20	6	44	24	65	15	6	28	9	27	32	64	46	35	92	528	18.5%
Malleus/Incus Fixation	7	4	0	5	0	1	3	1	3	3	4	2	5	13	2	3	56	2.0%
Incus Subluxation	5	0	4	0	0	0	0	4	0	0	0	0	0	7	3	10	33	1.2%
Ossicle Related	27	24	10	49	24	66	18	11	31	12	31	34	69	66	40	105	617	21.6%
Fixed Footplate	30	0	0	23	0	67	7	7	6	1	0	3	0	28	7	0	179	6.3%
Otosclerosis Regrowth	2	2	4	23	5	21	6	17	0	11	6	18	11	0	3	50	179	6.3%
Fibrous Adhesions	13	3	13	13	7	1	5	22	0	16	0	46	29	0	34	0	202	7.1%
Perilymphatic Fistula	5	1	3	41	3	21	7	2	8	2	4	4	15	17	5	0	138	4.8%
Reparative Granuloma	22	1	0	0	0	0	0	5	0	0	0	0	0	0	1	0	29	1.0%
Footplate Related	72	7	20	100	15	110	25	53	14	30	10	71	55	45	50	50	727	25.5%
Negative Findings	0	13	0	0	2	0	0	12	0	0	0	1	0	0	20	42	90	3.2%
Other Causes	5	2	2	0	17	20	4	12	13	0	0	0	28	0	0	0	103	3.6%
Total Findings	154	60	53	300	96	374	79	155	102	79	73	160	226	273	210	459	2853	100.0%

categorized the cause and rate of failures differently. This chapter groups the etiology of failures in three broad categories: prosthesis related, ossicle related, and footplate related. Negative findings at re-exploration and all other causes were pooled.

Causes of Failure of Primary Surgery

Patients who have hearing improvement after primary stapes surgery and who develop a recurrent conductive hearing loss, whether early or late, may be good candidates for revision stapes surgery, whereas patients with the same or worse hearing after the primary procedure have a lower revision success rate.[25] The type of stapes operation, prosthesis selection, and oval window management are important in anticipating the possible cause of failure.

Prosthesis-Related Failures

About 46% of failed primary stapedectomy surgeries are caused by prosthesis-related failures. The prosthesis-related failures can be divided into five main categories: prosthesis dislocation, a loose prosthesis, a short prosthesis, a long prosthesis, and a fractured prosthesis. Prostheses must fit onto the incus tight enough to efficiently conduct sound vibrations, but not too tight as to cause necrosis of the bone. The loose connection of the prosthesis to the incus may be due to inadequate crimping. Over time, the prosthesis may migrate from the oval window to create a recurrent conductive hearing loss or even a perilymphatic fistula (**Fig. 9.1**). Similar migration occurs when a prosthesis is too short to bridge the distance from the incus to the oval window. Accurate measurements help to avoid this complication, especially when stapedotomy is performed. In stapedectomies, there is a greater margin for error in determining the appropriate length for the prosthesis because the oval window tissue seal can effectively transmit vibrations at different levels in the oval window, just as long as it is in stable contact with the prosthesis. Inappropriate prosthesis length may result in inner ear dysfunction. A prosthesis that is too long may traumatize the saccule (**Fig. 9.2**); a short prosthesis may not occlude the stapedotomy opening and result in a perilymphatic fistula (**Fig. 9.3**).

Adhesions to the prosthesis may also cause fixation and prevent normal conduction of sound to the inner ear. Using lasers, these adhesions can be lysed without causing significant mechanical trauma to the inner ear (**Fig. 9.4**). A rare reason for prosthesis malfunction is fracture of the prosthesis itself.

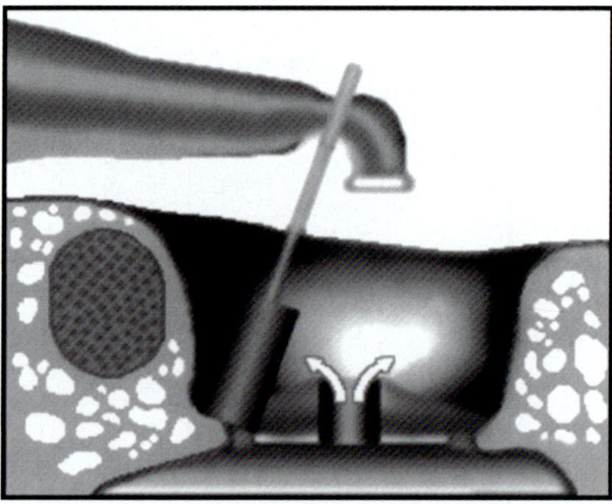

Fig. 9.1 Displaced stapes prosthesis. Note evidence of incus erosion at the crimping site. White arrows indicate a perilymphatic fistula.

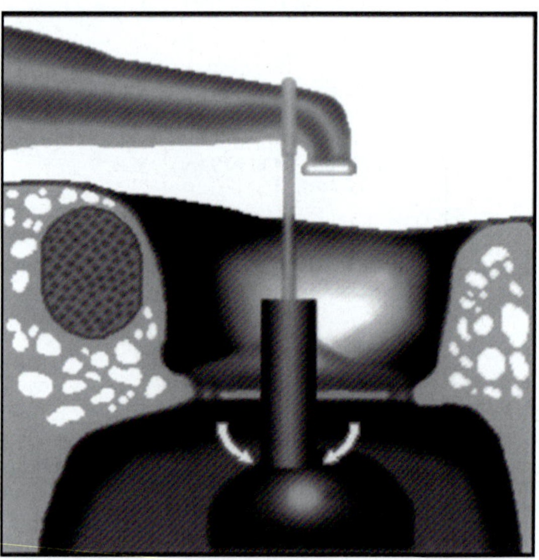

Fig. 9.2 A long stapes prosthesis may injure the saccule.

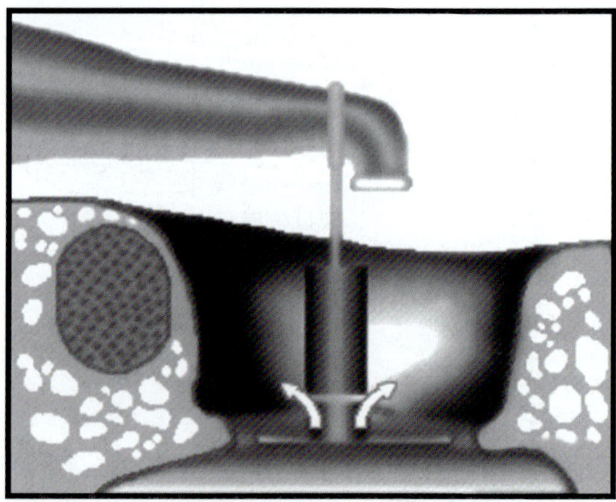

Fig. 9.3 A short piston prosthesis will not engage the stapedotomy and will result in a perilymphatic fistula (*white arrows*).

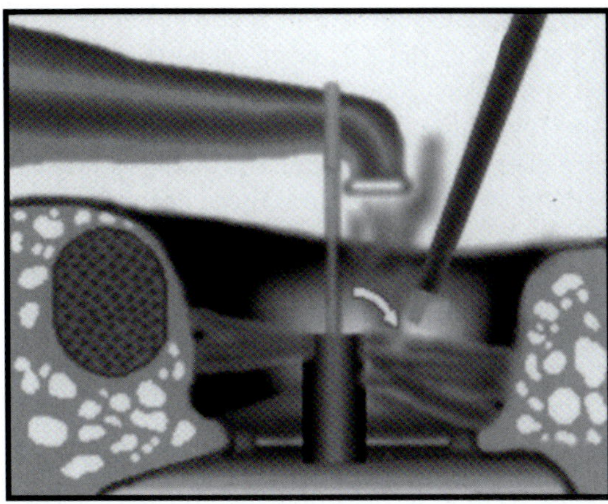

Fig. 9.4 Adhesions to the stapes piston may be vaporized with a laser to mobilize the prosthesis.

Ossicle-Related Failures

Incus Erosion and Necrosis

About one fifth of stapedectomy/stapedotomy failure is due to incus necrosis or erosion. The cause of incus necrosis may be due to one of two mechanisms. Lesinski proposed a theory of incus necrosis resulting from a prosthesis that has migrated out of the oval window (**Fig. 9.1**).[14] In this situation, the prosthesis becomes fixed against the otic capsule. The vibrating lenticular process is abraded by the immobile prosthesis crimped onto it, eventually leading to erosion and necrosis of the distal incus. Lesinski stated that the risk of complete erosion increases if there is a delay of revision following a recurrence of conductive hearing loss.[14] Incus necrosis can also result from an overtightened crimping of the stapes prosthesis, limiting the periosteal blood supply to the lenticular process and causing its ischemic necrosis.[1]

Malleus and Incus Fixation

An uncommon etiology for recurrent conductive hearing loss after an initially successful stapes operation is malleus or incus ankylosis or fixation. Ankylosis should be recognized by the primary surgeon when palpating the ossicular chain to assess its mobility and usually occurs in the epitympanum.[26] It is at least theoretically possible that ankylosis of the malleus or incus could occur after an initial surgery where these ossicles were found to be mobile. Etiologies for this acquired ankylosis include traumatic injury to the malleus or incus at the initial surgery and an intervening infection since the original surgery.[27] Both of these scenarios are probably less likely than an unrecognized fixation of the ossicles that was present prior to the first surgery.

Incus Subluxation

Traumatic iatrogenic incus subluxation or complete dislocation could occur as a result of an inadvertent injury to the incus when operating in the middle ear. It could also occur after a purposeful maneuver at the first surgery, including palpation of the incus to assess its mobility, or at the time of prosthesis crimping.

Footplate-Related Failures

Perilymphatic Fistula

A perilymphatic fistula may be suspected in patients soon after their primary operation if fluctuating vertigo, dysequilibrium, sensorineural hearing loss, aural fullness, tinnitus, or sound distortion develops. Audiograms should corroborate the clinical complaint of fluctuations in hearing. The hearing loss is usually sensorineural. Cases of immediate sensorineural hearing loss are less likely to be successfully treated.[25] In addition, patients who develop sensorineural hearing loss more than a year after stapes surgery that had used an oval window tissue seal should not be revised unless there is a history of trauma or dizziness.[15] In cases with immediate or delayed sensorineural hearing loss without an oval window seal, findings of oval window fistulas are more common. Repair with a tissue seal may result in an improvement in dizziness and occasionally an improvement in hearing.[25]

Granuloma

Postoperative granulomas were more common in the era when Gelfoam was used to seal the oval window instead of a tissue seal. When granulomas occur, they occur most often in the first 8 weeks postoperatively.[1] The symptoms are indistinguishable from a perilymphatic fistula with dysequilibrium, vertigo, and/or progressive sensorineural hearing loss. On physical examination, a red mass may be seen behind the tympanic membrane; however, the absence of this finding does not rule out the possibility of a granuloma being present. If a granuloma is suspected, high-dose steroids can minimize the inflammatory effect on the inner ear.[1] It is thought that the granuloma is a foreign body reaction to Gelfoam, glove starch, Teflon fragments, and refractile particles in irrigation solution.[26,28]

Indications for Revision Surgery

The primary indications for revision stapedectomy are to restore a previously successful conductive hearing loss closure, to close a conductive hearing loss when an initial attempt has failed, to stabilize or possibly improve a sensorineural hearing loss due to a perilymphatic fistula or granuloma, and to improve vestibular symptoms due to these same two etiologies. Patients may also complain of dysacusis, diplacusis, and tinnitus. Part of the decision regarding a patient's candidacy for revision stapes surgery is based on a review of the technique employed at the initial surgery and on the postoperative history after the primary stapes operation. An initial improvement of hearing with narrowing of the air–bone gap bodes well for a favorable result of a revision operation for a conductive hearing loss.[25] This is true for either early or late failure. Although persistent conductive hearing loss may be due to the inexperience of the primary surgeon, unsatisfactory outcomes may also result after an operation by an experienced stapes surgeon. Weber and Rinne tuning fork tests are integral in deciding if either ear should undergo revision stapes surgery in patients with profound bilateral mixed hearing loss.

Many patients with unsuccessful stapes surgery have a mix of both conductive and sensorineural hearing loss. The degree of sensorineural hearing loss is an important determinant in the decision regarding candidacy for repair of the conductive component. Attempting to repair a small conductive loss while a large sensorineural hearing loss is present is unwise, as these patients will still require aiding even if the conductive component of their hearing deficit is reduced. Also, revision surgery for minimal sensorineural hearing loss alone is not indicated. It is entirely appropriate to operate on a patient with a profound sensorineural hearing loss, if a perilymphatic fistula or a granuloma is suspected. Both of these complications are more common in patients who underwent reconstruction of the oval window without a tissue seal. Successful audiologic outcomes for surgery to address perilymphatic fistula or a granuloma, however, are rare.[25]

Decisions regarding the technique of reconstruction to be employed and if a reconstruction should be attempted or aborted must be made at surgery. For example, at the time that the middle ear is explored, revision stapedectomy should not be performed if the round window is obliterated by otosclerosis, or if the prosthesis is prolapsed entirely into the vestibule and the patient has no vestibular symptoms.

Lowering the Risk of a Second Failure

The laser provides an excellent method of dissection of the previously operated middle ear and oval window. The use of the laser allows for vaporization of soft tissue adhesions and bone without the risk of mechanical trauma. Several articles have studied the risk of laser thermal trauma to the inner ear, and debate continues as to which laser is safest for use in the oval window region.[29] Proponents of the CO_2 laser argue that the CO_2 laser power is well absorbed by the soft tissue of the oval window and that there is minimal perilymph temperature increase even when a laser pulse is inadvertently applied directly to an open vestibule. These proponents argue that visible lasers of a short wavelength, such as the potassium-titanyl-phosphate (KTP) and argon lasers, pass directly through clear perilymph. Accordingly, there is a risk of absorption of the laser energy by the saccule, found medially in the vestibule. Proponents of the CO_2 laser also argue that the KTP and argon lasers can cause a significant temperature rise that may, in turn, cause additional thermal trauma to the inner structures. Although the theoretical limitations of visible lasers have been cited, little clinical correlation of their risks has been documented in the literature.[30,31]

Visible lasers, such as the KTP-532 and argon lasers, have a distinct advantage over the CO_2 laser in that they may be used through flexible fiberoptic handheld probes that facilitate ease of use. These probes have a spot size of 100 microns (μ) and are highly precise.[29] CO_2 lasers cannot be employed by a handheld probe held several millimeters away from the target as with the visible lasers. Instead, the CO_2 laser is delivered through a microscope-mounted micromanipulator, increasing the working distance to 250 mm. Precision and accuracy may be accordingly affected.

The CO_2 laser is out of the visible range and so requires a separate helium-neon (HeNe) beam for targeting. For accuracy and safety, the two beams must be perfectly aligned, parfocal, and coaxial. This is inherently difficult in many CO_2 systems that employ a complex path of lenses and mirrors to transport the beam from its source to the target. Even in microscope-mounted lasers, the loss of alignment is of great concern and requires regular adjustments. If the two beams fall out of alignment, the otologic surgeon could be perfectly aimed on a target with the HeNe beam, while the CO_2 laser energy is delivered to a different nearby site, obviously resulting in unwanted consequences.

The smallest spot size to which the Laser Engineering (Nashville, TN) Model MD-75 CO_2 beam can focus is 300 μ.[32] The microscope-mounted CO_2 laser by IlMed (Walpole, MA) can focus to 150 μ at a focal length of 250 mm, compared with the 100 μ diameter of the KTP laser probe.[33]

Surgical Techniques for Revision Surgery

The revision otologic surgeon must identify the cause for the primary stapes surgery failure intraoperatively and determine whether it can be corrected. This determination requires surgical judgment but also the wisdom gained by an introspection of the surgeon's own capabilities and confidence in dealing with these complex and technically demanding surgical challenges.

Anesthesia

Revision stapes surgery is best performed under local anesthesia with intravenous sedation. The use of local anesthesia allows for interaction with the patient when palpating the mobility of the ossicular chain and the oval window. If dizziness, vertigo, or a sudden increase in tinnitus is encountered when the prosthesis is manipulated, the operation should be terminated. For children or when operating on adults who refuse local anesthesia, patient interaction at surgery is not possible. Although information regarding dizziness or tinnitus cannot be obtained, objective measurement of inner ear physiologic function can be gathered by brainstem auditory evoked response (BAER) audiometry while the patient is under general anesthesia.[34] Facial nerve monitoring can be used to reduce the risk of facial paralysis in stapes operations; however, there is currently no strong evidence showing a significant risk reduction.[35]

The Exploratory Tympanotomy

A speculum holder attached to the operative table can free the surgeon's hands and is often helpful. A tympanomeatal flap is raised to give access to the middle ear. The length of the flap should be adequate to cover the curettage defect in the posterosuperior aspect of the medial portion of the external auditory canal, as the curettage at the original surgery may have been overly generous. On the other hand, the revision stapes surgeon must be prepared to enlarge the curettage defect if the oval window cannot be adequately visualized. This can be accomplished with curets or a microdrill. The use of the laser in this instance is ineffective and slow.

If the chorda tympani had been preserved at the original surgery, efforts should be made to preserve and displace the nerve inferiorly. If the chorda tympani obstructs the access to the oval window despite efforts to reroute it, it may be divided. The risk of surgical trauma resulting in hearing loss and vertigo because of inadequate visualization of the oval window by an overhanging chorda tympani outweighs the clinical consequences of sharply dividing the chorda tympani nerve, a maneuver that usually results in no clinical deficits.

To improve exposure of the middle ear, adhesions that are encountered may be lysed with a laser, thereby limiting potential mechanical trauma to the conduction system.

Prior to proceeding, the round window region should be evaluated to exclude the possibility of an obliterative round window otosclerosis. This finding would make any further reconstructive surgery contraindicated.

Correction of Incus- and Malleus-Related Failures

The next operative dilemma involves the assessment of the mobility of the malleus and incus. If palpation of the incus reveals that it is subluxed or entirely dislocated, the incus and the prosthesis should be removed, and if the malleus is mobile, a repair from the malleus to the oval window can be attempted (techniques of prosthesis removal from the oval window region will be discussed later in this chapter).[27] If malleus fixation is present, it often has resulted from an ankylosis of the lateral aspect of the malleus head to the epitympanic wall.[14] This ankylosis may have been present prior to the primary surgery, or it may have developed subsequently. In this situation, the incus and prosthesis are removed, and the malleus head is separated from its long process. A portion of the malleus head should be removed so there is a gap between the residual malleus head and its long process, thereby minimizing the risk of refixation. This may be accomplished with the use of the laser. The tensor tympani attachment to the long process of the malleus should be maintained. Again, a repair from the malleus to the oval window can be attempted.[27] Depending on the type of prosthesis that is being employed, a portion of the distal long process of the malleus may need to be exposed. This can be achieved with a sharp myringotomy knife or with a laser with a small and precise spot size. With both techniques, efforts must be made to avoid creating a perforation at the site of the long process to the tympanic membrane interface. The prosthesis may need to be bent to accommodate the offset relationship between the malleus handle and the oval window.

Correction of Failures Related to the Incus-to-Prosthesis Interface

The proximal attachment of the prosthesis at the incus should be examined for looseness and for erosion or necrosis of the long process of the incus. If the proximal attachment of the prosthesis is loose, and if the distal prosthesis is in place and mobile, an attempt at recrimping the proximal attachment should be made. If there has been partial erosion of the long process of the incus, the stapes prosthesis should be removed (again, techniques of prosthesis removal from the oval window region will be discussed later in this chapter). A specially designed

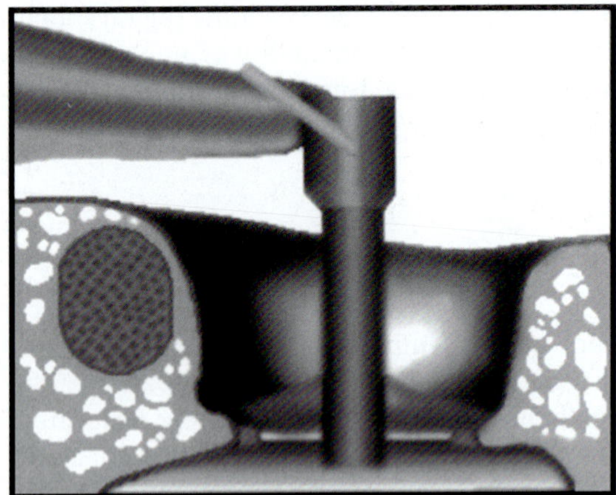

Fig. 9.5 Lippy-modified stapes prosthesis employed with distal incus erosion.

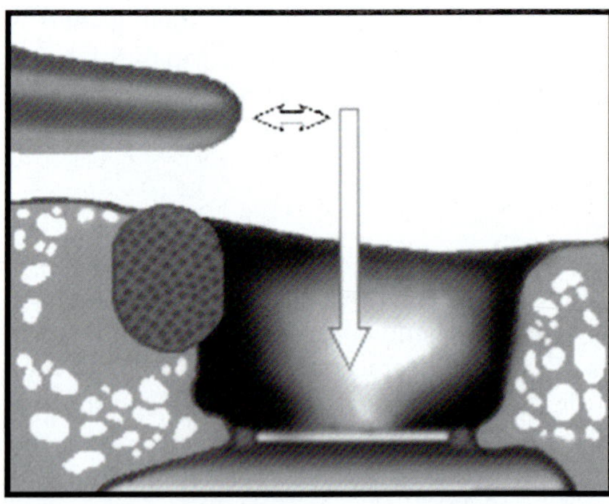

Fig. 9.6 Increased distal incus erosion or a dehiscent facial nerve may impede direct access to the oval window from the incus and require a malleus-to-oval window prosthesis.

prosthesis, such as the Lippy-modified stapes prosthesis (Model 14–2114; Smith & Nephew, Bartlett, Tennessee), should be employed (**Fig. 9.5**). If the erosion is greater, such that the posterior portion of the tympanic segment of the facial nerve impedes direct access to the oval window from the eroded long process, then the prosthesis and the residual incus should be removed (**Fig. 9.6**). The surgeon may proceed as when a mobile malleus alone is present.[27]

Correction of Failures Related to the Prosthesis-to-Oval Window Interface

The focus of revision stapes surgery is microdissection in the oval window, because it is at this time that permanent inner ear damage can occur. Direct penetration deeply

into the oval window and saccule is probably not the mode of injury in most surgeons' hands. Rather, injury probably occurs as a result of manipulation of the neomembrane or footplate. The elevated risk of manipulation in secondary stapes surgery is a result of the well-described saccular fibrosis that can occur on the medial aspect of these structures (**Fig. 9.7**).[14]

Risk may be minimized by the use of a laser, which can vaporize adhesions of a prosthesis to an oval window neomembrane, lyse adhesions around a stapedotomy piston, or vaporize portions of the bony footplate with extreme precision when used with the lowest possible effective wattage and duration. After the surgeon has used the laser to define the anatomy and pathology of the oval window region, and the distal aspect of the prosthesis has been freed by laser vaporization of adhesions of the distal prosthesis to the oval window neomembrane or retained footplate (**Fig. 9.8**), the

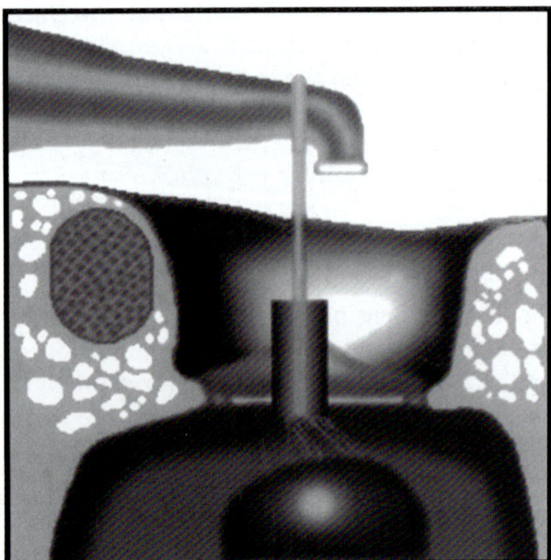

Fig. 9.7 When fibrosis from the prosthesis to the saccule occurs, removal of the prosthesis may incur injury to the saccule.

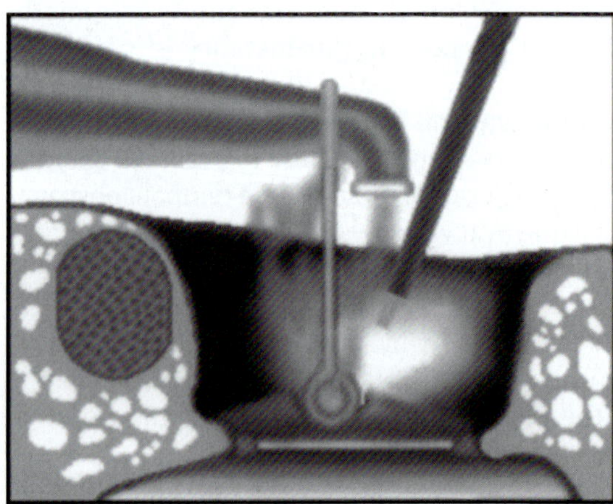

Fig. 9.8 Laser vaporization of obliterating soft tissue at the distal end of the wire loop prosthesis will allow for safe removal of the prosthesis.

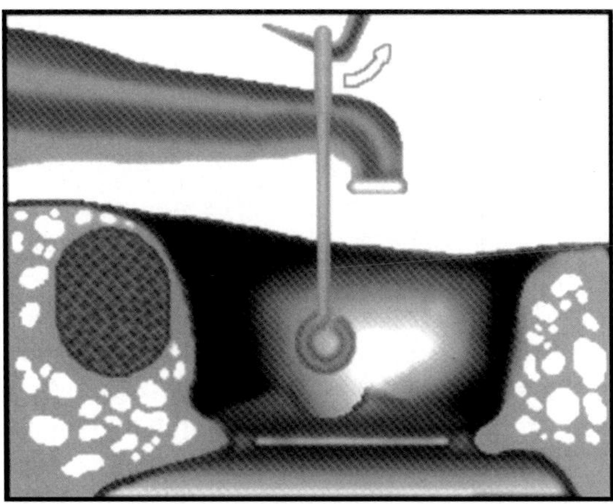

Fig. 9.9 Removal of a wire loop prosthesis.

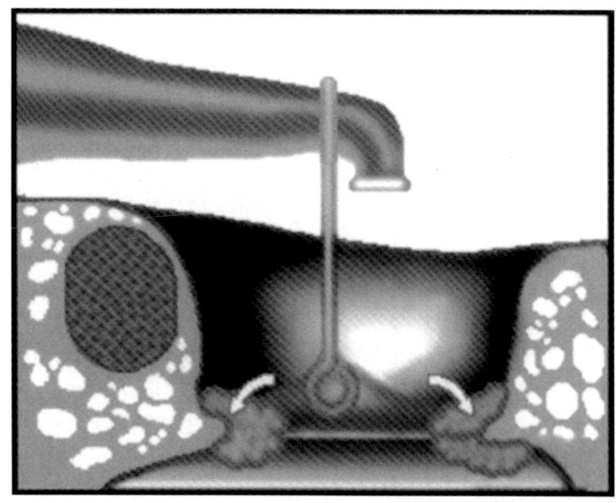

Fig. 9.10 Regrowth of otosclerosis fixing the stapes footplate.

prosthesis can be safely removed (**Fig. 9.9**). When lasers were not available, dividing the wire portion of the piston and leaving the distal portion of the piston in place was advocated to avoid manipulation of the oval window.[27] This necessitated working around the primary piston in the oval window and performing a stapedotomy or stapedectomy adjacent to it.

Gentle palpation of the prosthesis will demonstrate if it is mobile and if it is in the oval window. If the malleus and incus are in place and mobile, the stapes prosthesis to incus articulation is intact, and the stapes prosthesis is in the stapedotomy or on the neomembrane and is mobile, the surgeon should next determine if a perilymphatic fistula is present. When the characteristic clear fluid in the oval window is visible on palpation of the prosthesis, additional soft tissue graft should be placed at the fistula site and the procedure terminated. A perilymphatic fistula can also be present if the prosthesis has been displaced (**Fig. 9.1**) or when the prosthesis is too short (**Fig. 9.3**). Again, repair of the fistula is required.

Often, the location of a displaced prosthesis is obvious. If the prosthesis has migrated out of the oval window, the adhesions holding it in place should be vaporized with the laser or microdissected, and the prosthesis should be removed. Particular care should be exercised if the prosthesis has adhered to the tympanic segment of the facial nerve. Similarly, if a prosthesis is too short, its adhesions holding it in place should be lysed and the prosthesis removed. In general, unnecessary manipulation of the neomembrane or mobile footplate in the oval window should be avoided, and all other middle ear pathologies should be assessed before deciding to go forward with surgery on the footplate.[36]

If the neomembrane of the oval window is mobile, a new prosthesis can be placed directly on it. If the neomembrane is not mobile, it is possible that there is a fixed footplate beneath it. The fixed footplate could represent new otosclerosis or could represent a failure by the primary surgeon to address the original immobile footplate (**Fig. 9.10**). If an adjacent region of the neomembrane is mobile, an exploration of the footplate can be obviated, as the reconstruction can be performed at the mobile region. If an exploration is indicated, a laser on a low power setting is invaluable in vaporizing the neomembrane, thus allowing the surgeon to assess the fixation immediately beneath it. The surgeon then has the option to proceed with a revision stapedotomy or stapedectomy (**Fig. 9.11**), or the surgeon can decide to terminate the surgery at that point. If a stapedectomy is performed, a new soft tissue graft should be used to cover the oval window, and a prosthesis should be placed. If a

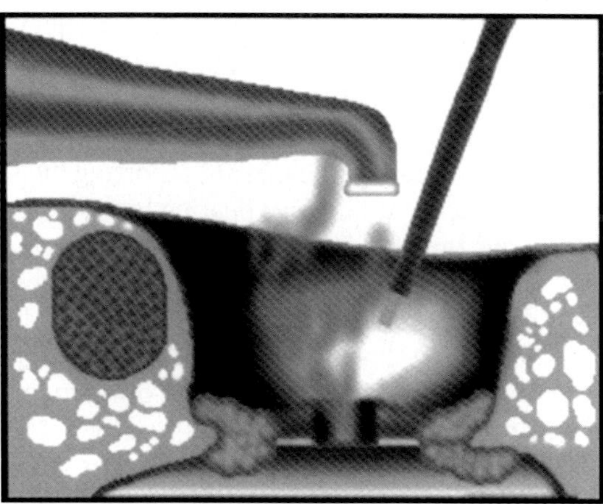

Fig. 9.11 Creation of a stapedotomy through a fixed stapes footplate with a handheld laser.

stapedotomy is performed, soft tissue or blood should be used as a seal around the stapedotomy piston. If at any time dizziness or tinnitus is reported by the patient while manipulating the oval window, the procedure should be terminated.

Because Gelfoam is rarely used any longer in the reconstruction of the footplate, foreign body granulomas of the oval window are also increasingly unusual. When encountered, the laser is a powerful tool in their management. The KTP and argon lasers have the capabilities for attaining hemostasis while vaporizing these lesions.

Once the secondary surgery on the footplate has been achieved, the tympanomeatal flap is laid back into position, and the external auditory canal can be packed with ointment, Gelfoam, or a wick sponge.

Outcomes

The choice of outcome measure becomes important to compare studies. Optimal objective measures of hearing continue to be debated.[37] The three common frequencies of 500, 1000, and 2000 Hz that traditionally have been selected for calculating pure tone averages (PTAs) correspond well to conversational speech. Guidelines were instituted in 1965 by the American Academy of Ophthalmology and Otolaryngology to standardize the reporting of hearing results for reconstruction of hearing due to chronic ear infection and to otosclerosis.[38] These guidelines required reporting data from 1 year after surgery and calculation of postoperative and preoperative air and bone conduction scores at 500, 1000, and 2000 Hz. Controversy arose when some studies used postoperative bone conduction after stapes surgery to minimize the Carhart effect, whereas others used preoperative bone conduction to evaluate success.[37,39] This lack of uniformity in reporting led to a comprehensive statistical study by Goldenberg that showed little difference in overall outcome when calculating PTAs using 3, 4, or 5 frequencies, and using either pre- or postoperative bone conduction levels to calculate air–bone gaps.[37] The American Academy of Otolaryngology–Head and Neck Surgery (AAO-HNS) in 1995 drafted guidelines for reporting hearing results in surgery for conductive hearing loss, recommending that the thresholds at 500, 1000, 2000, and 3000 Hz be averaged to calculate PTA and that air and bone conduction values determined on the same date be employed to determine the air–bone gap.[40] A minimum of 1-year follow-up before reporting was recommended. Measurements of success were further defined by a class system. Class A was defined as a postoperative air–bone gap of 0 to 10 dB at 1 year, class B as 11 to 20 dB, class C as 21 to 30 dB, and class D as an air–bone gap > 30 dB.

Most of the studies cited below were published before these guidelines, and thus used similar but not identical methods for calculating hearing results.

There is relatively little literature on revision stapes surgery. One study from the 1970s, seven studies from the 1980s, eight studies from the 1990s, and one study from 2000 have been identified that have adequate data to allow meaningful outcome analysis (**Table 9.2**).[2,3,7,12–24,41] There is a lack of uniformity in the method of revision stapes performed, the tissue employed, the hearing parameters assessed, and the length of follow-up studied. All of these factors limit the ability to accurately compare data from different studies. With that in mind, the studies whose patients had the best overall hearing do share some commonalties, such as the use of a laser and the use of stapedotomy. The two studies using this technique had 75 and 73% of their patients fall into the group with an air–bone gap of < 10 dB. In addition, there was no profound sensorineural hearing loss in either study. However, it must be noted that one study followed only 12 patients. There are inadequate data to identify an advantage of a specific prosthesis type or a type of tissue seal. It appears that laser stapedotomy for revision stapes surgery is superior to the techniques used in the other studies analyzed.

In several studies, it was shown that a progressive conductive hearing loss may develop in the frequency range 500 to 2000 dB that becomes clinically significant after 15 to 20 years.[42,43]

Complications

Patient counseling is essential when contemplating revision stapedectomy/stapedotomy, because the incidence of favorable hearing outcomes decreases with each additional revision surgery. In addition, the risks of complications in revision stapes surgery are inherently higher than in the primary stapes procedure. The incidence of significant sensorineural hearing loss > 15 dB was 0 to 20%, and the incidence of profound sensorineural hearing loss was up to 14% (**Table 9.2**). Anacusis occurs rarely (0.6%) with the first procedure, but increases to 2% in the first revision, 4% in the second revision, and 9% in the third revision.[7,44] The risk of anacusis approximately doubles with each additional revision.

About 25% of primary stapes surgery patients have transient postoperative dysgeusia, but < 5% have permanent chorda tympani nerve dysfunction.[1] Revision cases deserve special attention, because the nerve may have adhered to the posterior surface of the tympanic membrane. These risks increase with each additional revision procedure.

Table 9.2 Outcomes for Revision after Stapes Surgery

Authors	Feldman and Schuknecht, 1970 (12)	Lippy et al, 1980 (16)	Crabtree et al, 1980 (17)	Sheehy et al, 1981 (7)	Pearman and Dawes, 1982 (18)	Derlacki, 1985 (19)	Glasscock et al, 1987 (20)	Bhardwaj and Kacker, 1988 (21)	Bartels, 1990 (41)	Farrior and Sutherland, 1991 (3)	McGee et al, 1993 (22)	Langman and Lindeman, 1993 (15)	Han et al, 1997 (23)	Somers et al, 1997 (2)	Lesinski, 1997 (14)	Hammerschlag et al, 1998 (24)	De la Cruz and Fayad, 2000 (13)
Patient Nmber	154	63	35	258	74	217	79	120	12	102	185	66	74	226	200	308	356
Method	manual	manual	manual	manual	manual	manual	manual	manual	KTP	manual	CO_2/KTP/ manual	manual/CO_2	manual/ argon	manual	CO_2	manual	Argon/CO_2
Stapedectomy vs. stapedotomy	ectomy	ectomy	ectomy	ectomy	ectomy	ectomy	ectomy	ectomy	otomy	ectomy	ectomy	ectomy	ectomy	Both	otomy	ectomy	Both
Prosthesis type *	IRP, WL	HO, R	WL	IRP, TORP, WL	IRP, LP	HO, HW, LR, R	HW, TORP	HW, LP	LP	HO, HW, IRP, LP, TORP	MP, MOW	HW, IRP, LP, TORP	TP	HO,HW, LP, TP	LP, LR, MOW, TORP	TP	Piston
Oval window seal	Fat	Vein	Tissue	Tissue	Vein	Fascia	Tissue	Tissue	Vein, Blood	Fascia	Fat, Gelfoam	Fat	Gelfoam	Vein	Blood	None described	Blood, Fascia, Perichondrium
KHz used in ABG	0.5, 1, 2	0.5, 1, 2	0.5, 1, 2	0.5, 1, 2	0.5, 1, 2	0.5, 1, 2	0.5, 1, 2	0.5, 1, 2	0.5, 1, 2	0.5, 1, 2	0.5,1,2	0.5, 1, 2	0.5,1,2, 4	0.5, 1, 2	0.5, 1, 2, 3	0.5, 1, 2	0.5, 1, 2, 3
Bone conduction used for post-ABG	Pre-	Pre-	Pre-	Best	Pre-	Pre-	Pre-	Pre-	Post-	Best	Pre-	Post-	Post-	Post-	Pre-	Post-	Post-
ABG <10 dB	54%	49%	46%	44%	58%	60%	39%	33%	75%	57%	80.5%	61%	46%	40%	73%	80%	60%
ABG <20 dB	72%	54%	NR	71%	73%	72%	64%	43%	92%	83%	93.5%	84%	83%	64%	92%	85%	78%
>15 dB worse SNHL	NR	0.0%	20.0%	7.0%	0.0%	1.3%	3.0%	11.0%	0.0%	0.0%	1.3%	0.0%	4.1%	1.0%	0.0%	0.8%	7.7%
Profound SNHL	6.0%	0.0%	14.0%	3.0%	0.0%	1.3%	2.0%	2.2%	0.0%	0.0%	0.0%	0.0%	1.3%	NR	0.0%	4.9%	1.4%

Abbreviations: WL, wire loop; HW, House wire; LP, loop piston; TP, Teflon piston; R, Robinson; MP, McGee piston.

Facial palsy is also a recognized complication of stapes surgery, with the tympanic segment of the facial nerve the most often injured.[45] There are several articles that described a postoperative, delayed, temporary facial palsy.[35,46] Risks are 0.07% for facial nerve paralysis, 0.25% for inner ear, and 0.18% for tympanic membrane perforation.[44]

Conclusion

Experience and technological advances have brought revision stapes surgery into a new era marked by superior hearing results in the face of decreasing surgical risk.

References

1. Smith MFW, Roberson JB. Avoidance and management of complications. In: Brackmann DE, ed. Otologic Surgery. Philadelphia: WB Saunders; 1994:358–371.
2. Somers T, Govaerts P, De Varebeke SJ, Offeciers E. Revision stapes surgery. J Laryngol Otol 1997;111:233–239.
3. Farrior J, Sutherland A. Revision stapes surgery. Laryngoscope 1991;101:1155–1161.
4. McKenna MJ, Kristiansen AG, Haines J. Polymerase chain reaction amplification of a measles virus sequence from human temporal bone sections with active otosclerosis. Am J Otol 1996;17:827–830.
5. Shea JJ. A personal history of stapedectomy. Am J Otolaryngol 1998;19(5 Suppl):1–12.
6. Shambaugh GE Jr, Scott A. Sodium fluoride for arrest of otosclerosis. Arch Otolaryngol 1964;80:263–270.
7. Sheehy JL, Nelson RA, House HP. Revision stapedectomy: a review of 258 cases. Laryngoscope 1981;91:43–51.
8. Chandler JR, Rodriguez-Torro OE. Changing patterns of otosclerosis surgery in teaching institutions. Otolaryngol Head Neck Surg 1983;91:239–245.
9. Rosen S. Palpation of stapes for fixation: preliminary procedure to determine fenestration suitability in otosclerosis. AMA Arch Otolaryngol 1952;56:610–615.
10. Lempert J. Improvement of hearing in cases of otosclerosis: a new one stage surgical technic. Arch Otolaryngol 1938;28:42–97.
11. Shea JJ Jr. Fenestration of the oval window. Ann Otol Rhinol Laryngol 1958;67:932–951.
12. Feldman BA, Schuknecht HF. Experiences with revision stapedectomy procedures. Laryngoscope 1970;80:1281–1291.
13. De la Cruz A, Fayad JN. Revision stapedectomy. Otolaryngol Head Neck Surg 2000;123:728–732.
14. Lesinski SG. Revision stapedectomy with CO_2 laser. In: Carrasco VN, Pillsbury HC III, eds. Revision Otologic Surgery. New York: Thieme; 1997:3–21.
15. Langman AW, Lindeman RC. Revision stapedectomy. Laryngoscope 1993;103:954–958.
16. Lippy WH, Schering AG, Ziv M. Stapedectomy revision. Am J Otol 1980;2:15–21.
17. Crabtree JA, Britton BH, Powers WH. An evaluation of revision stapes surgery. Laryngoscope 1980;90:224–227.
18. Pearman K, Dawes JDK. Post-stapedectomy conductive deafness and results of revision surgery. J Laryngol Otol 1982;96:405–410.
19. Derlacki EL. Revision stapes surgery: problems with some solutions. Laryngoscope 1985;95:1047–1053.
20. Glasscock ME, McKennan KX, Levine SC. Revision stapedectomy surgery. Otolaryngol Head Neck Surg 1987;96:141–148.
21. Bhardwaj BK, Kacker SK. Revision stapes surgery. J Laryngol Otol 1988;102:20–24.
22. McGee TM, Diaz-Ordz EA, Kartush JM. The role of KTP laser in revision stapedectomy. Otolaryngol Head Neck Surg 1993;109:839–843.
23. Han WW, Incesulu A, McKenna MJ, Rauch SD, Nadol JB, Glynn RJ. Revision stapedectomy: intraoperative findings, results, and review of the literature. Laryngoscope 1997;107:1185–1192.
24. Hammerschlag PE, Fishman A, Scheer AA. A review of 308 cases of revision stapedectomy. Laryngoscope 1998;108:1794–1800.
25. Lippy WH. Special problems of otosclerosis surgery. In: Brackmann DE, ed. Otologic Surgery. Philadelphia: WB Saunders; 1994:348–355.
26. Dawes JDK, Curry AR, Rannie I. Post-stapedectomy granuloma of the oval window. J Laryngol Otol 1973;87:365–378.
27. Shea JJ. How I do primary and revision stapedectomy. Am J Otol 1994;15(1):71–73.
28. Burtner D, Goodman ML. Etiological factors in post-stapedectomy granulomas. Arch Otolaryngol 1965;100:171–173.
29. Lesinski SG, Palmer A. Lasers for otosclerosis: CO_2 vs. argon and KTP-532. Laryngoscope 1989;99(46 Suppl):1–8.
30. Gherini S, Horn KL, Causse JB, McArthur GR. Fiberoptic argon laser stapedotomy: is it safe? Am J Otol 1993;14(3):283–289.
31. Thedinger BS. Applications of the KTP laser in chronic ear surgery. Am J Otol 1990;11(2):79–84.
32. Haberkamp TJ, Harvey SA, Khafagy Y. Revision stapedectomy with and without the CO_2 laser: an analysis of results. Am J Otol 1996;17:225–229.
33. Vernick DM. A comparison of the results of KTP and CO_2 laser stapedotomy. Am J Otol 1996;17:221–224.
34. Selesnick SH, Victor JD, Tikoo RK, Eisenman DJ. Predictive value of intraoperative brainstem auditory evoked responses in surgery for conductive hearing losses. Am J Otol 1997;18(1):2–9.
35. Shea JJ. Thirty years of stapes surgery. J Laryngol Otol 1988;102:14–19.
36. Causse JB, Causse JR. Minimizing cochlear loss during and after stapedectomy. Otolaryngol Clin North Am 1982;15:813–835.
37. Goldenberg RA, Berliner KI. Reporting operative hearing results: does choice of outcome measure make a difference? Am J Otol 1995;16(2):128–135.

38. The Committee on Conservation of Hearing of the American Academy of Ophthalmology and Otolaryngology. Standard classification for surgery of chronic ear infection. Arch Otolaryngol 1964;81:204–205.

39. Berliner KI, Doyle KJ, Goldenberg RA. Reporting operative hearing results in stapes surgery: does choice of outcome measure make a difference? Am J Otol 1996;17(4):521–528.

40. Monsell EM. Draft guidelines for the evaluation of treatment of conductive hearing loss. AAO-HNS Bull 1994;13(4):14–15.

41. Bartels LJ. KTP laser stapedotomy: is it safe? Otolaryngol Head Neck Surg 1990;103:685–692.

42. Langman AW, Jackler RK, Sooy FA. Stapedectomy: long-term hearing results. Laryngoscope 1991;101:810–814.

43. Nilsson G. Long-term results after stapedectomy. Acta Otolaryngol 1977;84:260–265.

44. Shea JJ. Forty years of stapes surgery. Am J Otol 1998;19(1):52–55.

45. May M, Wiet RJ. Iatrogenic injury: prevention and management. In: May M, ed. The Facial Nerve. New York: Thieme; 1986.

46. Vernick DM. Stapedectomy results in a residency training program. Ann Otol Rhinol Laryngol 1986;95:477–479.

Decision tree for recurrent tumor after surgery

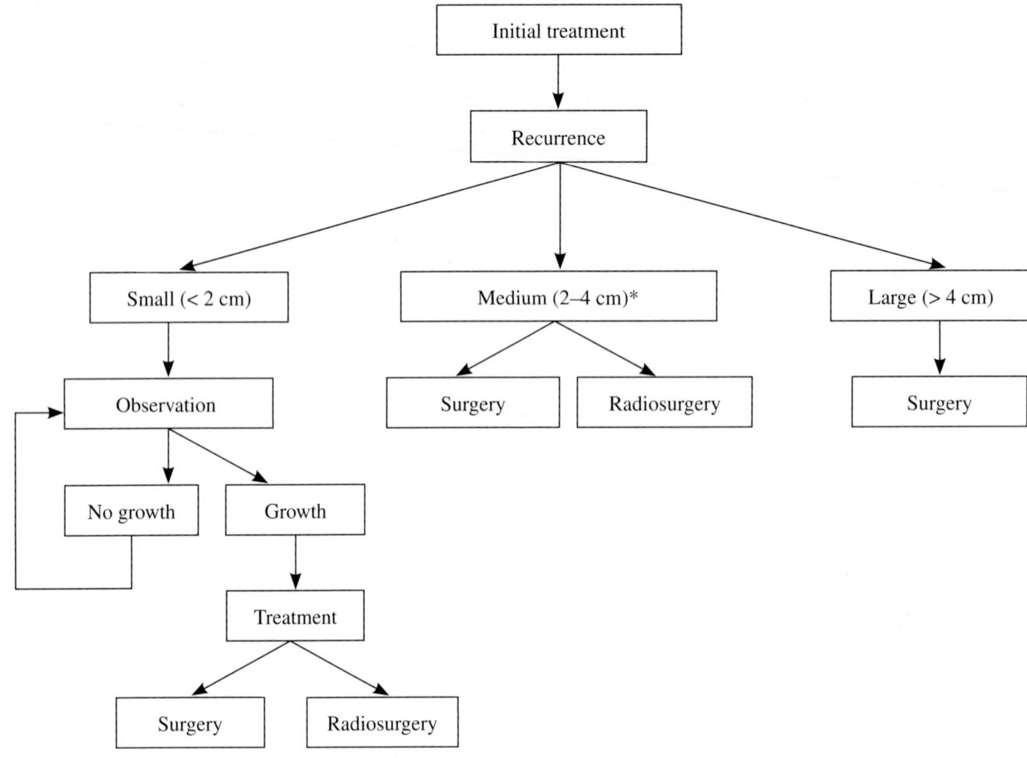

Decision tree for recurrent tumor after radiosurgery

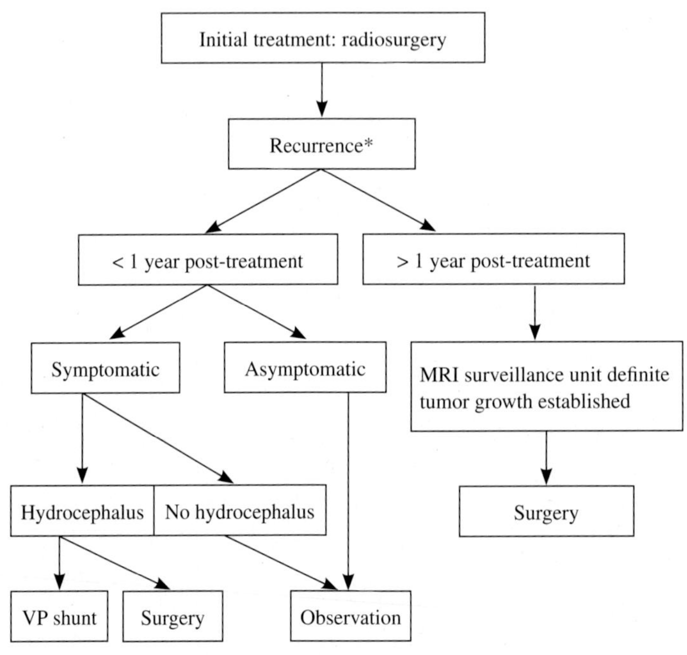

Revision Surgery for Acoustic Neuroma

Colin L. W. Driscoll and Robert K. Jackler

The goals of vestibular schwannoma (VS) treatment have differed at various times in history. In the early 1900s, Harvey Cushing recommended intracapsular enucleation with no effort made to achieve complete tumor removal.[1] Later, Walter Dandy, a former student of Cushing, proposed that complete tumor removal should be the goal.[2] After the introduction of the microscope, modern surgical techniques, and the concept of a skull base team, complete tumor removal became the objective, and virtually all tumors were operated soon after discovery. In general, the philosophy of complete tumor removal persists today but not without some important exceptions. The management of acoustic neuromas is becoming increasingly complex because of early identification (very small tumors), a better understanding of tumor growth (or lack thereof in some patients), hearing conservation operations, the concept of a near total removal, and the now widespread availability of stereotactic radiosurgery (SRS).

Recurrence of VS after apparently complete microsurgical resection with modern techniques is rare. SRS also appears to result in long-term tumor control in the majority of patients. When a recurrence is detected after microsurgical removal, or tumor progression occurs after SRS, the management paradigm is different than that for primary tumors. In this chapter, we will review the frequency of tumor recurrence after treatment by SRS and microsurgery, the causes of failure, treatment options, and surgical technique.

Microsurgery

Incidence of Recurrence after Microsurgery

The definition of *recurrent tumor* varies among studies. For some authors, only tumors that were thought to be completely resected at the primary surgery and then subsequently regrow are considered a true recurrence. Tumors that were knowingly incompletely removed (e.g., small residual in the fundus or along the facial nerve) are termed residual tumors. In this chapter, unless otherwise specified, we use the term *recurrence* broadly to include residual tumors and to describe tumor regrowth in the setting of what was thought to be complete removal. Because of the different pathophysiology, patients with neurofibromatosis type 2 (NF2) are not included by most authors in calculating recurrence rates.

The overall published recurrence rate after complete microsurgical tumor removal is quite low, 1 to 2% in most studies.[3] These studies, however, most likely underestimate the true recurrence rate for several reasons. First, there is a lack of sufficient long-term radiologic follow-up with magnetic resonance imaging (MRI) scans to exclude late or very small recurrences. Second, patients with recurrent tumors often seek care at an institution other than that providing the original surgery. Third, asymptomatic patients may not continue to return for follow-up. These patients may have radiographic evidence of recurrent or residual tumors but are without symptoms. The clinical presentation of recurrent tumors is different than that of primary tumors because the hearing that may have been present originally has most often been lost after the initial surgery. Although many tumors are discovered during routine postoperative surveillance, a significant number of patients are lost to follow-up or told they are cured after a short follow-up period. Beatty et al reported on 23 patients who underwent revision surgery for recurrent tumors; the most common symptoms at the time of reoperation were ataxia, facial paresthesias, and headaches.[4] **Figure 10.1** shows a large recurrence after a retrosigmoid resection in a patient who opted to avoid follow-up examinations or imaging for financial reasons.

Reasons for Tumor Recurrence following Microsurgery

A VS recurs either because the tumor was left unresected or because a new tumor has grown de novo. Patients with NF2 fall into this second category, and the tumor recurrence in these cases may not represent a technical failure with the primary treatment modality but may simply reflect the natural history of the disease. These patients should be considered separately. Most recurrences occur because the surgeon either chose to leave the tumor unresected (near-total or subtotal removal) or inadvertently failed to extirpate all tumor due to the inherent technical challenges of the operation.

A few general statements about recurrences can be made. First, if the surgical team is experienced and a complete gross tumor removal is achieved, the recurrence rate is very low. Second, if a tumor recurs after "complete removal," it will most likely do so in the lateral end of the

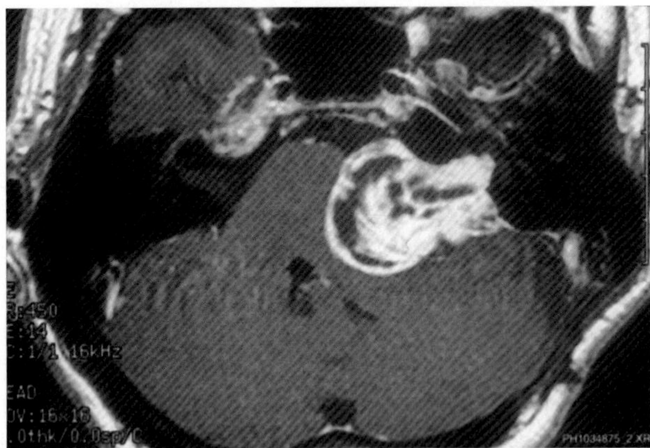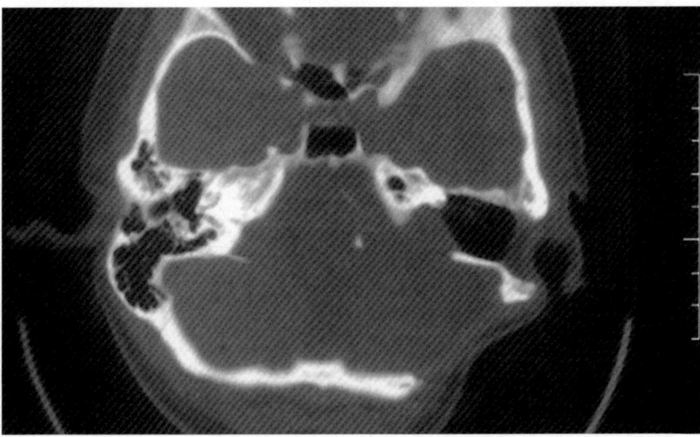

Fig. 10.1 **(A)** Axial T1 postgadolinium magnetic resonance imaging showing a large cystic recurrence approximately 10 years after "complete" removal via the retrosigmoid approach. The patient had refused any follow-up imaging after the primary surgery. She underwent a revision surgery again via the retrosigmoid approach. Subsequent postoperative imaging demonstrated another recurrence in the fundus of the internal auditory canal. **(B)** Axial computed tomography scan following resection of the second recurrence through the translabyrinthine approach. Because the tumor was restricted to the internal auditory canal, limited bone removal was needed to fully expose the tumor and achieve complete removal. Note the remaining bone along the posterior face of the petrous bone medial to the sigmoid sinus.

internal auditory canal (IAC). Third, subtotal resections often grow and require further treatment.[5,6]

The Impact of the Specific Surgical Approach on Risk of Recurrence

It appears from the literature that the recurrence rate may vary slightly depending on the surgical approach used. For surgeons familiar with all three common surgical approaches, the retrosigmoid (RS), translabyrinthine (TL), and middle fossa (MF), it is not surprising that the TL approach has the lowest apparent recurrence rate. There is little argument that this approach affords the best visualization of the lateral end of the IAC, the site of most recurrences. A large series from the House Ear Clinic (3123 patients) found a recurrence rate of 0.3%, excluding patients with NF2 and those with incomplete tumor removals.[7] The average time from the initial tumor removal to recurrence was 10 years, underscoring the importance of long-term follow-up. Although not specifically stated, it is probable many of these patients were followed radiologically with computed tomography (CT) scans. Had MRI technology been available, the elapsed time to identification of a recurrence would likely have been less. In a large series of 620 tumors removed via the RS approach, without an attempt to preserve hearing, three patients (0.5%) developed a recurrence.[8] The same authors reported a recurrence rate of 1.5% (4/260) when an attempt was made to preserve hearing through either an RS or MF approach. Many smaller studies with various follow-up ranges and inclusion criteria and surgical approaches report recurrence rates ranging from 0 to 7.5%.[3,5,8] The rate of 7.5% is in a series of 83 tumors thought to be completely removed via the MF or extended MF approach. Three of the six patients were reoperated,

and recurrences have been confirmed while the other three patients were being followed by serial imaging.

The lateral extent of the tumor is often not directly visible during the RS or MF approach. In the RS approach, the preserved overhanging bone of the otic capsule structures precludes direct visualization of the fundus of the IAC. The tumor remnants must be dissected blindly with angled instruments or with the use of an endoscope. Not surprisingly, the risk of recurrence is higher in this approach compared with the TL, where the entire distal IAC is routinely visualized.[9] If hearing preservation is not a priority during the RS approach, then the lateral end of the canal can be exposed completely, obviating the need for any blind dissection.

The MF approach provides its own unique exposure challenges. **Fig. 10.2** depicts a recurrence after the MF approach. In the MF approach, a tumor in the fundus may be obstructed from direct view by the transverse crest and by the facial nerve (**Figs. 10.3, 10.4**). Approximately 25% of the inferior wall of the IAC is not directly visible during the MF approach.[10] Awareness of this anatomy and proper instrumentation are essential to achieving complete tumor removal. Lastly, there will be occasional cases with tumor extension into the cochlea; even with the TL approach, this type of tumor may be left behind.[11,12]

In summary, all the approaches present anatomical limitations that may increase the risk of incomplete tumor removal. Because the risk of recurrence after microsurgery is overall very low, it is our opinion that this variable should not be a significant consideration in choosing a surgical approach. Other issues, such as tumor size and location, hearing status, facial nerve outcome, postoperative headache risk, and cerebrospinal fluid (CSF) leak, will have a greater impact on our choice of approach than the risk of recurrence.

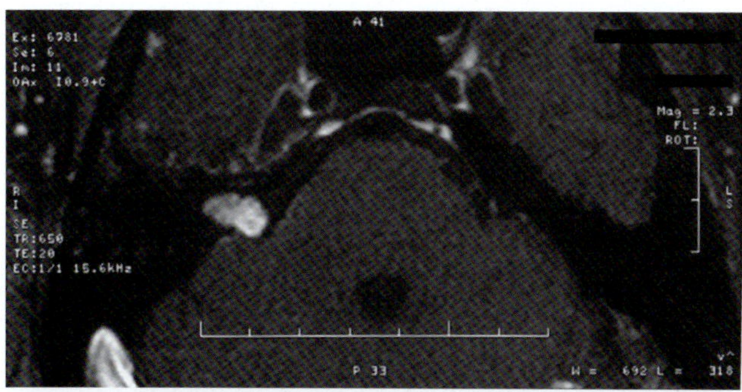

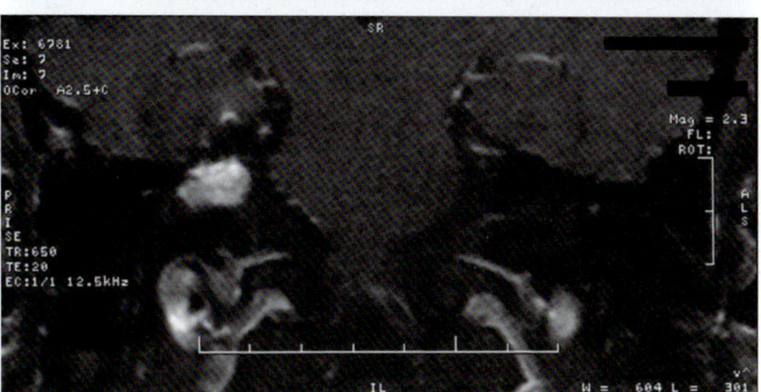

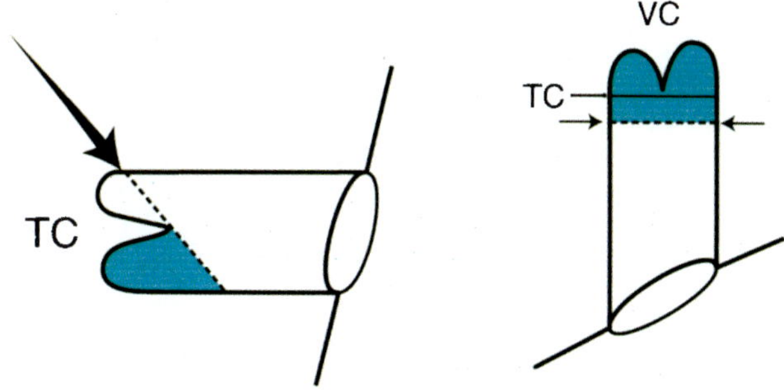

Fig. 10.3 (**A**) Arrow indicates the surgeon's angle of view to the internal auditory canal; shaded area indicates the tumor hidden from direct view by the transverse crest (TC). (**B**) View of the internal auditory canal from a superior position; shaded area represents a hidden tumor. VC, vertical crest. (From Driscoll CLW, Jackler RK, Pitts LH, Banthia V. Is the entire fundus of the internal auditory canal visible during the middle fossa approach for acoustic neuroma? Am J Otol 2000;21:382–388. Reprinted with permission.)

Fig. 10.2 (**A**) Axial and (**B**) coronal MRI scan postadolinium depicting a recurrence after the middle fossa approach. Occasionally, a muscle plug used to fill the defect after the primary surgery will enhance and be mistaken for recurrent tumor. We now use a small fat graft that can easily be distinguished from recurrent tumor using fat suppression algorithms. Serial images demonstrated tumor growth, confirming it as a true tumor recurrence.

Risk of Recurrence following Near-Total or Subtotal Tumor Removal

Increasingly, in the literature, there has been put forth the concept of a "near-total" tumor removal (**Fig. 10.5**). The idea is to leave a tiny fragment of tumor to limit the risk to cranial nerves and vascular structures. Most often this is a small remnant left on the facial nerve just proximal to the porus acusticus, where the tumor is typically most adherent. This fragment should be meticulously trimmed and coagulated with bipolar cautery, to the extent possible without injuring the facial nerve. This strategy is not a substitute for familiarity with the surgical techniques that are needed to achieve total tumor removal.

A vernacular, to help with reporting consistency, has been proposed to describe the tumor fragments that are sometimes left behind. Of course, visually quantifying residual tumor is imprecise. We suggest using the term *near-total removal* when the fragment left is < 5 mm in diameter and no more than 2 mm thick. Larger residuals should be termed subtotal removals.

The risk of developing a recurrence after a near-total tumor removal is low. In a recent series, only 1 (3%) of 33 patients who had a near-total removal developed a recurrence versus 6 (32%) of 19 who had a subtotal removal.[13] This experience is consistent with other reports summarized below.

Vanleeuwen et al reported results of subtotal removal in 73 patients of a total population of 106.[14] Of 106 patients, 23% underwent total removal, 8% near-total removal, and 69% a subtotal excision. The decision to leave tumor was made intraoperatively and was based on the perceived risk of injury to the facial nerve and surrounding structures. Follow-up revealed that 20% of the subtotally removed tumors continued to grow and required further surgical treatment. The

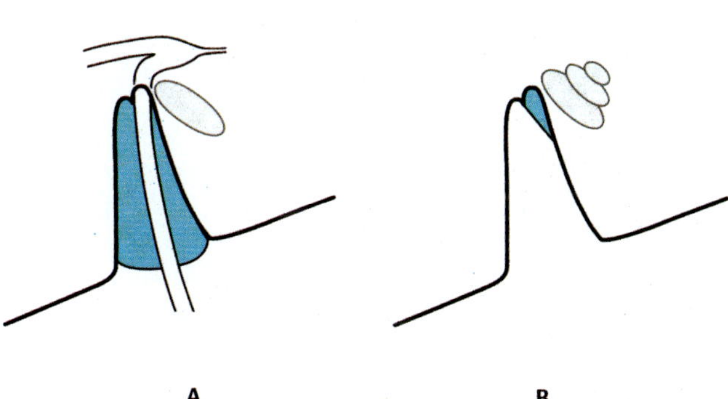

Fig. 10.4 (**A**) The facial nerve is in a relatively unfavorable location during the middle fossa approach, lying between the surgeon and the tumor (*shaded area*). However, the nerve in the midportion of the internal auditory canal can be moved from side to side to gain access to the tumor. (**B**) The shaded area is the tumor located under the immobile portion of the nerve as it exits the canal. Tumor in this location can be difficult to remove atraumatically from the overlying nerve. (From Driscoll CLW, Jackler RK, Pitts LH, Banthia V. Is the entire fundus of the internal auditory canal visible during the middle fossa approach for acoustic neuroma? Am J Otol 2000;21:382–388. Reprinted with permission.)

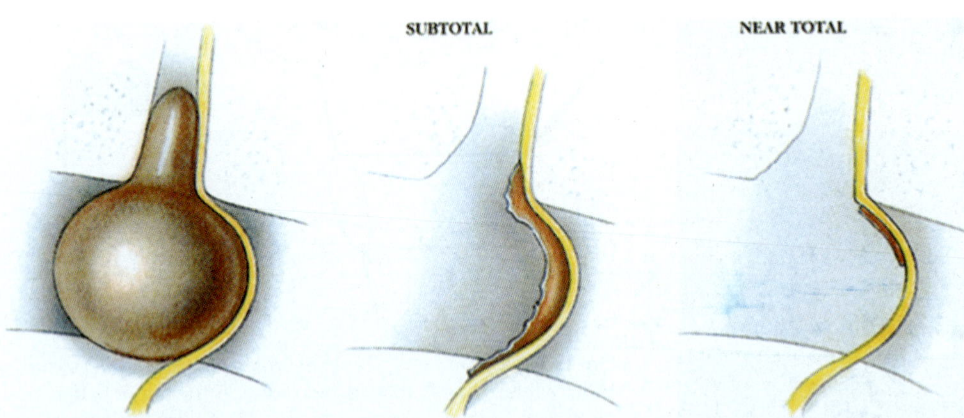

Fig. 10.5 The most difficult area of tumor removal is along the facial nerve just medial to the porus acusticus. Tumor may sometimes be left in this area as a compromise to preserve neural function. The resection is termed a near-total removal if the tumor fragment measures < 5 mm in width and 2 mm in thickness. If a larger remnant is left, then it is considered a subtotal excision. To minimize the risk of recurrence, it is important to coagulate the remnant with bipolar cautery. (From Jackler RK. Atlas of Neurotology and Skull Base Surgery. St. Louis: Mosby-Year Book; 1996:Fig. 1–24. Reprinted with permission.)

eventual complication rates in the patients requiring revision surgery were much higher than in the group of patients who underwent complete removal at the primary surgery. Subtotal resection is not recommended by this group as a viable method to achieve lower long-term morbidity.[14]

Another study that examined outcomes after near-total or subtotal resection found a very low incidence of tumor growth.[15] Out of 20 patients, 19 were followed by CT scan and 1 by MRI for a minimum of 3 years (mean = 5 years).

No tumor was visible in seven patients, despite known tumor to be present at the end of the case. Tumor regrowth occurred in only one patient, who had a subtotal removal and the highest estimated residual tumor volume of 5 to 7 cm^3. Because most of these patients are being followed with CT scans, longer follow-up is needed before definitive conclusions can be drawn. **Figure 10.6** is an example of long-term stability of a large residual tumor fragment after subtotal resection.

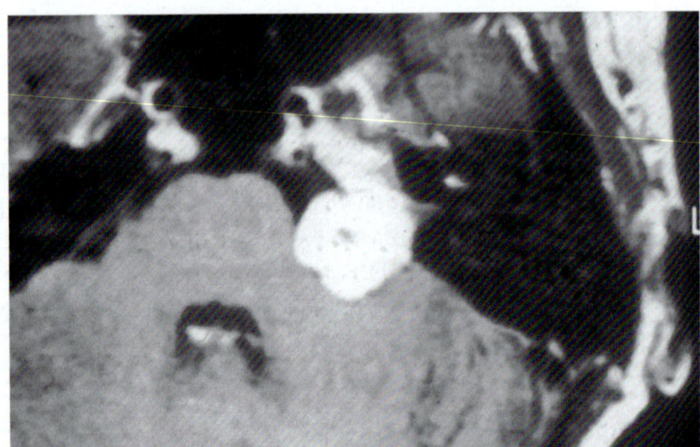

A

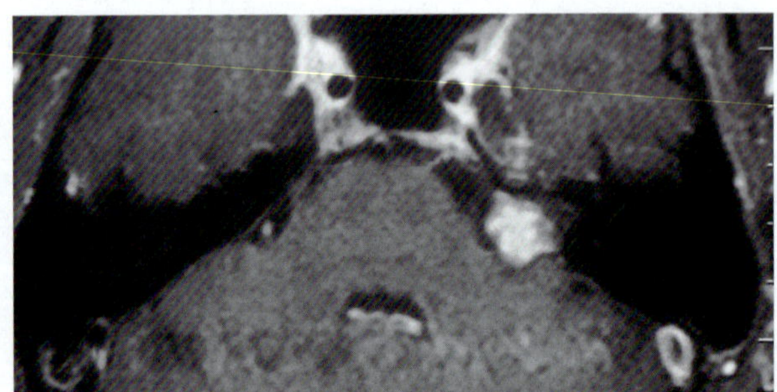

B

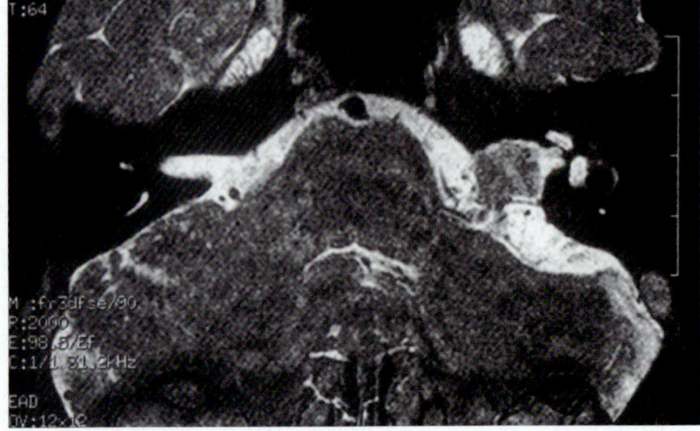

C

Fig. 10.6 **(A)** Preoperative axial postcontrast MRI showing a medium-sized acoustic neuroma. Unfortunately, this patient was congenitally deaf in the contralateral ear. She was operated at another institution via the retrosigmoid approach with the intent of performing a subtotal tumor removal. She lost most of her hearing at surgery (class D postoperatively), but the remaining hearing does help with her lip-reading ability. Her residual tumor has been followed for 12 years and has not grown despite its rather large size, as illustrated on a **(B)** T1 postcontrast MRI and **(C)** T2 image.

El-Kashlan et al reported on 39 patients who underwent incomplete resection of tumors and had a minimum follow-up of 3.5 years and a mean of 6.2 years (range 3.5–10.2 years).[16] Overall, 43.6% of incompletely removed tumors demonstrated continued growth, and 25.6% of patients required further treatment within 7 years. Eight patients had an estimated > 98% tumor removal, and none of these patients have shown tumor growth. Unfortunately, only 32 of the patients have had CT scans for postoperative imaging, and only 7 have been followed with MRI. Facial nerve morbidity was high with revision surgery.

Occasionally, tumors seem to shrink spontaneously, and there is one report of an apparent 18 mm recurrent tumor completely disappearing, at least to the extent that it was no longer visible on CT scans.[17]

Taken together, these and other reports suggest that subtotal resections are associated with high recurrence rates and that this strategy should be employed only in select cases. Some investigators argue that subtotal removal has a role in elderly patients or in cases where nerve preservation has a particularly high priority.[6,15] A strategy that has not yet been well studied is subtotal tumor removal followed by planned SRS.

Cystic Tumors and Recurrence Risk

Cystic tumors present a unique situation from a recurrence standpoint and need to be considered separately (**Fig. 10.7**). Subtotal resection of cystic tumors, in our experience, has been associated with a higher risk of recurrence with potential rapid expansion of residual cystic areas. These patients may present with acute and rapid deterioration due to brainstem compression and/or hydrocephalus. It is our opinion that cystic tumors should be totally removed at the initial operation.

Imaging Protocol after Microsurgical Tumor Removal

The majority of recurrent tumors are discovered during routine imaging after primary treatment. Post-treatment imaging protocols vary considerably and are often modified to fit the clinical circumstances. Following complete microsurgical removal, it is reasonable to obtain scans at 1, 4, and 10 years. If a near-total resection had been performed or there is concern of a remnant in the lateral end of the IAC or under the transverse crest, an MRI at 3 months is obtained to serve as a baseline study, followed by subsequent imaging at 1, 4, and 10 years. If there are concerns noted on an MRI, then interval scans could be obtained. A negative MRI scan at 10 years should be indicative of a cure. Patients should be forewarned that postoperative MRI reports will often contain phrases such as "small focus of enhancement, recurrence cannot be excluded." These are usually not representative of recurrent or residual disease, but the report can be quite unsettling for the patient. Accurate interpretation is facilitated by obtaining both pre- and postcontrast scans and by using fat suppression algorithms to help delineate graft material.

Radiosurgery

Incidence of Failure following Radiosurgery

Stereotactic radiation can be delivered using linear accelerator (linac) technology, Gamma Knife (Elekta AB Stockholm, Sweden) or Cyberknife (Accuray Inc., Sunnyvale, CA) systems. The radiation can be delivered as a single bolus or can be fractionated. No one system, or protocol, has proven to be superior to another.

The failure rate after radiosurgery with current dosing protocols is still not definitively established. Because the goal of treatment is tumor growth control, not elimination, there must be long-term follow-up to determine the efficacy of this treatment. An increasing number of patients are choosing radiosurgery as their primary treatment strategy; consequently, we are seeing an increasing number of treatment failures. As in the case of the microsurgical literature, the definition of a recurrence varies. Some may not even consider a growing tumor to be a treatment failure if it remains asymptomatic. Most radiosurgery studies quote a 93 to 97% tumor control rate, with a median follow-up typically ranging from 2 to 4 years.[18,19]

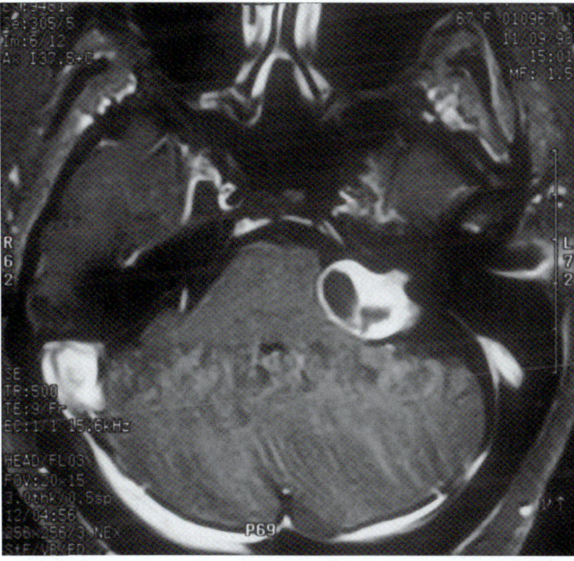

Fig. 10.7 Axial T1 postcontrast MRI showing a medium-sized cystic acoustic neuroma. In our experience, tumors with cystic components may rapidly recur after subtotal resection due to expansion of other cystic areas and should therefore be completely removed. Cystic tumors have also rapidly expanded after radiosurgery, resulting in severe brainstem compression.

Reasons for Failure following Radiosurgery

The two most common reasons for failure after radio-surgery are poor targeting and insufficient radiation dose. Because of the desire to limit radiation exposure to surrounding structures, there will be some tumor margins that receive inadequate therapy. The improved cranial nerve function with such a strategy is perceived as worth the risk of a probable increased likelihood of tumor recurrence. The same philosophy applies to the radiation dose delivered. High doses of radiation have a high likelihood of effectively controlling the tumor but carry an unacceptable complication rate. At the other extreme, a very low dose will result in no additional cranial neuropathies but will uniformly fail to control tumor growth. Proponents of radiosurgery feel that, with appropriate targeting strategies, current dosing regimens delivering ~12 to 14 Gy prescribed to the 50% isodose line at the tumor margin is sufficient to control tumor growth and has an acceptable complication profile.

It is critically important that the radiation be delivered accurately to the tumor. Failure to properly target the tumor leads to either persistent growth due to undertreatment or unnecessary radiation exposure to surrounding structures and subsequently higher complication rates. The ability to deliver the proper dose of radiation is improving with advances in MRI technology, targeting software, and the use of multiple isocenters. Despite these advances, there are still limits on how the radiation can be distributed across the tumor volume.

Cystic tumors have demonstrated a variable response to radiosurgery, with rapid expansion and pressure symptoms developing in some patients.[20,21] This may be transitory, but in some cases it requires acute surgical intervention.[22,23] In one study of 45 patients with solid tumors and 20 with cystic tumors treated with fractionated stereotactic radiosurgery, a higher rate of transient tumor enlargement was found in the cystic tumors, but this group had a better subsequent tumor size reduction rate over a mean follow-up period of 37 months (range 6–97 months).[24] Overall, the literature suggests caution should be exercised in applying radiosurgery to cystic tumors.

Imaging Routine after Radiosurgical Treatment

After radiosurgery, patients must be followed with imaging studies to assess for tumor growth and for other complications, such as hydrocephalus, or changes in the tumor consistent with malignant degeneration.[25] MRIs are commonly obtained every 6 months for 2 years, every year for 2 years, then once every other year thereafter. Until long-term data are available, the tumors should be reimaged throughout life.

Treatment Strategy for Residual and Recurrent Tumors following Failed Microsurgery

The otolaryngologist must be certain that what appears to be recurrent tumor is, in fact, just that. Postoperative enhancement may be due to several causes, including packing material (fat, fascia, muscle), cysts, scarring, traumatic neuroma, and dural inflammation.[26,27] Occasionally, surgeons operating on presumed recurrences have been surprised to find a fragment of bone wax or a muscle plug rather than tumor. Growth on serial imaging will exclude the possibility of some other etiology. If the prior surgery was done elsewhere, the operative note should be obtained for review.

The initial treatment strategy for most recurrent tumors is a period of clinical observation and serial imaging. Because most recurrences are identified on routine postoperative imaging, they are often found when they are small. Usually the only initial potential risk of the observation strategy is the loss of any residual hearing. Psychologically, the patient needs to understand that he or she may have a recurrent tumor and that it is reasonable to follow it for a period of time. For some patients, this is unacceptable. In these cases, early surgical removal is an alternative.

Once a tumor demonstrates definite growth on MRI, several treatment strategies can be considered. The treatment plan must be tailored to the specific patient. For example, a slowly growing 9 mm intracanalicular tumor in a 30-year-old woman with poor hearing may reasonably be removed by the TL approach to afford the best chance of normal facial nerve function. The same tumor in a 70-year-old diabetic male with a history of two myocardial infarctions should probably be followed radiographically or treated with SRS. One must consider the factors of tumor size, growth rate, cranial nerve function, patient age, overall health, and patient priorities, such as the importance of hearing and facial function, in planning treatment. After the patient establishes the priorities, and the tumor growth characteristics are identified, a course of action can be plotted.

Generally, SRS is considered the primary salvage therapy for a surgical failure, and surgery is recommended for SRS failures. Pollock et al reported on 76 patients who underwent SRS after failed microsurgery.[28] Tumor growth control was achieved in 94%, six patients underwent additional surgical resection a median of 32 months after SRS, and one patient had additional SRS to tumor outside the initial treatment field. Of the patients with House-Brackmann grade 1 to 3 facial nerve function before treatment, 23% developed progression of the weakness, and 14% developed new trigeminal nerve symptoms. The authors conclude that SRS should be considered in those patients who have previously undergone surgical resection(s).

Treatment Strategy for Residual and Recurrent Tumors following Failed Radiosurgery

Tumors that have failed treatment with SRS will require surgical removal unless the patient's life expectancy is short and the tumor is still small. As with failed microsurgery, it is important to establish tumor growth and not to mistake a transient swelling of the tumor due to radiation as a treatment failure. A significant number of tumors will show some enlargement during the first year.[29] This may be followed by subsequent diminution in size. Surgery at this time should be performed only if there is an impending life-threatening complication, such as severe brainstem compression.[28]

There are few reports documenting the outcome of surgical resection after radiation, but in general, the outcomes are worse than those associated with nonradiated tumors.[30,31] Although tumor removal has been reported to be similar to nonradiated VS by some surgeons, most often the arachnoid planes are obliterated and the tumor is more adherent to surrounding neural and vascular structures than in nonirradiated cases. To the best of our knowledge, there is yet to be reported a case of hearing preservation with complete tumor removal after SRS. The facial nerve outcomes are worse than what would be expected in a cohort of matched nonradiated patients.

The House Ear Clinic reported facial nerve function of 35 patients who required revision surgery for tumors ranging in size from 0.5 to 6 cm that failed after surgery or RT.[32] Before the revision surgery, 6 patients had a House-Brackmann facial nerve grade of 6, and none were grade 5. Two patients underwent an intraoperative cable graft nerve repair, and 10 more eventually had a hypoglossal-facial anastomosis. If we assume the original six patients with preoperative complete paralysis comprised part of this group, then an additional six patients developed either a grade 5 or 6 facial nerve function as the result of surgery. This rate of facial nerve dysfunction far exceeds that typically reported by this experienced team. Another group also found a markedly increased risk of facial nerve dysfunction after revision surgery, reporting permanent facial paralysis in five of eight patients.[16]

Preservation of auditory function is rarely attempted during revision surgery. If hearing preservation is a prime concern, such as in the setting of an only hearing ear, then the patient should be counseled that in an effort to maintain auditory integrity a near-total or subtotal resection might be necessary. Even then, the expectation should be that there is a high risk of losing hearing. If the cochlear nerve is preserved, the patient may be a candidate for a cochlear implant; if not, the patient could be considered for a brainstem implant.

The risks of injury to the lower cranial nerves and of CSF leak, headache, balance problems, or vascular injury do not appear to be any higher in revision surgery after failed microsurgery. This may in part be due to the fact that experienced teams perform most revision cases.

Because hearing preservation takes on a lower importance in these revision cases, either the TL or RS approach would be appropriate for removing the tumor. The choice of approach depends on the surgeon's experience, and it can be reasonably argued that either approach will allow for complete tumor removal and comparable outcomes. The TL approach offers the advantage of better access to the fundus of the IAC if the tumor extends far laterally. Also, if the facial nerve integrity is lost, access to the full course of the nerve facilitates reconstruction. Rerouting the nerve may permit a direct VII–VII anastomosis. Or, if there is not adequate nerve stump at the brainstem for reconstruction, the nerve can be mobilized for a direct facial-hypoglossal anastomosis or jump graft.

The Surgical Technique for Removal of Recurrent Tumors after Primary Treatment with Microsurgery or Radiosurgery

Tumors that have failed SRS should be removed through either the TL or RS approach based on the surgeon's preference. Unless the tumor is very large, our bias is to use the TL approach. This provides the best access to the facial nerve for the dissection. In addition, if the facial nerve continuity is lost, immediate reconstruction with direct repair, cable graft, or hypoglossal-facial anastomosis can be readily performed. The actual tumor removal is approached in the same manner as an untreated tumor. Depending on the extent of fibrosis, each step may be routine or extremely tedious and difficult.

The choice of surgical approach after prior surgery depends on tumor size, recurrence location, hearing status, previous surgical procedure, and surgeon experience. As a general principle, it is best to use an approach different than that used for the primary surgical procedure. This allows at least the initial dissection to be performed through tissues not previously operated. If the prior operation was either RS or MF, then we will use the TL approach. We recommend revising the TL with an RS, due to adhesion of the fat graft to the facial nerve in the IAC. The patient with a small tumor and good hearing who previously underwent an RS removal could be considered a candidate for revision surgery via an MF approach.

Revision surgery is often technically quite challenging due to the adhesions and scarring from the prior surgery or radiation. Even small, "routine" tumors can be deceptively difficult. The exception to this rule is when the tumor has been merely biopsied or minimally debulked and the tumor–nerve planes have not been previously dissected.

The actual tumor removal is performed in similar fashion to primary surgery. However, even the typically straightforward steps of identifying and protecting the lower cranial nerves and the anteroinferior cerebellar artery (AICA) and finding the facial nerve at the brainstem or in the lateral IAC can be arduous exercises. Intraoperative frozen section pathologic analysis of the tumor is important to confirm the tumor type and exclude the rare malignant lesion.

Translabyrinthine Approach

The TL approach begins with a curved postauricular incision initiated 1 cm above the ear and carried ~4 cm behind the ear, ending along the posterior aspect of the mastoid tip. It may be necessary to incorporate any prior incision or to modify the course somewhat to account for previous surgery. If the patient had a previous RS approach without replacement of the bone flap or a cranioplasty, then the dura or sigmoid sinus may be vulnerable during the skin incision. A full-thickness scalp, subcutaneous tissue, and periosteal flap is elevated anteriorly to the external auditory canal. Using a large cutting bur, the bone over the sigmoid sinus, mastoid, and middle fossa dura is removed. If the recurrence is small and just within the IAC, the incision and bone removal can be limited. Typically, bone is removed for 1 cm behind the sigmoid sinus, but much of this bone should have been removed at the prior surgery. **Figure 10.8** shows the usual bone removal needed for adequate exposure. **Figure 10.9** shows the dissection after a labyrinthectomy; the descending portion of the facial nerve, jugular bulb, and IAC have been identified. As the dissection is carried down to the IAC, the surgeon may encounter areas previously operated. Because the dura may be absent in some areas, it is important to stimulate for the facial nerve frequently and proceed cautiously. Also, because the patient has had prior surgery, the facial nerve may be displaced by tumor into an unusual location. Once all the bone work has been completed, the dura is opened. If possible, this is done away from the site where either the facial nerve stimulates or where the surgeon anticipates finding the facial nerve. Early release of CSF from the cisterna magna will facilitate the exposure. **Figure 10.10** shows the dural flaps

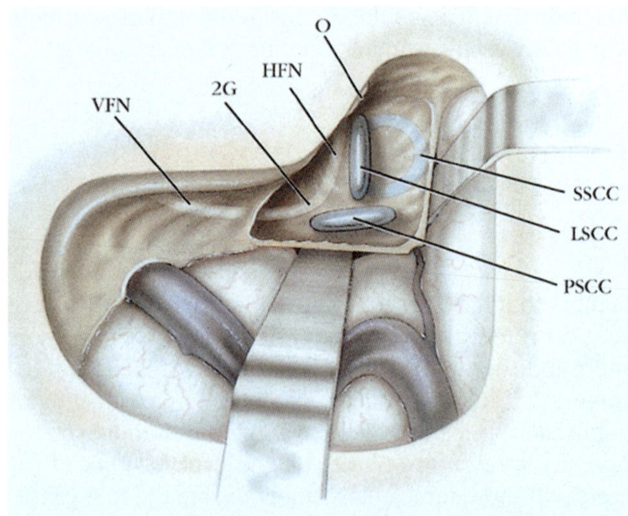

Fig. 10.8 Translabyrinthine approach. The retractors protect the sigmoid sinus and dural surfaces in addition to expanding the view. HFN, horizontal facial nerve; O, ossicles; SSC, superior, lateral, and posterior semicircular canals; 2G, second genu; VFN, vertical segment of the facial nerve. (From Jackler RK. Atlas of Neurotology and Skull Base Surgery. St. Louis: Mosby-Year Book; 1996:Fig. 2–7. Reprinted with permission.)

opened to expose a typical medium-sized tumor. A flexible tip nerve stimulator probe is helpful for locating the facial nerve because it can be used to stimulate atraumatically around structures obstructing direct vision. Tumor removal begins by incising the capsule and debulking the

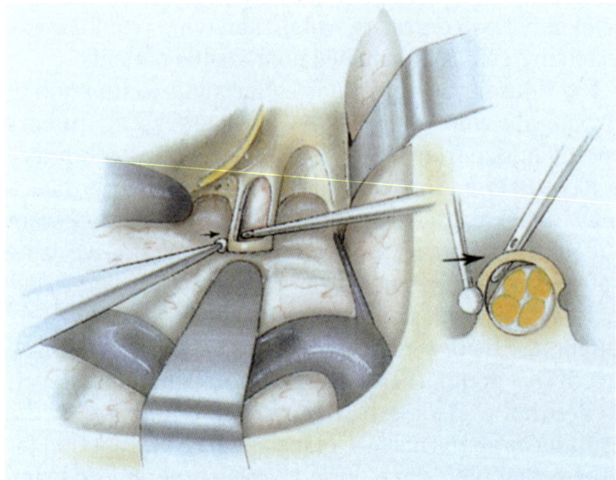

Fig. 10.9 After the labyrinthectomy is completed, the internal auditory canal is skeletonized, and deep troughs are created superiorly and inferiorly. Laterally, the transverse crest should be identified. Some surgeons also like to identify Bill's bar, separating the facial nerve from the superior vestibular nerve. If a retrosigmoid approach had been used previously, then much of the bone around the lateral part of the canal will still be present. Removal of this bone will allow for exposure of the nerve in a region that has not been previously dissected. (From Jackler RK. Atlas of Neurotology and Skull Base Surgery. St. Louis: Mosby-Year Book; 1996:Fig. 2–19. Reprinted with permission.)

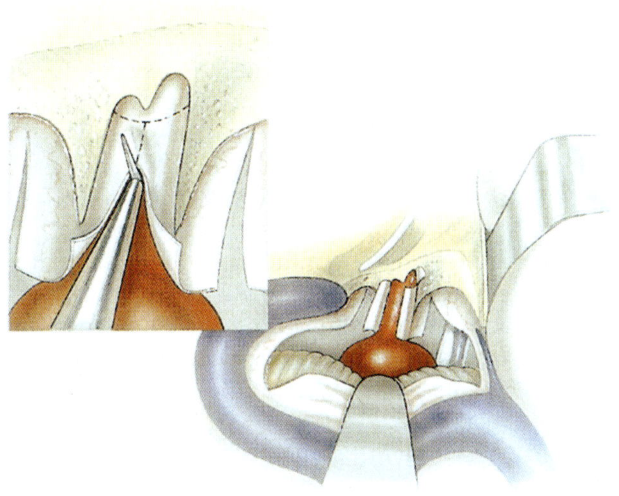

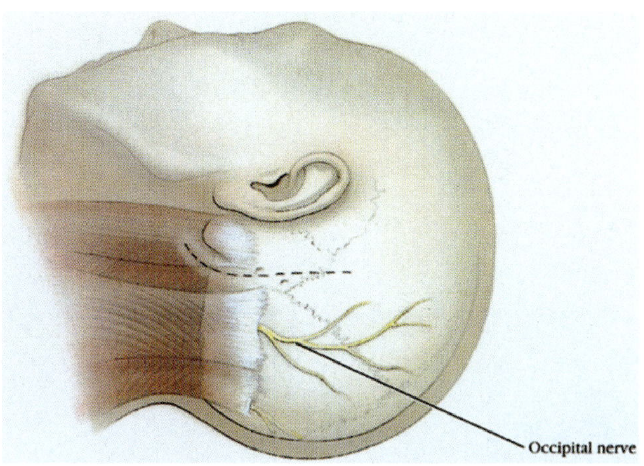

Fig. 10.11 The incision for the retrosigmoid approach is typically J-shaped to minimize trauma to the nuchal musculature and the occipital nerve. Prior surgeries may require that the incision be modified. If there is a prior postauricular incision, then the incision should be moved more posteriorly and oriented vertically to allow for good vascularization of the flaps. It should be kept in mind that the blood supply to this area arises primarily from posteriorly and inferiorly. If not previously sacrificed, the occipital artery should be preserved. (From Jackler RK. Atlas of Neurotology and Skull Base Surgery. St. Louis: Mosby-Year Book; 1996:Fig. 4–5. Reprinted with permission.)

Fig. 10.10 Following bone removal, the nerve stimulator is used to identify the location of the facial nerve. The facial and other cranial nerves may be in very unusual locations, depending on where the recurrence developed. Cranial nerve monitoring is extremely helpful. The dura is incised away from the facial nerve, and flaps are elevated to expose the tumor. Sharp dissection may be needed to develop surgical planes due to scarring from prior surgery or radiation. The tumor–brainstem interface may be ill defined; care must be taken to avoid developing a subpial dissection and brainstem injury. (From Jackler RK. Atlas of Neurotology and Skull Base Surgery. St. Louis: Mosby-Year Book; 1996:Fig. 2–27. Reprinted with permission.)

internal portion of the tumor with a cavitronic ultrasonic surgical aspirator (Valleylab, Boulder, Colorado). The suction level is typically set at 50%, and care is taken not to penetrate the capsule. Once debulked, the capsule can be folded inward and resected. The tumor is removed with the goal of identifying the facial nerve in the lateral end of the IAC and also at the brainstem. It is usually easiest to approach the root entry zone of the facial nerve inferiorly after first identifying and protecting the lower cranial nerves. Tumor removal is mainly done from a medial to lateral direction. If the facial nerve becomes neuropraxic from early dissection in the IAC, it can be extremely difficult to identify the nerve at the brainstem. Once the lower pole of the tumor has been removed and the facial nerve at the brainstem identified, the trigeminal nerve is identified, and the superior part of the tumor is removed. The last portion of tumor to remove, and the most difficult part, is usually the disease just medial to the porus acusticus. In tumors where there is extensive fibrosis, an alternative surgical technique can be employed. Rather than identifying all of the important neurovascular structures, the tumor is meticulously dissected from the thickened arachnoid. No attempt is made to clearly identify the facial nerve, but rather all nontumor tissue is preserved.

After the tumor has been removed, the closure is the same as for a primary case. Fascia is placed over the antrum and facial recess air cells, strips of abdominal fat are layered into the defect, and the wound is closed in layers to create a watertight seal. A mastoid dressing is placed to compress the fat graft and is left on for 3 days.

Retrosigmoid Approach

The RS approach usually begins with a J-shaped incision (**Fig. 10.11**). This incision avoids the occipital nerve, and by curving anteriorly, the surgeon can dissect off the nuchal musculature from the bone rather than transect these muscles, thus minimizing trauma and postoperative pain. The incision may need to be modified depending on the prior procedures. Although the scalp is quite vascular and generally forgiving regarding incision location, the primary blood supply to the area is from posteriorly and inferiorly. This blood supply should be preserved when possible. If the patient has previously had a TL approach, then the sigmoid sinus and dura may again be vulnerable during the incision. Regardless of prior treatments, the bone is removed inferior to the transverse sinus and posterior to the sigmoid sinus. The dura is then opened, the CSF released from the cisterna magna, the cerebellum retracted, and the lateral aspect of the tumor exposed (**Fig. 10.12**). Again, vigilance should be maintained when dissecting in the region of the facial nerve. Frequent stimulation with the nerve stimulator is helpful in a scarred field with few initial landmarks. The

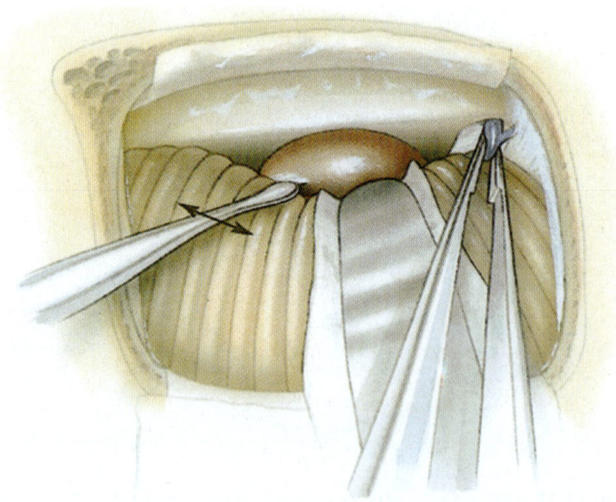

Fig. 10.12 After the craniotomy is completed, cerebrospinal fluid is released, and the cerebellum is retracted to expose the tumor surface. In larger tumors, the superior cerebellar (Dandy's) vein can be coagulated and divided to allow for better retraction of the cerebellum. There is a small risk of venous infarction; therefore, routine division is discouraged. If the patient previously had a translabyrinthine approach, then the plane between the cerebellum and fat graft may be difficult to dissect. It is often helpful to explore superiorly and inferiorly in this situation. (From Jackler RK. Atlas of Neurotology and Skull Base Surgery. St. Louis: Mosby-Year Book; 1996:Fig. 4–13. Reprinted with permission.)

intracranial portion of the tumor is removed, and then the IAC is opened as necessary (**Fig. 10.13**). If a TL approach has been performed previously, it may be difficult to dissect the tissue in the IAC. The facial nerve can be adherent to the fat graft. In some cases, it is best to meticulously remove the tumor, leaving all other tissue, in place rather than trying to identify the facial nerve specifically. If drilling of the IAC needs to be performed, Gelfoam should be placed in the posterior fossa to prevent dissemination of bone dust. Because hearing preservation is very rarely attempted in revision surgery, the bone removal over the IAC does not need to be limited by a concern for entering the labyrinth. It is more important to obtain adequate distal IAC exposure for tumor removal and facial nerve identification. After tumor removal, potential routes of CSF egress in the temporal bone are occluded with bone wax, fibrin glue, fascia, or free tissue grafts, as preferred. The dura is reapproximated and the bone flap replaced, or cranioplasty is performed.

Conclusion

The treatment of VS is becoming increasingly complex. Although the vast majority of tumors are successfully managed with primary SRS or microsurgery, some failures do occur. Treatment of recurrent tumors, or treatment failures, requires a different algorithm. In general, tumors that have failed primary SRS are treated with microsurgery, and those that have failed microsurgery are treated with SRS. Although these additional treatments carry a higher risk, most patients still have successful outcomes.

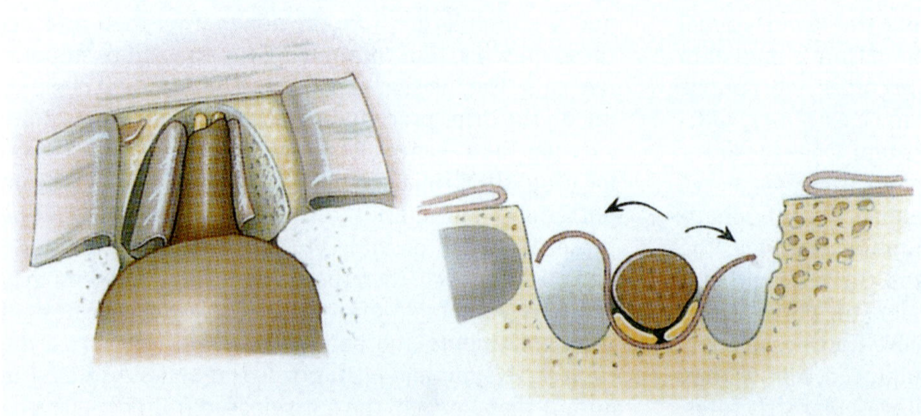

Fig. 10.13 Depending on the tumor location and prior surgery it may, or may not, be necessary to remove the posterior lip of the petrous bone to expose the internal auditory canal (IAC). If bone removal is needed, Gelfoam should be placed in the cerebellopontine angle to prevent the spread of bone dust into the posterior fossa. Bone should be removed widely around the IAC. This facilitates the use of angled instruments to develop the plane between the facial nerve and the tumor. Following tumor removal, closure proceeds in the same fashion as a primary case. (From Jackler RK. Atlas of Neurotology and Skull Base Surgery. St. Louis: Mosby-Year Book; 1996:Fig. 4–17. Reprinted with permission.)

References

1. Cushing H. Tumors of the Nervus Acusticus and the Syndrome of the Cerebello-pontile Angle. Philadelphia: WB Saunders; 1917.
2. Dandy WE. Exhibition of cases. Johns Hopkins Medical Bull 1917;28:96.
3. Harner SG, Beatty CW, Ebersold MJ. Retrosigmoid removal of acoustic neuroma: experience 1978–1988. Otolaryngol Head Neck Surg 1990;103(1):40–45.
4. Beatty CW, Ebersold MJ, Harner SG. Residual and recurrent acoustic neuromas. Laryngoscope 1987;97:1168–1171.
5. Charabi S, Tos M, Thomsen J, Borgesen SE. Suboccipital acoustic neuroma surgery: results of decentralized neurosurgical tumor removal in Denmark. Acta Otolaryngol 1992;112(5):810–815.
6. Lownie SP, Drake CG. Radical intracapsular removal of acoustic neuromas. J Neurosurg 1991;74(3):422–425.
7. Shelton C. Unilateral acoustic tumors: how often do they recur after translabyrinthine removal? Laryngoscope 1995;105(9 pt 1):958–966.
8. Samii M, Matthies C. Management of 1000 vestibular schwannomas (acoustic neuromas): hearing function in 1000 tumor resections. Neurosurgery 1997;40(2):248–260.
9. Haberkamp TJ, Meyer GA, Fox M. Surgical exposure of the fundus of the internal auditory canal: anatomic limits of the middle fossa versus retrosigmoid transcanal approach. Laryngoscope 1998;108(8 pt 1):1190–1194.
10. Driscoll CLW, Jackler RK, Pitts LH, Banthia V. Is the entire fundus of the internal auditory canal visible during the middle fossa approach for acoustic neuroma? Am J Otol 2000;21:382–388.
11. Green JD, McKenzie JD. Diagnosis and management of intralabyrinthine schwannomas. Laryngoscope 1999;109(10):1626–1631.
12. Green JD, Beatty CW, Czervionke LF, Reimer R, Benecke JE. Intracochlear vestibular schwannoma: a potential source for recurrence after translabyrinthine resection. Otolaryngol Head Neck Surg 2000;123:281–282.
13. Bloch DC, Oghalai JS, Jackler RK, Osofsky M, Pitts LH. The fate of the tumor remnant after less-than-complete acoustic neuroma resection. Otolaryngol Head Neck Surg 2004;130(1):104–112.
14. Vanleeuwen JPPM, Meijer E, Grotenhuis JA, Thijssen HOM, Cremers CWRJ. Suboccipital surgery for acoustic neuroma. Clin Otolaryngol Allied Sci 1996;21(3):244–251.
15. Kemink JL, Langman AW, Niparko JK, Graham MD. Operative management of acoustic neuromas: the priority of neurologic function over complete resection. Otolaryngol Head Neck Surg 1991;104(1):96–99.
16. El-Kashlan HK, Zeitoun H, Arts HA, Hoff JT, Telian SA. Recurrence of acoustic neuroma after incomplete resection. Am J Otol 2000;21:389–392.
17. Redleaf MI, McCabe BF. Disappearing recurrent acoustic neuroma in an elderly woman. Ann Otol Rhinol Laryngol 1993;102(7):518–520.
18. Flickinger JC, Kondziolka D, Niranjan A, Lunsford LD. Results of acoustic neuroma radiosurgery: an analysis of 5 years' experience using current methods. J Neurosurg 2001;94(1):1–6.
19. Hasegawa T, Kida Y, Yoshimoto M, Koike J, Goto K. Evaluation of tumor expansion after stereotactic radiosurgery in patients harboring vestibular schwannomas. Neurosurgery 2006;58(6):1119–1128.
20. Bertalanffy A, Aichholzer M, Reinprecht A, et al. An intramural macrocyst of an acoustic neurinoma rupturing after gamma knife radiosurgey: a case report. Minim Invasive Neurosurg 2001;44(2):110–113.
21. Gormley WB, Sekhar LN, Wright DC, Damerer D, Schessel D. Acoustic neuromas: results of current surgical management. Neurosurgery 1997;41(1):50–58, discussion 58–60.
22. Pendl G, Ganz JC, Kitz K, Eustacchio S. Acoustic neurinomas with macrocysts treated with gamma knife radiosurgery. Stereotact Funct Neurosurg 1996;66(1 Suppl):103–111.
23. Unger F, Walch C, Haselsberger K, et al. Radiosurgery of vestibular schwannomas: a minimally invasive alternative to microsurgery. Acta Neurochir (Wien) 1999;141(12):1281–1285, discussion 1285–1286.
24. Shirato H, Sakamoto T, Takeichi N, et al. Fractionated stereotactic radiotherapy for vestibular schwannoma (VS): comparison between cystic-type and solid-type VS. Int J Radiat Oncol Biol Phys 2000;48(5):1395–1401.
25. Shamisa A, Bance M, Nag S, et al. Glioblastoma multiforme occurring in a patient treated with gamma knife surgery: case report and review of the literature. J Neurosurg 2001;94(5):816–821.
26. Mueller DP, Gantz BJ, Dolan KD. Gadolinium-enhanced MR of the postoperative internal auditory canal following acoustic neuroma resection via the middle fossa approach. AJNR Am J Neuroradiol 1992;13(1):197–200.
27. Spiegelmann R, Lidar Z, Gofman J, Alezra D, Hadani M, Pfeffer R. Linear accelerator radiosurgery for vestibular schwannoma. J Neurosurg 2001;94(1):7–13.
28. Pollock BE, Lunsford LD, Flickinger JC, Clyde BL, Kondzioka D. Vestibular schwannoma management, I: Failed microradiosurgery and the role of delayed stereotactic radiosurgery. J Neurosurg 1998;89(6):944–948.
29. Limb CJ, Long DM, Niparko JK. Acoustic neuromas after failed radiation therapy: challenges of surgical salvage. Laryngoscope 2005;115(1):93–98.
30. Battista RA, Wiet RJ. Stereotactic radiosurgery for acoustic neuromas: a survey of the American Neurotology Society. Am J Otol 2000;21(3):371–381.
31. Roberson JB Jr, Brackmann DE, Hitselberger WE. Acoustic neuroma recurrence after suboccipital resection: management with translabyrinthine resection. Am J Otol 1996;17(2):307–311.

Decision tree for management of a symptomatic patient after a prior endolymphatic sac surgery

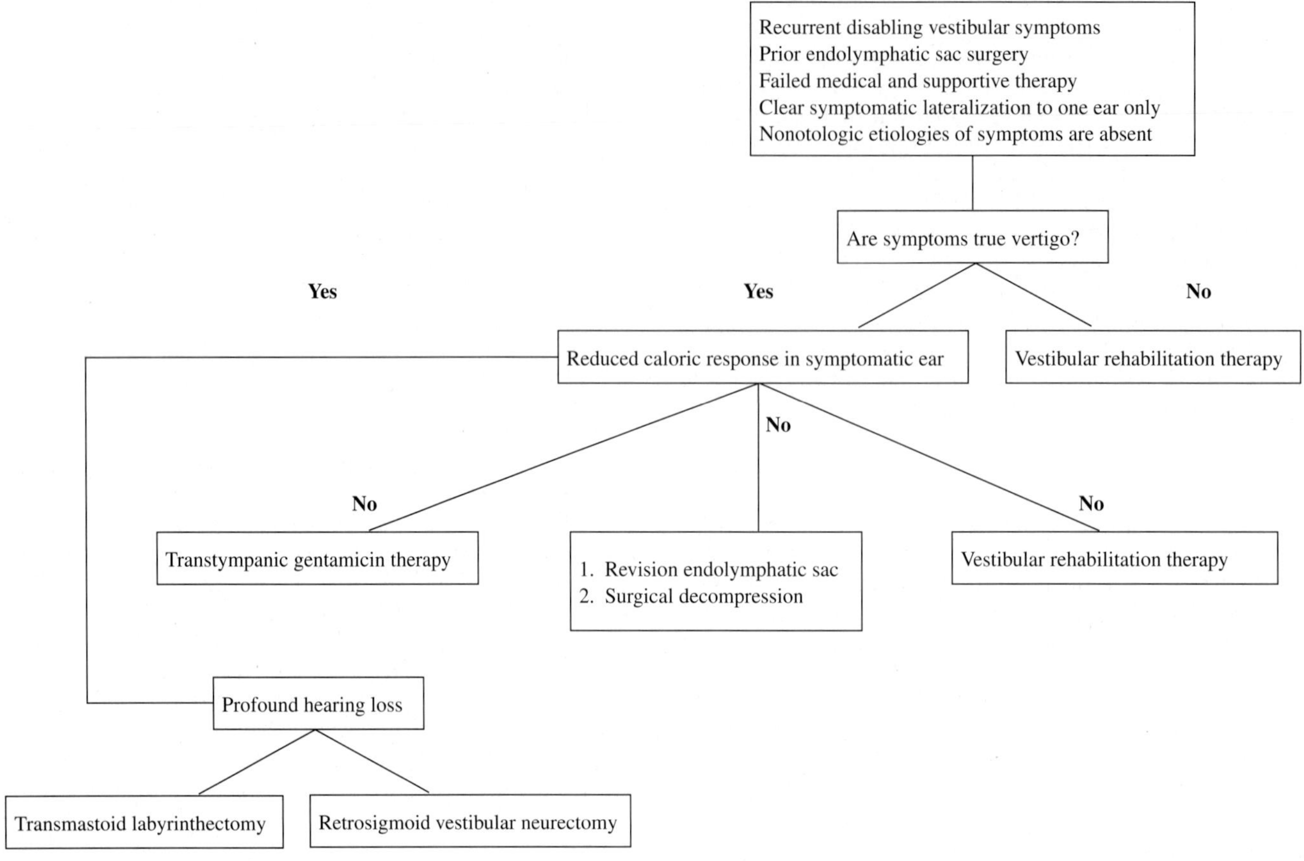

Revision Vestibular Surgery

Edwin M. Monsell

Vertigo and imbalance occasionally are symptoms of disease processes that can threaten a patient's health, such as acoustic neuroma, multiple sclerosis, and stroke. Once such conditions have been excluded, the goal in the management of vestibular disorders is to make patients as functional and comfortable as possible. Usually patients can be managed with counseling, vestibular exercises, and vestibular suppressant medications. Episodic vertigo will often abate. Infrequently, patients may become disabled enough by their symptoms to justify surgical treatment. Surgical treatments offer the best chance for controlling spells of vertigo due to otologic diseases. When properly selected and performed, surgical treatments are usually successful. Complications are uncommon; however, surgical treatments are not always successful and may even cause other problems for the patient. Adverse effects include dysequilibrium, motion intolerance, and hearing loss. Other complications include cerebrospinal fluid (CSF) leakage, facial palsy, and conductive hearing loss.

When the frequency and severity of episodic vertigo due to Meniere disease become disabling despite nonoperative measures, surgical treatments come into consideration (**Table 11.1**). Two things must be true before a person is a surgical candidate. First, the problem must be correctable by surgery. Second, the benefits must outweigh the risks. When patients are properly selected and counseled, and when the operation is properly performed, the surgeon has provided the best possible level of care. The results of some procedures, such as labyrinthectomy and selective vestibular nerve section, are predictable. The results of other procedures, such as endolymphatic sac operations and aminoglycoside treatments, are less predictable, though these procedures have other advantages.

Any procedure may fail to control vestibular symptoms. Determining what to do next may be the greatest of all clinical challenges to the otologist. This situation requires a thorough knowledge of vestibular physiology, pathophysiology, clinical assessment, psychological assessment, pharmacotherapy, counseling, and surgical technique. This chapter is an overview of some of the critical issues in revision vestibular surgery.

Meniere Disease

Definition and Clinical Features of Meniere Disease

Meniere disease is one of the most common vestibular disorders, and the one that most commonly results in the need for surgery. Meniere disease is defined as endolymphatic hydrops with the clinical manifestations of Meniere syndrome.[1] Meniere syndrome consists of recurrent, spontaneous vertigo, hearing loss, and tinnitus and/or aural fullness as defined by the Committee on Hearing and Equilibrium of the American Academy of Otolaryngology–Head and Neck Surgery (AAO-HNS).[1] Definitive spells of vertigo in Meniere disease are rotational and last 20 minutes or longer. They are by definition accompanied by imbalance. Nausea and vomiting are common. Hearing loss is present in the ear with active disease.[1] Early in the course of the disease, hearing levels often fluctuate, especially in the low frequencies. The hearing loss tends to progress to threshold levels of 40 to 70 dB hearing level (HL); speech discrimination scores commonly fall to levels of 70 to 50%. Hearing usually does not worsen beyond these levels in Meniere disease.[2] Tinnitus in Meniere disease is typically described as a buzzing or roaring sound. The

Table 11.1 Indications for Surgery or Intratympanic Gentamicin in Meniere Disease

The ear with active disease can be identified.
It is a unilateral disease.
There has been a failure of medical management.
As a result of the disease, the patient experiences disability affecting normal activities.
Disability is due to definitive spells of vertigo, typically a definitive attack once or more per month.
The patient is an acceptable risk for the proposed treatment and is able to give informed consent.

patient usually experiences a sense of fullness or pressure in the affected ear.

In addition to these defining features of Meniere disease, patients may experience less typical symptoms, such as milder or shorter spells of vertigo. A more or less constant sense of dysequilibrium may occur after several years with the disease. In most of these cases, there is evidence of some permanent loss of vestibular function in the form of a reduced caloric response on the affected side, or testing of the vestibulo-ocular reflex may show abnormality in phase, gain, or asymmetry. Otolithic crises of Tumarkin ("drop" attacks) occur rarely. In these episodes, there is an apparent sudden collapse of vestibulospinal tone without loss of consciousness.[3]

The full clinical syndrome of classic Meniere disease is nearly always unilateral. It is not unusual for a patient to experience an occasional sense of fullness or tinnitus in the opposite ear without developing the full clinical syndrome. (See discussion of autoimmune inner ear disease, below.)

Disability in Meniere Disease

Spontaneous vertigo can become disabling when it occurs with such frequency and severity that the patient cannot work, drive, take care of a family, or make plans for travel. In general, disability occurs when definitive spells occur about once a month or more, especially if accompanied by nausea and vomiting. Such a person is locked into a state of constantly suffering through an episode, recovery from an episode, or anticipation of the next episode.

Disability can also result from sensations of imbalance and motion intolerance if they are constant and severe enough. Presumably, these symptoms arise from the damaged vestibular system and its interactions with vision, perception of space and movement, proprioception, and the autonomic nervous system. Malfunction of the vestibular system is associated with feelings of malaise, nausea, vomiting, headaches, and anxiety. In most cases, it is more appropriate to treat constant dysequilibrium by patient education, anxiolytic medication, and vestibular exercises than by surgery.

Treatment of Meniere Disease

Currently, there is no treatment that is acknowledged to reverse the natural history of the underlying endolymphatic hydrops or to improve hearing. Consequently, the goal of treatment in Meniere disease is relief of symptoms and preservation of useful hearing, when present. The elements of initial management include counseling, reassurance, diet, vestibular exercises for dysequilibrium (if present), diuretics, and vestibular suppressant medication for temporary symptomatic relief from attacks of vertigo. This management is sufficient for nearly all patients and is renewed if attacks of vertigo occur after surgical treatment.

Surgery for Meniere Disease

Surgery can reasonably be proposed to control the definitive spells of vertigo in Meniere disease when several conditions have been met (**Tables 11.1**, **11.2**). First, to be a surgical candidate, a patient reaches a state of disability due to the frequency and severity of definitive spells (AAO-HNS functional level 4–6). It is not necessary or appropriate to offer surgery simply because a patient has the diagnosis of Meniere disease, because nonsurgical management is usually sufficient. Moreover, vestibular destructive procedures result in very troublesome dysequilibrium in 15% or more of patients.[4] It is best not to offer surgery unless the patient is ready to accept the risk of substituting one disturbing symptom for another.

Second, it must be possible to identify the ear that is the source of the definitive attacks. The active ear is the ear with the hearing loss and/or caloric weakness. Occasionally, it may be difficult to be certain which one is the active ear.

Reading the Clinical Literature

The literature on Meniere disease is plagued by methodological problems. One of the most significant is the difficulty of identifying stable, verifiable clinical end points to measure. Meniere disease is primarily a subjective disorder.

Table 11.2 Surgical Treatments for Meniere Disease, Including Intratympanic Gentamicin*

Intralabyrinthine shunts: cochleosacculotomy, Cody'tack procedure

Endolymphatic sac procedures, including decompression, with or without insertion of a drain, valve, or shunt to the posterior cranial fossa

Transmastoid labyrinthectomy, transcanal labyrinthectomy, translabyrinthine vestibular neurectomy

Lateral semicircular canal treatments with ultrasound or cryoprobe

Selective vestibular nerve section in the posterior cranial fossa or internal auditory canal via the middle cranial fossa

Aminoglycoside application via the middle ear (round window), lateral semicircular canal, or endolymphatic sac

*The four most commonly used procedures are in **bold italics**.

Although vertigo may precipitate a dangerous fall or traffic accident, Meniere disease is not in itself life threatening. Audiometry, vestibular laboratory tests, and imaging are useful in the assessment of patients, yet there is no standardized test with acceptable precision and accuracy that will confirm the diagnosis or indicate the status of the endolymphatic hydrops.

The symptoms of Meniere disease are particularly difficult to measure in a research setting, because patients vary enormously in the frequency, severity, and qualitative type of symptoms they experience. Emotional factors are highly prevalent, and the natural history of vestibular disorders is variable. Although the AAO-HNS has issued clinical research reporting guidelines,[1] these guidelines are not always followed or interpreted uniformly.[5] There is still a strong tendency for patients, and therefore some physicians, to consider any vestibular symptoms to be "vertigo." Finally, there are many sources of investigator bias, principally case selection.

Of the many procedures that have been proposed for Meniere disease (**Table 11.2**), four continue to be widely used. These are the various endolymphatic sac procedures (decompression, shunts), selective vestibular nerve section, surgical labyrinthectomy, and intratympanic application of a vestibulotoxic antibiotic, usually gentamicin.

Torok reported that 60 to 80% of patients improve regardless of the treatment used, confounding an analysis of surgical outcomes.[6] The phenomenon of regression to the mean, whereby patients present for care when they are at their worst and tend to recover spontaneously regardless of the treatment, must also be recognized. Another critical issue in surgery for Meniere disease has been the issue of the placebo, or nonspecific, effect, which has been studied mostly in relation to endolymphatic sac surgery.[7]

Surgery of the Endolymphatic Sac

Georges Portmann of Bordeaux, France, introduced endolymphatic sac (ELS) surgery in the 1920s. Portmann hypothesized that the sac has an important homeostatic function in the metabolism of the inner ear. ELS procedures consist of performing a mastoidectomy and exposing the endolymphatic sac. The sac exposure may be expanded by removing more of the bone over the posterior cranial fossa dura beyond the margins of the sac. Some authors have advocated probing the endolymphatic duct, performing the operation under electrocochleographic control, and placement of various drains, shunts, or other devices. Often the surgery can be performed as an outpatient procedure, and local anesthesia is possible.

The results of ELS surgery vary from 50 to 90% complete control of definitive vertigo attacks (**Table 11.3**).[8,9]

Table 11.3   Results of Surgical Treatment and Intratympanic Gentamicin for Meniere Disease

ELS	50–90%[8,9]
Labyrinthectomy	95–100%[10,11]
VNS	88–92%[22,23]
ITG	80–90%[29,30]

The variability seems to depend primarily on the criteria used to select patients for surgery, rather than on the technical skill of the surgeon or variables associated with the procedure itself. Realistically, 50 to 65% of patients will experience complete control of vertigo for a period of 1 to 2 years.[8] These results will suffice for many patients.

ELS procedures have the highest rate of failure to control vertigo of the four major procedural treatments (**Table 11.1**). However, they also have the lowest rate of complications, including the lowest rate of hearing loss. Especially when simple decompression is performed, ELS surgery is a nondestructive, extracranial procedure and poses little risk to hearing or balance. It can be performed as an outpatient procedure under local or general anesthesia.

If vertigo recurs following ELS surgery, medical management is resumed. If the patient becomes disabled again, he or she should have a comprehensive reevaluation. If the sac procedure was initially successful, it is reasonable to repeat it; however, the patient and surgeon may prefer to proceed to more definitive treatment, such as one of the other four procedures (**Table 11.1**).

Surgical Labyrinthectomy

Surgical labyrinthectomy is a procedure that removes the vestibular sensory tissue of the inner ear and is intended to eliminate the sensory conflict between the dysfunction of the inner ear and the otherwise concordant input of the normal inner ear, vision, proprioception, and touch. The sensory epithelia can be avulsed through a transcanal approach[10] or removed under direct vision through a transmastoid approach.[11] The expectation is that all vestibular function ceases in the operated ear, and all residual hearing is usually also lost.

Immediately following labyrinthectomy, patients experience a syndrome of acute unilateral vestibular loss, which consists of continuous vertigo, imbalance, and motion intolerance, all of which gradually cease as central nervous system (CNS) compensation occurs over 1 to 3 months. By 1 year nearly all patients after labyrinthectomy have compensated to the point where they have resumed all previous activities without significant impairment or disability. They typically will experience a mild sense of imbalance on sudden head movements, especially when tired or under stress.

Labyrinthectomy and translabyrinthine vestibular neurectomy are the gold standard for control of vertigo in Meniere disease. Complete control of definitive spells occurs in 95% of patients with classic Meniere disease (**Table 11.3**).[10,11] However, the diagnosis of vestibular disorders is often difficult. An uncommon cause of incomplete control of definitive spells is diagnostic error. The 5% rate of incomplete control of spells also reflects the problems of semantics and questionnaires in research design of some clinical studies.

Very troublesome and persistent dysequilibrium occurs in 15 to 50% of patients, presumably due to incomplete CNS compensation. Older patients may have more difficulty compensating. Often, postoperative testing confirms postural instability and/or abnormalities of the vestibulo-ocular reflex, though there are no reliable objective test indicators or tests for functional compensation. Infrequently, a patient may compensate satisfactorily initially but develop troublesome dysequilibrium later in life.

In some cases, patients are found to exhibit normal posture and gait examinations, suggesting that much postoperative dysequilibrium is subjective. Patients who receive prolonged disability compensation are less likely to get well. Persistent dysequilibrium is usually best treated by vestibular rehabilitation.

The incidence of incomplete labyrinthectomy when experienced surgeons use the transcanal approach has been shown to be as low as 5%.[10] When appropriate, a transcanal labyrinthectomy could be revised with transmastoid labyrinthectomy or translabyrinthine vestibular neurectomy.

When the vestibular nerve is completely removed through a translabyrinthine approach (translabyrinthine vestibular neurectomy), the rate of complete control of definitive spells is equivalent to the results from labyrinthectomy.[12] In addition, the translabyrinthine vestibular neurectomy requires exposing the vestibular nerve and hence CSF, increasing the risk of a postoperational CSF leak. The high rate of success of labyrinthectomy suggests that attacks of vertigo in Meniere disease arise within the membranous labyrinth, rather than within the vestibular nerve.

Rarely, a patient may have persistent spells of vertigo or even drop attacks following transcanal or transmastoid labyrinthectomy. When a patient has persistent spells of vertigo following labyrinthectomy, the patient must be evaluated carefully. There could be diagnostic error, coexistent CNS disease, or active peripheral vestibular disease on the opposite side. The persistence of dysequilibrium may lead the patient to report that spells of vertigo are continuing. Traumatic neuromas have been demonstrated in the vestibule following labyrinthectomy. It has been suggested that traumatic neuromas may cause a state of irritability in the vestibular nerve, which may cause persistent symptoms.[13] A controversy has arisen whether there is a role for translabyrinthine vestibular neurectomy as a secondary treatment for patients who fail labyrinthectomy.[12]

Selective Vestibular Nerve Section

Vestibular nerve sections were performed by McKenzie[13] and by Dandy[14] through a posterior fossa approach beginning in the 1930s.

William House proposed selective vestibular nerve section through a middle cranial fossa approach.[15] The advantage of the middle fossa approach is that the vestibular nerve is accessible lateral to the point where its fibers join with the fibers of the cochlear nerve to form a single nerve. Thus, a complete nerve section is anatomically possible without the risk of dividing auditory nerve fibers. When the middle fossa approach was first proposed, some surgeons divided only the superior vestibular nerve, because it is more difficult to reach the inferior vestibular nerve deep to the falciform crest of the internal auditory canal. Unfortunately, only ~75% of patients had complete control of vertigo following selective division of the superior vestibular nerve.[16] Higher rates of control were achieved when the entire nerve was divided.[4,17,18]

The middle fossa approach is relatively difficult technically. The geniculate ganglion is dehiscent in its position in the middle fossa approach in 5% of cases.[19] It may be damaged during elevation of the dura. For these reasons, Silverstein and others advocated returning to the practice of dividing the eighth cranial nerve (CN VIII) in the posterior fossa through a retrolabyrinthine approach,[20] a retrolabyrinthine/retrosigmoid approach,[22] or a similar posterior fossa approach.

Removing the posterior internal auditory canal was advocated in some studies to expose the medial parts of the CN VIII complex. This latter practice has not become universal because of the problems of postoperative headache associated with aseptic meningitis resulting from bone dust seeding the posterior fossa, extended operating time and risk, and the perception that there was little advantage to the additional exposure. Thus, selective vestibular nerve section in the posterior cranial fossa has become the preferred approach of selective vestibular nerve section by most neurotological skull base surgeons.[21] Some prominent surgeons have continued to prefer some form of the middle fossa approach.[22,23] Following selective vestibular nerve section in the posterior fossa, the rate of complete control of definitive spells of vertigo in classic Meniere disease is 88 to 92% (**Table 11.3**).[21,24] Several lines of evidence suggest that the different success rates between labyrinthectomy (~95%) and selective vestibular nerve section (92%) are due to incomplete destruction of the vestibular nerve in the latter case.[10] First, Rasmussen[25] and later Silverstein and

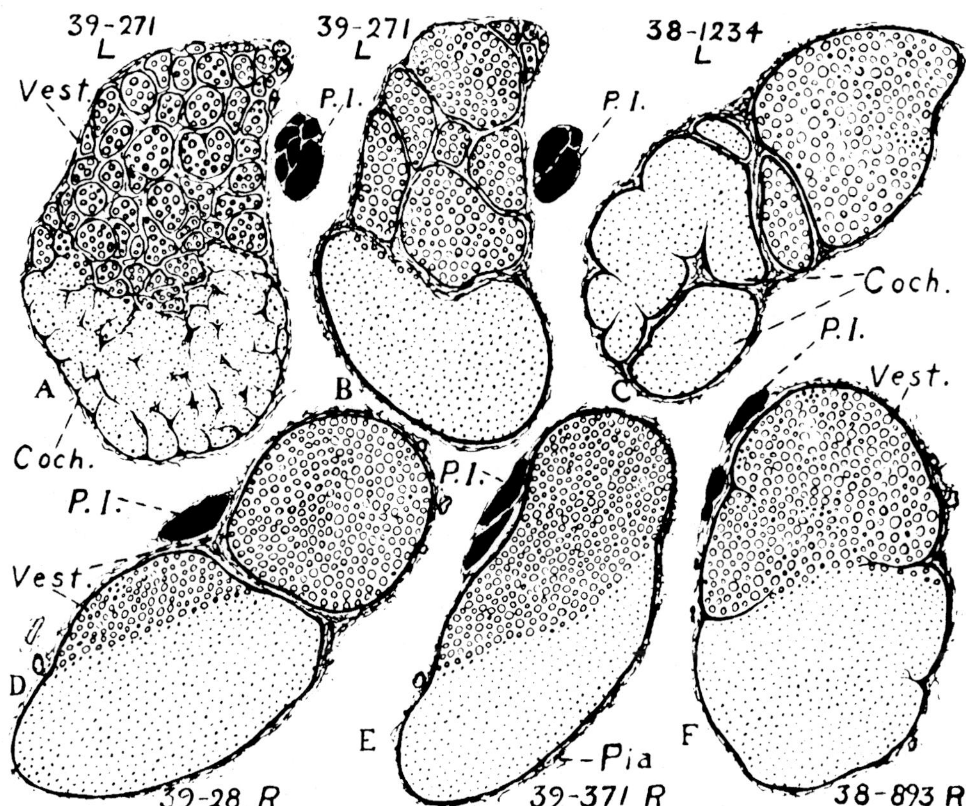

Figure 11.1 Anatomical variations of the human vestibulocochlear nerve. The small circles indicate the vestibular portion of the nerve; the stippling represents the cochlear portion. The three diagrams in the upper portion of the figure show how the structure of the nerve changes from lateral to medial regions. The three diagrams in the lower portion of the figure show variations in the plane of separation between the vestibular and cochlear divisions. There is no fascial plane or anatomical landmark that consistently corresponds to a natural division between the vestibular and cochlear divisions. (From Rasmussen G. Studies of the VIIIth cranial nerve of man. Laryngoscope 1940;50:67. Reprinted with permission.)

Rosenberg[24] pointed out how the orientation of the plane of demarcation between the vestibular and auditory divisions rotates as CN VIII courses between the inner ear and the brainstem (**Fig. 11.1**).

Second, the vestibular and auditory axons intermingle at their boundary zone in the posterior fossa (**Fig. 11.2**).[25,26] As much as 10% of vestibular fibers lie within the auditory division. Moreover, there is often no clear demarcation between the two divisions (**Figs. 11.1, 11.2**).

For the anatomical reasons just stated, any nerve section is likely to spare some vestibular axons. The author has demonstrated a case whereby a patient had a translabyrinthine vestibular neurectomy following a retrolabyrinthine vestibular nerve section. Ten percent of the normal number of vestibular axons survived the initial retrolabyrinthine vestibular nerve section. These fibers were sufficient in number to support enough labyrinthine activity to be disabling.[26]

These studies suggest that surgical anatomy and surgical techniques make a crucial difference in the results from vestibular nerve section. It is now accepted that selective vestibular nerve section in the posterior fossa will result in complete control of vertigo in ~92% of patients. There is little that the surgeon can do to improve

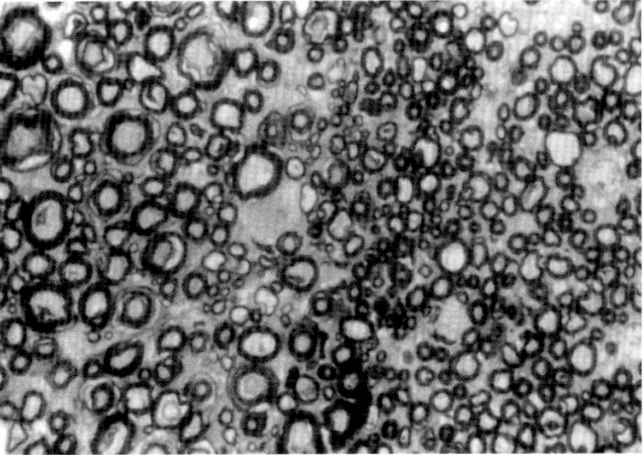

Figure 11.2 Histologic section of a human eighth cranial nerve (CN VIII) from the posterior cranial fossa. This specimen was fixed with osmium tetroxide, sectioned at 1 μm, and stained with toluidine blue. Note that the larger (vestibular) fibers seen on the left side of the figure (vestibular portion of CN VIII) intermingle with smaller (cochlear) fibers on the right side of the figure (cochlear portion of CN VIII). There is no distinct separation or fascial plane between the vestibular and cochlear portions of the nerve. Large fibers are not present in the cochlear division at greater distances from the boundary zone. Approximately 10% of the vestibular fibers are present in the cochlear division of the nerve. (From Monsell E, Brackmann D, Linthicum F. Why do vestibular destructive procedures sometimes fail? Otolaryngol Head Neck Surg 1988;99:472. Reprinted with permission.)

these results without dividing more of the nerve, increasing the risk of hearing loss.

If definitive spells of vertigo return following retrolabyrinthine or retrosigmoid vestibular nerve section, the patient should be reevaluated. Often it is the case that symptoms are relatively mild and are adequately controlled by symptomatic management.

Before a secondary vestibular procedure is considered, it may be valuable to determine whether and to what extent functional vestibular tissue might remain. Currently, there is no vestibular test that can confirm that all vestibular tissue has been functionally ablated. A positive prone caloric response may indicate the presence of functional tissue.[11]

In the standard caloric position, a cold stimulus will induce nystagmus, with the fast component beating toward the side opposite the test ear. Sectioning the vestibular nerve creates a peripheral vestibular lesion. Alerting such a patient, which is accomplished by the caloric irrigation, will tend to bring out a latent spontaneous nystagmus, which also beats toward the opposite side. Thus, a caloric test performed postoperatively with the patient in the standard caloric position may give a false-positive response.

A true caloric-induced nystagmus, if present, can be differentiated in this situation by performing a prone caloric test. If the subject is situated so that the head position is reversed by 180 degrees, a cold stimulus will induce a caloric nystagmus beating toward the test ear, whereas nystagmus from alerting alone would beat away from the test ear. It may be necessary to use ice water, which is the strongest caloric stimulus, because the strength of the response would be expected to be weak.

If an active caloric response is present, and possibly even if a response cannot be demonstrated, a revision surgical procedure can be considered if appropriate criteria are met (**Table 11.1**). If hearing is good, the best option for revision surgery is probably selective vestibular nerve section through a middle fossa approach (or Fisch's intratemporal approach).[27] If hearing is poor, a labyrinthectomy may be considered. Treatment with intratympanic gentamicin can also be considered (see below). If the patient is disabled by constant dysequilibrium, counseling and vestibular rehabilitation are appropriate.

Leakage of CSF may occur following selective vestibular nerve section through any of the approaches mentioned above. CSF leakage is best managed by prevention. Meticulous attention to the details of closure, including watertight closure of the dura and/or patching, and waxing exposed mastoid air cells will usually suffice. If postoperative CSF leakage occurs through the ear and nose, the patient is hospitalized, and a lumbar CSF drain is placed for several days. If drainage persists, revision of the closure may be needed. In some cases, it may be necessary to block the eustachian tube and perform a blind sac closure of the external auditory canal.

Intratympanic Gentamicin Treatment

The vestibulotoxic properties of streptomycin and gentamicin were discovered shortly after the drugs were introduced for antimicrobial therapy. Fowler, Schuknecht, and others applied streptomycin in the middle ear for unilateral vestibular ablation.[28] Some authors began to use gentamicin, hoping that it would preserve hearing more consistently than streptomycin.

Intratympanic gentamicin administration has been performed with either an unbuffered stock solution or a buffered solution injected into the middle ear. Fixed-dosage protocols, so-called titration protocols, and protocols calling for treatment until toxicity is reached have all been reported. Some authors have included an exploratory tympanotomy or myringotomy with or without placement of a tympanostomy tube, Gelfoam, or some other delivery device. Other authors have simply injected the solution one or more times through the intact tympanic membrane.[29]

Intratympanic gentamicin treatment has been reviewed by several authors.[29,30] In most series, 80 to 90% of patients have complete control of vertigo (**Table 11.3**). Hearing worsens in 25 to 50% of patients, and 5 to 15% become deafened by the treatment. Efforts to reduce the rate of hearing loss from the treatment by using a series of treatments separated in time have not been successful to date. Gentamicin exposure to cochlear hair cells is unavoidable. Intratympanic gentamicin treatment has the advantage of being a nonoperative treatment that can be performed in the outpatient setting. However, it is also difficult to control and causes a high rate of associated hearing loss. Moreover, disabling chronic dysequilibrium may result, as with any vestibular destructive procedure. This dysequilibrium may be particularly bothersome for older persons, who constitute the primary group for this mode of therapy.

If a patient with Meniere disease becomes disabled by definitive spells of vertigo following intratympanic treatment, the treatment can be repeated. Other options include vestibular nerve section and surgical labyrinthectomy.

The otolithic crises of Tumarkin are thought to arise from dysfunction of the utricle. Aminoglycoside treatments affect primarily the ampullae of the semicircular canals. Because of the risks of personal safety posed by otolithic crises, labyrinthectomy and vestibular nerve section are probably better treatment options for primary or revision surgical treatment than ELS procedures or intratympanic gentamicin. Aminoglycosides are appropriate for hydropic disorders but only rarely for nonhydropic disorders.[29]

Benign Recurrent Vertigo

Barber described a clinical syndrome that he called recurrent vestibulopathy. This syndrome consists of recurring spells of vertigo of the Meniere type, but without hearing loss. Others have called this syndrome benign recurrent vertigo (BRV) or vestibular neuritis of the recurrent type.[31,32] There may or may not be a caloric weakness.

This disorder usually runs a milder course than classic Meniere disease. BRV can usually be managed with vestibular suppressants and counseling. Recently, some authors have suggested that many patients with BRV have a form of vestibular migraine.[33] A trial of antimigrainous medication may be considered.

Disability from spells of vertigo is rare in BRV. If vertigo does become disabling, it is recommended that a series of steps be considered prior to recommending surgery (**Table 11.1**). A critical issue in surgery for BRV is determining which ear is responsible for the patient's symptoms. The most commonly performed procedure for disabling vertigo due to BRV is selective vestibular nerve section or neurectomy. Occasionally, this clinical syndrome may occur in a nonhearing ear, in which case labyrinthectomy should be considered. Failure of vestibular nerve section to control spells of vertigo is more common in BRV than in Meniere disease.[32] For failure after selective vestibular nerve section in the posterior cranial fossa for BRV, surgical options include selective vestibular nerve section or neurectomy in the internal auditory canal via a middle fossa approach, surgical labyrinthectomy, and translabyrinthine vestibular neurectomy. Intratympanic gentamicin may be attempted if hearing is poor, but such treatment is likely to fail, because nonhydropic ears are more resistant to the effects of intratympanic gentamicin.[29]

Benign Paroxysmal Positioning Vertigo

Benign paroxysmal positioning vertigo (BPPV) occurs when a person moves in the provocative manner. This movement is reproduced by the Dix-Hallpike maneuver. The sitting patient briskly reclines in the supine position with the head turned 45 degrees to one side. There is a characteristic torsional nystagmus whose onset, peak, and decline parallel the patient's experience of vertigo. The most effective stimulus for BPPV is not head position, but movement in the plane of the posterior semicircular canal (PSCC). BPPV is due to otoconia from the maculae becoming dislodged and ultimately resting on the ampulla of the PSCC (cupulolithiasis) or disturbing flow of endolymph within the lumen of the PSCC (canalithiasis). Once the movement has stopped, the vertigo runs its course and stops in

~30 seconds. BPPV is paroxysmal, brief, and intense, and exhibits latency characterized by a few seconds' lapse between the acceleration and the vertigo. It is also fatigable; the response wanes as the maneuver is repeated. BPPV may be confused with generalized motion intolerance.

BPPV is very common but rarely disabling. The disorder is self-limited; most cases resolve spontaneously in 8 to 12 weeks. Positioning maneuvers or habituation exercises are remarkably effective in controlling symptoms. In a few patients, most of whom are elderly, BPPV continues indefinitely.

The procedures that have been widely used for disabling vertigo due to BPPV include singular neurectomy,[34,35] PSCC occlusion,[36,37] and other treatments to the PSCC.[38]

These procedures prevent the PSCC from provoking the sensation of vertigo when patients move in the plane of that canal. Consequently, although most patients will no longer have positioning vertigo, some head motions may not be well tolerated after this procedure. Postoperative motion intolerance is best addressed by vestibular exercises.

BPPV may occur in association with episodic vertigo from disorders, such as Meniere disease. Singular neurectomy or procedures on the PSCC would not be expected to control spontaneous spells of vertigo.

A syndrome of positioning vertigo due to dysfunction of the lateral semicircular canal has recently been recognized.[39] Successful surgical treatment of the lateral canal syndrome would require an anatomically appropriate treatment; however, this syndrome usually resolves spontaneously.[37]

Surgery is only infrequently needed for BPPV, because so-called particle positioning maneuvers are usually successful in controlling spells of positioning vertigo.[37] Should PSCC occlusion or singular neurectomy fail and the patient remain disabled by positioning vertigo, selective vestibular nerve section may be considered as a revision procedure.

Bilateral Meniere Disease and Autoimmune Inner Ear Disease

Bilateral Meniere disease is defined as the presence of the full clinical syndrome of Meniere disease in both ears.[1] It has been estimated to occur in 2 to 47% of cases, depending on the duration of follow-up and the criteria for diagnosis used by the author.[2] This is similar to another syndrome, autoimmune inner ear disease.[40] This latter syndrome is characterized by progressive, stepwise deafness in both ears over weeks to months. Although vertigo may occur in autoimmune inner ear disease, it is not characteristic, and it is rarely disabling. In recent years, some experts have suggested that there is an indistinct clinical boundary between bilateral Meniere disease and autoimmune inner ear disease. When the diagnosis of bilateral Meniere disease is considered, autoimmune inner ear disease should also be considered.

Vertigo due to bilateral Meniere disease can often be controlled with intramuscular streptomycin.[28] Patients are usually grateful for the relief of their severe vertigo, even if they are not able to work again due to severe dysequilibrium. Some authors have advocated a graduated or "titrated" treatment approach when using intramuscular streptomycin to try to avoid disabling the patient from severe bilateral vestibular ataxia and oscillopsia. However, there does seem to be a trade-off between reduced rates of disabling dysequilibrium and an increased risk for return of episodic vertigo when long-term follow-up is considered. It is possible to retreat a patient years after treatment with intramuscular streptomycin, though it would be unlikely to have a functional improvement in the patient.[29]

The Perilymphatic Fistula Hypothesis

A perilymphatic fistula (PLF) may lead to disabling vertigo and dysequilibrium from spontaneous or traumatic leakage of perilymph from the inner ear to the middle ear.[41,42] The paths of fluid leakage have been proposed to be primarily the fissula ante fenestram or the round window membrane. Repairing such fistulas results in a high rate of success for control of vertigo. The presence of PLF has been supported by histopathological and anecdotal clinical evidence.

The otologic surgical community at large has remained skeptical of the presence of PLF as a frequent cause of vertigo, especially in patients who do not have an adequate inciting cause. Despite vigorous advocacy by some for more than 20 years, the practice of finding and repairing spontaneous fistulas has remained the activity of a minority of otologists. It has been suspected that many patients with the diagnosis of PLF have symptoms from other causes, such as classic Meniere disease, labyrinthine fibrosis, superior semicircular canal dehiscence syndrome, other peripheral vestibular problems, anxiety disorders, or purely emotional causes.

The Vascular Loop Hypothesis and Microvascular Decompression

Hemifacial spasm may be caused by compression of the root entry zone of the facial nerve by a loop of an intracranial artery, such as the anteroinferior cerebellar artery.[43] Ephaptic transmission between nerve fibers has been demonstrated to occur reversibly when the vessel impinges against the facial nerve. It has been argued that there may be an analogous syndrome of episodic vertigo, aural fullness, and tinnitus when such a vessel impinges on CN VIII. Confirmatory evidence is lacking for this hypothesis, however,

and microvascular decompression of CN VIII has not become widely practiced by neurotological surgeons.

Revision for Other Causes

In hearing preservation surgery for the treatment of vertigo, such as ELS surgery, conductive hearing loss due to ossicular fixation resulting from a complication of the prior surgery such as the accumulation of bone dust, adhesions, or dislocation of the ossicles can occur. Management options include amplification and exploratory tympanotomy, lysis of adhesions, and ossicular reconstruction.

The facial nerve can be injured during mastoidectomy, labyrinthectomy, or surgery of the internal auditory canal and cerebellopontine angle. Following well-defined bony landmarks and identification of the facial nerve early in the procedure can usually prevent injuries.[44] Electrical monitoring may be a useful adjunctive measure, but it should not be depended upon.

The tympanic segment of the facial nerve may be injured when approaching the lateral semicircular canal during transmastoid labyrinthectomy. The labyrinthine segment of the facial nerve may be injured when approaching the ampulla of the superior semicircular canal. The mastoid segment may be injured when approaching the ampulla of the PSCC, which lies medial to the facial nerve. The mastoid segment may also be injured when approaching the endolymphatic sac. If the injury is severe, exploration, decompression, primary anastomosis, cable interposition grafting, or substitution grafting of the facial nerve may be necessary.

Avoiding a Second Failure

Examining the Causes of Failure

No patient or surgeon wants a treatment to fail. The discomfort and life disruption of disabling vertigo are bad enough to experience once. Avoiding a second failure requires careful conceptual thinking about the cause of the disorder and the cause of failure of the original procedure.

The claim that a procedure has failed begs a list of compelling questions. Was the diagnosis correct? What was the diagnosis based on? Was the correct ear selected? Was surgery appropriate in the first place? Did the surgery actually fail, or were the patient's expectations inappropriate? Was the operation successful in controlling the vertigo, but the patient is uncomfortable or disabled by adjunctive symptoms, such as dysequilibrium or tinnitus? Is the patient having vertigo, but the attacks are so infrequent or mild that nonoperative treatment is sufficient? Is the patient embellishing because of fear of returning to work or fear that symptoms will return? Is the patient experiencing so much anxiety about the symptoms that the anxiety itself is the predominant symptom?

There are three categories of failure to consider. Biological failure may be due to the wrong diagnosis, operating on the wrong ear, or incomplete ablation of functional vestibular tissue. Functional failure may be due to a continuing sense of imbalance or motion intolerance from incomplete CNS compensation. Psychosocial failure may be due to continued suffering by the patient as a result of chronic disruption of social and economic functions, such as loss of a job, disruption of a career, or effects on interpersonal relationships.

Testing

Vestibular testing may be very useful in guiding decisions about revision vestibular surgery. As discussed above, the various caloric tests may help determine whether active vestibular function remains after selective vestibular nerve section or intratympanic gentamicin treatment. Rotational chair testing is a measure of compensation of the vestibulo-ocular reflex, though it should be interpreted as only a guide to vestibular compensation in general. Computed dynamic posturography is a measure of postural stability. It may identify functional embellishment of symptoms and is a guide to vestibular rehabilitation.[45]

The degree of lifestyle impairment and coping styles can be assessed with questionnaires, such as the functional level scale of the AAO-HNS,[4] the Dizziness Handicap Inventory,[46] and the Minnesota Multiphasic Personality Inventory.[47]

Conclusion

Although usually successful, any procedure to control vertigo can fail. Initial and revision treatment decisions must be weighed carefully, because it is possible for some

Table 11.4 Questions to Ask When Surgical Treatment of Meniere Disease Fails

What was the goal of treatment?
In what way was that goal not achieved?
Was the goal realistic and appropriate?
Why was that goal not achieved?
How functionally impaired is the patient now?
What are the management options?
What could be gained and what could be lost by pursuing further treatment?
Are the patient's expectations appropriate and realistic?

treatments to be worse than the disease, especially if patients have only mild symptoms. When treatment failure occurs, the causes and consequences should be carefully examined (**Table 11.4**). Causes of failure include incorrect diagnosis, inappropriate procedure, incomplete ablation of vestibular tissue, failure of CNS compensation, inappropriate or exaggerated psychological reactions, and the normal shortcomings or anatomical limitations of some procedures. It is prudent to consider a period of symptomatic management to determine whether disabling symptoms will improve and to weigh the emotional consequences of vestibular disorders. In most cases, something can be done to improve function.

Since this chapter was prepared, the importance of migraine-related vertigo (MRV) has been more widely and clearly recognized.[48] First, MRV is important in the differential diagnosis of any vestibular disorder. The symptoms and findings of MRV overlap with those of Meniere's disease and benign recurrent vertigo. Second, MRV may coexist with Meniere's disease, benign paroxysmal positioning vertigo, and other vestibular disorders, intensifying symptoms and making them resistant to treatment. Third, anti-migraine therapy can be dramatically effective and obviate the need for primary or revision surgery. Surgery for superior semicircular canal dehiscence[49] is still evolving and is outside the scope of this chapter.

References

1. Committee on Hearing and Equilibrium. Committee on Hearing and Equilibrium guidelines for the diagnosis and evaluation of therapy in Meniere's disease. American Academy of Otolaryngology–Head and Neck Foundation. Otolaryngol Head Neck Surg 1995;113:181–185.

2. Friberg U, Stahle J. The epidemiology of Meniere's disease. In: Harris JP, ed., Meniere's Disease. The Hague: Kugler Publications; 1999:17–28.

3. Tumarkin A. The otolithic catastrophe. BMJ 1936;2:175–177.

4. Fisch U. The vestibular response following unilateral vestibular neurectomy. Acta Otolaryngol 1973;76:229–238.

5. Cass S. Staging and outcomes for Meniere's disease. In: Harris JP, ed., Meniere's Disease. The Hague: Kugler Publications; 1999:239–253.

6. Torok N. Old and new in Meniere's disease. Laryngoscope 1977;87:1870–1877.

7. Bretlau P, Thomsen J, Tos M, et al. Placebo effect in surgery for Meniere's disease: a three-year follow-up study of patients in a double blind placebo controlled study on endolymphatic sac shunt surgery. Am J Otol 1984;5:558–561.

8. Monsell EM, Wiet RJ. Endolymphatic sac surgery: methods of study and results. Am J Otol 1988;9:396–402.

9. Ress B, Harris J. Endolymphatic sac surgery. In: Harris J, ed., Meniere's Disease. The Hague: Kugler Publications; 1999:355–360.

10. Nadol J, McKenna M. Transcanal labyrinthectomy. In: Brackmann DE, Shelton C, Arriaga C, eds., Otologic Surgery. Philadelphia: WB Saunders; 2001.

11. Vernick D. Labyrinthectomy. In: Nadol J, Schuknecht H, eds., Surgery of the Ear and Temporal Bone. New York: Raven Press; 1993.

12. Nelson R. Translabyrinthine vestibular neurectomy. In: Brackmann D, Shelton C, Arriaga C, eds., Otologic Surgery. Philadelphia: WB Saunders; 2001.

13. McKenzie KG. Intracranial division of the vestibular portion of the auditory nerve for Meniere's disease. Can Med Assoc J 1936;34:369–381.

14. Green R. Surgical treatment of vertigo, with follow-up on Walter Dandy's cases: neurological aspects. Clin Neurosurg 1958;6:141.

15. House WF. Surgical exposure of the internal auditory canal and its contents through the middle cranial fossa. Laryngoscope 1961;71:1363–1385.

16. Glasscock ME. Vestibular nerve section: middle fossa and translabyrinthine. Arch Otolaryngol 1973;97:112–114.

17. Glasscock ME III, Kveton J, Christiansen S. Middle fossa vestibular neurectomy: an update. Otolaryngol Head Neck Surg 1984;92:216–220.

18. Fisch U. Vestibular and cochlear neurectomy. Trans Am Acad Ophthalmol Otolaryngol 1974;78:ORL252–ORL255.

19. House WF, Crabtree JA. Surgical exposure of the petrous portion of the seventh nerve. Arch Otolaryngol 1965;81:506–507.

20. Silverstein H, Norrell H. Retrolabyrinthine surgery: a direct approach to the cerebellopontine angle. Otolaryngol Head Neck Surg 1980;88:462–469.

21. Silverstein H, Wanamaker H, Flanzer J, Rosenberg S. Vestibular neurectomy in the United States—1990. Am J Otol 1992;13:23–30.

22. Garcia-Ibanez E, Garcia-Ibanez J. Middle fossa vestibular neurectomy: a report of 373 cases. Otolaryngol Head Neck Surg 1980;88:486–490.

23. Fisch U, Chen J. Middle cranial fossa: vestibular neurectomy. In: Brackmann DE, Shelton C, Arriaga C, eds., Otologic Surgery. Philadelphia: WB Saunders; 2001.

24. Silverstein H, Rosenberg S. Retrolabyrinthine/retrosigmoid vestibular neurectomy. In: Brackmann DE, Shelton C, Arriaga C, eds., Otologic Surgery. Philadelphia: WB Saunders; 2001.

25. Rasmussen G. Studies of the VIIIth cranial nerve of man. Laryngoscope 1940;50:67.

26. Monsell EM, Brackmann D, Linthicum F. Why do vestibular destructive procedures sometimes fail? Otolaryngol Head Neck Surg 1988;99:472–479.

27. Fisch U. Transtemporal supralabyrinthine approach. In: Fisch U, Mattox D, eds., Microsurgery of the Skull Base. New York: Thieme Medical Publishers; 1988.

28. Schuknecht HF. Ablation therapy for the management of Meniere's disease. Acta Otolaryngol Suppl 1957;132:1–42.

29. Monsell EM, Cass S, Rybak L, Nedzelski J. Chemical treatment of the labyrinth. In: Brackmann DE, Arriaga C, Shelton C, eds., Otologic Surgery. Philadelphia: WB Saunders; 2001.

30. Blakley BW. Clinical forum: a review of intratympanic therapy. Am J Otol 1997;18:520–526.

31. Leliever WC, Barber HO. Recurrent vestibulopathy. Laryngoscope 1981;91:1–6.

32. Nadol JB Jr. Vestibular neuritis. Otolaryngol Head Neck Surg 1995;112:162–172.

33. Baloh R, Andrews JC. Migraine and Meniere's disease. in: Harris J, ed., Meniere's Disease. The Hague: Kugler Publications; 1999.

34. Gacek RR. Singular neurectomy update, II: Review of 102 cases. Laryngoscope 1991;101:855–862.

35. Gacek R, Gacek M. Posterior ampullary nerve section for benign paroxysmal positional vertigo. In: Brackmann D, Shelton C, Arriaga C, eds., Otologic Surgery. Philadelphia: WB Saunders; 2001.

36. Parnes LS, McClure J. Posterior semicircular canal occlusion in the normal hearing ear. Otolaryngol Head Neck Surg 1991;104:52–57.

37. Parnes LS. Posterior semicircular canal occlusion for benign paroxysmal positional vertigo. In: Brackmann D, Shelton C, Arriaga C, eds, Otologic Surgery. Philadelphia: WB Saunders; 2001.

38. Anthony PF. Partitioning the labyrinth for benign paroxysmal positional vertigo: clinical and histological findings. Am J Otol 1993;14:334–342.

39. Fife TD. Recognition and management of horizontal canal benign positional vertigo. Am J Otol 1998;19:345–351.

40. Harris JP, Tomiyama S. Immunology/virology of Meniere's disease. In: Harris J, ed., Meniere's Disease. The Hague: Kugler Publications; 1999.

41. Gulya A. Perilymphatic fistulas. In: Nadol J, Schuknecht H, eds., Surgery of the Ear and Temporal Bone. New York: Raven Press; 1993.

42. Singleton G, Slattery W. Perilymphatic fistula. In: Brackmann DE, Shelton C, Arriaga C, eds., Otologic Surgery. Philadelphia: WB Saunders; 2001.

43. Janetta P, Moller M. Operations for microvascular compression syndromes. In: Brackmann DE, Shelton C, Arriaga C, eds., Otologic Surgery. Philadelphia: WB Saunders; 2001.

44. Monsell E. Iatrogenic facial nerve injury: prevention and management. In: Jackler R, Brackmann D, eds., Neurotology. St. Louis: Mosby; 1994:1333–1343.

45. Monsell EM, Furman J, Herdman S, Konrad H, Shepard N. Technology assessment: computerized dynamic platform posturography. Otolaryngol Head Neck Surg 1997;117:394–398.

46. Barin K, Durrant J. Applied physiology of the vestibular system. In: Canalis R, Leliever W, eds., The Ear: Comprehensive Otology. Philadelphia: Lippincott Williams & Wilkins; 2000:113–140.

47. Jacobson GP, Newman C. The development of the dizziness handicap inventory. Arch Otolaryngol Head Neck Surg 1990;116:424–427.

48. Neuhauser HK, Radtke A, von Brevern M, Feldmann M, Lezius F, Ziese T, Lempert T.: Migrainous vertigo: prevalence and impact on quality of life. Neurology 2006 26;67(6):1028–1033.

49. Carey JP, Migliaccio AA, Minor LB. Semicircular canal function before and after surgery for superior canal dehiscence. Otol Neurotol 2007; 28(3):356–364.

Revision Cochlear Implant Surgery

Ravi N. Samy and Jay T. Rubinstein

Cochlear implantation is an effective therapeutic option for selected deaf adults and children. By improving speech perception and production skills, cochlear implants may lead to a significant gain in a patient's sensory and social environment and overall improvement in quality of life. As the worldwide experience in this procedure has increased and will continue to do so, numerous reports have emerged describing the need for and techniques of reimplantation. When an individual undergoes cochlear implantation for rehabilitation of deafness, it is natural for the expectations of the patient, his or her family, and the community to be high; a failed implant procedure is a disappointment to all concerned and can be a setback to a cochlear implant program.[1] A functioning implant requires substantial financial and personal investment and can be considered the equivalent of an only-hearing ear.[2]

Reimplantation

Numerous reports exist about the success of reimplantation. Over 250 patients have had single-channel implants replaced with multichannel devices at multiple centers.[3] In addition, by the end of the 1980s, the Nucleus 22 from Cochlear Corporation (Englewood, Colorado) had a 2.8% incidence of reimplantation. Other devices have had a reimplantation rate varying from 3 to 7%.[4] The first reported experience with scala tympani electrode reinsertion was in 1985.[5] In that report, two patients had their 3M-Vienna cochlear implants replaced (please note that this implant is no longer being made). After reimplantation, the patients continued their improvement in auditory performance over many months, with no impairment caused by revision surgery. This report showed that reimplantation was technically feasible and successful.[5]

Experience with reimplantation at the University of Iowa was first reported in 1989.[6] In five patients who had device failure ranging from 6 weeks to 4 years after implantation, all had improved performance on a uniform battery of audiologic tests after reimplantation. Replacements of electrodes did not appear to induce any clinically detectable degeneration of auditory performance. This has been confirmed in several other reports.

Numerous indications for reimplantation exist,[2,7,8] including

- Device failure (e.g., from static/electric shocks, high temperatures, trauma to the receiver/stimulator, or percutaneous pedestal fracture)
- Wound infection/dehiscence
- Need for device upgrade
- Need for electrode repositioning (due to facial nerve stimulation, electrode compression, or electrode displacement)
- Device migration/extrusion

Device Failure

Some types of device malfunction may be addressed by reprogramming. Early experience with cochlear implants in children demonstrated a higher failure rate than in adults who used the same device.[8] In addition, in the pediatric population, as more receive cochlear implantation, there may be increasing numbers of device failures because many patients may outlive the finite life span of their implants.[8] The body's extracellular fluid may also breach the protective casing.[4] Consultation with the implant manufacturer may be appropriate, and the old implant should be returned to the manufacturer for analysis as to the cause of the device failure.[9]

Wound Infection/Dehiscence

Delayed cochlear implant infections are a rare but potentially devastating complication.[2] Removal of an infected device can lead to cochlear fibrosis and ossification, potentially requiring a "drill-out" of the cochleostomy if the replacement procedure is delayed. The expense of these devices can also make replacement difficult if financial resources are not available.[2] Occasionally, functional integrity of the electronic components of the original device, documented intraoperatively, can allow reinsertion using the same device, avoiding the expense of a new receiver/stimulator.[1] In fact, one implant was reported as being inserted into the cochlea on three separate occasions without detriment to auditory performance.[2]

Decision tree for revision cochlear implant surgery

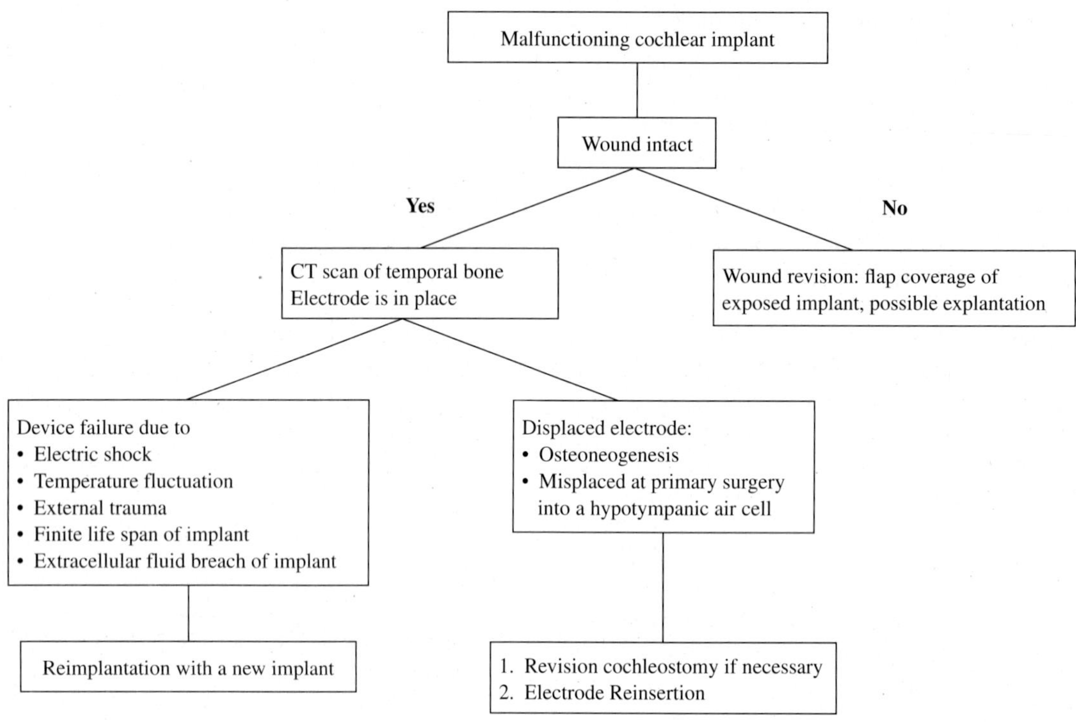

Need for Device Upgrade

The newer devices often incorporate the necessary technology to allow some speech-processing improvements to be incorporated without requiring revision surgery.[3] However, as implant technology and coding strategies continue to evolve, reimplantation to improve performance may be a consideration.[8] This does pose a risk-versus-benefit question for both the patient and the surgeon.[4]

Need for Electrode Repositioning

Intraoperative radiography, in addition to impedance testing, may be helpful in proper positioning of the electrode. Ongoing growth of new bone may gradually displace the electrode, resulting in an observed deterioration of performance.[1] Sudden changes in electrode position can dramatically alter speech recognition without changing threshold or dynamic range.[2] The most frequent error in electrode placement is inadvertent implantation of a hypotympanic air cell. This is more likely to occur if the round window niche is not clearly identified but may even occur in experienced hands if the round window niche is obliterated by fibrous or bony tissue overgrowth.[9]

Device Migration/Extrusion

Overall, problems with the newest cochlear implants are much less common than with first-generation devices. Improvements in design and technical innovations gained from increased knowledge and experience have led to a corresponding reduction in the failure rate.[8,10] Newer devices have a smaller thickness and size of the internal receiver compared with older models, which is especially helpful in children in preventing device extrusion as well as skin flap or wound breakdown.[11]

In a retrospective review of the experience with revision cochlear implant surgery, Rubinstein et al examined five patients who required surgery for delayed implant infections or extrusion.[2] Three of the patients had skin erosion to expose an Ineraid (Cochlear Corp., Englewood, CO) pedestal with secondary infection, and one had migration and extrusion of a cochlear nucleus CI-22 receiver with secondary infection. Split pericranial–temporalis muscle flaps and rotation skin flaps were used for the coverage of the Ineraid pedestal implants (**Figs. 12.1, 12.2**). Of key importance was the use of well-vascularized skin and muscle flaps to prevent wound dehiscence/infection and implant exposure. Based on our experience, we felt that limited infections could be treated in a limited but aggressive manner. Low-grade flap/skin infections could be treated with systemic (either intravenous or oral) antibiotics and local wound care,

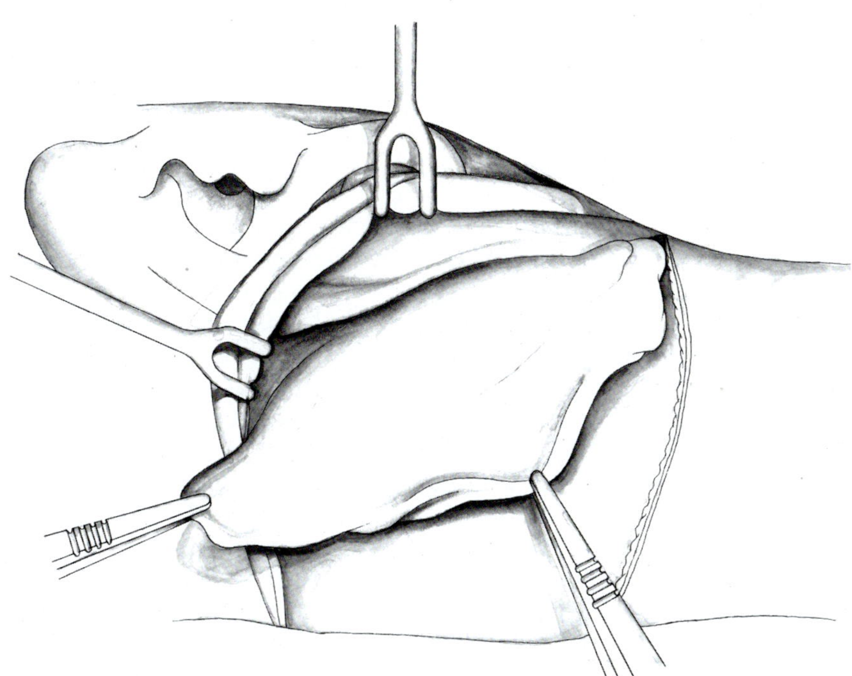

Fig. 12.1 Temporalis muscle and fascia are used as a rotational flap over the cochlear implant.

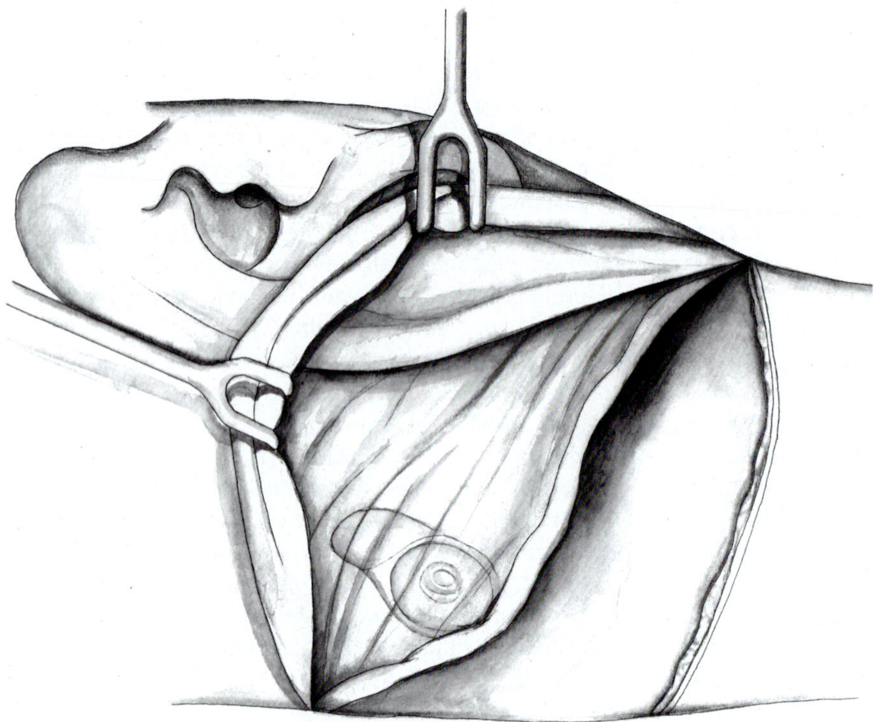

Fig. 12.2 The location of the cochlear implant is seen under the flap.

which could avoid explantation. However, if there is any evidence of systemic infection, such as meningitis, the infected implant must be removed.[2]

Auditory Brainstem Implants

A related topic is that of reimplantation of auditory brainstem implants (ABIs). Brainstem implants have benefited patients with bilateral cochlear nerve loss. An ABI stimulates the central auditory pathways in patients with deafness due to damage, resection (e.g., bilateral acoustic neuroma resection NF-2), or congenital absence of the auditory nerves.[12] The first ABI implanted by William House was in 1979; the patient continues to use it today.[13] These implants assist with environmental sounds, increase lip-reading skills, and possibly may relieve tinnitus.

These implants are the only successful medical/surgical aural rehabilitation for these patients. The overall worldwide experience with ABI patients is much smaller than with cochlear implant patients.[12] Conceptually, the ABI is similar to a multichannel cochlear implant. The differences lie in the electrode's design and the fact that the array of electrodes is placed on the cochlear nucleus complex rather than in the scala tympani. Electrical stimulation of the cochlear nucleus evokes auditory sensations different than those evoked by electrical stimulation of the cochlea. The devices may cause extra-auditory effects due to activation of somatosensory or motor pathways. Fortunately, surgical repositioning has still allowed satisfactory results.[12]

Speech recognition improves more slowly in patients with an ABI than with a cochlear implant. Also, scores for open-set words and sentences without lip reading and contextual cues are poorer. Although the results with an ABI are not as good as with a cochlear implant, the quality of life is still often improved.[12] The ABI is a relatively new device, so little exists in the literature on revision surgery for device complication or malfunction.

Patient Selection

Patient selection for revision cochlear implantation requires careful consideration of many factors that are similar to those of primary implantation. A patient should undergo a thorough otologic history, physical, audiovestibular, and psychological assessment.[9] The assessment may include radiologic evaluation of the cochlea. The precise etiology of implant/device failure is determined whenever possible. Although the audiologic assessment is the primary means of determining suitability for revision cochlear implant surgery, there should be no medical contraindications. Reimplantation remains an elective surgical procedure. The patient should demonstrate a continued high level of motivation and appropriate expectations. He or she should be counseled that there is no certainty that performance will improve with reimplantation. In fact, performance may actually become worse.

A psychological evaluation may be helpful in reimplantation. The evaluation may provide information related to the management of the patient in rehabilitation. Occasionally, an exclusionary factor is identified, such as a previously undetected psychosis, organic brain dysfunction, or mental impairment. In addition, some patients may determine that they are not interested in the time and expense of reimplantation.

On physical examination, routine microscopic evaluation of the tympanic membranes is performed. Absence of detectable middle ear and external canal pathology should be present prior to reimplantation.[14] The ear proposed for reimplantation must be free of infection, and the tympanic membrane must be intact. Reimplantation performed only after a short period of time following the initial implantation has been associated with a greater degree of middle ear inflammation.[4] Because children are more prone to otitis media than adults, concern exists that a middle ear infection could cause an implanted device to become an infected foreign body, requiring removal. Another possibility is that an infection might extend along the electrode into the inner ear, resulting in a central complication such as meningitis or further degeneration of the auditory nerve. To date, although the incidence of otitis media in children who received cochlear implants parallels that seen in the general pediatric population, no serious complications of reimplantation have been documented.[15] Although the risk of meningitis is elevated in cochlear implant recipients relative to the normal-hearing population, there is no evidence yet that reimplantation modifies this risk. Chronic otitis media (with or without keratoma) must also be successfully addressed prior to reimplantation using routine otologic techniques.

Radiologic examination of the cochlea may be performed to determine the position of the primary implant and whether the implant is physically intact. High-resolution temporal bone computed tomography (CT) scans in the axial and coronal planes are the scans of choice. CT scans can also demonstrate bone growth.[1] Intracochlear ossification does not contraindicate cochlear reimplantation, but it can limit the type and length of the electrode array that can be inserted into the scala tympani. When a temporal bone fracture has resulted in implant failure, CT scanning may provide helpful information predicting the integrity of the cochlear nerve. Plain films may also assist with determination of incorrect positioning or implant/electrode migration.[1,9]

Surgical Reimplantation

Reimplantation is usually accomplished without adverse physical or audiologic consequences. Device-specific surgical techniques for replacement of an intracochlear electrode array are required. Oftentimes, reimplantation is no more difficult than the primary procedure. In general, removal of single-channel implants is easier than removal of multichannel devices. Also, some implants are easier to remove than others due to design.[3] Although device removal and replacement may not always be simple, it usually is technically feasible.[3,9] Avoidance of wound and flap complications is of great concern in cochlea implant replacement surgery, as with primary surgery. The same skin incision is used to prevent flap ischemia tissue loss and subsequent exposure of the implant package. Wound-related problems leading to explanation of the device can be avoided by careful planning of the incision, meticulous handling of the flap, and closure of the incision without tension.[10] The postauricular skin and scalp superior to the auricle are widely shaved and prepped. A facial nerve monitor is used to assist in the identification and protection of the facial nerve. (During surgery for replacement of an ABI, intraoperative monitoring of the 9th and 10th cranial nerves is performed. Postoperatively, an electrically evoked auditory brainstem response is recorded to evaluate the correct position of the electrodes on the cochlear nucleus complex.[12]

The use of traditional monopolar electrocautery is prohibited in revision or replacement surgery because of the concern for device and/or end-organ tissue damage.[7] Electrical current spread to the malfunctioning device could interfere with an accurate cause-of-failure analysis. Also, heat produced by the current could spread to spiral ganglion cells. Hemostasis can be achieved with either bipolar cautery or use of the Shaw heated scalpel (Hemostatix Medical Technologies, Bartlett, Tennessee). This specially designed scalpel utilizes a sharp, heated blade for simultaneous cutting and coagulation and was used as an alternative to bipolar cautery in one study.[7]

Prophylactic antibiotics, such as a first-generation cephalosporin with good skin microbial coverage, are administered. A Palva flap is elevated. The mastoidectomy is revised due to bone regrowth that invariably has occurred.[8] At the time of reoperation, one may note a capsule of smooth fibrous tissue around the receiver with a foreign body/granulation tissue reaction. Fibrosis and granulation tissue may involve the posterior tympanotomy and facial recess; careful dissection is needed to avoid damage to the tympanic membrane annulus and facial nerve in this area, especially if the fallopian canal has been inadvertently opened at the primary procedure. The presence of granulation tissue may be related to the use of absorbable gelatin sponge.[4] The facial recess also allows comfortable introduction of the instruments used in the subsequent steps of the procedure.[11] The cochleostomy and primary electrode are then identified through the facial recess. The primary electrode is removed sometimes with slight difficulty, particularly if the indwelling electrode does not have a smooth external surface. Electrode contact surfaces that protrude from the wire bundle may become encased by fibrosis and may even shear off and remain behind following electrode extraction.[4] The cochleostomy may need to be enlarged. A laser is used by some to ablate soft tissue in the cochleostomy. Dense reactive scar tissue and/or new bone growth is often noted at the site of cochlear fenestration from previous connective tissue grafts as well as within the scala tympani around the electrode capsule.[8]

The intracochlear electrode is surrounded by a fibrous sheath; this sheath remains in situ when the original electrode is removed and facilitates insertion of the new array, as long as the new array is implanted immediately.[4,10] However, if reimplantation is delayed after explantation, the sheath can collapse and create a luminal restriction. Thus, in those instances where reimplantation needs to be delayed, the surgeon should cut the electrode at the level of the round window, which leaves the intracochlear portion in place as a lumen keeper.[4] Reports do exist describing difficulty with replacing a short-electrode of a single-channel implant with the longer electrode of a multichannel device, due to the presence of the fibro-osseous cuff in the scala tympani.[13] Cochlear ossification may need to be drilled out. The osteoneogenic bone is a chalky white color, lighter than the color of the surrounding otic capsule.[1] The presence of ossification within the scala tympani following initial implantation often occurs and may be due to a variety of causes, including the etiology of the deafness (e.g., meningitis), cause of device failure, and type of implant initially inserted.[8] The degree of occlusion within the scala tympani is variable and results from both a fibrous and an osseous component. Reactive bone growth associated with trauma to the endosteum or introduction of bone dust drilling remnants into the cochlea may also contribute to the osteoneogenesis. Care must be taken so as not to injure the internal carotid artery in its location anterior to the cochlea. The electrode array is then inserted as far as possible. One should avoid forceful attempts to insert the electrode to avoid damage to the cochlea or the electrode itself.[4] Although the length of electrode insertion may be slightly reduced without compromising auditory benefit,[1,8] all electrodes ideally should be fully inserted.[4] The cochleostomy is closed with a plug of temporalis fascia.

The bone surrounding the internal receiver is purposely drilled without saucerized edges to decrease the chance of receiver movement/displacement. A suture is passed through the cortex surrounding the receiver for its final stabilization. Overlying temporalis muscle also aids in preventing receiver movement. A loop of the electrode is left in the mastoid in the hope of avoiding withdrawal of the electrode from the cochlea that could occur with skull growth in the pediatric population. After implantation, the Palva flap is sutured closed and used to protect the electrodes and prevent a postauricular depression. Before closure of the skin incision in layers, impedance testing is performed to confirm accurate device placement and proper function. Of note, care must be taken to avoid placement of the receiver near the site where eyeglasses are worn. This will allow for a behind-the-ear processor to be used.[2]

Complications

Surgical complications of reimplantation may include those associated with any surgical procedure (e.g., bleeding and anesthetic risks), as well as those related to otologic procedures and that of primary implantation in particular. The complication rate is slightly higher than that for primary implantation. Fortunately, complications are infrequent in experienced hands and can be largely avoided by careful preoperative planning and meticulous surgical technique. The most frequently encountered problem involves the incision and postauricular skin flap. The risks of performing the mastoidectomy and opening the facial recess are no greater than for any other revision otologic procedures. Care must be exercised to avoid facial nerve injury by direct bur movement or thermal injury secondary to friction heat generated from the shaft of the bur or the bur itself.[14] Adequate irrigation will usually dissipate the heat generated during drilling. Cerebrospinal fluid (CSF) leaks are usually managed intraoperatively without postoperative sequelae.[8]

Histopathology

Representative human temporal bone histopathologic sections and an experimental animal study involving cat temporal bones show interesting histopathologic changes associated with reimplantation.[3,4] The two distinct electrode tracks noted with reinsertion may be displaced into the scala vestibuli by reactive osteoneogenesis in the scala tympani. Usually, insertion results in stria vascularis, spiral ligament, and basilar membrane disruption, as well as damage to the organ of Corti and peripheral dendrites, yet overall function of the implant is not affected.[10] There exists a risk of increased hair cell and spiral ganglion damage with reimplantation.[9] In fact, there is often a partial loss of spiral ganglion cells; however, there are usually a substantial number of spiral ganglion cells remaining that are present in all turns. Whether the spiral ganglion cell loss occurs because of the original injury necessitating a cochlear implant, primary implantation, reimplantation, or a combination of these is unknown. Histological examination of the cochlea also shows fibrous tissue growth, possible granulation tissue growth, and bone formation, all to varying degrees.[9] Endolymphatic hydrops has also been noted to occur with distension of the Reissner's membrane.[4]

Performance Results

The primary role of a cochlear implant is to make speech sounds accessible to the auditory system. However, if cochlear implants are to make a significant impact upon deafened adults and children, they must also serve as aids to speech production. The scores for reimplanted subjects showed gradual improvement over time. However, there are large between-subject differences in implant benefit.[14] Because the perceptual mechanism varies among individuals, each implantee incorporates auditory, visual, linguistic, and nonlinguistic information to varying degrees. For any given implant system, scores on sentence recognition tasks in quiet can vary from 0 to 100%; implantees who exhibit the same psychological results can have very different speech recognition abilities. Unfortunately, reimplantation benefit cannot be reliably predicted. Duration of deafness and residual hearing before implantation, educational setting, and age at onset of deafness are independent variables that may also explain performance differences.[2,14]

Reimplantation benefit is measured using a battery of audiological tests that assess sound and speech reception with the implant and is compared with the patient's preoperative performance with the initial implant. The least difficult tests are those that assess identification of environmental sounds and recognition of certain characteristics of speech, such as temporal or intonation patterns. Speech-reading enhancement is measured by assessing recognition of sentences or connected discourse with the implant turned off and is compared with the performance with the implant turned on. Auditory word identification is assessed using a "closed-set" and an "open-set" response format. Of significance is that data from numerous studies evaluating reimplantation of cochlear implants demonstrate that even with trauma to the peripheral auditory structures, the speech-understanding performance is usually as good as or better than the original implant.[3,7,8,10]

Patients undergoing reimplantation may have a single-channel implant removed and replaced with a multichannel device. Initially, at our institution, we did not feel it appropriate to remove functioning single-channel devices; in particular, we had concerns that reimplantation with multichannel units would not necessarily result in improved performance in any specific patient.[3] We have since changed our approach to implant upgrades because our clinical experience has shown significantly improved speech recognition scores after reimplantation. Except in the unusual circumstance that the contralateral ear is audiometrically superior, we now recommend reimplantation rather than primary implantation of the contralateral ear in any adult patient with a single-channel device who desires improved performance. Multichannel devices lead to significantly higher scores on tests that assess recognition. Reimplantation with multichannel implants definitively improves auditory performance when compared with the primary single-channel implants in the same ear in adults.[3]

Patients may initially show an immediate decrement in performance after reimplantation with a subsequent improvement over time.[3] Implant candidates with residual hearing may suffer a comparable initial decrement in speech perception before learning the code of electrical stimulation. It appears that the central auditory pathways "learn" a specific processing strategy and that a strategy richer in information content can cause an initial decrement in performance until this new strategy is learned. Candidates for either reimplantation or processor upgrade should be warned of this possibility.[3]

The largest review of cochlear reimplantation was done by Parisier et al.[8] The authors retrospectively reviewed the outcome of 27 consecutive multichannel reinsertions performed in 25 children. There was a minimum follow-up of 6 months for both surgical and audiological performance. In all patients, the need for reinsertion was device failure. Two patients suffered an intraoperative CSF leak, and two had a flap breakdown. Open-set speech recognition scores and speech reception abilities remained stable or improved compared with results before reimplantation in 96% of patients, regardless of age at initial implantation or the time interval to reimplantation. Although concern regarding changing coding strategies may exist with difference devices, the results of this study did not show any adverse effect with changing the type of implant device or coding strategy. The authors stated that additional time of follow-up may show continued improvement in performance.[8]

Conclusion

Cochlear implants offer a proven alternative for selected deaf children and adults. Improvements have been manifested in both speech perception and production skills. The full impact of implantation and reimplantation will be further refined with detailed longitudinal studies. Multichannel systems that provide spectral information in addition to temporal and intensity cues have demonstrated performance advantages over single-channel systems. Continued improvements in signal coding and processing will continue to push the envelopes of performance and benefit.[14] The continuing evolution of cochlear implant design and reliability, coupled with advances in surgical technique, should reduce the incidence of device replacement. However, should the need for reimplantation arise, the current evidence suggests that a revision procedure can be accomplished without great technical difficulty, and a favorable outcome can be expected in terms of the patient's audiologic performance.

References

1. Telian SA. Successful revision of failed cochlear implants in severe labyrinthitis ossificans. Am J Otol 1996;17(1): 53–60.
2. Rubinstein JT, Gantz BJ, Parkinson WS. Management of cochlear implant infections. Am J Otol 1999;20:46–49.
3. Rubinstein JT, Parkinson WS, Lowder MW, et al. Single-channel to multi-channel conversions in adult cochlear implant subjects. Am J Otol 1998;19(4):461–466.
4. Jackler RK. Cochlear implant revision: effects of reimplantation on the cochlea. Ann Otol Rhinol Laryngol 1989;98(10):813–820.
5. Hochmair-Desoyer I, Burian K. Reimplantation of a molded scala tympani electrode: impact on psychophysical and speech discrimination abilities. Ann Otol Rhinol Laryngol 1985;94(1 pt 1):65–70.
6. Gantz BJ, Lowder MW, McCabe BF. Audiologic results following reimplantation of cochlear implants. Ann Otol Rhinol Laryngol Suppl 1989;142:12–16.
7. Roland JT Jr. Shaw scalpel in revision cochlear implant surgery. Ann Otol Rhinol Laryngol Suppl 2000;185:23–25.
8. Parisier SC, Chute PM, Popp AL, et al. Outcome analysis of cochlear implant reimplantation in children. Laryngoscope 2001;111:26–32.
9. Saeed SR, Ramsden RT, Hartley C, et al. Cochlear reimplantation. J Laryngol Otol 1995;109(10):980–985.
10. Woolford TJ, Saeed SR, Boyd P, et al. Cochlear reimplantation. Ann Otol Rhinol Laryngol Suppl 1995;166:449–453.
11. Filipo R, Barbara M, Monini S, et al. Clarion cochlear implants: surgical implications. J Laryngol Otol 1999;113(4): 321–325.
12. Di Nardo W, Fetoni A, Buldrini S, et al. Auditory brainstem and cochlear implants: functional results obtained after one year of rehabilitation. Eur Arch Otorhinolaryngol 2001;258(1):5–8.
13. House WF, Hitselberger WE. Twenty-year report of the first auditory brain stem nucleus implant. Ann Otol Rhinol Laryngol 2001;110:103–104.
14. Miyamoto RT, Osberger MJ, Kessler K. Cochlear implants in aural (re)habilitation of adults and children. In: Ballenger JJ, Snow JB Jr, ed. Otorhinolaryngology: Head and Neck Surgery. 15th ed. Philadelphia: Williams and Wilkins; 1996:1142–1152.
15. Gyo K. A case of revision of a cochlear implant. Nippon Jibiinkoka Gakkai Kaiho 1994;97(11):2113–2116.

Revision Surgery for Congenital Aural Atresia

Mark C. Witte and Paul R. Lambert

Learned otologists have stated that the surgical repair of congenital aural atresia is among the most difficult tasks in otology. It follows, then, that revision atresia surgery represents an even more daunting task. As is so often true in otologic surgery, the key to success in this enterprise resides in the details. In revision atresia surgery, the preoperative assessment and planning require great circumspection, and the operative technique must be meticulous. In the common scenario of revising another surgeon's first repair attempt and in situations where the cause of the previous surgical shortfall is not immediately apparent, the operative repair is best undertaken in a stepwise fashion. Finally, conscientious and thorough care is required in the early postoperative period to optimize the course of healing and to avoid incipient complications.

The difficulty of atresia surgery is perhaps best illustrated by the high revision rate that may be anticipated even in the hands of the most experienced otologist. It is expected that up to one third of surgical atresia repairs will require some greater or lesser degree of revision surgery to achieve optimal results in hearing rehabilitation and freedom from infection.[1] In various series, revision rates were 34% (17 of 50 primary surgeries),[1] 30% (21 of 69),[2] 32% (20 of 63),[3] 30% (6 of 20),[4] and 33% (8 of 24 major atresia repairs).[5] Later series involving some of the same primary surgeons demonstrated decreases to 19% (3 of 16 primary repairs)[6] and 22% (13 of 58),[7] perhaps a reflection of refinements of technique.

Indications for Revision

When discussing revision surgery for congenital aural atresia with the patient, the option of a bone anchored hearing aid must be considered. Indeed, this device must be mentioned at the time of the initial assessment for aural atresia, just as a hearing aid is for otosclerosis. In this chapter, however, the focus will be on surgical management of the ear canal and middle ear.

In the initial consideration of surgical revision, the reasons for failure of the primary repair must be determined, if possible. When infection and otorrhea are the primary patient concern, the history will immediately make this apparent. When the principal issue is suboptimal hearing rehabilitation, clinical clues may be valuable in determining the origin of the ongoing conductive hearing loss (CHL). The patient's failure to achieve marked subjective hearing improvement in the immediate postoperative period (from packing removal to about 2 months postoperatively) is suggestive of an immediately displaced prosthesis or an occult ossicular chain abnormality that was not addressed. The gradual onset of CHL over months or years implicates the healing mechanism in the cause of hearing loss; if the patient also has undergone a columella-type reconstruction using either artificial or autologous materials, the possibility of adhesions causing ossicular chain disarticulation or ankylosis is high. Lateralization of the tympanic membrane graft or thickening due to chronic inflammation is also consistent with this time course and should be evident to the careful microscopic ear exam. One would not expect a severe conductive hearing loss solely from external canal stenosis until the stenosis is very advanced (opening ≤ 2 mm). Although otitis media is not a frequent concern in children with congenital atresia (perhaps due to selection bias against operating on the hypopneumatized middle ear cleft), the possibility of middle ear fluid, which may not be apparent through the reconstructed tympanic membrane, must be considered. Rarely, a patient may note daily hearing fluctuations in the context of barometric or body positional changes, suggesting a partially reversible ossicular chain discontinuity as might occur in repairs employing a stapes piston or a nonbiointegratable artificial prosthesis.

In the patient whose chief complaint is residual CHL, the decision to perform revision surgery should be compared with expected hearing results in successful atresia repairs. In the numerous series of atresia repairs, a variety of methods have been used to report hearing results, making comparisons difficult. Nevertheless, review suggests that in candidates for reconstruction, it is reasonable to expect a gain in pure tone average (PTA) of 25 to 30 dB,[2,4,6,8] for 40% of patients to achieve a postoperative PTA of $\leq$ 20dB, and 60% overall to achieve a PTA of $\leq$ 30dB,[2,4,9] with comparable speech reception thresholds (SRTs).[6] This translates to a residual air–bone gap of $\leq$ 20 dB in ~50% of patients and of $\leq$ 30 dB in 70% of selected patients.[3,7,10] Equally interesting to the surgeon considering revision are data concerning the odds of successful

133

Decision tree for aural atresia revision surgery

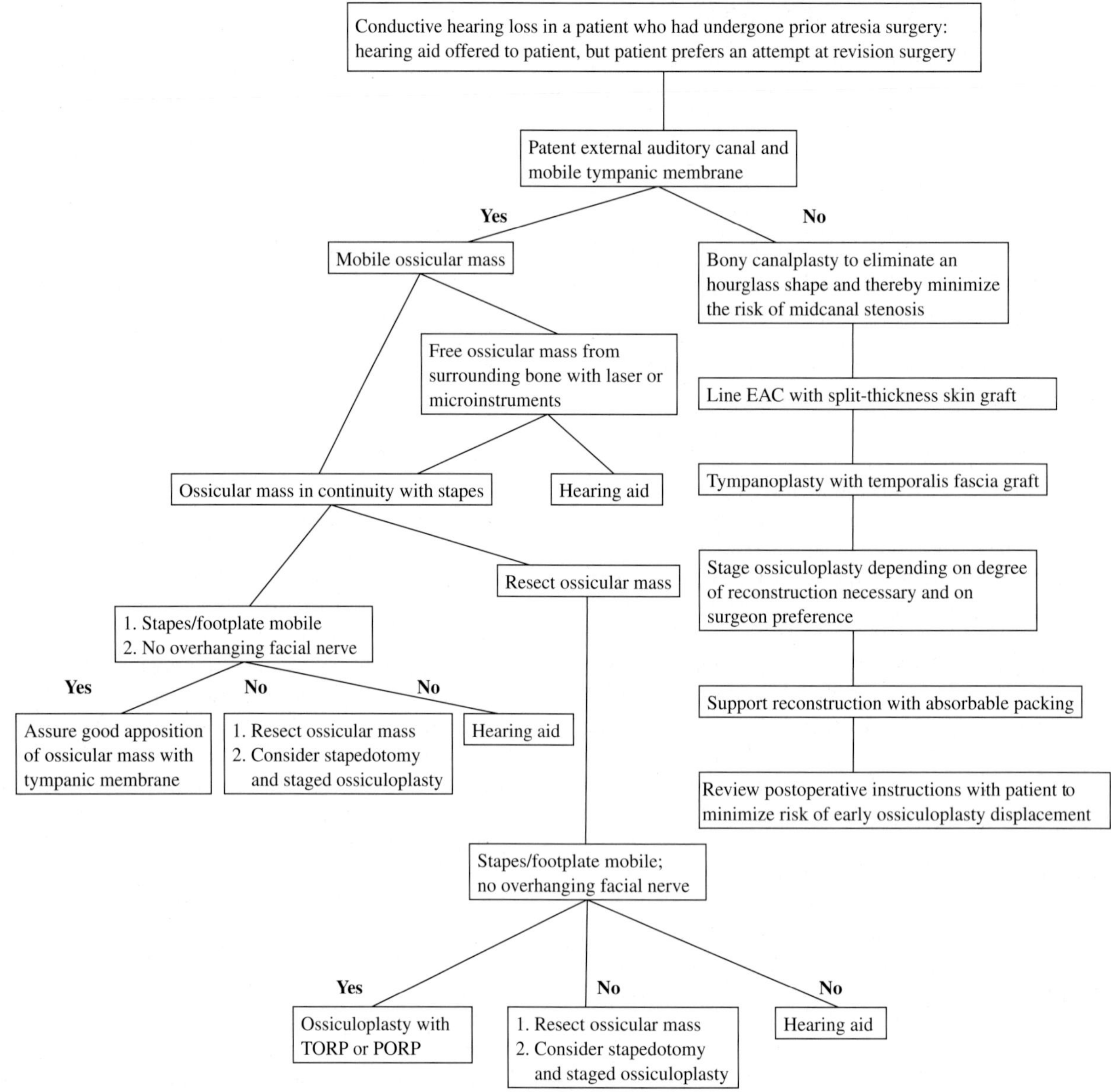

hearing rehabilitation in revision repairs. Provided the expectations are appropriately restrained, as in any revision surgery, the prognosis for well-selected patients is quite reasonable. In one revision series of the surgeon's own primary repairs, 12 of 20 of the patients were able to achieve a < 20 dB residual air–bone gap;[3] in another series, four of four revisions obtained a patent external auditory canal (EAC) and achieved "serviceable" hearing (PTA ≤ 40 dB).[8] In another series, 53% (8 of 15) of patients undergoing revision attained an SRT of ≤ 30 dB.[6] A final factor in decision making is an awareness of the mild progressive CHL that occurs in a large percentage of successful atresia repairs; in such a patient, a revision procedure may be unlikely to yield significant long-term improvement. In a typical series, the natural history of hearing decrement in repairs deemed successful was 19%; this averaged a 20 dB loss over an average 2.6-year follow-up.[7]

Individual patient factors are of paramount importance when considering whether to undertake a revision operation for hearing. Numerous surgeons have alluded to subsets of patients with both favorable and unfavorable indicators. For example, in one series an initial very good hearing result was found to be an excellent prognostic sign, whereas the need to use an artificial prosthesis for ossicular chain reconstruction was identified as a significant unfavorable sign.[6] As in primary atresia repair, it is prudent to attempt to limit elective surgery to patients with normal or near-normal cochlear function and middle ear anatomy conducive to a repair attempt. Largely through the labors of Jahrsdoerfer and colleagues,[11] marked advances have been made in characterizing the anatomical features critical to successful reconstruction of the conductive hearing apparatus. The two most important features appear to be the presence of the stapes and the size of the middle ear cleft. The detection of a stapes on a temporal bone computed tomography (CT) scan simultaneously implies the existence of a patent oval window with a mobile footplate and a facial nerve that does not obstruct the oval window to a degree prohibiting ossicular chain reconstruction. The existence of a middle ear cleft of at least 50% normal area in both coronal and axial CT views[6] (compared with age-matched controls or the opposite ear in unilateral atresia) implies that recognizable mesotympanic landmarks exist to guide the surgeon to the otic capsule and the oval window. This "50% criterion" probably further implies that enough mediolateral depth exists in the middle ear cleft to allow reconstruction of the transformer apparatus without subsequent middle ear collapse, a feature long considered critical to lasting hearing rehabilitation in chronic ear surgery. The middle ear cleft is so critical that its absence is an absolute contraindication to a surgical attempt at hearing rehabilitation, whether primary or revision.

Causes of Surgical Failure

Canal Stenosis

In the atresia ear requiring reoperation, a knowledge of the frequency of various types of malfunction is informative in both initial and intraoperative assessment. Soft tissue stenosis of the reconstructed external auditory canal (neo-EAC) is such a common postoperative problem that one surgeon affirmed that more failures occur due to graft and canal healing problems than ossicular chain problems.[10] In accordance with this assertion, many series have cited soft tissue stenosis as the most frequent problem necessitating revision, typically affecting 10 to 25% of patients who have undergone primary repair. In one large series, this rate was 18% (9 of 50 primary repairs),[6] in another, 26% (18 of 69).[2] Factors important in reducing soft tissue stenosis include the use of split-thickness versus full-thickness skin grafts, meticulous coverage of all exposed bone,[10] a generous meatoplasty,[12] and the recognition that the more severe grade III microtias have a significantly higher rate of meatal stenosis due to reduced conchal cartilaginous support.[6] In a single series, bony restenosis was cited as a complication in 12% of cases (7 of 58 primary surgeries) and a factor in revision in 35% (9 of 26) cases.[7] One factor the authors considered important in this adverse occurrence was the youthfulness of their average atresia patient; the presumed higher metabolic bone activity in younger patients predisposed them to "exuberant bone growth."

Tympanic Membrane Lateralization

Nearly as common as the complication of soft tissue stenosis is lateralization of the grafted neo-tympanic membrane (neo-TM). In one large series, this occurred in 8% of cases (4 of 50 primary repairs).[6] In another series of 56 primary repairs, lateralization was the most common cause of a poor hearing result, occurring in 14 (25%).[3] This complication was noted to ensue most commonly within the first 12 months postoperatively. In a later series from the same group, neo-TM lateralization was a significant factor in 42% (11 of 26) of cases selected for revision.[7] It is perhaps noteworthy that this complication occurred in only 9% of primary cases but in 15% of revision cases.[7] In another series, TM lateralization requiring revision occurred in only 6% (1 of 16 cases), yet lateralization recurred despite reoperation.[6] Such data suggest that either prior surgical trauma or particular anatomical or physiologic patient characteristics may increase the risk of recurrent lateralization during further repair attempts. One anatomical characteristic, the severity of the malleus deformity, has been implicated as a factor in lateralization. Specifically, it has been noted that an absent or rudimentary malleous makes medial fixation of the fascia graft more difficult and less predictable.[6]

Ossicular Chain Malfunction

Ossicular chain malfunctions are another significant cause of failure of primary surgical repair. Ossicular fixation is perhaps the most common problem of this type; in one series this rate was 3.4% (2 of 58 primaries).[7] Again, it is noteworthy that this rate climbed to nearly 8% in the revision cases in this series, suggesting that, like lateralization, this problem may be exacerbated by particular patient anatomical factors or by operating in previously violated territory. Certainly the patient with a low tegmen would seem to be at higher risk for bony or fibrotic refixation of the lateral ossicular mass to the epitympanum. The anatomical abnormalities common to atresia ears may also predispose to medial ossicular chain fixation. In 11% (8 of 71) of one surgeon's series, the stapes was found to be small and fixed to the fallopian canal.[7] He noted that severe stapes deformities were usually associated with a poorly developed middle ear space and an aberrant facial nerve. Because of the anatomical distortion of the middle ear in many atresia cases, the surgeon not uncommonly will be unable to clearly visualize either the stapes footplate or the round window. Therefore, in patients who by history never achieved a significant postoperative hearing improvement, unrecognized stapes fixation must be strongly considered. As alluded to previously, fibrotic attachment to an encroaching horizontal facial nerve segment may result in a delayed hearing loss. An uncommon possibility in a patient who has previously undergone oval window drill-out is bony reclosure. In support of this possibility, Bellucci has described osseous reclosure of surgical fenestrations in "a few cases" in his atresia series, while Shambaugh alludes to the osteogenic potential of periosteal (but not enchondral) otic capsule bone.[9,13] Again, the young age of the patient with very metabolically active bone may be a contributory factor to this scenario.

Risks of Surgery

Other vital considerations in revision surgery are the risks that, although not unique to this type of surgery, are disproportionately high compared with those in other otologic procedures. In primary atresia surgery, removal of the bony atresia plate is associated with a risk of high-frequency sensorineural hearing loss (SNHL) as high as 15%; therefore, if revision will entail drilling, this risk must be assumed in the secondary procedure as well. In one series the risk of broad-frequency SNHL is 4 to 5%, where SNHL was defined as an average "pure tone drop of 30 dB" or a 30% decrement in speech discrimination score (SDS).[7] An earlier series cited an incidence of 11% (2 of 19 primary cases) related to drill trauma; the typical pattern was a loss $\geq$ 2000 Hz accompanied by a marked drop in SDS.[8] The risk of a total or profound loss (i.e., a "dead ear")

is cited as 0.6 to 3.0%.[6] In one series 1 of 56 patients (1.8%) undergoing primary revision experienced a total SNHL after a fenestration attempt; this increased to 5% (although only 1 of 20 cases) in the author's revision series.[3] This latter patient lost sensorineural function after an attempted oval window drill-out, suggesting this risk is most pronounced if otic capsule drilling is anticipated.

Perhaps the greatest concern in atresia surgery is the risk to the facial nerve. In an earlier series, a temporary palsy rate of 11% was cited.[2] Whatever the baseline risk in primary atresia repair, in revision cases the risk may be even higher because postoperative scarring and fibrosis along the surgical approach tract obscure anatomical details, require more forceful dissection, and transmit higher traction forces to the nerve.

Timing of Surgery

Once the surgeon and patient (or parents) have decided to perform an elective revision, the timing of the surgical intervention must be determined. First, if the external pinna repair is incomplete or unsatisfactory, plastic surgical consultation is advisable, as the further compromise to the lateral scalp blood supply from a second otologic procedure can only increase the difficulty of cosmetically improving an already compromised field. As in plastic surgical procedures, in otologic revision it may be advisable to delay revision for 6 to 12 months to allow stabilization of tissues that have been manipulated in the previous operation. Finally, because revision surgery entails increased risk to the inner ear and facial nerve, in some children with unilateral atresia it may be prudent to consider delaying a significant reoperation until adolescence or adulthood when the patient can assume some of the risks of the procedure.

In some situations the timing of surgery is a subordinate consideration. Prompt revision is mandated in the presence of cholesteatoma, whether residual/recurrent or acquired in the context of stenosis of the neo-EAC. Because soft tissue stenosis is a frequent complication of primary atresia repair, cholesteatoma is not an uncommon indication for surgery. In one series, 2 of 26 (8%) of revisions were performed for acquired cholesteatoma, ~3% (2 of 58) of the primary surgeries.[7] Also, infection and chronic drainage, if not responsive to conservative measures, should be considered indications for timely revision. If not addressed, such problems may over time lead to local or regional tissue compromise and/or stenosis. Due to its lack of natural self-cleaning, the grafted skin of the neo-EAC is susceptible to epithelitis, which, if not treated promptly, can become refractory to conservative measures. Once sloughing of the majority of the graft has occurred, surgical revision is probably inevitable, compelled because the exposed bone of the EAC will granulate and stenose. Finally, acute facial palsy[7] and impending intracranial complication (of otologic infection or cholesteatoma) would be indications for urgent surgery.

Other Considerations

Prior to revision of the conductive hearing apparatus, preoperative testing is necessary to ensure the presence of and to document the level of sensorineural hearing. Auditory brainstem response (ABR) testing in unilateral atresia and bone conduction ABR or sensorineural acuity level (SAL) testing in bilateral atresia can estimate the sensorineural reserve of the candidate ear and help the surgeon decide how aggressively to pursue hearing reconstruction. Finally, a current CT scan of the temporal bones should be obtained and reviewed in detail prior to considering further surgical intervention. If infection or cholesteatoma obscures the middle ear findings, the most recent scan that preceded the first operation may be helpful as well.

Surgical Techniques

Although the current techniques of atresia repair have been described in detail,[4,6,8,10] several points are worth reviewing as relevant to atresia surgery in general and revision surgery in particular. In the following section, these issues will be approached in the approximate order in which one might expect to encounter them during the operation, beginning with anesthetic induction. In his review of 83 atresia surgeries, Gill remarked that all atresia patients should be considered higher than average intubation risks, as it was his impression that nearly all had some degree of mandibular hypoplasia, described as an "underslung jaw."[5] In this context, it is appropriate to ensure that the anesthesiologist is aware of the potential risk in this category of patient even if no mandibular abnormalities are apparent.

A facial nerve monitor is always recommended in revision atresia cases. The need for monitoring is self-evident when one anticipates revision of the bony ear canal or middle ear, as the literature indicates that the majority of facial nerve encounters occur while drilling the medial canal.[2,14] Less apparent are the possible risks to the extratemporal facial nerve, which not uncommonly runs an aberrant course and is prone to tethering to the soft tissues by postoperative scarring. The use of the monitor also allows for the use of an evoked electromyogram (EEMG) nerve stimulator for identification, should a nervelike structure encroach upon the reconstructive field. A further, more subtle advantage to the use of the facial nerve monitor is the additional assurance it gives to the parents during preoperative counseling.

The surgical approach typically proceeds through careful removal of the skin incision created at the previous atresia surgery. Removal of the scar with a very narrow cuff of normal tissue (1 mm) rather than through the scar allows for the optimal cosmetic closure. One uncommon exception to this approach would be to plan a postauricular incision in the patient who has an unobtrusive and mature preauricular skin incision from the previous surgery.

Once the temporal bone is exposed and tissues retracted, the anterior approach is recommended, as previously described.[1,4] Even when the planned procedure is primarily replacement of the canal skin graft, this wide exposure through a postauricular incision is recommended, as the careful placement of the graft is difficult in a transcanal approach. As in the primary procedure, the bony EAC and soft tissue meatus should be widened until they are ~2 times the normal diameter or at least 10 to 11 mm, while maintaining whatever conchal cartilaginous support is present. This canalplasty aids in reducing postoperative stenosis and improves subsequent middle ear exposure. The drill is used to remove any remaining atretic plate or regrowth of bone ankylosing the ossicular chain. Any fibrous attachments to the lateral ossicular mass are sharply dissected to avoid excursion or rotation of the ossicular chain. An interesting modality that was described for this use is the CO_2 laser.[7] Assuming appropriate precautions are taken to avoid generation of that and possible ossicular necrosis, this "no touch" technique may confer significant advantages for this stage of the procedure.

Because of the aforementioned likelihood of significantly poorer hearing results in prosthetic reconstruction, a conservative approach to the native ossicular chain is recommended. If examination indicates that the lateral ossicular chain is not functionally connected to the stapes footplate, it should be removed. If the patient undergoing revision has a large conductive loss and the surgeon has confidently excluded other conductive apparatus pathology (e.g., TM lateralization), the lateral ossicular mass must be removed. This maneuver allows a direct approach to the oval window for an attempt at repair of the hearing mechanism. Finally, in the exceptionally deformed ear in which the lateral ossicular mass lies directly medial to the temporomandibular joint, one may need to remove the lateral chain to allow neo-TM reconstruction.[3,4]

Following evaluation of the lateral ossicular chain, attention is turned to the stapes. In assessing the ossicular chain, an apparent developmental paradox has been noted by several atresia surgeons, namely, that stapes abnormalities are more commonly seen in patients with a relatively less abnormal appearing lateral conductive apparatus (i.e., EAC patent and TM present).[4] This variant conforms to Gill's type IV abnormality (7% of his cases), in which the patient has a "nearly normal" pinna and EAC and normal-appearing TM and malleus handle, yet has a grossly deformed or absent incus and stapes.[5] Again, this corresponds to Colman's group I patients, characterized by the presence of an EAC and TM but abnormality of the stapes.[12] Embryologically, this phenomenon may represent a primary failure of the second arch in the context of relatively normal first arch development; empirically, it suggests that if the lateral sound conduction apparatus appears fairly normal, it likely functions fairly normally, and the primary conductive problem resides in the medial ossicular chain.

In the event that the lateral ossicular chain must be removed and the stapes is functional, several options exist for reconnection of the ossicular chain to the tympanic membrane. The direct myringostapediopexy of neo-TM to the capitulum has a well-documented association with inferior hearing results and is not recommended.[2] At various times a columella has been sculpted from the incus remnant,[2] built out of conchal cartilage blocks,[3] or supplied premade in the form of a partial or total ossicular replacement prosthesis (PORP or TORP),[6] all with similar hearing results. As previously mentioned, the need to reconstruct with a columella, at least in the form of an artificial prosthesis, has been significantly related to suboptimal correction of the CHL. In part this may relate to a commonly seen distortion of the stapes superstructure. From the footplate to the capitulum, the stapes superstructure often demonstrates a significant inferior cant, which, with PORP placement on this type of stapes, leads to significant angulation (from the 180 degree optimum) at the prosthesis–capitulum interface. This angulation may result in suboptimal sound transmission and a propensity for PORP displacement. Therefore, when the stapes is considerably angled, it is preferable to reconstruct with a TORP, leaving the stapes superstructure intact and placing the TORP shaft in the pocket formed between the stapes crura (**Fig. 13.1**).

A much more challenging situation arises when the stapes footplate is determined to be fixed or absent. If the ear is "sterile," one can consider an exposure of the labyrinth. A well-exposed and easily identified footplate invites a stapedotomy-type fenestration procedure if the incus long process can accommodate a piston. More commonly, the incus long process is deficient, and a TORP or similar columella must be used for reconstruction. In the absence of an oval window, a fenestra into the vestibule may be attempted using the external genu of the facial nerve as a guide. With a low-speed drill and appropriate care, it is possible to remove bone while leaving the endosteum intact. If, however, the vestibule is opened, reconstruction requires the placement of a TORP on a membrane overlying the perilymph space. This scenario

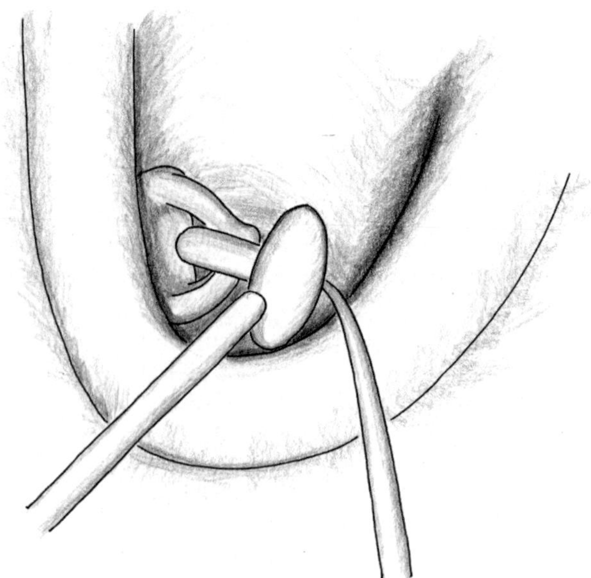

Fig. 13.1 Placement of a total ossicular replacement prosthesis (TORP) between the crura of the inferiorly canted stapes superstructure.

entails some inner ear risk. As the neo-TM heals, a small lateral or medial shift of an attached prosthesis could occur, causing a perilymph leak or injure the membranous labyrinth. Accordingly, some surgeons maintain that any procedure that involves exposing the vestibule is best performed in two stages over 6 to 12 months, with TM grafting during the initial procedure. Such reconstructions have an excellent chance of restoring near-normal hearing in the short term; however, the conductive deficit tends to return over time.[15] This deterioration is likely due to adhesion or displacement of the medial contact point of the TORP or bony regrowth of the periosteal layer of the otic capsule. If such factors can be controlled, the drill-out procedure may allow marked hearing improvement in the patient who is otherwise not surgically improvable. If the patient declines a second-stage procedure after the TM has been reconstructed, an ear-level air conduction hearing aid may be employed to minimize the hearing deficit.

Due to the close interaction of the facial nerve and the second branchial arch structures during middle ear development, one commonly finds that the problem of the missing stapes or absent footplate connection is compounded (and most likely induced) by an overhanging facial nerve. In some series, such a situation was grounds for terminating the hearing reconstruction procedure.[7,8] More frequently, a horizontal canal fenestration procedure was performed. In theory this situation seems to be an ideal indication for the procedure, particularly when the middle ear space is directly medial to the transmandibular joint (TMJ), placing the fenestra in the center of the neo-EAC. Unfortunately, however, in the atresia population, the hearing results postfenestration are frequently unsatisfying. In one series, one of three patients undergoing fenestration achieved normal hearing, whereas the other two averaged a 42 dB conductive deficit, prompting the authors to abandon fenestration in atresia cases.[7] Other series report one patient obtaining no improvement in his 55 dB conductive deficit following fenestration,[4] and a second patient improving to a 43 dB PTA.[8] Bellucci was able to achieve somewhat better results, stating that the hearing results following autograft reconstruction to the stapes head and fenestration were "approximately the same."[9] The number of fenestrations in Bellucci's series, 26, is far higher than the other atresia surgeons surveyed and is perhaps a reflection on his comparative familiarity with the procedure. Of his patients, 15 (57%) maintained a PTA of ≤ 30 dB for 2 years postoperatively. Two patients (8%) had no hearing improvement, and in 8% the PTA regressed to the 40 dB level over the first 2 postoperative years, a phenomenon attributed to bony reclosure of the fenestra. With the exception of this last series, the results of fenestration in atresia repair have been generally disappointing compared with those in otosclerosis. Reports of senior otosclerosis surgeons indicate that with the fenestration procedure, they were able to consistently reduce the conductive deficit to 20 to 25 dB, allowing near-normal hearing levels to be achieved.[15,16] Possibly differences in the patient populations (one mostly adults with essentially normal, undiseased ears; the other largely children with metabolically active bone and a juvenile propensity for ear infections) are factors critical to the disparity in results.

Occasionally, one may find the facial nerve inferiorly displaced and completely obstructing the oval window. In such cases, the stapes superstructure is usually deformed and rudimentary. Access to the oval window to assess patency and for reconstruction can be achieved by transposition of the nerve at the external genu (**Fig. 13.2**). In Jahrsdoerfer's 12 published cases, only 1 patient suffered any facial weakness, a temporary paresis that resolved after 1 month.[14,17] In the first four patients who underwent this procedure, reconstruction of one was deferred because of excessive footplate mobility, but two of the three that were reconstructed averaged a 30 dB postoperative gain (in one of these, the prosthesis ultimately extruded).[17] The criteria for consideration of the procedure are bilateral atresia (with poor contralateral hearing performance), CT evidence of a patent oval window, lack of large feeder vessels to the external genu, and the use of facial nerve monitoring. Given the excellent initial success of this procedure and these patient selection guidelines, the atresia surgeon has the opportunity to construct a transformer mechanism to a functional stapes footplate, a

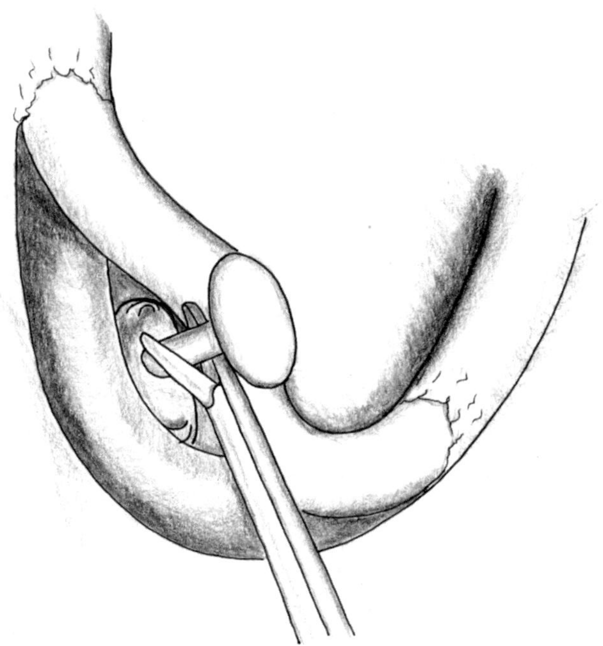

Fig. 13.2 TORP placement on the stapes footplate following anterior transposition of the external genu of the facial nerve.

potentially significant advantage over a fenestration approach. Furthermore, this reconstruction method avoids some problems related to the anatomy of the fenestration: the potential for endosteal "ballooning,"[15] the risk of serous or purulent labyrinthitis following otitis media, the need for careful postoperative cleaning and strict water precautions, and the occasional vertiginous episode.

After appropriately addressing the ossicular chain concerns, closure is performed in the manner previously published,[6] with special attention to the following details. The neo-TM is reconstructed with a temporalis fascia scaffold, taking care to tuck the anterior and superior edges into the middle ear space to inhibit lateralization. If no anterior sulcus is present, one may be fashioned with diamond burs and the fascia graft carefully laid onto it with minimal overlap of the anterior canal wall. The external meatus is constructed using a short anteriorly pedicled "tragal" skin flap, which does not compromise the conchal cartilaginous rim. By swinging this flap medially for use as the anterolateral neo-EAC covering, a staggered "stairstep" suture line is created, inhibiting the tendency for meatal stenosis (**Fig. 13.3**). A 0.008 inch skin graft is used to line the ear canal; the thin edge that typically occurs following harvest with the electric dermatome is placed medially to cover the neo-TM with the thinnest possible skin. As stressed by virtually every atresia surgeon, article, meticulous coverage of all surfaces of the neo-TM/neo-EAC complex is critical to avoid

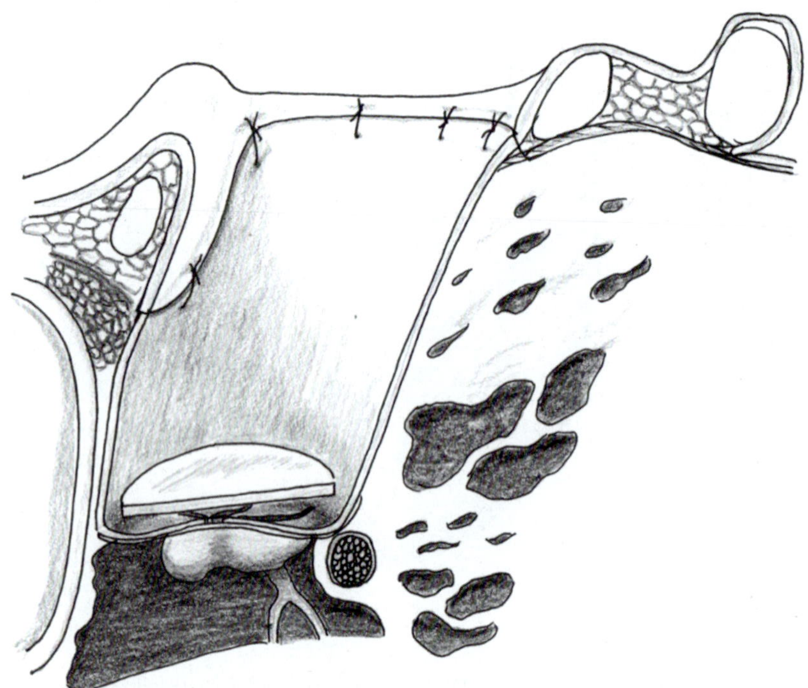

Fig. 13.3 Schematic transverse cross section through a reconstructed atresia ear. Note the anteriorly pedicled skin flap and the Silastic disk placed on the reconstructed tympanic membrane. Merocel wicks have been omitted from the drawing for clarity.

postoperative granulations and stenosis. A 0.040 inch thick Silastic disk 2 to 3 mm smaller in diameter than the neo-TM is placed directly over the skin-grafted eardrum and tucked against the anterior sulcus. This disk helps to minimize trauma to the thin skin during postoperative pack removal and to enhance drum attachment to the anterior sulcus. To hold the medial skin graft in position, the bony ear canal is packed with polyvinyl alcohol formaldehyde foam (Merocel) ear wicks trimmed to an appropriate length and hydrated with neomycin-polymyxin-cortisone suspension. After suture fixation of the lateral edge of the skin graft, the lateral (membranous) ear canal is similarly packed. All packing is removed 7 to 10 days postoperatively.

Early stenosis of the neo-EAC typically occurs at the external meatal suture line, where it is accessible for injection of small amounts (0.3–0.5 mL) of triamcinolone 40 mg/mL suspension. This may be repeated several times at 3 to 4 week intervals. Uncommonly, anterior enlargement of the ear canal during surgery results in penetration of the parotid capsule. This in turn may allow the development of a small but annoying parotid-EAC fistula. Conservative treatment, including a canal stent to lightly apply pressure and short-term glycopyrrolate (Robinul) use, is usually effective in resolving this complication. To minimize the possibility of this development, one should cover all but the smallest breaches of the parotid capsule with fascia to reinforce the skin graft–tragal flap suture line.

Future Directions

In the future, technological advances may allow a surgical approach to patients with deformities now considered too severe for operative intervention. Refinement in implantable materials and local application of biological modifiers of healing may reduce postoperative adhesions, fibrosis, and stenosis. Improved imaging sensitivity and refinement of real-time image-guided surgery may allow a substantial breakthrough in atresia surgery, allowing the surgeon to confidently drill through the nonpneumatized middle ear in an approach to the labyrinth. Bellucci's "experimental" approach to the severely constricted temporal bone, constructing an ear canal by raising the dura, awaits further elaboration.[9] The selective revival of the fenestration procedure, the refinement of the oval window drill-out, and the appropriate use of facial nerve transposition are techniques that may allow the continued advancement of the art of atresia surgery.

Conclusion

Revision atresia surgery, in distinction even to other forms of revision surgery, requires meticulous assessment and planning. It also necessitates extensive counseling to ensure that the patient has realistic expectations and a reasonable understanding of the surgical risks, and to allow the surgeon a confident sense of patient preferences.

This, in turn, allows the revision atresia surgeon the flexibility in intraoperative decision making that is necessary for the best attempt at hearing rehabilitation. A methodical, stepwise surgical approach is counseled to avoid neglecting significant details, with appropriate exercise of caution and maintenance of adequate exposure. Finally, scrupulous attention to postoperative care, particularly in the immediate postoperative period and for the first 1 to 2 years thereafter, is necessary to give each patient the optimal chance for healing and hearing rehabilitation.

References

1. Lambert PR. Major congenital ear malformations: surgical management and results. Ann Otol Rhinol Laryngol 1988;97:641–649.
2. Schuknecht HF. Congenital aural atresia. Laryngoscope 1989;99:908–917.
3. De la Cruz A, Linthicum FH Jr, Luxford WM. Congenital atresia of the external auditory canal. Laryngoscope 1985;95:421–427.
4. Jahrsdoerfer RA. Congenital atresia of the ear. Laryngoscope 1978;88(13 Suppl):1–48.
5. Gill NW. Congenital atresia of the ear: a review of the surgical findings in 83 cases. J Laryngol Otol 1969;83:551–587.
6. Lambert PR. Congenital aural atresia: stability of surgical results. Laryngoscope 1998;108:1801–1805.
7. Chandrasekhar SS, De la Cruz A, Garrido E. Surgery of congenital aural atresia. Am J Otol 1995;16:713–717.
8. Crabtree JA. Tympanoplastic techniques in congenital atresia. Arch Otolaryngol 1968;88:63–70.
9. Bellucci RJ. Congenital aural malformations: diagnosis and treatment. Otolaryngol Clin North Am 1981;14(1):95–124.
10. Molony TB, De la Cruz A. Surgical approaches to congenital atresia of the external auditory canal. Otolaryngol Head Neck Surg 1990;103:991–1001.
11. Jahrsdoerfer RA, Yeakley JW, Aguilar EA, Cole RR, Gray LC. Grading system for the selection of patients with congenital aural atresia. Am J Otol 1992;13:6–12.
12. Glasscock ME III, Schwaber MK, Nissen AJ, Jackson CG. Management of congenital ear malformations. Ann Otol Rhinol Laryngol 1983;92:504–509.
13. Glasscock ME III, Shambaugh GE Jr. Surgery of the Ear. 4th ed. Philadelphia: WB Saunders; 1990:408–418.
14. Jahrsdoerfer RA, Lambert PR. Facial nerve injury in congenital aural atresia surgery. Am J Otol 1998;19:283–287.
15. Shambaugh GE Jr, Wiet RJ. The fenestration operation in 1979. Am J Otol 1979;1:1–6.
16. Masciotra NJ, Caparosa RJ. A comparison of fenestration of the horizontal canal and stapedectomy in the opposite ear. Laryngoscope 1978;88:1725–1731.
17. Jahrsdoerfer RA. Transposition of the facial nerve in congenital aural atresia. Am J Otol 1995;16:290–294.

Decision tree for revision facial nerve injury

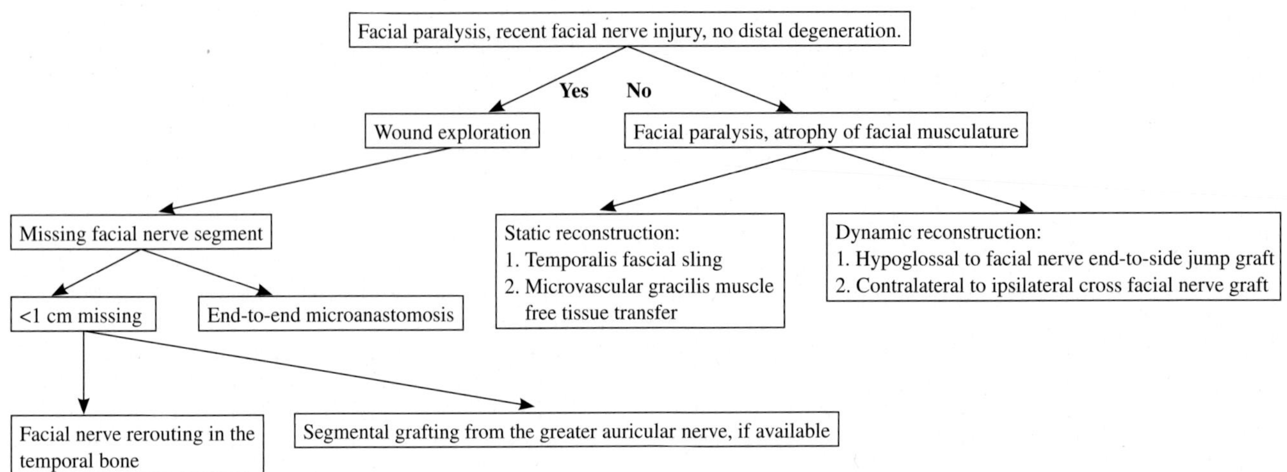

Revision Facial Nerve Surgery

Simon Ellul and Clough Shelton

Most revision otologic and neuro-otologic surgery requires some attention to the facial nerve. Revision surgery on and around the facial nerve is particularly challenging because the landmarks that guide the surgeon to the location of the facial nerve in primary surgery have often been altered or are completely absent in the revision case. This may be compounded by fibrosis, scar, or the recurrence of disease closer to the nerve than before. Surgeons experienced with revision surgery involving the facial nerve are aware of these difficulties, so in primary procedures where revision may be a possibility at some later time, all attempts are made to preserve the normal architecture.

An essential requirement to perform revision surgery and avoid injury to the facial nerve is a thorough knowledge of temporal bone anatomy at those landmarks, which can be used to pinpoint the location of the facial nerve. Continuous electromyography (EMG) facial nerve monitoring is a valuable adjunct in this difficult surgery.

Review of the Anatomy of the Facial Nerve

The seventh cranial nerve (CN VII) exits the brainstem at the pontomedullary groove medial to the root entry zone of the vestibulo-cochlear nerve. It joins the nervus intermedius and eighth cranial nerve (CN VIII) traveling through the pontine cistern before passing into the porus of the internal auditory canal. A loop of the anteroinferior cerebellar artery (AICA) often passes into the medial portion of the internal auditory canal, where it gives off the labyrinthine artery to the inner ear. In this region the loop of the AICA may lie in the plane between the facial nerve anteriorly and the vestibular nerve posteriorly. The facial nerve then courses in the anterosuperior position of the internal auditory canal to pass above the transverse crest and anterior to Bill's bar before passing through the meatal foramen at the lateral end of the internal auditory canal. At the meatal foramen, the dura continues as the epineurial sheath of the facial nerve and contains portions of the arterial supply, including branches of the superior petrosal artery from the AICA and the stylomastoid artery, a branch of the postauricular artery supplying the distal portion of the nerve. In addition, venous plexuses are found within the epineurium. The intracranial portion, in contrast, lacks an epineurium and is therefore less resistant to mechanical manipulation. The labyrinthine portion distal to the meatal foramen courses over the cochlea to the geniculate ganglion, where it gives off the greater superficial petrosal nerve, which carries parasympathetic secretomotor fibers ultimately destined for the lacrimal gland. The facial nerve then turns posteriorly and courses along the medial wall of the middle ear, passing superior to the cochleariform process and over the superior margin of the oval window. Dehiscence of the bony canal has a reported incidence of up to 50%, with the most common area of dehiscence being located over the oval window.[1] The nerve then turns inferiorly, passing inferior and medial to the lateral semicircular canal to run down to the stylomastoid foramen. In this vertical segment it gives off (in order from superior to inferior) the motor branch to the stapedius muscle, a sensory branch to the skin of the external auditory canal, and the chorda tympani nerve. Upon exiting from the temporal bone through the stylomastoid foramen, it gives off motor branches to the auricularis posterior muscle and the posterior belly of the digastric muscle. It then passes into the substance of the parotid gland, where it divides into three upper divisions and two lower divisions to form the pes anserinus.

Facial Nerve Monitoring

Currently, facial nerve monitoring is used commonly when the surgical dissection directly involves the facial nerve, or when the nerve is at risk because of unusual location or other factors. There is no consensus regarding its role in revision middle ear or mastoid surgery,[2] nor are there any data supporting its efficacy in these situations. EMG-based facial nerve monitoring offers crucial scrutiny when compared with sonar-based systems.

Some experts advocate use of facial nerve monitoring in revision middle ear and mastoid surgery when there were problems with the facial nerve at the initial surgery, such as a postoperative paralysis. During revision of these cases, care should be taken to avoid inadvertently anesthetizing the facial nerve with injections of lidocaine and epinephrine, which would not only render the facial nerve monitoring useless, but turn it into a liability and potentially put the facial nerve at higher risk for injury. In revision cases requiring external auditory canal injections or cases where there is a mastoid cavity, we use injections of epinephrine diluted to 1:100,000 without lidocaine for hemostasis. This avoids the problem of inadvertent anesthesia to the facial nerve.

If facial nerve monitoring is to be used in a patient with a preoperative partial facial weakness, one must place the monitoring electrodes in areas of the face with the maximal amounts of facial nerve movement. In these cases, higher than usual levels of current may be required when stimulating the nerve.

Lastly, it cannot be overstressed that the anesthetic staff understand that a facial nerve monitor is being used and that they avoid the use of paralyzing drugs, except for a short activity agent at the time of induction of anesthesia.

Revision Surgeries in which the Facial Nerve May Be at Risk

Mastoid Surgery for Chronic Otitis Media

In revision mastoid surgery for chronic otitis media, preoperative computed tomography (CT) scanning to identify the facial nerve may not be very helpful, because the soft tissue that is invariably present can make it difficult to determine if the facial nerve is dehiscent. Recurrent or residual cholesteatoma in a previous intact canal wall mastoidectomy is not unusual and may be removed at the planned second stage (12 months after the primary surgery) via the tympanotomy and facial recess. Although the facial nerve is usually at risk in the area of the facial recess and epitympanum (**Fig. 14.1**), the tympanic segment of the facial nerve has the highest incidence of iatrogenic facial nerve injury during mastoid surgery.[3] Areas of dehiscence created by either the disease process (cholesteatoma) or the surgery should be noted at the primary procedure so that care may be taken in those areas at the second stage or during revision surgery.

Risk to the facial nerve is more significant when revising a canal wall down mastoidectomy. For example, canal incisions should be made lateral to the location of the facial nerve to avoid injury. To achieve this, the bulge of the lateral semicircular canal should be used as a guide to the location of the facial nerve and the incisions made posterior and to this region. The tympanomeatal flap should be elevated carefully over the lateral semicircular canal and forward over the facial ridge. Initial elevation of the flap over the inferior aspect of the facial ridge generally avoids the facial nerve, as the residual bone is usually thicker at that point.

The bone over the facial nerve should be palpated with a blunt instrument, such as a gimmick elevator or the side of a sickle knife. Skin over a dehiscent facial nerve should

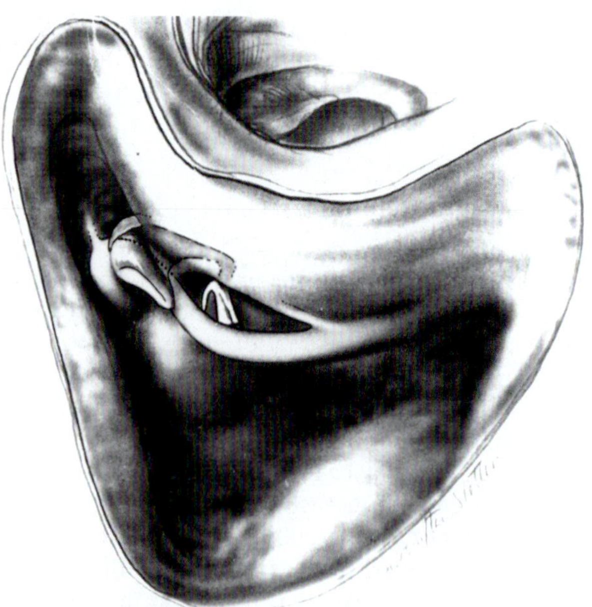

Fig. 14.1 The course of the facial nerve is depicted for a right canal wall up mastoidectomy with the facial recess open. Recurrent cholesteatoma involving the mastoid tends to occur in areas of the facial recess and epitympanum and therefore adjacent to the facial nerve through its course in these areas. (From Brackmann DE, Shelton C, Arriaga MA, eds. Otologic Surgery. Philadelphia: WB Saunders; 2001. Reprinted with permission.)

readily dissect away from the sheath of the nerve unless the sheath and/or nerve had been injured during the previous surgery. In this situation a facial nerve monitor and stimulating probe are very useful to aid identification of the nerve. Once the middle ear cleft is entered, secondary landmarks, such as the oval window (immediately inferior to the facial nerve) and cochleariform process (immediately inferior and anterior to the facial nerve), are used to pinpoint the course of the facial nerve. Once the course of the nerve is appreciated, the recidivistic cholesteatoma can be safely removed.

Middle Ear Surgery

The facial nerve may be vulnerable during revision stapedectomy or ossiculoplasty surgery if dehiscent and/or prolapsed over the oval window.

It is important to recognize early in the operation if the facial nerve is dehiscent. This can be determined by palpation (**Fig. 14.2**). Facial nerve identification can be difficult in revision cases due to the distortion of the anatomy by fibrous tissue. The cochleariform process is a useful landmark to locate the anterosuperior aspect of the oval window. The facial nerve will be directly superior and posterior to the cochleariform process. Initial identification of the inferior margin of the oval window can allow for its identification in a circumferential fashion, which

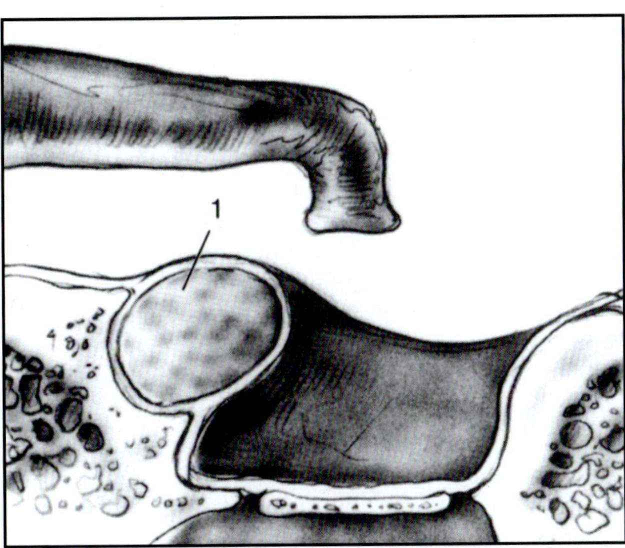

Fig. 14.2 Dehiscent facial nerve shown overhanging the oval window. In this situation, identification of the facial nerve is important, but it is generally possible to work past it to complete the operation. (From Brackmann DE, Shelton C, Arriaga MA, eds. Otologic Surgery. Philadelphia: WB Saunders; 2001. Reprinted with permission.)

will also allow identification of the facial nerve. Particularly in revision stapedectomy surgery, adequate removal of the bone of the scutum will permit adequate visualization of the anatomy in this area.

Before using a laser in the oval window, it is important to determine whether it is dehiscent and what its location is in relationship to the previously placed prosthesis. Laser facial nerve injury is very rare, but it is a potential pitfall best avoided.

Glomus Tumors

Revision surgery for glomus tumors is particularly difficult when an infratemporal fossa approach was used during the primary surgery, as this involves closure of the ear canal and transposition of the facial nerve. Furthermore, the facial nerve may be surrounded by a fat graft. After making skin incisions, the surgeon should try to identify the margins of the bony defect. The mastoid tip is absent, as it is typically removed during the initial procedure. The superior bony margin is usually intact, and one can follow it forward to the root of the zygoma and temporomandibular joint. With these landmarks, the middle fossa dural plate (or dura) is traced medially. Once the labyrinth is identified, the facial nerve can be found just superior to the cochleariform process (**Fig. 14.3**). The nerve is typically in the normal anatomical position in this area, and may also be found in the remnant of the fallopian canal in its horizontal portion, if it was replaced in that location at the previous procedure. The facial nerve usually separates from the surrounding fat graft and can be verified using the facial nerve monitor. Inferior to the mastoid genu, there is no bony support for the nerve, and it tends to be surrounded by fat and fibrous tissue. It is necessary to mobilize the facial nerve enough

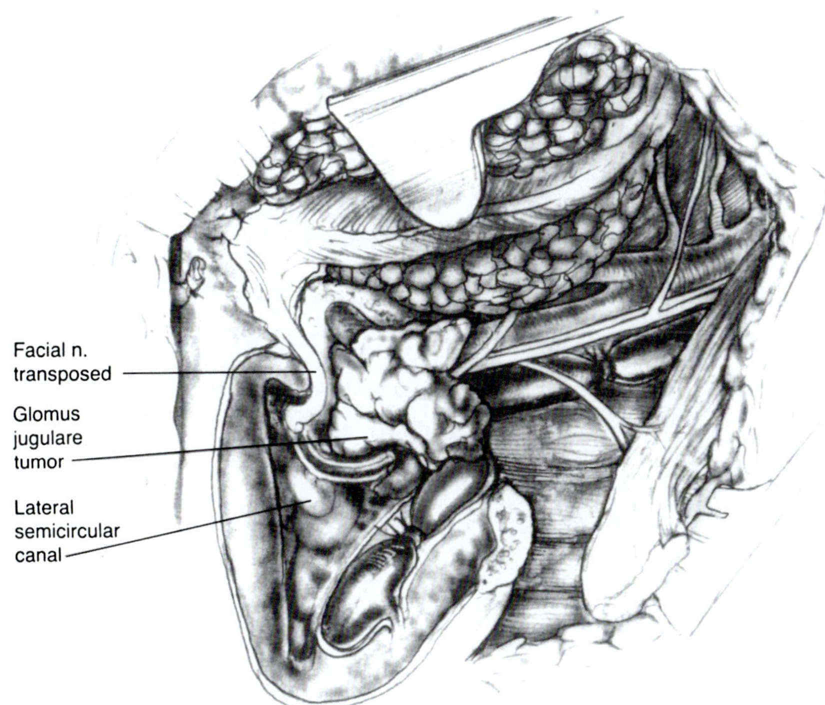

Fig. 14.3 Infratemporal fossa approach for a right ear. Note the bony margin of the mastoid cavity superiorly along the middle fossa dural plate. The facial nerve is shown transposed, but it remains in the normal anatomical position adjacent to the cochleariform process and can be identified in this area. (From Brackmann DE, Shelton C, Arriaga MA, eds. Otologic Surgery. Philadelphia: WB Saunders; 2001. Reprinted with permission.)

to transpose it anteriorly, but it does not have to be skeletonized, and some fat and fibrous tissue can be left attached, as long as its bulk does not impede visualization.

More commonly, recurrent glomus jugulare tumors occur when the initial surgeon has been timid in exposing the tumor. In these situations, the facial nerve has not been transposed, and much of the normal bony anatomy remains. Typically, a full infratemporal fossa approach is required at revision, but the surgeon must be aware of areas of facial nerve exposure from the previous surgery.

Recurrence of glomus tympanicum tumors is typically related to inadequate exposure during an initial transcanal removal. Removal of these tumors through an extended facial recess approach usually provides the adequate access.[4]

Acoustic Tumors

Recurrent acoustic tumors are uncommon, with the majority reported after initial retrosigmoid removal.[5] Residual tumor left behind in the internal auditory canal is generally felt to be responsible for these recurrences.[6] Tumor recurrence after initial complete translabyrinthine removal is very rare and occurs in less than 1% of cases.[7,8] After middle fossa removal, there have only been scattered reports of recurrences identified.

For removal of recurrent acoustic tumors, we prefer the translabyrinthine approach, as it provides positive intratemporal facial nerve identification in a location not involved with previous scar tissue and with very predictable anatomy.

Scar tissue in the posterior fossa can obscure the proximal facial nerve location and make its identification more difficult. Facial nerve monitoring is very helpful in these cases as well. The facial nerve is identified laterally at Bill's bar (**Fig. 14.4**), and the dissection can proceed medially into the posterior fossa, although the manipulation of the facial nerve should be in a lateral direction to prevent neuropraxia due to traction. Sharp dissection is required at times to separate the facial nerve from fibrous tissue, which can also obscure important posterior fossa blood vessels. In a series of five recurrent acoustic tumors reported in 1995 and removed through the translabyrinthine approach, all patients with preoperatively intact facial nerves had preservation of the nerves postoperatively.[7]

When surgery is performed to treat cerebrospinal fluid (CSF) leaks following acoustic tumor surgery, careful repacking with fat can usually be performed without having to expose the intracranial portion of the nerve.

Congenital Aural Atresia

Congenital aural atresia is due to the absence of the development of the tympanic portion of the temporal bone.

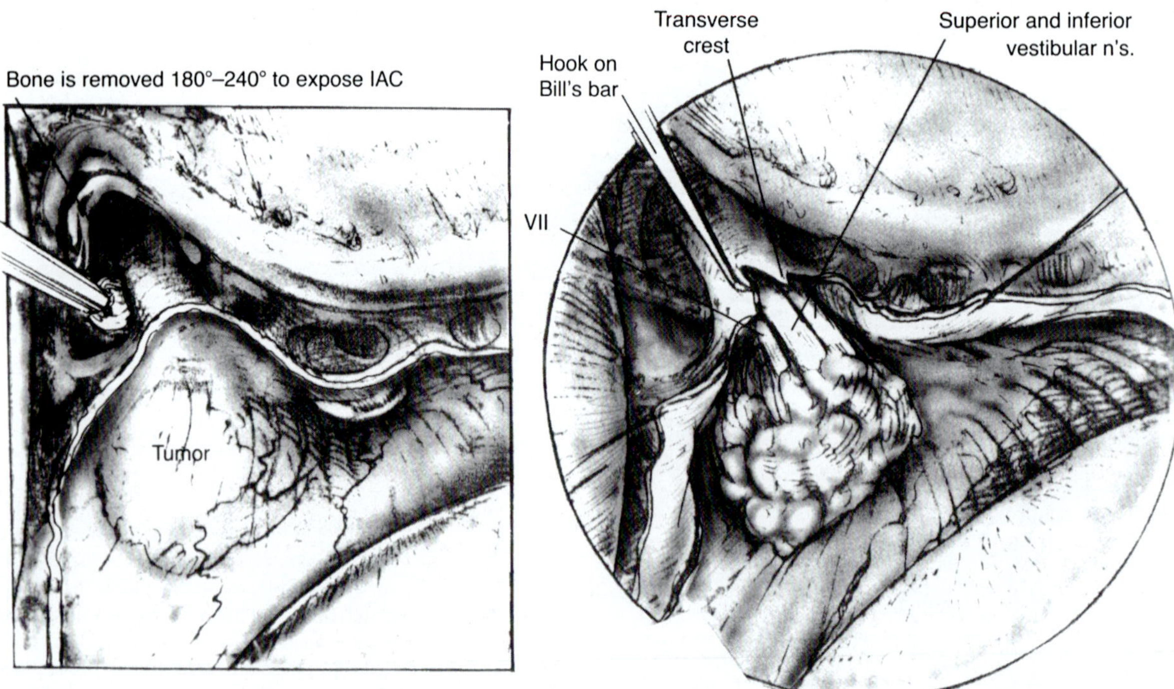

Fig. 14.4 Translabyrinthine approach with Bill's bar identified adjacent to the facial nerve. In this drawing, the vestibular nerves are still intact. For recurrent acoustic tumors, these nerves may or may not be present at the revision operation. IAC, internal auditory canal. (From Brackmann DE, Shelton C, Arriaga MA, eds. Otologic Surgery. Philadelphia: WB Saunders; 2001. Reprinted with permission.)

Normally, the facial nerve can be thought to turn or "genu" around the tympanic bone when transitioning from its tympanic to its ventral segment. With an absent tympanic bone portion of the temporal bone, the facial nerve turns anteriorly after making its second genu and often exits the temporal bone near the temporomandibular joint.

Revision surgery may be required following previous atresia surgery. The most common indication will be lateralization of the tympanic membrane and stenosis of the external auditory canal.[9] In revision congenital atresia cases, the facial nerve is particularly vulnerable along its vertical segment, especially if the nerve has an anterior and/or lateral course. Great care must be taken in this situation, as the facial nerve may lie very close to the surface of the bony external auditory canal. High-resolution computed tomography (CT) of the temporal bone may be useful to demonstrate the course of the facial nerve and determine its proximity to the posterior canal wall. Continuous facial nerve monitoring will be valuable to prevent injury during elevation and excision of the stenotic canal skin. Furthermore, radiologic evaluation may identify an unfavorable facial nerve location that may have been responsible for failure of the initial procedure, and may preclude successful revision.

Cochlear Implants

At revision surgery for a cochlear implant in the area of the facial recess, one should assume the facial nerve is exposed in this area from previous surgery. Often there is typically soft tissue in the recess, due to either postoperative fibrosis or muscle placed there at the first surgery in conjunction with closure of the cochleostomy. The soft tissue should be separated from the margins of the recess, but even if the facial nerve is dehiscent, the soft tissue usually separates easily, as long as the epineurium of the nerve is intact. The dissection should proceed parallel to the course of the facial nerve.

If the cochleostomy must be enlarged, care must be taken not to allow the rotating shaft of the drill to contact the facial nerve directly or to heat the bone covering it (**Fig. 14.5**).

Surgeries Primarily Involving the Facial Nerve

Bell Palsy

The need for revision surgery in Bell (or Bell's) palsy is unusual and is usually manifest as recurrent facial palsy in a patient who had previously undergone an inadequate

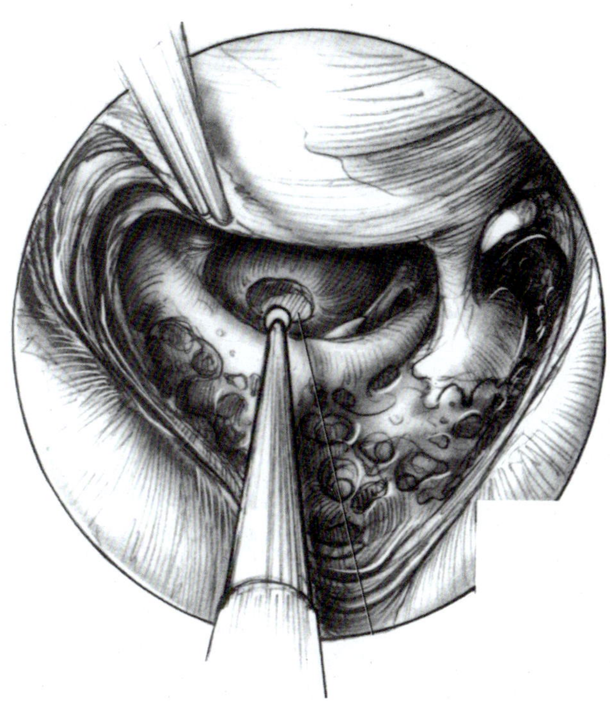

Fig. 14.5 When the cochleostomy is enlarged through the facial recess, care must be taken not to allow the rotating shaft of the bur to contact a dehiscent facial nerve or to heat up the bone of the intact fallopian canal over the facial nerve. (From Brackmann DE, Shelton C, Arriaga MA, eds. Otologic Surgery. Philadelphia: WB Saunders; 2001. Reprinted with permission.)

decompression. Commonly, the previous decompression was limited to the mastoid and tympanic segment only; it can be verified by the presence of a postauricular incision and also by temporal bone CT imaging.

Current recommendations are for middle fossa decompression of the labyrinthine portion of the facial nerve for the patient with acute onset Bell palsy and who reaches > 90% deinnervation on electroneuronography (ENoG) within 14 days of onset.[10] For the typical revision case, surgery has not been performed on the labyrinthine segment of the facial nerve, which is therefore found undisturbed at revision surgery. However, when performing revision surgery in this instance, one must be careful upon elevating the temporal lobe, as there may be a dehiscence of the tegmen from the previous surgery, and the dura can be adherent to the exposed facial nerve in the proximal tympanic segment or the geniculate ganglion. The previously decompressed facial nerve will be abnormal in appearance if the nerve sheath was opened at the earlier operation. The nerve in this case is larger in diameter and looks more like fibrous tissue than the typical appearance of the nerve. Opening the tegmen and finding the heads of the ossicles can be a useful adjunct in determining facial nerve location (**Fig. 14.6**). The geniculate ganglion will be directly anterior to the cochleariform process.

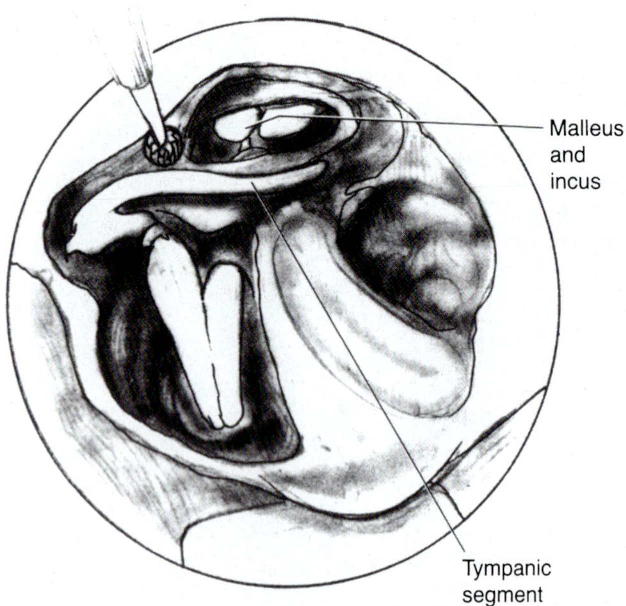

Fig. 14.6 The ossicular heads are exposed through the middle fossa approach. The facial nerve is exposed from the internal auditory canal through the tympanic segment. The geniculate ganglion lies just anterior to the cochleariform process. (From Brackmann DE, Shelton C, Arriaga MA, eds. Otologic Surgery. Philadelphia: WB Saunders; 2001. Reprinted with permission.)

Facial Nerve Trauma

Revision surgery following trauma to the facial nerve usually amounts to some form of reanimation procedure, rather than an attempt to further decompress the nerve. Facial paralysis following temporal bone fracture is more likely with transverse or oblique fractures, but it is seen most frequently in association with longitudinal fractures, because of the much higher frequency of longitudinal fractures compared with transverse fractures. Immediate or complete paralysis with evidence of poor electrical activity on ENoG (degeneration > 90%) is an indication for a primary exploration of the nerve, bony decompression, and appropriate repair of the injured segment.

Indications for reexploration of the nerve are much more poorly defined and may lead to little clinical benefit.

Should these patients recover facial nerve function poorly, the time required to pass to allow for recovery also usually precludes further direct surgery on the facial nerve itself. In these cases, typically a secondary reanimation procedure is performed, such as a hypoglossal-facial nerve anastomosis.

Facial Nerve Tumors

The most common facial nerve tumors are facial nerve neuromas and hemangiomas.[11] Facial nerve neuromas are intrinsic to the facial nerve and usually require resection and repair of the facial nerve for treatment. Hemangiomas are extraneural in nature, and in some cases, the facial nerve can be preserved after tumor resection.

Techniques for facial nerve repair will be discussed below. Causes of failure of return of facial nerve function after facial nerve repair at final nerve tumor resection include issues involved in the repair itself, such as poor approximation of the nerve ends and tension at the nerve anastomosis. Residual tumor at a nerve end can also be responsible for failure of the nerve repair. Frozen section examination of each nerve stump is necessary not only to validate complete tumor removal but also to ensure no tumor remains at the anastomotic site that would impede axonal regrowth.

Patients with preoperative facial nerve dysfunction tend to have worse facial nerve recovery after repair than those who have normal preoperative facial function.[12,13] Facial nerve repair results are adversely correlated with the duration and the severity of preoperative facial nerve weakness.[14] It is likely that the facial nerve nucleus loses trophic strength with prolonged paralysis, leading to poor facial nerve repair results in patients with long-standing dysfunction. Facial nerve tumor patients with long-standing complete paralysis are not likely to have facial nerve recovery with primary repair and may best be reconstructed with an alternative technique such as a hypoglossal-facial nerve anastomosis at the time of tumor resection.

Indications for Revision Surgeries

Revision of surgery done primarily on the facial nerve is rarely indicated, with the exception of decompression of the labyrinthine portion of the facial nerve through the middle fossa approach for a patient with a recurrent Bell palsy, if this had not been done previously (see above).

When Not to Operate

In cases involving facial nerve repair, when sufficient time has been allowed to pass for assessment of recovery (typically 6–12 months), revision of the nerve repair itself is not effective, because of the loss of neural trophism. In patients with long-standing facial paralysis, little recovery is expected from a revision procedure, and the patient is best reanimated by hypoglossal–facial nerve anastomosis. Revision surgery of facial nerve anastomoses is not effective for amelioration of synkinesis or hyperkinesis. These aberrances of facial nerve regeneration are best treated by facial nerve rehabilitation (physical therapy) and by injections of botulinum toxin to hypergenetic regions.

Identification of Causes of Failure That Are Not Correctable

Failure to improve hearing in cases of stapedectomy, ossiculoplasty, and congenital atresia may be due to abnormal location of the facial nerve. If the oval window is covered by the facial nerve, either due to prolapse or an anomalous location of the nerve, it may not be possible to place a prosthesis and achieve hearing improvement. The vagaries of previous operative reports and the ambiguity of high-resolution CT scanning may preclude an accurate determination of the facial nerve anatomy in the area of the oval window preoperatively. This anatomy may best be determined at exploratory tympanotomy.

In some cases of facial nerve prolapse, it may be possible to displace the nerve to place a prosthesis. However, if the facial nerve location is not favorable, the procedure should be terminated.

Delineation of Increased Risk for Revision Surgeries

Patients who experience facial nerve dysfunction after a previous operation are at high risk for facial nerve injury at subsequent surgeries. This generalization pertains particularly to operations of the middle ear and mastoid. Postoperative palsy in this setting would indicate that the facial nerve is at least exposed and that it may have been partially injured at the previous surgery. Mucosa, cholesteatoma, and granulation tissue tend to dissect easily and cleanly from the facial nerve, if the epineurium is intact. A nerve with violated epineurium may have fibrous tissue in the area of injury that is adherent to the surrounding tissues, making clean dissection of surrounding diseased tissues very difficult. In some cases, there may be a traumatic neuroma, which may appear as a mass of fibrous tissue on the nerve and may be difficult to identify intraoperatively. The traumatic neuroma is best left undisturbed. Intraoperative facial nerve monitoring is a useful adjunct.

The intracranial facial nerve has no epineurium, so adhesions at these sites directly involve the nerve fascicles. Dissection of these adhesions poses a high risk to the nerve.

Surgical Techniques to Lower Risk of Failure

Decompression

As mentioned above, for facial nerve decompression to be effective in the treatment of Bell palsy, it must be performed through the middle fossa approach to decompress the labyrinthine segment of the facial nerve. The fallopian canal is narrowest in this area, and this is felt to be the site of involvement in Bell palsy cases. Recent data indicate that this decompression should be performed within the first 14 days of onset if diagnostic criteria are met.[10] The nerve should be exposed as fully as possible; however, in the labyrinthine segment, because of the juxtaposition of the cochlea, wide exposure must be minimized. In this setting, incision of the epineurial sheath is performed, taking care to cut the fibrous bands at the meatal foramen (**Fig. 14.7**). A disposable microblade (Beaver 59–10) is used to perform this neurolysis.

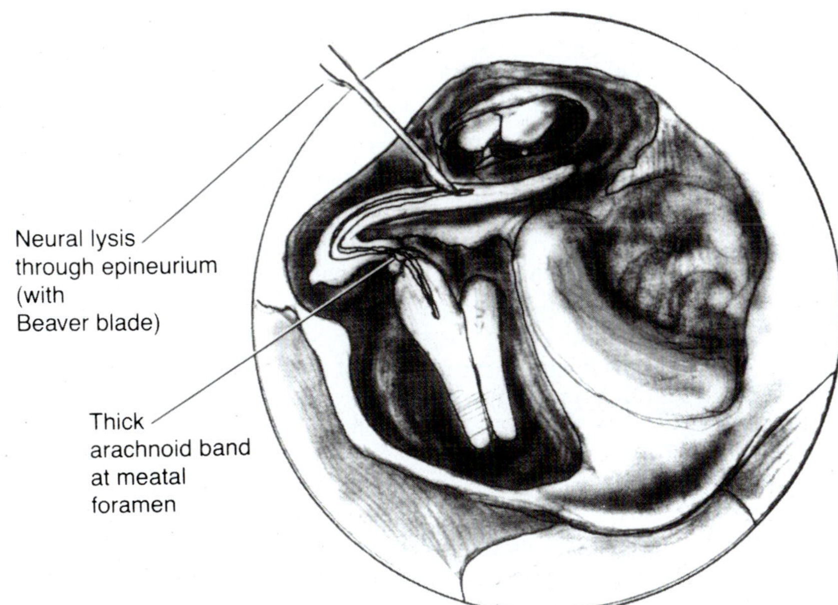

Fig. 14.7 The nerve sheath is incised from the internal auditory canal through the tympanic portion of the facial nerve. (From Brackmann DE, Shelton C, Arriaga MA, eds. Otologic Surgery. Philadelphia: WB Saunders; 2001. Reprinted with permission.)

In cases of trauma to the temporal bone, the role of facial nerve decompression is to explore for neural injury and, if present, to treat. Unlike Bell palsy, decompression for trauma is aimed at the area of injury, not specifically the labyrinthine segment. If the facial nerve is intact and pinned between two displaced bone fragments, decompression will aid in facial nerve recovery. For trauma, incision of the epineural sheath is not routinely performed, but done to explore for intraneural injuries, such as intraneural hematoma, or to extract penetrating bony spicules.

Nerve Anastomosis

The standard technique for intracranial or intratemporal facial nerve repair involves either suture neurorraphy or sutureless approximation of the nerve ends in the trough of the remnant fallopian canal. The foreign body reaction of sutures can adversely affect the anastomotic site, so suturing should be kept to a minimum. Because the intratemporal and intracranial facial nerve is monofascicular, an epineural suture technique is used when indicated. Many sutureless techniques have been tried in the past, including fibrin glue.[15,16] Unfortunately, its adhesive strength is low, and the glue tends to be washed away by pulsating CSF.

A tensionless anastomosis is critical to the success of the nerve repair. When there is doubt regarding the presence of tension at the nerve repair, a nerve graft should be interposed. The results of facial nerve repair using a graft and those of primary anastomosis are similar.

Graft Material

The most common donor nerve for facial nerve grafting is the greater auricular nerve. The donor deficit is minimal, and the diameter match is appropriate. It is adjacent to the operative field, and adequate length can be obtained to graft the facial nerve from the internal auditory canal to the stylomastoid foramen. The greater auricular nerve is located on the lateral surface of the sternocleidomastoid muscle, just posterior to the external jugular vein. It can be found between the angle of the mandible and the tip of the mastoid process (**Fig. 14.8**). Ample length can be obtained by dissecting the nerve from its emergence from the posterior aspect of the sternocleidomastoid muscle.

Another option for a donor nerve is the medial antebrachial cutaneous (MAC) nerve.[17] This nerve is located on the medial surface of the upper arm and is a branch of the medial cord of the brachial plexus. It is found between the junction of the biceps and triceps muscles and parallel to the basilic vein (**Fig. 14.9**). The diameter match is good for the facial nerve, and it has adequate length to graft from the posterior fossa to the extratemporal portion of the nerve. The distal branching pattern of the MAC nerve

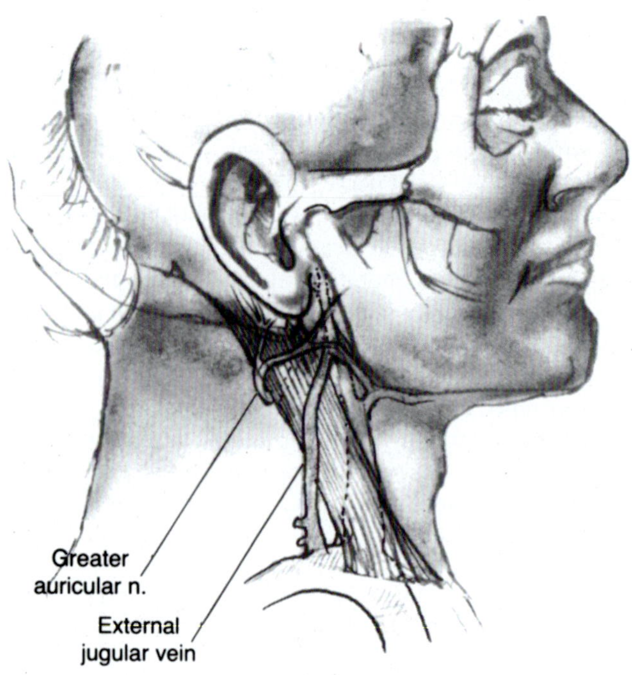

Fig. 14.8 The greater auricular nerve is found on the lateral surface of the sternocleidomastoid muscle between the tip of the mastoid and the angle of the mandible. (From Brackmann DE, Shelton C, Arriaga MA, eds. Otologic Surgery. Philadelphia: WB Saunders; 2001. Reprinted with permission.)

is helpful when nerve grafting must be performed distal to the pes anserinus. Because it is not directly adjacent to the operative site, it can be used in cases involved in the treatment of malignancy.

The sural nerve is another option for a donor grafting nerve (**Fig. 14.10**). It has excellent length but is larger in diameter than the facial nerve. The nerve is found on the lateral aspect of the ankle and can be turned proximally.

When harvesting the donor graft, it is important not to crush it with forceps or exert excessive traction on it. Excessive fibrous tissue and epineurium are trimmed from the nerve stumps, and the nerve ends are cut sharply. A wet tongue blade works well as a surface to prepare the nerve graft. When placing the graft, the nerve direction is reversed to prevent axons from growing out of branches of the graft not involved in the anastomosis. The length of the graft is cut longer than the length of the deficit to ensure a tensionless repair.

Anastomotic Technique

For intratemporal repair, the remnant of the fallopian canal can serve as a trough. The nerve graft can be placed in approximation to the nerve stump, and a sutureless repair can be accomplished (**Fig. 14.11**). Avitene is used to

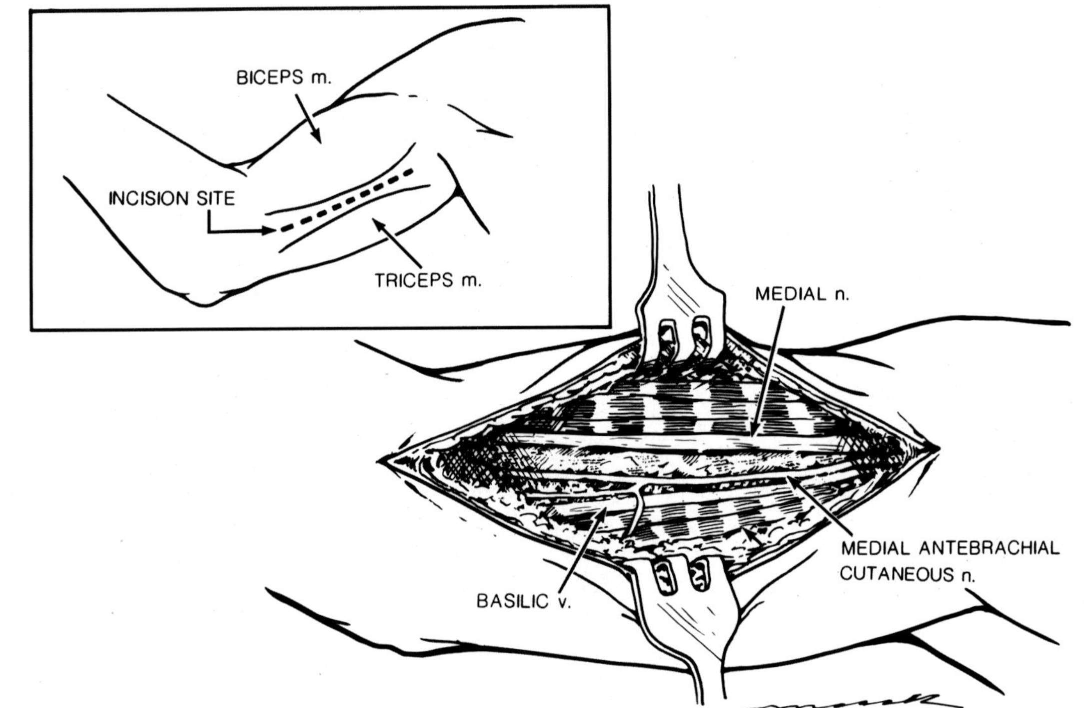

Fig. 14.9 (**A**) For harvesting the medial antebrachial cutaneous nerve, a longitudinal incision begins 2 to 3 cm proximal to the epicondyle and extends between the junction of the biceps and triceps medially. (**B**) The medial antebrachial cutaneous nerve is found running adjacent to the basilic vein. Notice the median nerve running through the dissection site. (From Brackmann DE, Shelton C, Arriaga MA, eds. Otologic Surgery. Philadelphia: WB Saunders; 2001. Reprinted with permission.)

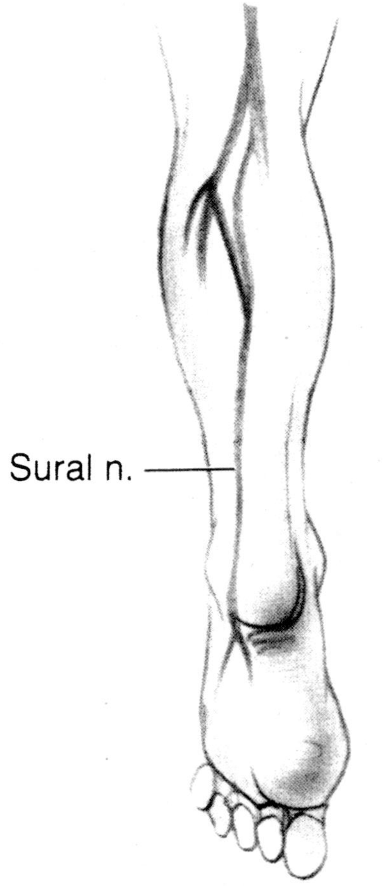

Fig. 14.10 The sural nerve is found at the ankle, just posterior to the lateral malleolus. (From Brackmann DE, Shelton C, Arriaga MA, eds. Otologic Surgery. Philadelphia: WB Saunders; 2001. Reprinted with permission.)

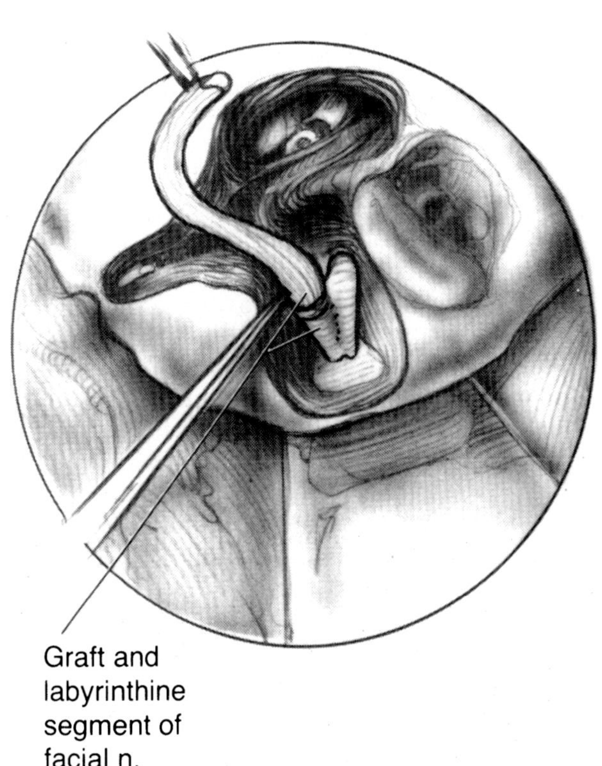

Fig. 14.11 The nerve graft can be approximated to the facial nerve stump using the remnant of the fallopian canal to stabilize the anastomosis. (From Brackmann DE, Shelton C, Arriaga MA, eds. Otologic Surgery. Philadelphia: WB Saunders; 2001. Reprinted with permission.)

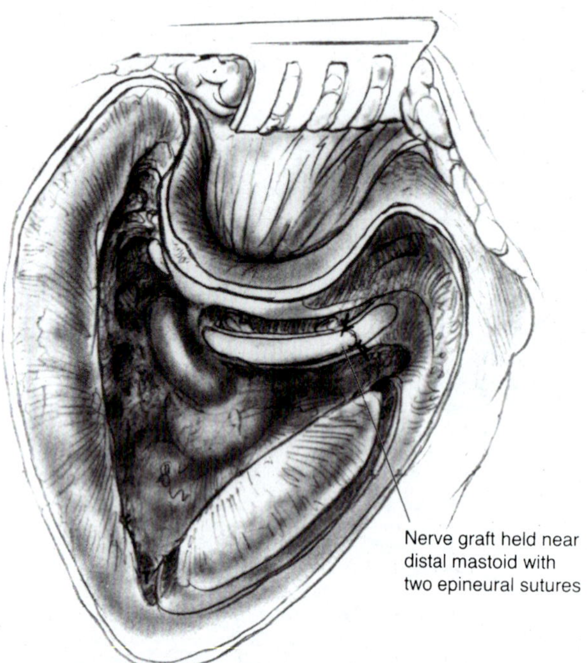

Fig. 14.12 When the fallopian canal trough is not available, the anastomosis is approximated by several epineural sutures. (From Brackmann DE, Shelton C, Arriaga MA, eds. Otologic Surgery. Philadelphia: WB Saunders; 2001. Reprinted with permission.)

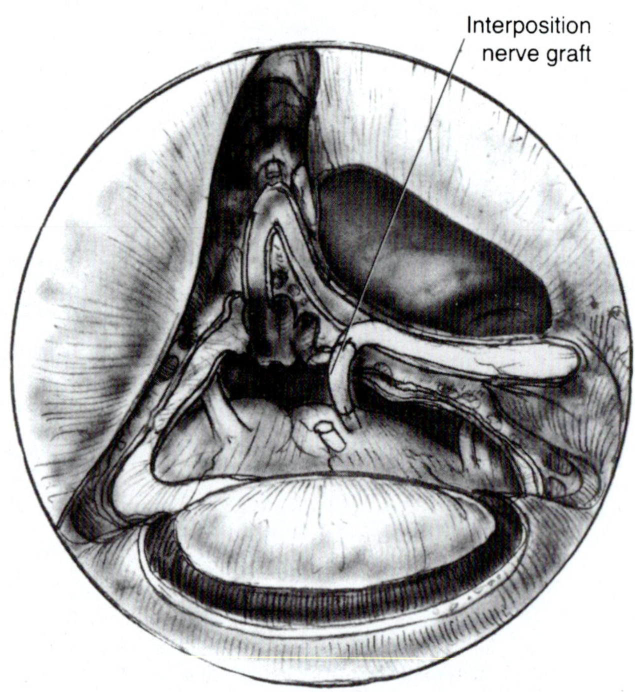

Fig. 14.13 Facial nerve graft placed from the nerve stump in the posterior fossa to the mastoid segment of the facial nerve. (From Brackmann DE, Shelton C, Arriaga MA, eds. Otologic Surgery. Philadelphia: WB Saunders; 2001. Reprinted with permission.)

pack over the anastomosis, forming a blood clot to help stabilize it. When sutures are required, two or three nonabsorbable epineural sutures of 9–0 monofilament work well (**Fig. 14.12**). By trimming the suture length to 4 or 5 inches, it is much easier to work with it under the microscope. Commercially available plastic background material is moistened and placed beneath the anastomosis to give a smooth working surface. When possible, the nerve graft is placed as part of the normal course of the facial nerve.

Because the intracranial facial nerve has no epineurium, the placement of an anastomosis in the internal auditory canal or posterior fossa is more difficult than that performed within the temporal bone (**Fig. 14.13**). Usually, a single through-and-through suture is used for this anastomosis.[18] The distal anastomosis is performed first to stabilize the nerve graft, then a suture is placed through the nerve graft and proximal end. When placing the suture through the intracranial facial nerve stump, a fenestrated suction can be used to support the facial nerve, and the needle is passed into the side hole of the suction (**Fig. 14.14**).[19]

It is possible to gain extra length of the facial nerve by removing it from its course in the fallopian canal and rerouting it. The amount of rerouting can vary, as can the length gains by this maneuver, but rerouting may allow for a primary anastomosis rather than require the use of a nerve graft (**Fig. 14.15**).

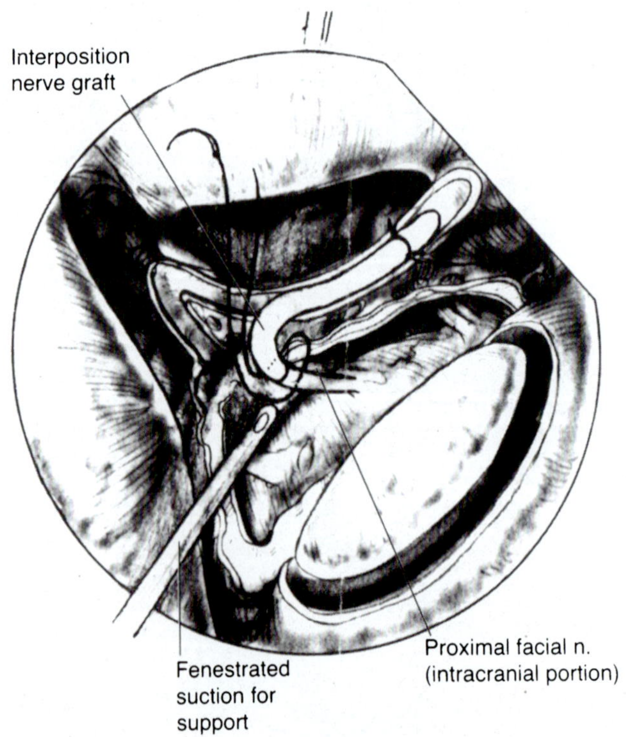

Fig. 14.14 A single through-and-through suture is used for the posterior fossa nerve anastomosis. A fenestrated suction tip is useful to stabilize a graft when placing the suture. (From Brackmann DE, Shelton C, Arriaga MA, eds. Otologic Surgery. Philadelphia: WB Saunders; 2001. Reprinted with permission.)

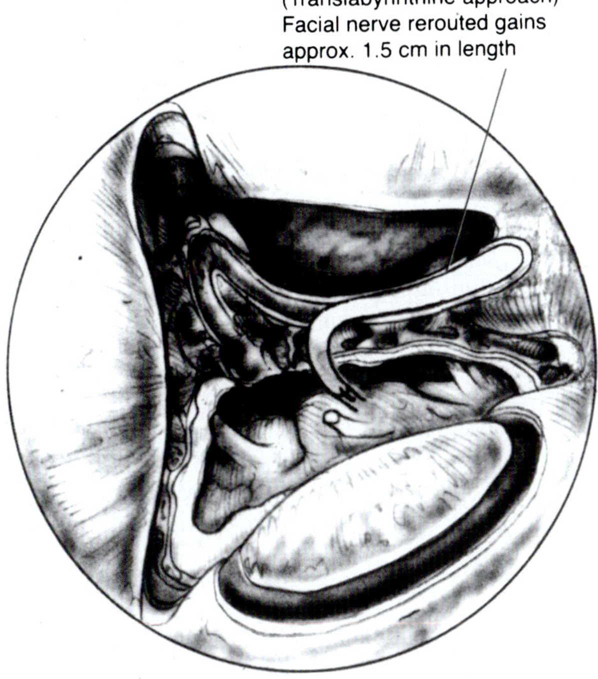

Fig. 14.15 Approximately 1.5 cm of additional facial nerve length can be obtained by removing the facial nerve from its intratemporal course and transposing it into the posterior fossa for a nerve repair. (From Brackmann DE, Shelton C, Arriaga MA, eds. Otologic Surgery. Philadelphia: WB Saunders; 2001. Reprinted with permission.)

Rerouting does disrupt the local blood supply to the nerve and so may be as detrimental as using an interposition graft.

Surgical Alternatives

There exists a wide variety of alternative methods of facial reanimation. The best results can be obtained through direct facial nerve repair. This is the only method of reconstruction that gives both voluntary facial movement and emotional expression. When facial nerve reconstruction is not possible, or if the previous facial nerve repair has not been successful, these alternative methods are very useful.

Nerve substitution surgery provides for excellent tone and symmetry at rest, along with a very robust range of voluntary motion.

The most common nerve substitution used for this purpose is the hypoglossal–facial nerve anastomosis.[20] There has been recent interest in performing a partial hypoglossal–facial nerve anastomosis using an end-to-side nerve graft.[21] This partial technique has the advantage of avoiding tongue atrophy that is associated with the full hypoglossal–facial nerve anastomosis, but it has much less power than that of the full anastomosis. It should be performed very shortly following the onset of the paralysis, possibly in conjunction with an additional reanimation technique.

Reanimation of the eye is an important aspect to rehabilitation of patients with facial paralysis. Several techniques are available, although the two most common are the placement of eyelid weight and an eyelid spring.[22] Both provide for good eye closure and are easily reversible when there has been facial nerve recovery and they are no longer needed.

Muscle transfer techniques, such as temporalis muscle transfer and microvascular free flap reanimation,[23] are typically indicated when the opportunity for a nerve repair or a hypoglossal–facial nerve anastomosis has passed. These techniques are used to reanimate the lower face and provide symmetry at rest and some voluntary motion, although they are not typically as robust as that obtained after a nerve substitution procedure.

References

1. Baxter A. Dehiscence of the fallopian canal: an anatomical study. J Laryngol Otol 1971;85:587–594.
2. Roland P. Intraoperative monitoring: is it the standard of care? In: Shelton C, ed. 12th Annual Cherry Blossom Conference—Facial Nerve Disorders: Update 1999. Alexandria, VA: American Academy of Otolaryngology-Head and Neck Surgery Foundatoin: 1999.
3. Green JD Jr, Shelton C, Brackmann DE. Iatrogenic facial nerve injury during otologic surgery. Laryngoscope 1994;104:922–926.
4. O'Leary MJ, Shelton C, Giddings NA, et al. Glomus tympanicum tumors: a clinical perspective. Laryngoscope 1991;101:1038–1043.
5. Dew LA, Shelton C, Hitselberger WE. Partial vs. total removal of acoustic tumors. In: House WF, Luetje CM, Doyle KJ, eds. Acoustic Tumors Diagnosis and Management. San Diego: Singular Publishing; 1997.
6. Roberson JB Jr, Brackmann DE, Hitselberger WE. Acoustic neuroma recurrence following suboccipital resection: management with translabyrinthine resection. Am J Otol 1996;17:307–311.
7. Shelton C. Unilateral acoustic tumors: how often do they recur after translabyrinthine removal? Laryngoscope 1995;105:958–966.
8. Thedinger BA, Glasscock ME, Cueva RA, et al. Postoperative radiographic evaluation after acoustic neuroma and glomus jugulare tumor removal. Laryngoscope 1992;102:261–266.
9. De la Cruz A, Linthicum FH Jr, Luxford WM. Congenital atresia of the external auditory canal. Laryngoscope 1985;95:421–427.
10. Gantz BJ, Rubinstein JT, Gidley P, Woodworth GC. Surgical management of Bell's palsy. Laryngoscope 1999;109:1177–1188.

11. Shelton C, Brackmann DE, Lo WW, Carberry JN. Intratemporal facial nerve hemangiomas. Otolaryngol Head Neck Surg 1991;104:116–121.

12. O'Donoghue GM, Brackmann DE, House JW, Jackler RK. Neuromas of the facial nerve. Am J Otol 1989;10:49–54.

13. King TT, Morrison AW. Primary facial tumors within the skull. J Neurosurg 1990;72:1–8.

14. Shelton C. Facial nerve tumors. In: Brackmann DE, Shelton C, Arriaga MA, eds., Otologic Surgery. Philadelphia: WB Saunders; 2001.

15. Sames M, Blahos J Jr, Rokyta R, Benes V Jr. Comparison of microsurgical suture with fibrin glue connection of the sciatic nerve in rats. Physiol Res 1997;46:303–306.

16. Maragh H, Meyer BS, Davenport D, Gould JD, Terzis JK. Morphofunctional evaluation of fibrin glue vs. microsuture nerve repair. J Reconstr Microsurg 1990;6:331–337.

17. Haller JR, Shelton C. Medial antebrachial cutaneous nerve: a new donor graft for repair of facial nerve defects at the skull base. Laryngoscope 1997;107:1048–1052.

18. Barrs DM, Brackmann DE, Hitselberger WE. Facial nerve anastomosis in the cerebellopontine angle: a review of 24 cases. Am J Otol 1984;5:269–272.

19. Arriaga MA, Brackmann DE. Facial nerve repair techniques in cerebellopontine angle tumor surgery. Am J Otol 1992;13:356–359.

20. Luxford WM, House JR. Hypoglossal facial anastomosis. In: Brackmann DE, Shelton C, Arriaga MA, eds. Otologic Surgery. Philadelphia: WB Saunders; 2001.

21. May M, Sobol SM, Mester SJ. Hypoglossal-facial nerve interposition-jump graft for facial reanimation without tongue atrophy. Otolaryngol Head Neck Surg 1991;104:818–825.

22. Julian GG, Hoffmann JF, Shelton C. Surgical rehabilitation of facial nerve paralysis. Otolaryngol Clin North Am 1997;30:701–726.

23. Fong B, Shindo M. Dynamic facial reanimation using free tissue transfer. Facial Plast Surg Clin North Am 1997;5:247–254.

III
Head and Neck Surgery

Decision tree for revision thyroidectomy

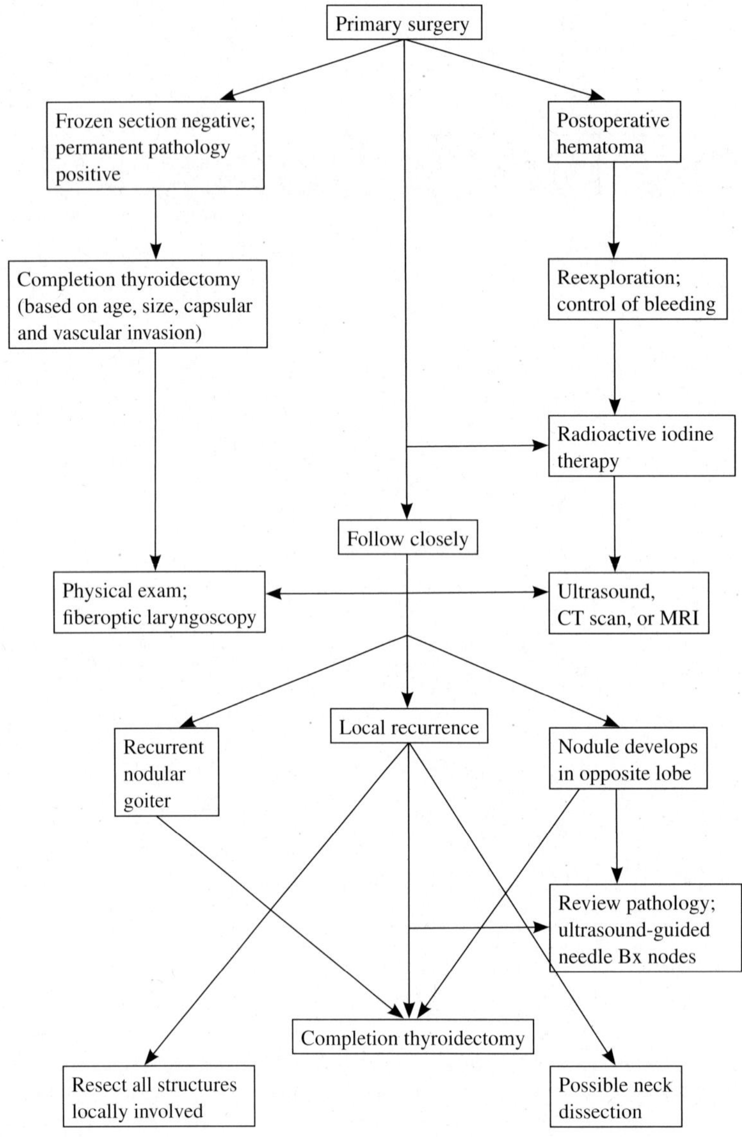

15 Revision Thyroidectomy

Ashok R. Shaha

In February 1974, *Otolaryngology Clinics of North America* devoted the entire volume to the symposium on revision surgery in otorhinolaryngology.[1] Dr. Jerome C. Goldstein was the guest editor for this volume. Dr. Goldstein describes in his foreword,

> We all know that not every operation is successful, and failure can assume different forms. Perhaps the primary disease was not eradicated or complication ensued. In those procedures done for traumatic or cosmetic reasons, the patient or the surgeon may not be satisfied with the result. Anyone faced with the further management of a patient in this difficult situation soon becomes aware of the paucity of information in the literature. Human nature being what it is, people are naturally more eager to publicize their successes than to discuss the management of failures.

The subject of revision thyroidectomy is very interesting, with a variety of indications and several controversial issues related to completion thyroidectomy. For a head and neck surgeon, this is a challenging surgical procedure in relation to certain adverse complications related to recurrent laryngeal nerve injury or permanent hypoparathyroidism. Although there are no definite data suggestive of increased complication in revision thyroidectomy, it is the general consensus that there is definitely a higher risk of complications, both wound-related problems and injury to the surrounding vital structures due to scarring and fibrosis. Obviously, the incidence of complications is related to the indications for which revision thyroidectomy is performed. In this chapter, we will describe the indications, the complications, and the special technical issues related to revision thyroidectomy.

Indications for revision thyroidectomy are enumerated in **Table 15.1.** The most common is completion thyroidectomy performed after ipsilateral thyroid lobectomy where the final pathology report reveals thyroid cancer. The other most common indication is recurrent thyroid cancer in the thyroid bed or metastatic disease in the cervical lymph nodes. The surgical procedures and the concerns regarding the complications are minimal if the surgical procedure is performed for metastatic nodes as compared with recurrent disease in the thyroid bed or in the tracheoesophageal groove area. Recurrent hyperthyroidism is a rare indication nowadays, as most patients with Graves disease are treated with radioactive iodine; a few who undergo surgical intervention mostly undergo total thyroidectomy, or very small residual thyroid tissue is left that is unlikely to result in recurrent hyperthyroidism. The surgical procedure in recurrent hyperthyroidism is very complex, and the residual thyroid tissue may be entangled in severe scar tissue, leading to a surgical procedure being most difficult with high incidence of injury to the recurrent laryngeal nerve and parathyroids. In such patients, due consideration may be given to treating them with radioiodine rather than reoperative surgery.

Postoperative Hematoma and Bleeding

Thyroid surgery is generally considered to be a safe procedure; however, postoperative wound hematoma and bleeding can be serious complications, generally seen within the first 24 hours following surgery. The overall incidence of postoperative hematoma ranges between 1 and 2%, generally requiring surgical exploration. The most common cause for wound hematoma is slipping of a ligature. This is more common in patients who have recovered from anesthesia bucking and coughing. The small venous tributaries in the thyroid bed may start bleeding due to increased intrathoracic pressure. After thyroidectomy, patients should be observed closely in the postoperative period as expanding hematoma may cause

Table 15.1 Indications for Revision Thyroidectomy

1. Reoperation for bleeding or hematoma

2. Completion thyroidectomy with a diagnosis of carcinoma in the ipsilateral thyroid lobe

3. Nodularity in the opposite lobe after ipsilateral thyroid lobectomy for thyroid nodule

4. Recurrent thyroid cancer in the thyroid bed

5. Recurrent bilateral nodular goiter after previous subtotal thyroidectomy

6. Recurrent Graves disease

7. Reoperation for cervical lymphadenopathy in well-differentiated thyroid cancer

8. Surgical exploration for persistent hypercalcitoninemia for medullary cancer of the thyroid

airway compression and severe difficulty in breathing, requiring opening of the wound at the bedside to avoid airway distress. Generally, the patient should be brought back to the operating room for surgical exploration and ligation of the bleeding vessel. Quite often no bleeding vessel is noted, and the hematoma is evacuated. The wound is irrigated, and fresh drains are placed in the thyroid bed.

Completion Thyroidectomy

One of the major indications for completion thyroidectomy is the patient presenting with a solitary thyroid nodule and having undergone thyroid lobectomy reported to be benign at the time of frozen section. The permanent section is reported as either follicular carcinoma or follicular variant of papillary carcinoma of the thyroid (**Table 15.2**). There continues to be considerable controversy regarding completion thyroidectomy. Obviously, the decisions related to completion thyroidectomy should be based on the risk group of the initial thyroid tumor. If the patient belongs to the low risk group—with the tumor being < 4 cm, the patient's age < 45 years, and a low-grade thyroid cancer—there is very little justification to proceed with completion thyroidectomy. However, there appears to be a consensus among many endocrinologists to consider completion thyroidectomy for a cancer > 1.5 cm in size. The surgeon will be asked to proceed with completion thyroidectomy to facilitate radioactive iodine dosimetry and possible ablation and routine serial thyroglobulin follow-up. In a low-risk thyroid cancer patient, the overall long-term outcome is so good that the role of completion thyroidectomy remains controversial and questionable. However, the general indications for completion thyroidectomy are a tumor > 4 cm in size or aggressive histology (e.g., poorly differentiated carcinoma; tall cell, insular, trabecular, or undifferentiated carcinoma of the thyroid; older patients or patients with major capsular or vascular invasion who are at high risk for development of distant metastasis). Some of the major

indications for completion thyroidectomy are the fear of development of distant metastases and the need for consideration of radioactive iodine dosimetry and ablation. This is because radioactive iodine cannot be used in the presence of normal thyroid tissue. Although a medical thyroidectomy can be performed with low-dose radioactive iodine, it takes a long time and is generally not satisfactory. Most of the time, the radioactive iodine will be absorbed by the normal thyroid rather than used to detect distant metastases.

Thyroid Nodule in the Opposite Lobe after Ipsilateral Thyroid Lobectomy

Many times after an ipsilateral thyroid lobectomy, the patient is followed closely, and a thyroid nodule is identified either clinically or by ultrasound. Obviously, it would be appropriate to proceed with a standard work-up, which would include a fine-needle aspiration biopsy of the opposite lobe. If this is suspicious or shows atypical cells, then a completion thyroidectomy may be undertaken. The incidence of microscopic thyroid cancer in the opposite lobe varies from 30 to 60%, depending on the careful serial sectioning of the thyroid lobe by the pathologist in an effort to identify microscopic carcinoma of the thyroid. It is vitally important that the initial operating surgeon evaluate the contralateral lobe for any gross abnormality. If there is gross nodularity in the opposite lobe at the time of surgery, it would be appropriate to proceed with total thyroidectomy, even though it will most likely be a benign problem. It would be very difficult to keep the thyroid nodules under follow-up and observation for fear that the thyroid nodules increase in size or a microscopic thyroid carcinoma is present. Quite often the patient is kept under thyroid suppressive therapy to prevent the growth of tiny nodules in the opposite lobe or benign nodular goiter in the opposite lobe after ipsilateral thyroid lobectomy.

Locally Recurrent Thyroid Cancer

One of the most distressing problems facing a thyroid surgeon is the difficulty in managing locally recurrent thyroid cancer. The subject is quite complex and revolves mainly on the initial presentation of locally advanced thyroid cancer involving the surrounding structures, such as strap muscles, esophageal musculature, the tracheal wall, and the recurrent laryngeal nerve. Considering that the patient has had an appropriate and adequate initial surgical procedure (including gross removal of the tumor), the recurrent tumor in the thyroid bed is a surgical challenge. In a majority of cases, the surgical procedure is unsatisfactory,

Table 15.2 Recurrent Thyroid Cancer

1. Recurrence in the opposite lobe (which was not removed previously)

2. Recurrence in the thyroid bed

3. Recurrence in the tracheoesophageal groove (with or without vocal cord palsy)

4. Recurrence with involvement of the trachea, esophagus, or cricoid cartilage area

5. Recurrence in the neck nodes

6. Inoperable recurrent thyroid cancer

and gross removal of the entire tumor is unlikely. At that time, adjuvant therapy may be used, including appropriate radioactive iodine ablation and possibly external radiation therapy in selected cases. The patients presenting initially with locally aggressive thyroid cancer may have a tumor adherent to the tracheal wall or surrounding structures. In most cases the tumor is shaved off the surrounding structures. Clearly, there is a high incidence of local recurrence in this group, particularly with adherence of the tumor to the tracheal wall or involvement of the trachea directly. It is vitally important in these cases to evaluate the initial extent of the disease. The pathology should also be re-reviewed to see if this is either a low- or a high-grade tumor or a poorly differentiated histology. This is important information and is vital to ascertain prior to any surgical intervention. It is also very important for the operating surgeon to find out the details regarding the extent of the surgery and the exact location of the gross residual tumor during the first surgery. The goal of the second surgery is to remove all gross tumor. The surgeon should be prepared (depending on the extent of the disease clinically, radiologically with imaging studies, and endoscopically) to resect the structures that are directly involved by the tumor. These may include strap muscles, the recurrent laryngeal nerve, the trachea, and/or the esophagus. If the tracheal lumen is directly involved by the tumor and there is a narrowing of the tracheal lumen, segmental resection of the trachea and end-to-end anastomosis are appropriate considerations. If the tumor directly involves the esophagus and the trachea, it is vitally important to evaluate whether it would be technically feasible to resect all gross tumor without a laryngectomy. In such situations, laryngectomy is necessary in most cases. Preoperative evaluation of the laryngeal function is extremely important, as is the proximity of the tumor to the cricoid cartilage. Obviously, laryngectomy is a very high price to pay, and many patients refuse the surgical intervention. At that time, alternate treatment approaches may be considered in a palliative effort. In rare circumstances, a patient may require total laryngopharyngectomy with reconstruction of the hypopharynx with jejunal free flap or gastric pull-up.

Recurrent Nodular Goiter after Subtotal Thyroidectomy

This is a common situation in areas afflicted by endemic goiter, particularly iodine-deficient areas such as the Himalayas and the Alps. It is very rare in the United States, as the incidence of colloid goiter or iodine-deficient endemic goiter has decreased with iodinization of table salt for the past 50 years. The incidence of recurrent goiter

after subtotal thyroidectomy is ~20%. Obviously, the second surgical procedure is high risk. In light of this, Reeve[2] suggested a routine total thyroidectomy for bilateral nodular disease. Although this may be a controversial issue (as to the indication of total thyroidectomy in benign nodular goiter), if there is a gross nodularity in both lobes of the thyroid, it would be appropriate to proceed with total thyroidectomy in an effort to reduce the incidence of recurrent nodular goiter. The indications for surgery in what appears as a benign recurrent nodular goiter have to be weighed against the risks of complications related to recurrent laryngeal nerve injury and permanent hypoparathyroidism.

Recurrent Graves Disease

This is one of the most difficult problems in thyroid surgery when operating on a patient who has previously undergone subtotal thyroidectomy for Graves disease. The Graves thyroid is extremely vascular, and with previous subtotal thyroidectomy, there is generally intense scarring, fibrosis, and adherence of the surrounding tissues, as well as scarring around the recurrent laryngeal nerves. Generally, patients who present with recurrent Graves disease are treated with radioactive iodine, but there may be rare situations where one may have to consider surgical intervention. Surgery in these cases can be fraught with increased complications, and I would strongly recommend treating these patients with appropriate radioactive iodine rather than reoperative thyroid surgery. Exceptions include cases where there is a gross amount of thyroid tissue left behind or regrowth of a substantial amount of thyroid tissue.

Preoperative Evaluation

Preoperative evaluation includes detailed information about the previous surgery, a review of the appropriate pathology, complete evaluation of the extent of the disease with proper imaging studies, and preoperative evaluation of the vocal cord function. The vocal cord evaluation is very important because the patient may have normal voice with a paralyzed vocal cord during the first surgery. If it is not documented preoperatively, the second operative surgery may be blamed for the nerve injury. Also, if the vocal cord is paralyzed preoperatively, resection of the tumor can be performed along with recurrent laryngeal nerve and sacrifice of the nerve for better oncologic clearance. If possible, it is very helpful to discuss with the previous operating surgeon the extent of the disease, intraoperative findings, status of the parathyroid glands, and any concerns about the reoperative surgery. Preoperative evaluation with computed tomography (CT) scans (without contrast) or ultrasound will help define the extent of the disease. The avoidance of contrast will help minimize any issues related to radioactive iodine ablation (if necessary) after the surgery. A magnetic resonance imaging scan may be better at evaluating the extent of the soft tissue disease and involvement of the tracheal lumen. Preoperative evaluation in the operating room with direct laryngoscopy, pharyngoscopy, esophagoscopy, and tracheoscopy is vitally important. If the tumor directly involves the trachea, then a segmental resection is mandatory. However, if the tumor does not involve the trachea, a shave procedure may be considered. Depending on the extent of the disease, the surgeon should be prepared for total laryngectomy or laryngopharyngoesophagectomy—although both are rare surgical procedures in recurrent thyroid cancer. If the surgeon is going to consider laryngopharyngoesophagectomy, it is vitally important to review the pathology of the initial surgical procedure or the previously operated thyroid specimen to rule out poorly differentiated thyroid cancer. This is because the chances of local control in poorly differentiated thyroid cancer are quite low. This issue needs to be considered in view of functional and quality of life issues related to total laryngectomy.

Treatment

The treatment of recurrent goiter or recurrent thyroid tumor depends on the extent of the disease and the indications.[3,4] In a recurrent thyroid cancer, the treatment goal should be the removal of all gross tumor. Under these circumstances, the patient will invariably require adjuvant therapy—including appropriate radioactive iodine ablation and possibly external radiation therapy. The main indications for the latter are inability to remove all gross tumor, tumor in critical areas such as tracheoesophageal groove or the esophageal musculature, and aggressive histology (e.g., tall cell, solid, or insular type). In nodular goiter, the goal should be the removal of all gross nodularity, essentially performing total thyroidectomy. In patients presenting for completion thyroidectomy after ipsilateral thyroid lobectomy, the time of surgery generally remains a controversial issue. A majority of surgeons would consider surgical intervention within a period of 3 to 5 days when the surgical planes are still well defined and there is no major scarring. However, after approximately 2 weeks, the wound becomes indurated, scarred, and phlegmonous. At this time, most surgeons prefer to wait ~8 to 12 weeks for the inflammation and scarring to subside before considering completion thyroidectomy.

The treatment decisions in revision thyroidectomy can be divided into revision thyroidectomy for either benign or malignant disease. They also can be divided according to type of patients: those in whom the thyroid lobe remains undisturbed and those where the opposite lobe has been explored and operated, such as in subtotal thyroidectomy. The revision thyroidectomy is generally easier in patients undergoing completion thyroidectomy, as the opposite lobe is generally undisturbed and there is no intensive scarring. Fifty percent of patients who have undergone previous surgery for either subtotal thyroidectomy or Graves disease invariably develop intense scarring, especially in the midline of the neck, with strap muscles adherent to the thyroid bed. In such patients the best approach is lateral, medial to the sternomastoid muscle, where generally there is a virgin plane. The dissection first exposes the lateral portion of the thyroid lobe and the tracheoesophageal groove, with subsequent identification of the recurrent laryngeal nerve and dissection of the remaining thyroid tissues. The recurrent laryngeal nerve may be identified low in the neck in the tracheoesophageal groove and traced superiorly if there is extensive scarring in the lateral aspect of the thyroid gland. The superior laryngeal nerve should be carefully preserved by dissecting on the substance of the thyroid gland. The thyroid lobe is retracted laterally and inferiorly with opening of the plane between the superior pole of the thyroid gland and the cricoid cartilage. The superior thyroid vessels are exposed after transecting the sternothyroid muscle; injury to the superior laryngeal nerve may be avoided by carefully ligating the superior thyroid vessels. In approximately two thirds of patients, the recurrent laryngeal nerve may be identified by careful dissection parallel to the superior thyroid vessels. The decision regarding the extent of the thyroidectomy in revision surgery is generally completion or total thyroidectomy. In patients with suspected recurrent cancer, appropriate resection of the recurrent tumor should be performed. The tumor is invariably adherent to the trachea or the esophageal musculature, and dissection should be performed carefully to avoid any residual tumor. The tumor may be shaved off the trachea. Preoperative evaluation of the recurrent laryngeal nerve function is extremely important. If the nerve has been paralyzed either due to tumor or previous surgical procedure with recurrent thyroid cancer, it should be sacrificed, and dissection should be performed in the tracheoesophageal groove. Occasionally, the tumor may be stuck to the cricoid cartilage or extend between the trachea and the esophagus, where complete resection may be unsatisfactory. Some patients with recurrent thyroid cancer exhibit poorly differentiated tumors with previous extrathyroidal extension, and complete surgical resection may be unsatisfactory. If the tumor is adherent to the esophageal musculature, the musculature of the esophagus may need to be sacrificed, with careful preservation of the mucosa needed to avoid any tear into the esophageal musculature, which may lead to subsequent esophageal fistula. Occasionally, tumor in the tracheoesophageal groove may extend into the superior mediastinum, where inferior dissection may be very difficult. In extensive recurrent disease in the superior mediastinum, one may need a sternal split. However, such occasions are quite rare in the reoperative thyroid surgical practice.

Issues, Concerns, and Complications in Revision Thyroidectomy

The decisions regarding revision thyroidectomy should be made critically based on the previous surgical procedure, as well as the status of the recurrent laryngeal nerve, vocal cord function, and the parathyroids. The previous operative note should be studied in detail, including the pathology report. Recurrent benign nodular goiter may be observed, and the indications for surgery in these patients may be limited. If the patient has mild enlargement of the thyroid with what appears to be benign nodularity, he or she may be observed rather than rushed into a surgical procedure. However, if there is a tracheal compression or any airway problems, reoperative thyroid surgery should be considered. In patients with recurrent thyroid cancer, surgery is definitely indicated; however, due consideration must be given to whether all tumor can be removed and whether the tumor is adherent to the trachea. If the tumor appears to be invading the trachea with intraluminal disease, tracheal resection should be planned. It is rare that the tumor involves the esophageal mucosa; however, if there is extensive tumor in the cricothyroid groove with involvement of the esophagus, due consideration must be given to total laryngopharyngoesophagectomy, and appropriate reconstruction should be planned with either a jejunal free flap or a gastric pull-up. If one recurrent laryngeal nerve is paralyzed, extreme care should be taken to avoid injury to the opposite recurrent laryngeal nerve, which may lead to bilateral vocal cord paralysis, requiring lifelong tracheostomy. In patients undergoing completion thyroidectomy with one paralyzed vocal cord on the ipsilateral side, the decision regarding completion thyroidectomy should be weighed against a paralyzed recurrent laryngeal nerve. Generally, a lateral approach is advised because there may be extensive scarring in the midline with adherence of the thyroid capsule to the sternothyroid muscle. Invariably, the sternothyroid requires resection for proper exposure of the thyroid lobe. The medial side of the thyroid lobe may be adherent to the trachea, where the dissection may be difficult. Even though there is no general consensus regarding recurrent laryngeal nerve monitoring, this may be one surgical

indication for such monitoring. Most of the time finding the nerve is not a difficult problem in the tracheoesophageal groove; instead, the most difficult problems are addressing the nerve in the region of the Berry ligament and avoiding injury to the recurrent laryngeal nerve where it enters the larynx. Careful dissection should be performed on the thyroid capsule in benign nodular goiter to avoid injury to the parathyroids. The surgeon must be familiar with the anatomy and blood supply to the parathyroid glands. The parathyroid glands receive blood supply from the inferior thyroid artery, and the branches of the inferior thyroid artery should be ligated very close to the thyroid gland to avoid devascularization of the parathyroid glands. Either the parathyroids are devascularized, or there is surface hematoma. They should be autotransplanted after confirming the tissue to be parathyroid gland with a small piece sent for frozen section. Most of the time in revision thyroidectomy, parathyroid autotransplantation can be performed in the sternomastoid muscle. There is no need to autotransplant the parathyroid glands in the forearm, which is generally routinely performed for parathyroid surgery in renal failure patients. Approximately two thirds of the autotransplanted parathyroid glands will regain function within 10 to 12 weeks. The overall incidence of complications in reoperative surgery is between 2 and 3%, compared with 1 to 2% in primary surgical procedures. Obviously, the complications are more related to the indications for surgery in patients with recurrent thyroid cancer. The incidence of complications, including hypoparathyroidism and nerve injury, is very high. However, sincere attempts should be made to preserve the parathyroid function in reoperative thyroid surgery.

In patients undergoing surgery for neck disease, due consideration should be given whether the neck disease is clinically apparent or not. Recently, with the routine use of thyroglobulin in the follow-up, an increasing number of patients are noted to have hyperthyroglobulinemia, where the disease is invariably present in the lymph nodes in the neck. Ultrasound and ultrasound-guided needle biopsy will assist in evaluating the extent of the disease in the neck. If the disease is clinically apparent and ultrasonographically noted, modified neck dissection is generally indicated. For most well-differentiated thyroid cancer patients, modified neck dissection includes removal of the lymph nodes at levels II, III, IV, and V with preservation of the sternomastoid, internal jugular vein, and accessory nerve. In patients with medullary thyroid cancer and persistent hypercalcitoninemia, invariably the disease is present in the cervical lymph nodes. However, there may be extensive metastatic disease in the mediastinum, lungs, or liver. Again, generally a modified neck dissection is performed with preservation of the sternomastoid, jugular vein, and accessory nerve. If the tumor is extensive in the neck, the sternomastoid and jugular veins may need to be sacrificed; however, every effort should be made to preserve the accessory nerve, which is important for functional outcome. The surgical procedure can be considered relatively safe with an overall low incidence of complication. Patience during surgery, meticulous dissection, and an attempt to preserve the parathyroid glands are extremely crucial in optimizing surgical outcomes. The safe thyroidectomy can be assisted with the use of loops, bipolar cautery, and microdissecting clamps to avoid injury to the recurrent laryngeal nerve and blood supply to the parathyroid glands.

Reference

1. Edmunds SL, Goldstein JC. Allergy and the refractory otorhinolaryngology patient. Otolaryngol Clin North Am 1974;7:145–151.
2. Reeve TS, Delbridge L, Cohen A, Crummer P. Total thyroidectomy. The preferred option for multinodular goiter. Ann Surg. 1987 Dec;206(6):782–786.
3. Chao TC, Jeng LB, Lin JD, Chen MF. Reoperative thyroid surgery. World J Surg. 1997 Jul–Aug;21(6):644–647.
4. Levin KE, Clark AH, Duh QY, Demeure M, Siperstein AE, Clark OH. Reoperative thyroid surgery. Surgery. 1992 Jun; 111(6):604–609.
5. Harness JK, Fung L, Thompson NW, Burney RE, McLeod MK. Total thyroidectomy: complications and technique. World J Surg. 1986 Oct;10(5):781–786.
6. Wilson DB, Staren ED, Prinz RA. Thyroid reoperations: indications and risks. Am Surg. 1998 Jul;64(7)674–678; discussion 678–679.
7. Reeve TS, Delbridge L, Brady P, Crummer P, Smyth C. Secondary thyroidectomy: a twenty–year experience. World J Surg. 1988 Aug;12(4):449–453.

Revision Surgery in Parathyroid Disease

Arnold Komisar

Revision surgery for hyperparathyroidism can best be summarized by three questions: Is the diagnosis correct? Can the abnormal glands be found? and How can they be removed surgically with minimal morbidity?

Patient Evaluation

Is the Diagnosis Correct?

Whenever a surgeon is referred a patient with suspected recurrence of hyperparathyroidism, the basic principle of making a diagnosis applies. Is this truly a recurrence of hyperparathyroidism, or is this a different disease? Was the original diagnosis correct? What were the patient's symptoms before the first operation, and have they recurred? Symptoms such as renal colic, abdominal pain, fatigue, and bone pain are commonly seen in parathyroid disease; however, they may also be seen with other syndromes. Signs may include nephrolithiasis, weakness of the proximal muscles of the lower extremities, mental changes, peptic ulcer disease, and chondrocalcinosis in some joints, commonly the knee and pseudogout. Patients can also have nephrolithiasis and hypertension and not have parathyroid disease. Laboratory studies should show elevations of serum calcium, intact parathyroid hormone (PTH), and elevated urinary calcium excretion, the latter requiring the 24-hour creatinine clearance be within the normal range. Supplementary studies may include bone density studies and plain radiographs. Patients with primary PTH may have pain in their long bones, clavicles, hands, and dentition; however, this is more commonly seen with secondary hyperparathyroidism. The physician should inquire if there is any family history or significant endocrine history. Entities that need to be considered include familial hyperparathyroidism, both the autosomal dominant pattern (four-gland hyperplasia) and the recessive (adenoma), and the multiple endocrine neoplasia syndromes, both type 1 (> 90%) and type 2 and their subtypes. One usually sees four-gland hyperplasia in these disease states. Familial hypocalciuric hypercalcemia is another entity that may at times lead the best of clinicians astray. Of paramount importance in diagnosing this disease is the evaluation of renal function and calcium excretion.

What Was Done Previously?

One of the most important aspects in evaluating the patient is obtaining old records. These should include old operative reports, pathology reports, slides, and old localization studies. Direct communication with the prior surgeon can be invaluable in performing an operation with minimal morbidity. Were any markers left in the patient to identify residual parathyroid tissue, such as a suture or clip? To what were these markers attached? Patients can also be very helpful by their recollection of prior surgery. What were they told after the surgery? How many glands were left? Were the glands in an ectopic location, and were their symptoms and signs improved after surgery? It can be extremely helpful to know if there were any complications after prior surgeries, including hoarseness and hypocalcemia. Did the patient need to take calcium or vitamin D after prior parathyroid exploration? Was the thyroid gland removed as well? How long was the patient symptom free?

What Needs to Be Done Now?

The diagnostic work-up should rest on the history and physical exam, with confirmation by ancillary studies. Often in parathyroid disease physical signs may be lacking, and the history may be nonspecific. Diagnostic chemistry should include the serum calcium, phosphate, serum protein, thyroid function studies, intact parathyroid hormone (iPTH) level, and urinalysis. A 24-hour urine test for calcium and creatinine clearance is mandatory to confirm the diagnosis of hyperparathyroidism and not familial hypocalciuric hypercalcemia (FHH). Hypercalcemia from an occult malignancy should be excluded as well. Radiological testing can include ultrasound, radioisotope studies, computed tomography (CT), magnetic resonance imaging (MRI), and angiography. Selective venous sampling of the arm can help determine the status of implanted glands. Selective internal jugular catheterization for comparative PTH can be helpful in localizing a recurrent lesion (**Fig. 16.1**).

Planning the Operation

It is understood that the operative procedure must be planned down to the last detail. These patients have had many procedures leading up to this one and, it is hoped,

Decision tree for revision surgery in parathyroid disease

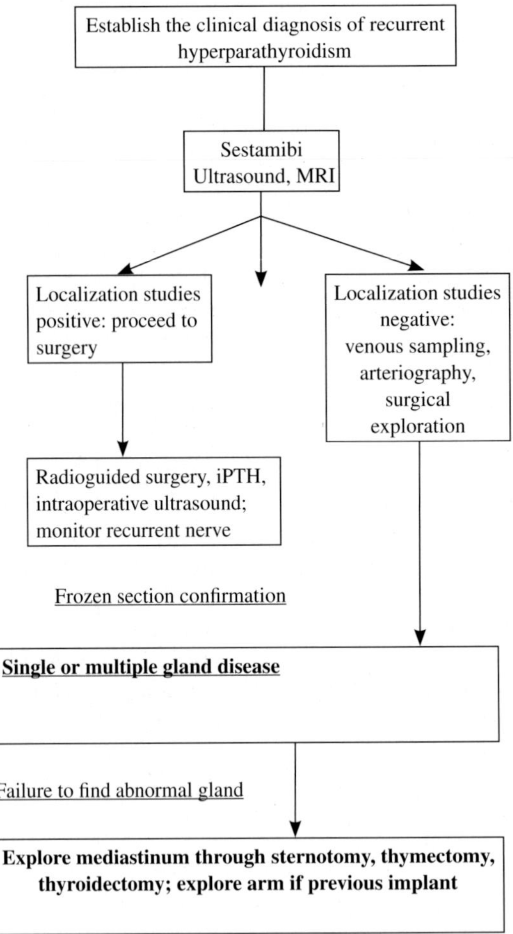

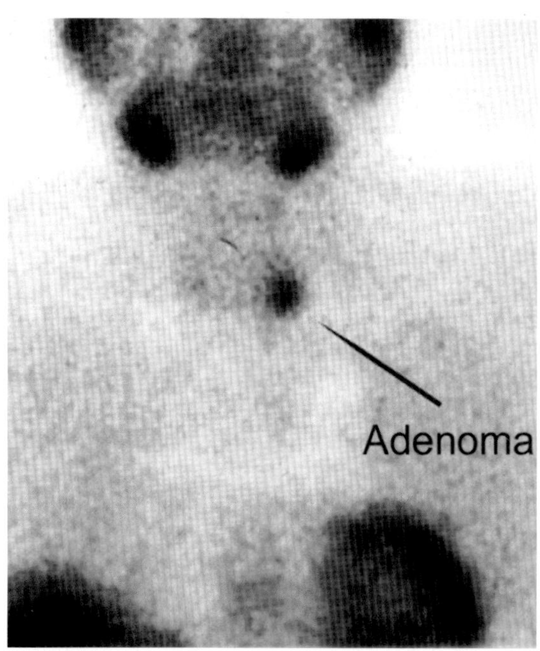

Fig. 16.1   Sestamibi scan showing parathyroid adenoma (2 hours after injection of isotope).

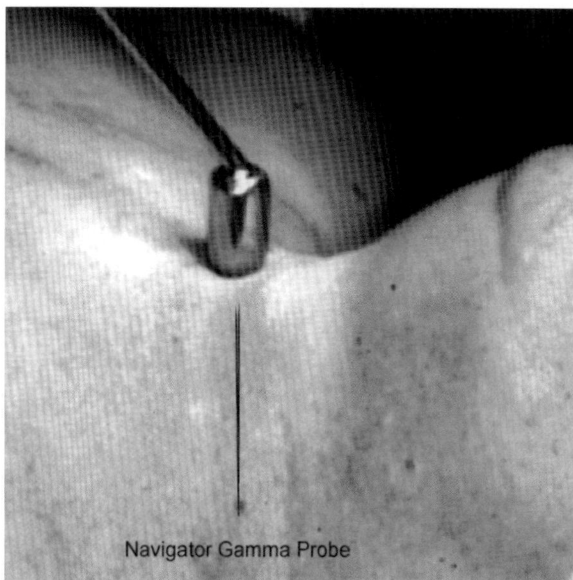

Fig. 16.2   Gamma probe applied to neck before incision is made (90 minutes after injection of isotope).

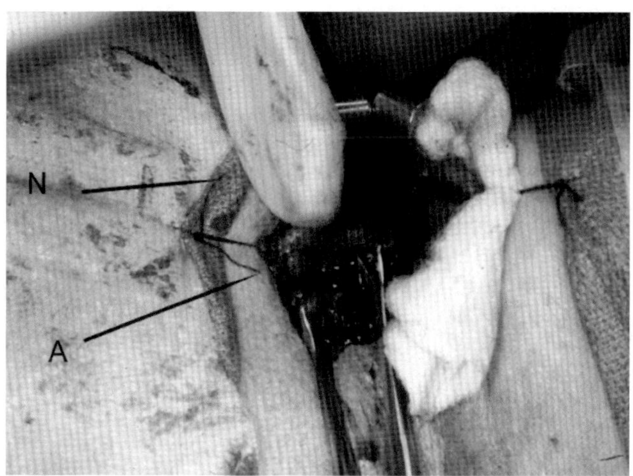

Fig. 16.3   Gamma probe used during operative procedure. A, adenoma; N, navigator.

will not have many more. Apart from the localization studies used to help guide the surgical approach, other ancillary procedures, many of which are perioperative, should be thought about and preparations made before the surgery begins. Some of these might include the following: recurrent nerve monitoring, intraoperative PTH assay, gamma probe localization, intraoperative ultrasound, thoracic surgical assistance, arterial access, appropriate permissions, and the ability to store parathyroid tissue long term.

Recurrent nerve monitoring is useful in cases where the scaring from previous surgery suggests a significant risk to the recurrent nerve. The device used is a special endotracheal tube with electromyography (EMG) sensors to pick up action potentials from the intrinsic laryngeal musculature. An audible or graphic warning alerts the operative surgeon to the proximity of the nerve. This is very useful for recurrent nerve localization when there is extensive scarring. The nerve can be a highly reliable landmark to the position of the parathyroid glands.

Intraoperative PTH assay, although costly and often not reimbursable, can be invaluable in establishing the removal of abnormal parathyroid tissue. The surgeon can, with relative certainty, stop the operative procedure when the iPTH has dropped to < 50% of the pre- or perioperative value, markedly lowering the complication rate.

Likewise, the gamma probe can save time, enabling the surgeon to rapidly locate the emitting abnormal gland. The probe is especially helpful in confirming removal of parathyroid tissue as it often emits even normal glands. This test is best used when the abnormal gland has been localized by a preoperative sestamibi scan (**Figs. 16.2, 16.3**).

If a significant drop in serum calcium is anticipated postoperatively, preparations such as an arterial or triple-lumen catheter should be made before the operative procedure begins. This will enable precise monitoring of the serum calcium without the need for multiple needle sticks.

Methylene blue may also be effective in identifying parathyroid tissue. A dose is given 1 to 2 hours before the proposed surgery. Proponents of this technique feel the dye localizes in parathyroid tissue, making identification easier.

Intraoperative ultrasound, although not used as widely, has been shown to be of some benefit in gland localization during surgery.

If the lesion appears to be in the chest, services of a thoracic surgeon should be arranged before the operation and a rational approach agreed upon between the two surgical teams. Who does what should be decided outside the operating room, not during the procedure.

"Banking" of parathyroid tissue can be performed in cases where it is anticipated that there will be minimal or no functioning tissue left in situ. This must be arranged in advance, with proper technique and facilities to preserve tissue long term.

The Operative Procedure

The surgeon must think about the surgical approach before the incision is made. Will the neck be explored based on a midline dissection? Will the sternothyroid muscle be identified and dissected off the thyroid gland from medial to lateral, exposing the tracheoesophageal (TE) groove? Although this is the standard of care for the primary operation, significant scarring may preclude this approach. The surgeon may be required to divide the strap muscles for added exposure, with the muscles being divided high in the neck and reflected down, preserving their neural and arterial blood supply. Another approach is to come in lateral to the TE groove, between the sternocleidomastoid muscle and the sternohyoid/thyroid muscles. This has the advantage of permitting surgery in a previously unoperated field, enabling normal structures to be found and preserved more easily. However, this approach may require reorientation to the anatomy and may prevent dissection medial to the recurrent nerve. We have seen recurrent lesions attached to the medial strap muscles, which may make this approach difficult (**Fig. 16.2**).

Is there a chance that the abnormal gland is in a superior ectopic location, such as the submaxillary triangle? Will the old incision permit exposure of this structure, or is a new or second incision necessary?

The surgical team has to decide the best way to approach a suspected mediastinal lesion. Although a cervical approach is effective in primary surgery for lesions in the thymus and high mediastinum, recurrent lesions may be scarred to vital structures, such as the innominate vein or artery and recurrent nerves. To avoid dissecting from superior to inferior in a scarred field, it may be better to perform a partial or complete sternotomy. A partial sternotomy through the second interspace often gives enough exposure; however, the best exposure is achieved with a full sternotomy, exposing the entire mediastinum. This gives the surgical team complete access to the anatomy and pathology of this anatomical unit. Scarred

reoperations are not the preferred venue for a thoracscopic approach.

Whatever approach is used, the surgeon should establish a rhythm and time limit to the exploration. All known anatomical regions where normal parathyroid glands are found should be explored, if possible. Finding these can be helped dramatically by finding the recurrent nerve and using this as a landmark. If the nerve is scarred in the TE groove, it often can be found lower in the neck and traced superiorly, or it can be found where it enters the cricothyroid muscle superiorly and traced inferiorly. Normally, the upper parathyroid gland will lie lateral to the nerve and the lower gland medial. Unfortunately, significantly enlarged parathyroid glands may displace or obscure the nerve, making its identification difficult. Sometimes the nerve may be attached to the abnormal parathyroid glands capsule, increasing the chances of nerve injury. After the normal locations are evaluated, the posterior, retropharyngeal, and retroesophageal regions should be explored. Palpation and ballottement of fatty, fibrous tissue can be very helpful in this situation. A previously placed nasogastric tube or esophageal temperature probe can help the surgeon identify where the esophagus is, preventing injury. If these maneuvers fail to identify the abnormal gland, one should look at the lower pole of the thyroid by the superior mediastinal region for glands in a perithymic location. This dissection is usually medial to the recurrent nerve. Next to be evaluated are the carotid sheath and carotid bifurcation region. One should also try to expose the submaxillary triangles to look for ectopic glands; other locations, which are more superficial, are within the sternohyoid or sternothyroid muscles. Gland remnants from previous surgery may have regrown in these locations. The thyroid gland should be evaluated for a recurrent or intrathyroid gland. If a thyroidectomy is necessary to aid in the exploration or to remove suspected intrathyroid parathyroid glands, it should be performed.

If the abnormal glands are not found after a suitable period of looking in the neck, the surgeon should consider stopping and reassessing the plan. Often fatigue can compromise further exploration, leading to more complications. If a neck exploration has been thoroughly done, the mediastinal exploration should be scheduled for another day, with a fresh team (**Figs. 16.4, 16.5, and 16.6**).

Managing the Patient Postoperatively

Hypocalcemia

Patients who have had reoperative parathyroid surgery are at great risk to develop postoperative hypocalcemia. This is especially true of those with chronic renal failure and secondary hyperparathyroidism. All of these patients

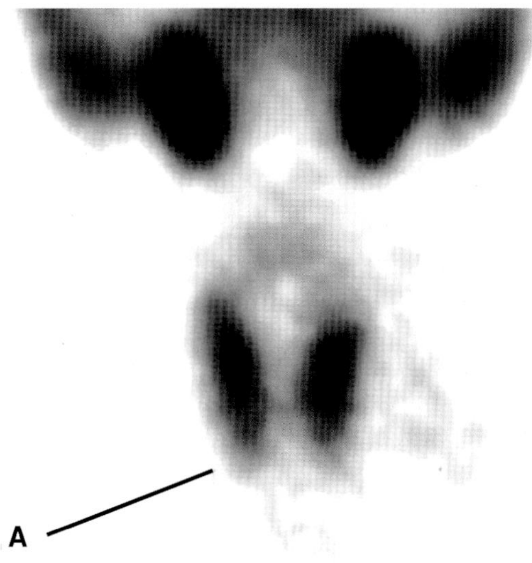

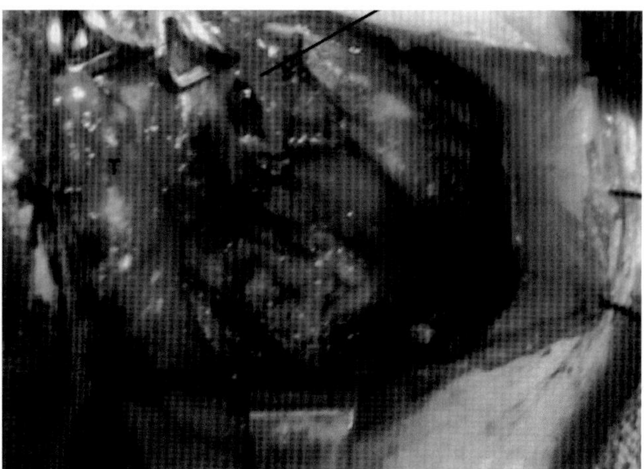

Fig. 16.5 Reoperation for hyperparathyroidism. T, thyroid.

Fig. 16.4 Sestamibi scan showing right lower adenoma (A).

must be monitored aggressively postoperatively to detect symptoms and signs of falling calcium. Symptoms may appear within the first 24 hours, or they may take up to 72 hours to develop. It is very helpful to have good vascular access such as an arterial line so that bloods can be drawn with a minimum of discomfort to the patient. Conversely, symptoms such as tetany, muscular spasms, and electrocardiogram (EKG) changes can develop rapidly, requiring immediate calcium infusion. The patients are observed postoperatively for signs such as Chvostek or Trousseau. Symptoms of perioral tingling and numbness in the hands and feet should immediately raise suspicion of hypocalcemia.

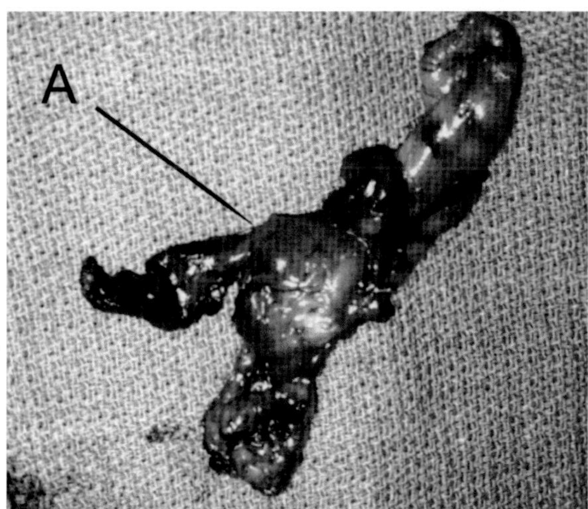

Fig. 16.6 Thymus gland with adenoma (A) approached via a median sternotomy.

It is best to treat patients if they are symptomatic when their serum calcium level is below 8.0 mg/dL. Patients with calcium levels below 7.5 mg/dL should be very closely observed, even if they are not symptomatic. Concurrent serum albumin and serum magnesium levels should be checked as well, as they can affect the ionized calcium and thus the patient's symptoms.

In an acute situation with significant symptoms, 10 to 20 mL of 10% calcium gluconate should be administered over a 5- to 10-minute period through an intravenous (IV) line. One can also add 1 or 2 ampules of calcium gluconate to 1 L saline and infuse this over 12 to 24 hours. This should be enough to prevent serious symptoms, except in those patients with hungry bone syndrome. We have seen patients after reoperative secondary hyperparathyroidism require 2 or 3 ampules of calcium gluconate 3 times a day to maintain a low normocalcemic state. If magnesium levels are low, one can start correction with an intramuscular injection or ampule of 1 g magnesium sulfate IV. The physician needs to be aware of any other drug interaction or medical condition that may affect calcium metabolism. While the patient is being stabilized on IV therapy, oral calcium and vitamin D replacement may be instituted. Oral calcium can be given in doses of 500 mg to 1 g t.i.d. We like to use calcitriol, a vitamin D analogue in doses of 0.25 to 1.0 mcg per day. The clinician should be aware, however, that the calcitriol can suppress the resumption of PTH secretion and should be used only when simple oral calcium replacement and low-dose oral vitamin D fails to raise serum calcium.

Finally, mention should be made of the patient with hypercalcemia after a second or third operation. This can be extremely frustrating to the patient and the surgeon. Full explanation of future directions for diagnosis and management can help assuage some of the patient's fears.

Conclusion

Reoperative parathyroid surgery can be both challenging and extremely rewarding to both the patient and the surgeon. A correct diagnosis, a well thought out surgical plan, and technical expertise can help mitigate some of the consequences of this disease.

Suggested Reading

Carter WB, Carter D, Cohn HF. Cause and current management of reoperative hyperparathyroidism. Am Surg 1993; 59(2):120–124.

Eastwood JB, Pazianas M, Moriniere P, Fournier A. Indications for surgery in secondary hyperparathyroidism. In: Lynn J, Bloom SR, eds Surgical Endocrinology. Oxford: Butterworth-Heinemann Publishers; 1993:31.

George EF, Komisar A, Blaugrund S, Ferucci A, Scharf S. The use of sestamibi scans in hyperparathyroidism: a case study. Laryngoscope 1998;108:627–629.

Irvin GL III, Molinari AS, Figueroa C, Carneiro DM. Improved success rate in reoperative parathyroidectomy with intraoperative iPTH assay. Ann Surg 2004;239(6):704–708.

Jarhult J, Nordenstrom J, Perbeck J. Reoperation for suspected primary hyperparathyroidism. Br J Surg 1993;80:453–456.

Kacker A, Scharf S, Komisar A. Reduced time window sestamibi scanning for nonlocalized primary hyperparathyroidism. Otolaryngol Head Neck Surg 2000;123:456–459.

Netterville JL, Aly A, Ossoff R. Evaluation and treatment of complications of thyroid and parathyroid surgery. Otolaryngol Clin North Am 1990;23(3):529–551.

Norman J, Denham D. Minimally invasive radioguided parathyroidectomy in the reoperative neck. Surgery 1998; 124:1088–1093.

Norton JA. Reoperation for missed parathyroid adenoma. In: Advances in Surgery. St. Louis: Mosby Year Book; 1998: 273–297.

Sullivan DP, Scharf S. Komisar A. Minimally invasive radioguided parathyroid surgery. Laryngoscope 2001;111:912–917.

Thompson GB, Grant CS, Perrier ND, et al. Reoperative parathyroid surgery in the era of sestamibi scanning and intraoperative parathyroid hormone monitoring. Arch Surg 1999;134:699–705.

Yu I, DeVita M, Komisar A. Long-term follow-up after subtotal parathyroidectomy in renal failure. Laryngoscope 1998; 108:1824–1828.

Decision tree for recurrent oral cavity carcinoma

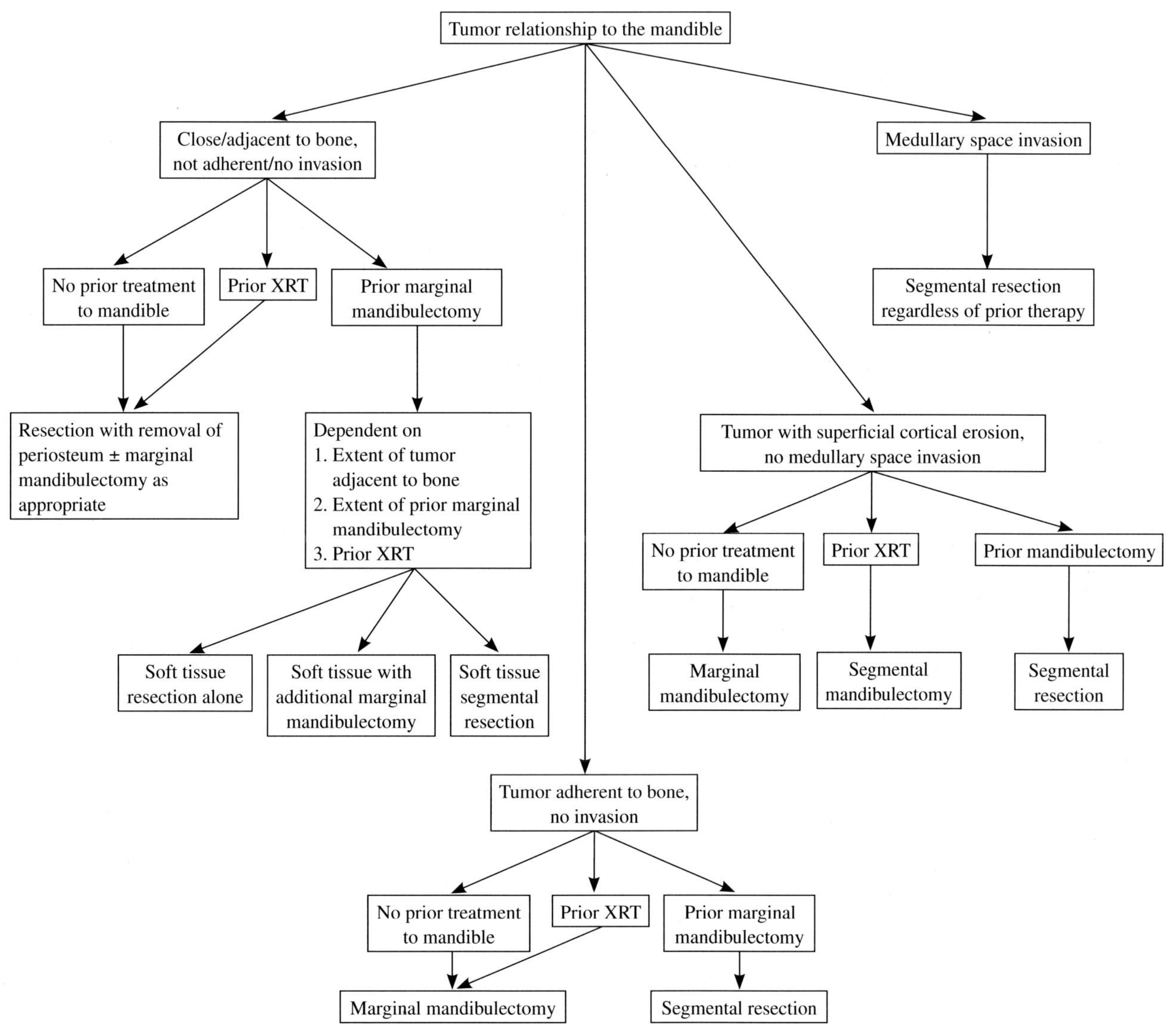

Decision tree for reconstruction options after resection of recurrent oral cavity cancer

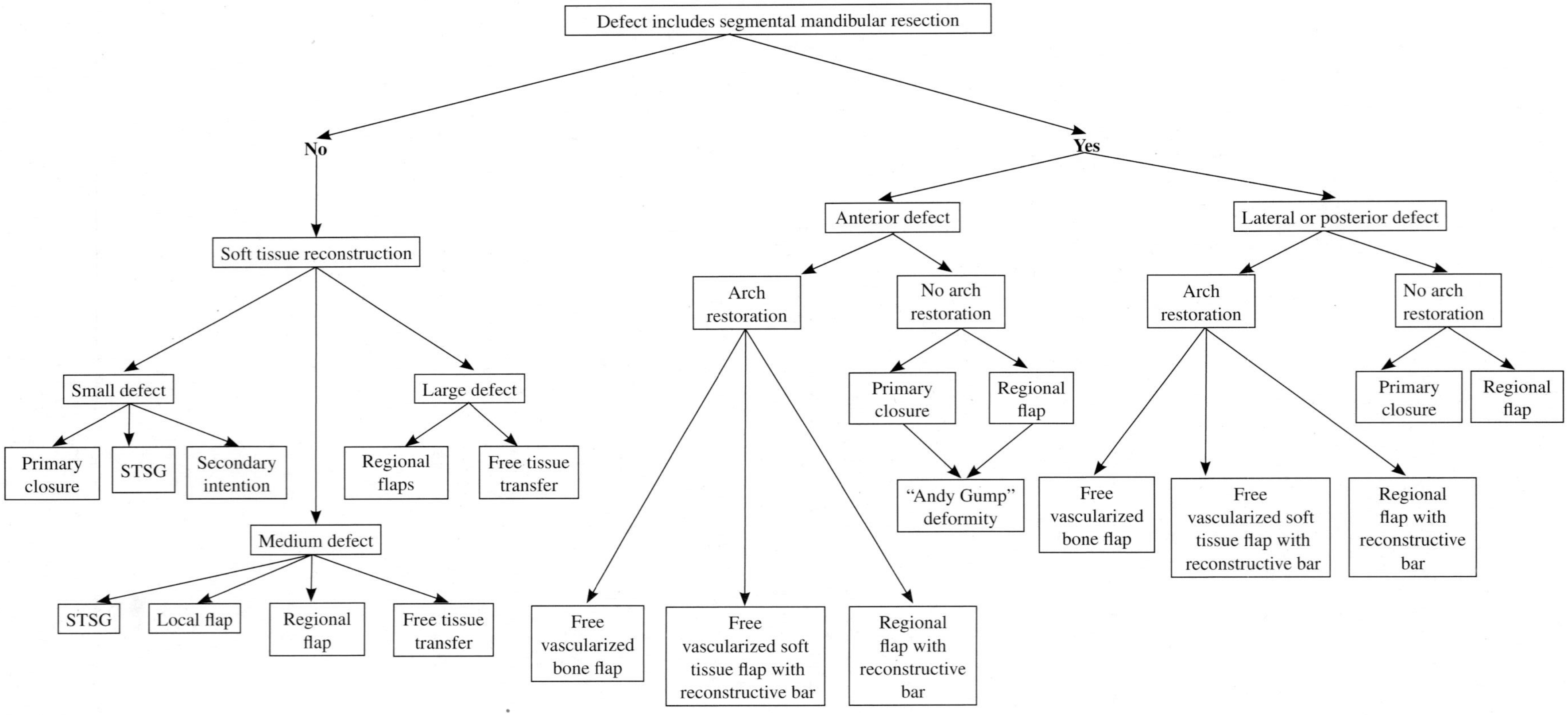

Recurrent Squamous Cell Carcinoma of the Oral Cavity

Russell B. Smith, Gerry F. Funk, and Henry T. Hoffman

Of all the new malignancies affecting the head and neck each year, 30% will involve the oral cavity.[1] Squamous cell carcinoma will be the predominant histopathology in these cases.[2] Treatment of oral cavity carcinoma is determined by many factors but is influenced most notably by the anatomical extent of the lesion and the preference of the treating institution. In general, similar cure rates for early-stage disease (stage I or II) result following initial treatment with either surgery or radiation therapy.[1,2] Despite the similar cure rates obtained with surgery and radiation therapy, most early oral cavity carcinomas are treated by surgical excision to avoid the long-term complications associated with primary radiation therapy of the oral cavity, which include xerostomia and osteoradionecrosis. Advanced-stage disease (stage III or IV) is usually treated with combined modality therapy using surgery and postoperative radiation therapy.[1,2] Nonsurgical therapy consisting of chemoradiation for advanced oral cavity carcinomas at this point has not been routinely employed. Recurrences often occur despite appropriate initial therapy, especially with advanced-stage disease. We will review the evaluation and management of locally recurrent squamous cell carcinoma of the oral cavity.

Recurrences

The appearance of tumor within the oral cavity after previous cancer therapy can be classified into three categories: persistent disease, recurrent disease, and a second primary. Persistent disease is defined as tumor that had an incomplete response to definitive therapy or tumor that appears within 6 months of definitive therapy after a brief disease-free interval. Recurrent disease is defined as tumor that occurs after at least a 6-month disease-free interval. A second primary is a tumor that is identified in a distinctly separate location from the original tumor. These lesions may be difficult to differentiate from recurrent disease if the lesion is adjacent to an area of previous tumor. Time is also an important consideration when classifying a tumor as a recurrence or a new primary in that most recurrences will occur within 18 to 24 months post-treatment, and lesions that occur 4 to 5 years after initial therapy, even if in the same location, are more

likely a second primary tumor. Literature on recurrent oral cavity carcinomas rarely differentiates persistent from recurrent disease, and both are reported as recurrent disease.

Recurrence rates for squamous cell carcinoma of the oral cavity have been reported to be between 20 and 73% when all stages are included.[3–7] These recurrences may occur locally, regionally, distantly, or as a combination of locations. The reported patterns of recurrence vary, with some reporting local recurrences occurring in nearly 60% of cases, whereas others note regional recurrences as being most common.[4–7] Fu et al reported an even distribution between local, locoregional, and regional recurrences.[8]

Multiple risk factors for local recurrence have been identified for oral cavity carcinomas. Yuen et al noted a linear increase in local recurrences based on advancing T-classification, with 16% of T1 lesions and 46% of T4 lesions developing local recurrences.[5] In a series of 51 patients with predominantly early-stage tongue carcinomas that had been treated by surgery with or without adjuvant therapy, Kirita et al found tumors with an endophytic growth pattern, grade 4 histologic pattern (diffusely infiltrating) of invasion, and surgical margins < 5 mm/positive margins to have a higher local recurrence rate.[3] El-Husseiny et al noted that in addition to positive margins, T4 tumors and tobacco use were associated with a higher recurrence rate.[9] It was also noted that the small cohort of patients with T3 and T4 tumors treated with irradiation alone had a high local recurrence rate. This is similar to the results of Leung et al.[10] Jones et al determined positive margins and tumor depth > 5 mm each independently increased recurrences by 3-fold, whereas tumor differentiation and the presence of desmoplasia, perineural spread, capillary lymphatic space invasion, and inflammatory response had no impact on recurrence.[11] Van Es et al noted that tumor parameters, such as tumor differentiation, tumor depth, pattern of invasion, and perineural spread, were not important prognostic factors for local recurrence in surgically treated early oral cavity carcinomas when clear margins were obtained.[12] Despite the variability noted for some prognostic factors, the impact of clear surgical margins is well defined. Shingaki et al reported a 3% local recurrence rate in early-stage oral cavity carcinomas treated with negative margin surgery alone.[13] Byers et al noted local recurrences in 80% of cases with positive margins in comparison to 20% in cases in which clear margins were obtained even if obtained by serial frozen sections.[14]

Patient Evaluation

Meticulous post-treatment surveillance is crucial in the care of patients with head and neck cancer. Variability in presentation exists among patients with recurrent oral cavity carcinomas. Most patients will experience pain and have obvious findings on physical examination. Some patients are asymptomatic but have obvious clinical findings of recurrence, and other patients will complain of pain without obvious clinical findings. By far the symptomatic patient without clinical findings is the most problematic for the head and neck oncologist.[15,16]

Depending on the previous treatment given for the initial tumor, the clinical exam may be of limited value. This is especially true in cases that were initially treated with combined modality therapy and significant post-treatment fibrosis has developed. The use of a flap reconstruction can further complicate the evaluation, especially if a bulky flap was used. In these instances, imaging studies become critical in the evaluation to exclude recurrence. Typically, computed tomography (CT) and magnetic resonance imaging (MRI) are used to delineate postoperative changes from disease. In recent years, positron emission tomography (PET) using 2-fluoro-2-deoxy-D-glucose (FDG) has also become a useful tool in detecting post-treatment recurrence.

A multitude of characteristics can be evaluated on post-treatment CT scans to help determine the presence or absence of recurrent disease. Some would argue that the only reliable CT criteria to discriminate post-treatment change from tumor are stable masses or gradually decreasing masses on serial scans.[17] Chikui et al reviewed CT scans on post-treatment oral cavity carcinomas to assess which radiographic findings were most predictive of recurrence.[18] Enhancement was found to be a nonspecific finding before 6 months post-treatment. Not only was enhancement demonstrated in all the recurrent cases, but it was also noted in 60% of the cases that never demonstrated recurrence. After 6 months post-treatment, all patients with recurrences demonstrated enhancement, whereas only 20% of the cases that remained disease free were noted to have enhancement. The enhancement in these cases was classified as not suggestive of recurrence and eventually did resolve in one case. Similarly, low-density areas were present in a majority of recurrent cases but rarely noted in disease-free cases after 6 months post-treatment. Finally, adipose

infiltration and adipose disappearance were almost exclusively noted in cases of recurrence.

The use of PET with FDG allows evaluation for tumor recurrence not by analysis of distorted anatomy, but by assessment of functionality of the tissue in question. In a prospective analysis, Anzai et al found a markedly improved diagnostic accuracy of PET over CT/MRI. In their cohort of 12 patients evaluated for recurrence, the sensitivity and specificity of PET versus CT/MRI were 88% and 100% versus 25% and 75%, respectively.[19] Fischbein et al reported slightly different results in their study of 35 patients, with sensitivity and specificity for primary and nodal recurrences being 100%/64% and 93%/67%, respectively, using PET imaging.[20] The slight differences in results were attributed to slightly different guidelines used to determine a positive or negative scan. When compared with imaging with CT or MRI, PET was again noted to be much more reliable in the assessment of recurrence. As with CT/MRI, a period of time to allow for post-treatment changes to resolve must occur before imaging for recurrence. Greven et al noted that post-treatment PET scans for various head and neck cancers were unreliable at 1 month, but by 4 months they had a high positive predictive value and a negative predictive value of 100%.[21]

Staging of Recurrent Oral Cavity Carcinomas

The tumor, nodal, and metastases (TNM) staging system established by the American Joint Committee on Cancer (AJCC) is routinely applied to new oral cavity carcinomas. Staging of tumors has many benefits, including planning treatment, discussing prognosis, exchanging information between treating physicians, and stratifying patients for research purposes. Unfortunately, this system has limitations when applied to recurrent oral cavity carcinomas, especially after previous surgical therapy.[22,23] Specifically, some primary (T) staging is not possible after previous resections, and regional status (N) is not accurately reportable after previous neck dissections. Other patient factors not directly linked to the tumor's anatomical extent, which may play a role in overall survival, are also not taken into account with the TNM staging system.[23,24] Because of these shortcomings, other staging systems have been developed in an attempt to better stratify patients with recurrent carcinomas.

Two such systems exist for staging recurrent oral cavity carcinomas. Both systems have been designed to be applicable to both oral cavity and oropharyngeal sites. Lacy et al based their staging system on a cohort of 249 patients with recurrent oral cavity and oropharyngeal carcinoma treated at Washington University.[22] Within this population, histologic differentiation, TNM status of the index tumor, initial treatment, time to recurrence, extent of recurrence, and recurrence treatment all have an impact on 2-year survival. Further multivariant analysis identified only initial tumor stage and extent of recurrence as predictors of survival. From this information, a staging system named Composite Oral Cavity and Oropharynx Recurrence Staging System (CORSS) was designed. Stage I represents initial AJCC stage I patients with local recurrences, and stage IV disease represents all distant recurrences regardless of initial stage. Two-year survival by stage ranged from 54% for stage I to 3% for stage IV. Yueh et al, using a similar technique, designed a staging system based on a cohort of 162 patients with a revised TNM system, weight loss, and deep muscle invasion as the prognostic factors.[23] Stage A disease represented early revised TNM disease without other poor prognostic factors, and stage D disease represented patients with muscle invasion or metastases. One-year survival with this system ranged from 88% for stage A to 4% for stage D.

Treatment

Many factors must be taken into consideration for treatment planning in recurrent oral cavity carcinoma. The characteristics of the recurrent tumor, the initial primary tumor, and its treatment, as well as patient comorbidities, will affect further cancer-directed therapy. Patients with recurrent oral cavity carcinomas overall have a poor prognosis. Almost all cases of recurrent oral cavity carcinomas that are treated for cure will involve surgery as a major component of the salvage therapy. Yuen et al reported a significantly longer salvage time for those treated with surgery for locally recurrent oral cavity carcinoma following initial surgery or combined modality therapy, but only had 9% of the patients experienced long-term disease-free survival after salvage.[5] In a second study of surgical salvage of primary radiation failures, Yuen et al noted a 39% 5-year disease-free survival rate for local recurrences and a 27% 5-year survival rate for locoregional recurrences with surgical salvage.[25] Sun et al also found 15% improvement in 3-year survival when surgery was included in the salvage regimen.[26] Finally, Schwartz et al noted that those salvaged with surgery had an improved salvage time and total survival time and a trend toward improved overall salvage cure.[4]

Surgical therapy of recurrent oral cavity carcinoma must include decision making regarding resection margins and management of the adjacent bone. Given the importance of obtaining clear margins during surgical excision of an initial oral cavity carcinoma, one would assume that the same premise would hold true for excision

of a recurrent tumor. Unfortunately, none of the literature that reports on prognostic factors for treatment of recurrent oral cavity carcinoma addresses this issue. Despite the lack of supporting data, clear margins need to be obtained. Most would agree that a 5 mm cuff of normal tissue around a lesion is the minimum to consider the margins to be clear. The amount of normal tissue that needs to be excised to obtain this is obviously more, given that contraction will occur after tumor removal. Johnson et al addressed the issue of tissue contracture after excision of oral cavity lesions in a canine model.[27] The tongue and labiobuccal mucosal excisions demonstrated a 30 to 47% shrinkage of margins from the time of excision to the final paraffin slide preparation. Their recommendations were to take at least 8 to 10 mm margins around the lesion to ensure clear margins. These guidelines, however, do not take into account nonpalpable microscopic disease that may be seen in infiltrating lesions. Additionally, in cases of recurrent oral cavity carcinoma, multiple confounding factors, such as scar from previous surgery, postradiation fibrosis, and soft tissue changes related to previous flap reconstructions, affect one's ability to detect tumor extent and the ultimate goal of clear margins. Subsequently, initial margins of 2 cm are appropriate and should be followed by frozen sections to confirm clear margins.

The management of the mandible in oral cavity carcinoma continues to be controversial even in previously untreated patients. Because of concerns related to periosteal lymphatics, the use of segmental mandibular resection is no longer practiced, but marginal and segmental mandibular resections are critical in cases in which tumor abuts or invades the bone. A multitude of methods have been evaluated for their ability to determine bone invasion preoperatively. Each technique has its merits, but no one test alone has proved to be the panacea to this difficult question. A combination of techniques, including clinical exam and radiographic evaluations, will provide the best information for clinical decision making.[28]

In cases in which previous therapy has not affected the mandible, the same guidelines can be used for previously untreated and recurrent oral cavity carcinomas. Current recommendations are if tumor abuts but is not felt to invade the bone, a marginal resection is acceptable, but if significant bone invasion through the cortex is present, segmental resection is required. In some instances, the tumor is adherent to the periosteum, or superficial cortical bone erosion is noted. Most would argue that, in this scenario, a marginal resection is still adequate.[28]

If previous irradiation or surgical excision has altered the mandible, a separate set of guidelines is incorporated in the management of tumor adjacent to the mandible. In the face of previous irradiation, if tumor abuts but does not invade the bone, a marginal mandibulectomy is required, whereas any bone erosion regardless of depth of invasion should be treated with a segmental mandibulectomy.[29] For a case in which previous marginal resection has been performed and the recurrence is adherent to the residual bone, segmental resection should be used for salvage.[30]

Despite these guidelines, situations do exist in which segmental resection is necessary to ensure clear margins despite the lack of bone invasion. The two locations for which this is most often encountered are the anterior floor of the mouth and the retromolar trigone region. In the floor of the mouth, especially in patients with an acutely angled anterior mandible, larger lesions with deep invasion into the floor of the mouth musculature are difficult to adequately resect with clear margins unless a segmental mandibulectomy is utilized. Similarly, if tumors of the retromolar trigone invade posteriorly into the pterygoid musculature, a segmental mandibular resection may be necessary to obtain adequate margins because the thin bone of the ramus may prohibit marginal resection.

The role of radiation therapy in the treatment of recurrent oral cavity carcinomas is difficult to ascertain. Most would administer postoperative radiation therapy after surgical salvage of patients with recurrence after primary surgery.[4,26] The use of radiation alone for recurrences of surgical failures has not been recommended and is viewed by some as a palliative intervention.[5] The results from radiation therapy as single modality salvage is slightly skewed in that only nonresectable recurrences are for the most part treated with radiation alone. Regine et al noted postoperative radiation therapy for recurrent head and neck carcinomas to be less effective than when given for initial therapy, but this study did not control for stage, other prognostic factors, or specific indications for the radiotherapy.[31] In patients with recurrence after primary irradiation or combined modality therapy, re-irradiation theoretically could also be advantageous after surgical salvage. Re-irradiation in the head and neck has mostly been administered for recurrent nasopharyngeal carcinoma and unresectable recurrent disease.[32,33] Conventional radiation therapy techniques are associated with severe morbidities in the previously irradiated patient.[34] Some of these morbidities can be minimized without compromise of effect using advanced techniques, such as intensity modulated radiation therapy (IMRT) in these situations. Postoperataive re-irradiation with IMRT has only recently been used, and long-term follow-up of this technique has yet to be reported.

Reconstruction

After resection of recurrent squamous cell carcinoma of the oral cavity, a multitude of defects may exist. The complexity of such defects is affected not only by the size and location of the recurrence but also by the previous therapy and its resultant alterations of the head and neck anatomy. Regardless of the complexity of the defect, the goal of reconstruction should still be restoring oral function such that the patient has efficient airway, speech, and swallowing. The reconstruction should also provide acceptable external cosmesis whenever possible.

The use of a reconstruction paradigm facilitates the decision process for defects of the oral cavity. The typical paradigm follows a logical progression of primary closure, healing by secondary intention, skin grafting, local flaps, regional flaps, and free tissue transfer. With the success and advantages of free tissue transfer in the reconstruction of the head and neck after ablative surgery, one may quickly proceed to this form of reconstruction, especially in these previously treated patients. Most experts, however, would agree that when primary closure can be obtained without compromise of function, this should be first employed. In recurrent oral cavity carcinomas, salvage surgery is radical, and the residual defect usually requires tissue transfer for closure. In this situation, either regional flaps or free tissue transfer can be used. The disadvantages of excessive flap bulk, limited pedicle length, and marginal flap necrosis associated with the regional flaps favor the use of free tissue transfer in these cases.

The ability to use free tissue transfer in the reconstruction of recurrent oral cavity cancer may potentially be limited by the previous therapy. Previous surgery, especially radical neck dissections, may limit the availability of recipient vessels in the neck for the free tissue transfer. Despite these concerns, the success of free tissue transfer in reconstruction of defects resulting from surgical excision of recurrent oral cavity carcinoma is high. Demirkan et al reported on the use of second free flap reconstruction for recurrent oral cavity carcinomas in 35 patients, with 94.6% flap survival.[35] This rate was comparable to the 97.3% success rate of the initial reconstruction. The rate of reexploration was noted to be slightly higher in the second flap cases at 13.5% in comparison to the 7.9% noted with the first reconstruction. In one half of the cases, the contralateral neck had to be entered to find suitable recipient vessels.

Prognosis

Despite the feasibility of salvage surgery for locally recurrent squamous cell carcinoma of the head and neck, prognosis remains poor. Salvage rates of 15 to 20% have been reported in most series.[4,22,26] Others have reported salvage rates from 3 to 55%.[5,11] Any improvements in survival for treatment of recurrent oral cavity carcinoma are probably related to the advances in reconstruction that allow more radical salvage resections and advances in radiation therapy that allow re-irradiation.

Several factors have been noted to affect the outcome of salvage therapy for recurrent oral cavity carcinomas. The impact of surgery as part of salvage therapy on survival has been discussed previously, but other factors, especially time to recurrence, are known to affect survival with recurrent oral cavity carcinoma. Lacy et al and Yueh et al incorporated factors found to significantly impact survival into revised staging systems, which have been previously discussed.[22,23] Most recurrent oral cavity carcinomas present within the first 12 months after curative therapy.[3,5] In 38 patients treated with curative intent for recurrent disease, Schwartz et al noted that recurrences occurring within 6 months of initial therapy and recurrences after treatment of advanced-stage primary disease had a much worse salvage time and total survival time.[4] Llewelyn and Mitchell analyzed 58 patients treated with salvage surgery after primary irradiation and also noted that most who failed salvage therapy had experienced early recurrences at a median time of 5 months, whereas those who survived after salvage therapy had their initial recurrences later, at a median of 12 months.[36] Sun et al had limited success with salvage therapy for recurrent oral cavity carcinoma, but they noted that patients who experienced recurrence after 6 months following initial therapy and who developed isolated local recurrences had slightly improved 2-year survival. Most who did survive were noted to have significant treatment-related complications.[26]

Conclusion

Recurrence of oral cavity carcinoma occurs frequently, regardless of initial therapy. Most patients who have recurrences will present within 2 years of their treatment. Subsequently, regular surveillance after initial therapy is valuable and may allow early detection of a recurrence. Despite the overall poor prognosis for patients with recurrent oral cavity carcinoma, salvage therapy is possible. The inclusion of surgery in the salvage regimen improves the chance of long-term disease-free survival, but the role of radiation therapy, especially re-irradiation, is still poorly defined. Radical resections for recurrent disease frequently result in complex defects, and free tissue transfer for reconstruction of these complex defects can be performed safely. Multiple factors have been identified that affect the prognosis of patients with recurrent oral cavity carcinoma and should be considered prior to initiating salvage therapy. Despite advances in salvage therapy, most patients with recurrent oral cavity carcinoma will succumb to their disease, and this needs to be considered by both the treating physician and the patient before initiating salvage therapy.

References

1. Alvi A, Myers EN, Johnson JT. Cancer of the oral cavity. In: Myers EN, Suen JY, eds. Cancer of the Head and Neck. Philadelphia: WB Saunders;1996:321–360.

2. Shah JP, Lydiatt WM. Buccal mucosa, alveolus, retromolar trigone, floor of mouth, hard palate, and tongue tumors. In: Thawley SE, Panje WR, Batsakis JG, Lindberg RD, eds. Comprehensive Management of Head and Neck Tumors. Philadelphia: WB Saunders;1999:686–694.

3. Kirita T, Okabe S, Izumo T, Sugimura M. Risk factors for the postoperative local recurrence of tongue carcinoma. J Oral Maxillofac Surg 1994;52:149–154.

4. Schwartz GJ, Mehta RH, Wenig BL, Shaligram C, Portugal LG. Salvage treatment for recurrent squamous cell carcinoma of the oral cavity. Head Neck 2000;22:34–41.

5. Yuen APW, Wei WI, Wong SHW, Ng RWM. Local recurrence of carcinoma of the tongue after glossectomy: patient prognosis. Ear Nose Throat J 1998;77:181–184.

6. Boysen M, Lovdal O, Tausjo J, Winther F. The value of follow-up in patients treated for squamous cell carcinoma of the head and neck. Eur J Cancer 1992;28:426–430.

7. Whitehurst JO, Droulias CA. Surgical treatment of squamous cell carcinoma of the oral tongue: factors influencing survival. Arch Otolaryngol 1977;103:212–215.

8. Fu KK, Lichter A, Galante M. Carcinoma of the floor of the mouth: an analysis of treatment results and the sites and causes of failure. Int J Radiat Oncol Biol Phys 1976;1: 829–837.

9. El-Husseiny G, Kandil A, Jamshed A, et al. Squamous cell carcinoma of the oral tongue: an analysis of prognostic factors. Br J Oral Maxillofac Surg 2000;38:193–199.

10. Leung TW, Lee AW, Chan DK. Definitive radiotherapy for carcinoma of the oral tongue. Acta Oncol 1993;32:559–564.

11. Jones KR, Lodge-Rigal R, Reddick RL, Tudor GE, Shockley WW. Prognostic factors in the recurrence of stage I and II squamous cell cancer of the oral cavity. Arch Otolaryngol Head Neck Surg 1992;118:483–485.

12. van Es RJJ, van Nieuw Amerongen N, Slootweg PJ, Egyedi P. Resection margin as a predictor of recurrence at the primary site for T1 and T2 oral cancers. Arch Otolaryngol Head Neck Surg 1996;122:521–525.

13. Shingaki S, Kobayashi T, Suzuki I, Kohno M, Nakajima T. Surgical treatment of stage I and II oral squamous cell carcinomas: analysis of causes of failures. Br J Oral Maxillofac Surg 1995;33:304–308.

14. Byers RM, Bland KI, Borlase B, Luna M. The prognostic and therapeutic value of frozen section determinations in the surgical treatment of squamous cell carcinoma of the head and neck. Am J Surg 1978;136:525–528.

15. Wong JK, Wood RE, McLean M. Pain preceding recurrent head and neck cancer. J Orofac Pain 1998;12:52–59.

16. Smit M, Balm AJM, Hilgers FJM, Tan IB. Pain as sign of recurrent disease in head and neck squamous cell carcinoma. Head Neck 2001;23:372–375.

17. Som PM, Urken ML, Biller H, Lidov M. Imaging the postoperative neck. Radiology 1993;187:593–603.

18. Chikui T, Yuasa K, Inagaki M, Ohishi M, Shirasuna K, Kanda S. Tumor recurrence criteria for postoperative contrast-enhanced computed tomography after surgical treatment of oral cancer and flap repair. Oral Surg Oral Med Oral Pathol Oral Radiol Endod 2000;90:369–376.

19. Anzai Y, Carroll WR, Quint DJ, et al. Recurrence of head and neck cancer after surgery or irradiation: prospective comparison of 2-deoxy-2-[f-18]fluoro-d-glucose PET and MR imaging diagnoses. Radiology 1996;200:135–141.

20. Fischbein NJ, Assar SA, Caputo GR, et al. Clinical utility of positron emission tomography with [18]f-fluorodeoxyglucose in detecting residual/recurrent squamous cell carcinoma of the head and neck. AJNR Am J Neuroradiol 1998;19:1189–1196.

21. Greven KM, Williams DW III, McGuirt WF Sr, et al. Serial positron emission tomography scans following radiation therapy of patients with head and neck cancer. Head Neck 2001;23:942–946.

22. Lacy PD, Spitznagel EL, Piccirillo JF. Development of a new staging system for recurrent oral cavity and oropharyngeal squamous cell carcinoma. Cancer 1999;86:1387–1395.

23. Yueh B, Feinstein AR, Weaver EM, Sasaki CT, Concato J. Prognostic staging system for recurrent, persistent, and second primary cancers of the oral cavity and oropharynx. Arch Otolaryngol Head Neck Surg 1998;124:975–981.

24. Piccirillo JF. Purposes, problems, and proposals for progress in cancer staging. Arch Otolaryngol Head Neck Surg 1995;121:145–149.

25. Yuen AP, Wei WI, Lam LK, Ho WK, Kwong D. Results of surgical salvage of locoregional recurrence of carcinoma of the tongue after radiotherapy failure. Ann Otol Rhinol Laryngol 1997;106:779–782.

26. Sun LM, Leung SW, Su CY, Wang CJ. The relapse patterns and outcome of post-operative recurrent tongue cancer. J Oral Maxillofac Surg 1997;55:827–831.

27. Johnson RE, Sigman JD, Funk GF, Robinson RA, Hoffman HT. Quantification of surgical margin shrinkage in the oral cavity. Head Neck 1997;19:281–286.

28. Politi M, Costa F, Robiony M, Rinaldo A, Ferlito A. Review of segmental and marginal resection of the mandible in patients with oral cancer. Acta Otolaryngol 2000;120:569–579.

29. McGregor AD, McDonald DG. Patterns of spread of squamous cell carcinoma within the mandible. Head Neck 1989;11:457–461.

30. Dubner S, Heller KS. Local control of squamous cell carcinoma following marginal and segmental mandibulectomy. Head Neck 1993;15:29–32.

31. Regine WF, Valentino J, Sloan DA, et al. Postoperative radiation therapy for primary vs. recurrent squamous cell carcinoma of the head and neck: results of a comparative analysis. Head Neck 1999;21:554–559.

32. Cho JH, Kim GE, Cho KH, et al. Hyperfractionation re-irradiation using a 3-dimensional conformal technique for locally recurrent carcinoma of the nasopharynx. Yonsei Med J 2001;42:55–64.

33. McLean M, Chow E, O'Sullivan B, et al. Re-irradiation for locally recurrent nasopharyngeal carcinoma. Radiother Oncol 1998;48:209–211.

34. Stewart FA. Re-treatment after full-course radiotherapy: is it a viable option? Acta Oncol 1999;38:855–862.

35. Demirkan F, Wei FC, Chen HC, Chen IH, Hau SP, Liau CT. Microsurgical reconstruction in recurrent oral cancer: use of a second free flap in the same patient. Plast Reconstr Surg 1999;103:829–838.

36. Llewelyn J, Mitchell R. Survival of patients who needed salvage surgery for recurrences after radiotherapy for oral carcinomas. Br J Oral Maxillofac Surg 1997;35:424–428.

Revision Surgery for Oropharyngeal Cancer

William M. Lydiatt and Daniel D. Lydiatt

In 2006, 8950 cases of pharyngeal carcinoma were expected to occur in the United States.[1] Approximately one half of oropharyngeal malignancies occur in the base of the tongue, one fourth in the tonsil, and the remainder in the soft palate or posterior pharyngeal wall. Definitive treatment consists of either surgery or radiation therapy for early-stage disease. Later-stage disease usually requires combination therapy, typically using radiation and concomitant chemotherapy or in selected cases surgery followed by radiation and chemotherapy for adverse pathologic findings. The role of combinations of chemotherapy and radiation therapy for stage III and IV disease has come about in an effort to improve the quality of life without compromising survival. Unfortunately, local and regional failure continues to be a major determinant of morbidity and mortality. Local and locoregional failure following initial therapy occurs in 11 to 58% of cases, depending on the stage at presentation.[2,3] This is true for all primary treatment modalities. Recurrent or persistent disease following aggressive initial treatment presents a challenge to the head and neck surgeon. This chapter will concentrate on the evaluation of the patient with recurrent or persistent malignancy of the oropharynx following initial surgical or nonsurgical therapy.

In the untreated patient, the chief goal is to provide an individualized treatment to maximize survival and minimize functional loss. The evaluation for salvage surgery is the same, but the options are more limited. The goal of the chemoradiotherapy approach is to eradicate disease and preserve the primary site function. Therefore, in the initial assessment of this patient, a decision was made that the anticipated functional deficit from an operation would be greater than with radiation. Salvage surgery is likely to result in the same or greater morbidity than the initial operation. Typically, the resection is bigger and the need for reconstruction greater. A realistic evaluation of the chances for local and regional control and a sense of the functional deficit resulting must be accomplished. Only then can one know how to do the operation, when to do the operation, whether to do the operation, and whether there is a realistic expectation to achieve palliation or cure. It is important that the patient and the physician understand and agree upon the goals of therapy.

Patient Evaluation

A multidisciplinary approach involving head and neck surgical oncology, radiation oncology, plastic surgery, dental oncology, medical oncology, and others is important to address all aspects of treatment. Decisions must be made on a continual basis and start with the initial decision of whether the therapy is intended to be curative or palliative. Local and regional failure of head and neck cancer has consistently been shown to be one of the most devastating afflictions due to the high degree of pain, functional loss, disfigurement, and reduction in quality of life. Therefore, either cure or palliation can be reasonable goals of surgical therapy. Pain relief may be better achieved by surgical therapy.[4] The presence of distant metastases does not necessarily exclude surgery as a treatment modality if an operation can be done with a reasonable expectation of recovery, a diminution in the likelihood for pain and uncontrolled local growth, and a life expectancy that is long enough to make the short-term recovery from surgery worth the longer-term benefit. This is typically at least 6 months. Although recurrent laryngeal cancer frequently meets these criteria, oropharyngeal cancer surgery, due to the cancer's lack of clear anatomical barriers and the morbidity associated with the operation, is less likely to be an option for palliative treatment. Thus, a more extensive evaluation for distant metastases should be done prior to salvage surgery to get an estimate of survival. A more extensive work-up individualized to the patient may include a chest and abdomen computed tomography (CT) scan, bone scan, or positron emission tomography (PET) scan. Similarly, patients who have persistent disease after treatment or who recur within 6 months after the completion of treatment tend to have a much worse prognosis and limited life expectancy and are less likely to be candidates for salvage surgery.

The surgeon must weigh the surgical options and likely sequelae against the alternatives. Consideration of the following issues will be important in determining operability and the extent of resection, which will best define the likely sequelae from the operation and be very important in predicting intermediate and long-term quality of life. Each case is carefully individualized and depends on factors

Decision tree for recurrent oropharyngeal cancer

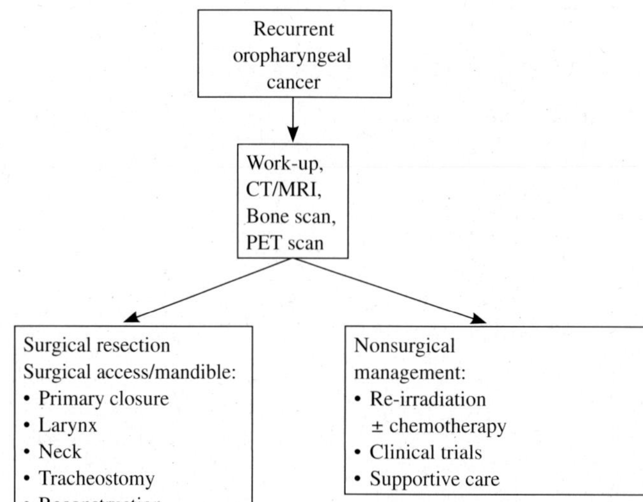

related to the patient, the tumor, and what options are available to the treating physician.

Determining the Extent of Resection

Physical examination coupled with CT and/or magnetic resonance imaging (MRI) is necessary to define the extent of disease and aid in determining operability. Disease that persists or recurs following radiation and chemotherapy is harder to assess clinically due to the fibrosis that accompanies such treatment. The role of PET scanning is currently being defined. At present, it appears that PET may yield important information with respect to the neck but is less accurate in predicting primary recurrence in the oropharynx.[5] Ultimately, clinical judgment and biopsies obtained during an exam under anesthesia may be the best way of outlining the extent of recurrence. Even more than with untreated disease, margins are often deceptive, with clinically normal-appearing tissue often harboring infiltrative carcinoma. Frozen section is vital to achieve clearance of disease. Subclinical disease found at frozen section often makes the extent of resection larger than anticipated. This possibility should be taken into account when planning reconstruction so that several options are available.

Assessment of the Mandible

Bone invasion following radiation therapy is more likely and proceeds along less predictable routes than in the untreated setting (**Fig. 18.1**).[6] Bone margins need to be more generous in the postirradiation setting. Marginal mandibulectomy may be hazardous in the postirradiation setting due to the unpredictable nature of invasion, the risk of mandibular fracture, and the potential increased risk of osteoradionecrosis.

Assessment of the Carotid Artery

It is important to determine in advance if the carotid artery is likely to be involved by tumor and have a preoperative management strategy mapped out (**Fig. 18.2**). If one is going to leave tumor on the artery, it is not likely that the operation will result in significant success, and a radical resection of the oropharynx is probably not warranted. If the artery is to be resected, then one should be prepared

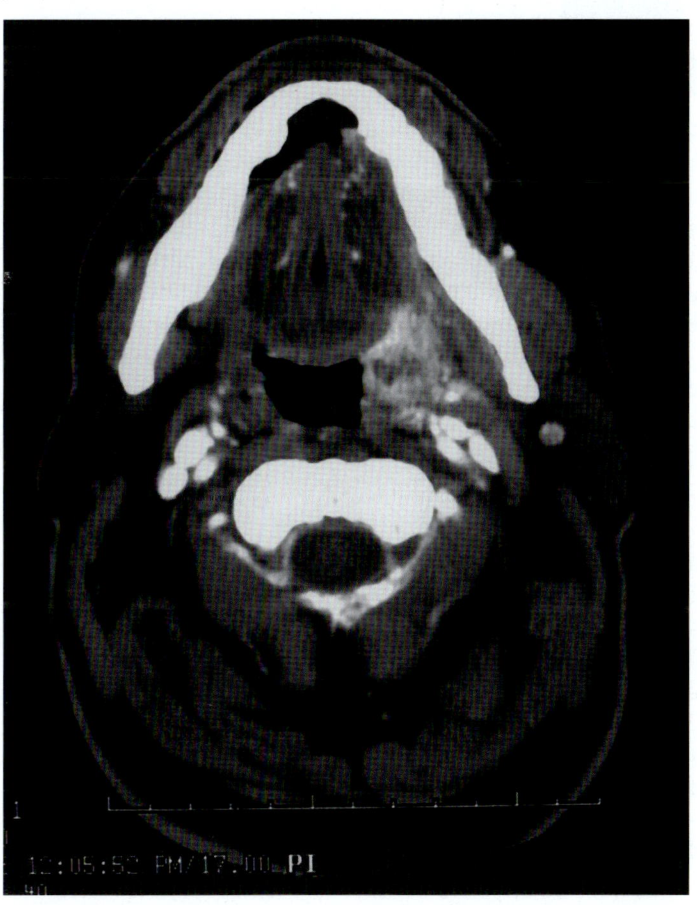

Fig. 18.1 Computed tomography scan demonstrating recurrent squamous cell carcinoma following concomitant chemotherapy and radiation. Tumor extends to the mandible without obvious involvement. Pathologically, the tumor extended into the bony cortex.

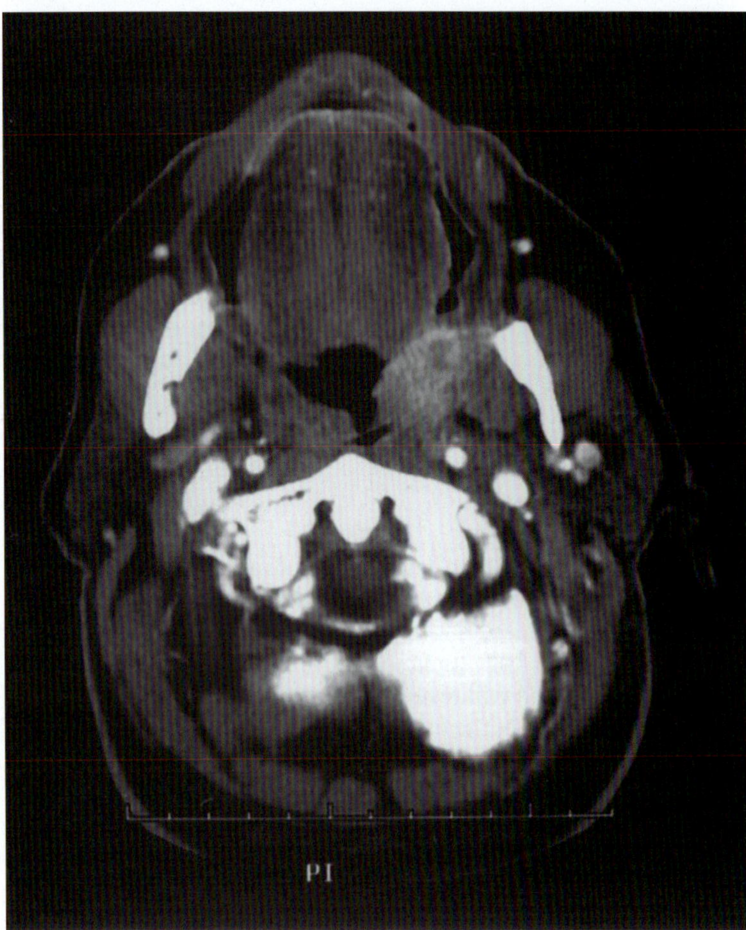

Fig. 18.2 Tumor extends to, but does not appear to involve, the carotid. No involvement was found at the time of the operation.

for reconstruction at the time. This can be very difficult with oropharyngeal cancers because involvement of the carotid is typically high near the skull base. Ligation of the artery without prior balloon occlusion studies imparts a significant risk of neurological injury and thus is probably not a reasonable palliative procedure. Similarly, clearance of disease from the skull base can be assessed preoperatively; if the expectation is low, other options should be considered.

Assessment of the Larynx

Lesions that track inferiorly through the tonsillar fossa and down to the lateral pharynx, particularly those that invade the base of the tongue, place the supraglottic larynx at high risk. Performing a supraglottic laryngectomy is hazardous in the postirradiated patient. Supraglottic swelling makes tracheal decannulation very difficult. Inhibition of laryngeal motion by radiation fibrosis further compounds aspiration problems that are usually present with supraglottic laryngectomy. Very serious consideration to completing the laryngectomy should be given, and the patient should be aware of this possibility.

If the larynx is preserved, aspiration continues to be a risk, particularly in the short term. Placement of a gastrostomy tube in the perioperative period should be strongly considered. A full discussion with the patient about the need for subsequent conversion to total laryngectomy for aspiration must also accompany this approach.

Operative Approaches

Once the above factors have been assessed, the operative approach can be selected. Specific attributes and detriments of each approach can be weighed to maximize exposure and minimize morbidity. The reconstructive options discussed below should also be considered in this decision.

Peroral Resection

Peroral resection is excellent for lesions of the soft palate. It is less useful for lesions of the tonsil and base of the tongue in the revision setting. The extent of resection is often greater than what clinically appears necessary, and exposure in the postirradiated setting can be more difficult due to fibrosis resulting in trismus. This method should only be selected with an option for conversion to a more open approach.

Composite Resection

The operative approach will hinge on the site of disease and the likelihood of resection of the mandible or larynx. For a tonsil resection, because of the infiltrative nature of the lesion and the unpredictability of bony invasion, as well as the need for a reliable form of reconstruction, one should typically err on the side of resecting posterior bone and approaching the tonsil through a standard segmental composite resection. This approach facilitates exposure to the base of the tongue, supraglottic larynx, and lateral and posterior pharyngeal wall and also provides access to the nasopharynx, a frequent site of extension of disease. Complex reconstruction is typically required and makes this a lengthier and potentially morbid approach. This is our preferred approach when mandibular resection is required.

Mandibular Swing

If the surgeon is quite confident that the mandible is not invaded or closely involved, a paramedian osteotomy with mandibular swing achieves excellent exposure to the base of the tongue, posterior wall, and tonsillar region.[3] The mucosal incision is carried lateral to the tongue in the glossal lingual fold. A midline glossotomy can also be accomplished from this approach, which may help preserve hypoglossal and lingual nerve function in small midline base of tongue carcinoma. By performing the mandibulotomy in the parasagittal area, one should avoid the previously irradiated portion of the mandible and preserve the mental nerve. With intensity modulated radiation therapy (IMRT), however, the anterior mandible does receive irradiation, although at a much lower dose, ~1000 cGy. This low dose is not likely to prove a detriment to this approach. The need for facial incisions and mandibular nonunion are potential complications of this approach.

Tongue Drop

Approaching the oropharynx through the neck has many advantages. By releasing the geniohyoid and mylohyoid muscles and incising the floor of the mouth, the entire tongue can be dropped into the neck, providing excellent visualization with fairly high short-term, but lesser long-term, morbidity (**Fig. 18.3**). Avoiding osteotomies in the

postirradiated mandible is a considerable advantage. A long mucosal suture line and the potential for devascularization are potential disadvantages, with the potential for fistula formation. Avoidance of the osteotomy and lip-splitting incision make this another option for surgical salvage in this population.

Lateral Pharyngotomy

The lateral pharyngotomy approach provides minimal exposure but at much less morbidity. It is useful for smaller lesions, particularly of the posterior pharyngeal wall. Like peroral resections, it is rarely used in the postirradiation setting, given the insidious nature of recurrent tumor. This approach can be converted to a composite resection, if operative findings dictate.

Suprahyoid or Transhyoid Pharyngotomy

This approach may be useful for small tumors of the tongue base or posterior wall.[7] The hyoid can be either preserved or resected. The utility of this approach is less compelling in the postirradiation patient due to limited exposure and blind entry into the vallecula.

Reconstruction

Primary Closure

It is not likely that primary closure will be achievable in most revision cases, but occasionally for a base of tongue lesion, this remains a viable option. Because the tissue has been previously irradiated or resected, the vascularity will be poor to marginal. Wound breakdown is therefore more likely, and what would have been a good primary closure becomes an open wound with disastrous implications. Similarly, allowing a wound to heal by secondary intent or placement of a split-thickness skin graft may be a more risky proposition. The threshold for bringing in nonirradiated vascularized tissue is lowered in revision surgery of the oropharynx in the postirradiation setting.

Free Fibula Microvascular Reconstruction

The osseocutaneous free fibula flap provides good soft tissue coverage with the ability to reconstruct the posterior aspect of the mandible in composite resections. It provides several advantages, such as nonirradiated tissue, replacement of bone stock, and pliable soft tissue.[8] Bony reconstruction is especially important in the dentate patient to maintain occlusion. Cosmetically, the contour appears better, and it is a reliable flap, with a 95% or better

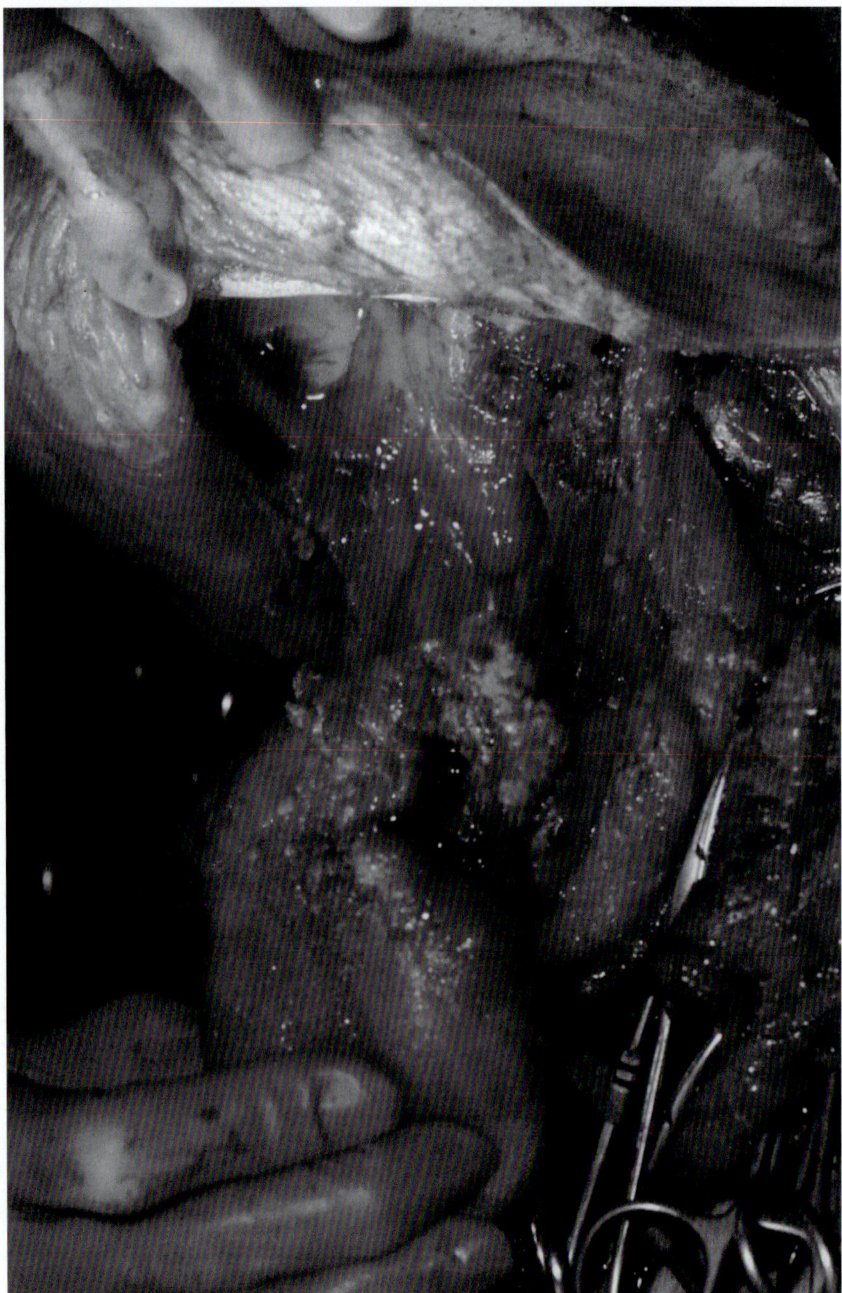

Fig. 18.3 Operative photo demonstrating exposure of base of the tongue recurrence utilizing the tongue drop. Neurovascular pedicles remain intact on the contralateral side.

flap success rate. It does carry somewhat more morbidity and may prolong hospital stay and recovery, especially when a large cutaneous paddle is necessary and the patient is not able to ambulate as quickly. As with most flaps, it is an insensate flap, making postoperative deglutition somewhat more difficult. The free fibula flap has the advantage of bringing vascularized bone and soft tissue into the previously irradiated area. Osseointegrated implants for dental rehabilitation can also be considered. If the segmental mandibulectomy extends to the anterior mandible, reconstruction of the bone should be performed whenever feasible, regardless of the patient's dental status.

Radial Forearm Free Flap

The fasciocutaneous radial forearm flap makes an outstanding choice for soft tissue reconstruction. A large volume of area can be covered, and it is a very reliable flap. It provides nonirradiated tissue with a healthy blood supply into the compromised area. It does not provide much soft tissue bulk if a significant amount of the base of the tongue has been resected. It is also an insensate flap, and aspiration can be a significant problem.[9]

Pectoralis Major Myocutaneous Flap

This flap provides skin and muscle bulk. It works well for a large resection of the base of the tongue with or without composite resection of the posterior mandibular bone and can be a less morbid alternative to a microvascular flap. There is a relatively high rate of at least partial flap loss, typically due to loss of the internal mammary perforators, which provide a good portion of the blood supply to the skin. This flap, therefore, has a high fistula rate, prolonging hospitalization and recovery.

With most operations for oropharyngeal carcinoma, a tracheostomy should be considered. This will protect against the effects of upper airway swelling. Postoperative nutrition is critical and may be a long-term issue. If the patient can take nutrition per os, supplementation may be beneficial, and a consultation with a dietitian is helpful. Lesions involving a significant amount of the tonsil and base of the tongue are likely to need prolonged enteral nutrition. A gastrostomy tube (G-tube) provides an excellent route. The G-tube may be placed at the same time as the resection or subsequently, either via a laparoscopically placed G-tube or a percutaneous endoscopic gastrostomy (PEG) or by interventional radiology through a percutaneous technique.[10] One advantage of the laparoscopic and percutaneous nonendoscopically placed tubes is that in the postoperative setting, there is no manipulation of the pharynx by an endoscope. Similarly, if done intraoperatively, there is less risk of tumor seeding compared with a PEG done endoscopically prior to resection.

Alternatives to Surgery

It is important for the physician to consider all options of therapy that may achieve the same goal as surgical resection. Broadly, the options include surgical resection, re-irradiation with or without chemotherapy, clinical trials of innovative therapies, and comfort or supportive care.

Re-irradiation

The role of re-irradiation with chemotherapy is evolving, particularly with the use of IMRT and sensitizing chemotherapy. Data are currently accruing as to whether this is a feasible approach (Radiation Therapy Oncology Group [RTOG] 99–11). One must consider the time from failure from previous radiation therapy. If it has been less than 1 year and certainly less than 6 months, it is highly unlikely that additional radiation therapy will be of any significant benefit. Similarly, because oropharyngeal carcinoma typically involves irradiation of the mandible or spinal cord, re-irradiation would likely encompass the same areas, making the morbidity potentially significant.

Clinical Trials

Clinical trials are beneficial to society because knowledge is advanced. Patients may benefit as well, but this is not necessarily true, particularly in early-phase trials. Subjects enrolled in clinical trials may feel they are contributing to future improvements in health care and thus helping others if not themselves. Clinical trials utilizing innovative treatment options or therapies should at least be considered.

Supportive Care

Finally, the best supportive care must also be considered. The primary goal is to achieve comfort, dignity, hygiene, nutrition, and spiritual assistance in the last phase of life. Pain will be controlled through a multipronged attack, using narcotics, non-narcotics, benzodiazepines, antibiotics, and antidepressants. This may be coupled with a recommendation for hospice care and a clear definition of end-of-life issues. Although arguably the most difficult task for a surgical oncologist, providing supportive care is crucial. The patient must have close and aggressive follow-up, lest he or she feel abandoned in this final treatment phase. Often the decision not to intervene is the most difficult to make.

Making the decision whether to operate or choose one of the nonsurgical alternatives must include a very frank discussion with the patient as to his or her expectations and understanding of the risks, complications, and expected sequelae balanced against the benefits associated with operating. On the one hand, the patient must understand what local disease progression will inflict upon him or her. On the other hand, the patient must understand the limitations to the proposed resection. Included in this discussion should be a plan for treatment of comorbid diseases, such as depression.

Depression

Depression is common among patients with head and neck cancer, with incidence rates of up to 40 to 50%.[11,12] Suicide rates are the highest among any cancer patients, with one study demonstrating up to 19% of all cancer-related suicides occurred in head and neck cancer patients.[13] Depression complicates recovery and has a detrimental effect on quality of life. Investigation into symptoms and signs of depression is important to maximize perioperative and postoperative recovery in patients with recurrent oropharyngeal cancer. Because much of the speech and swallowing rehabilitation occurs as a result of diligent work on behalf of the patient, depression can have a profoundly negative impact.

Effective treatment can be done using either pharmacologic or psychotherapeutic measures. Most head and neck surgeons are more familiar and comfortable with pharmacologic measures. First-line therapy using selective serotonin reuptake inhibitors (SSRIs) is effective in 50 to 70% of medically ill patients and should be strongly considered in patients who exhibit signs and symptoms of depression. An atypical antidepressant such as bupropion or mirtazapine could also be considered. Bupropion is helpful in smoking cessation, and mirtazapine has the advantage of stimulating appetite. The tricyclic antidepressants are equally effective, though typically not as well tolerated,

and can be more problematic in the medically ill patient. Support groups may also provide assistance. Local and/or national chapters exist, and recommendations should be made to the patient and his or her family or caregiver to participate if they have the inclination. If the head and neck surgeon is uncomfortable with psychiatric treatment, a referral pattern should be available for psychiatric and psychological treatment.

Conclusion

Failure following primary treatment for oropharyngeal carcinoma is a devastating problem. Treatment options must balance the devastating effects the tumor inflicts, such as pain, loss of function, and ultimately death, against the morbidity of the treatment. Honest and frank discussions are essential. All aspects of patient care must be considered to maximize outcome.

References

1. Jemal A, Seigel R, Ward E, et al. Cancer statistics 2006. CA Cancer J Clin 2006;56:106–130.
2. Clark JR, Busse PM, Norris CM Jr, et al. Induction chemotherapy with cisplatin, fluorouracil, and high-dose leucovorin for squamous cell carcinoma of the head and neck region: long-term results. J Clin Oncol 1997;15:3100–3110.
3. Spiro RH, Gerold FP, Shah JP, Sessions RB, Strong EW. Mandibulotomy approach to oropharyngeal tumors. Am J Surg 1985;150:466–469.
4. Weymuller EA Jr, Yueh B, Deleyiannis FW-B, Kuntz AL, Alsarraf R, Coltrera MD. Quality of life in head and neck cancer. Laryngoscope 2000;110(94 Suppl):4–7.
5. Wong RJ, Pfister DG, Lin DT, et al. 18-fluordeoxyglucose position emission tomography for the detection of recurrent squamous cell carcinoma of the head and neck. Paper presented at: Annual Meeting of the American Head and Neck Society; May 11, 2002; Boca Raton, FL.
6. McGregor AD, MacDonald DG. Routes of entry of squamous cell carcinoma to the mandible. Head Neck Surg 1988;10:294–301.
7. Zeitels SM, Vaughan CW. Suprahyoid pharyngotomy for oropharynx cancer including the tongue base. Arch Otolaryngol Head Neck Surg 1991;117:757–760.
8. Lydiatt DD, Lydiatt WM, Hollins RR, Friedman A. Use of the free fibula flap in patients with prior failed mandibular reconstruction. J Oral Maxillofac Surg 1998;56:444–446.
9. Lydiatt WM, Kraus DH, Cordeiro PG, Hidalgo DA, Shah JP. Posterior pharyngeal carcinoma resection with larynx preservation and radial forearm free flap reconstruction: a preliminary report. Head Neck 1996;18:501–505.
10. Lydiatt DD, Murayama KM, Hollins RR, Thompson JT. Laparoscopic gastrostomy versus open gastrostomy in head and neck cancer patients. Laryngoscope 1996;106:407–410.
11. List MA, Mumby P, Haraf D, et al. Performance and quality of life outcome in patients completing concomitant chemoradiotherapy protocols for head and neck cancer. Qual Life Res 1997;6:274–284.
12. Morton RP, Davies ADM, Baker J, Baker GA, Stell PM. Quality of life in treated head and neck cancer patients: a preliminary report. Clin Otolaryngol 1984;9:181–185.
13. Farberow NL, Ganzler S, Cutter F, Reynolds D. An eight-year survey of hospital suicides. Life Threat Behav 1971;1:184–202.

Revision Surgery for Early Carcinoma of the Larynx

Harvey M. Tucker

This chapter will explore the indications for and the special problems associated with attempts to surgically salvage a functioning larynx following local failure of primary surgery and/or radiotherapy/chemotherapy for the cure of early carcinoma of the larynx. With the advent of better and more widely available radiotherapy and, in some circumstances, the application of adjuvant chemotherapy, conservation surgery has been employed less frequently in recent years as the primary modality for early or moderately advanced carcinoma of the larynx. Even when conservation (subtotal) laryngeal surgery was used more commonly than it is now, radiotherapy was usually incorporated into planned pre- or postoperative management for all but the earliest malignancies.[1]

Local persistence of disease is relatively uncommon following planned, combined surgery and radiotherapy for even moderately advanced cancers of the larynx (i.e., most failures are in the neck) and almost unheard of after partial laryngectomy for early glottic lesions. More often, head and neck surgeons are called upon to attempt to salvage larynges with persistent cancers after failed radiotherapy and/or chemotherapy were used in an attempt to achieve a single-modality cure. When it is still possible in such cases, subtotal laryngectomy can be considered a form of revision surgery.

Conservation Laryngectomy

Conservation surgery may be defined as resection of tissue adequate to remove all apparent carcinoma with clear margins, while "conserving" enough tissue to permit functional reconstruction. Conservation surgery should not be confused with conservative surgery. This approach is *not* conservative, because all eventual surgical cure rates for any given lesion must be compared with those that can be achieved with total laryngectomy. When a physician elects to attempt surgical cure by a procedure less extensive than total laryngectomy, the onus is upon him or her to ensure that the lesion does not eventually persist in the laryngeal remnant "conserved" for functional reconstruction.

In the larynx, conservation procedures may be classified according to the location of the original lesion and/or the portion of the larynx that must be removed and reconstructed in an attempt to cure it. Generally, these procedures are referred to as (1) vertical partial laryngectomy (hemilaryngectomy), (2) horizontal partial laryngectomy (supraglottic laryngectomy), or (3) near-total laryngectomy. Any of these procedures may be applicable after persistence of carcinoma treated either by radiotherapy or previous partial laryngectomy, provided that the lesion can be removed with clear margins, leaving sufficient tissue to permit eventual functional reconstruction.

Principles and Precautions

Certain principles must be observed, and, particularly after failed radiotherapy, special precautions must be taken to increase the likelihood of eradication of tumor as well as successful reconstruction when subtotal laryngectomy procedures are attempted for salvage.

Adequate Tissue Removal

In the days when subtotal laryngectomy was often undertaken following planned preoperative radiotherapy, it was understood that the excision of tissue necessary to achieve reliable cure rates was that which would have been appropriate to the extent of the original lesion, before any tumor reduction that might have occurred as a result of radiotherapy.[2] Therefore, the decision to attempt conservation salvage surgery following failed radiation/chemotherapy for cure must follow the same principle.[3]

Moreover, the surgeon must remember that the pathologist's ability to accurately evaluate frozen section tumor margins may be compromised by previous radiotherapy. This is particularly true within the 3 to 4 months immediately following completion of radiotherapy/chemotherapy, during which period individual cells are often distorted and may mask the criteria needed to evaluate the extent of residual disease.

It is possible, however, to safely explore larynges with residual disease with the intent of carrying out a conservation procedure. In the study by Tucker, there was no difference in local tumor control rate among a

Decision tree for recurrent early larynx cancer

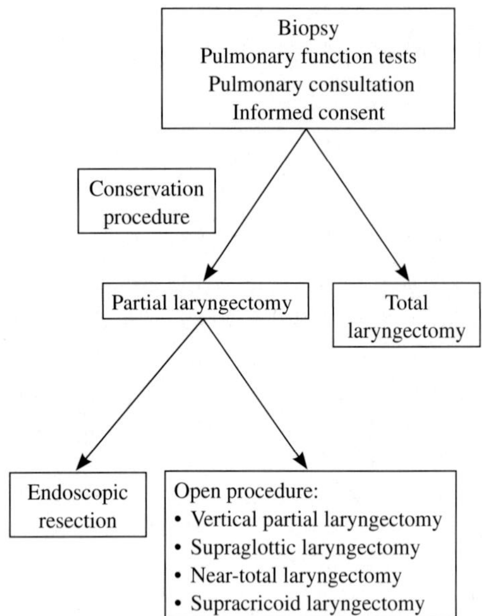

group of patients with T2 and T3 cancers of the larynx when subjected to initial en bloc total laryngectomy versus attempted partial laryngectomy, some of whom were then converted to total laryngectomy when intraoperative findings indicated that subtotal laryngectomy would have been inadequate.[4] Local control was comparable to total laryngectomy, as well, in the subgroup of patients who could be resected successfully by conservation technique. Because many patients with persistent disease following failed radiotherapy/chemotherapy and most of those who have failed initial attempted subtotal laryngectomy will have lesions that are "borderline" for salvage by partial laryngectomy, it is essential that permission for total laryngectomy be obtained in every case.

Reconstruction

Most classic partial laryngectomies are reconstructed with local tissues preserved for that purpose.[5] However, this residual tissue must not be "saved" at the expense of tumor resection sufficient to obtain local control. In cases where previous radiation/chemotherapy or partial laryngectomy have failed, residual local tissue that can be preserved after further resection will be, at best, strictly limited and, at worst, inadequate for safe functional reconstruction. Although it is seldom necessary to employ local or regional flaps in reconstruction of primary partial laryngectomy, it is very often necessary when secondary conservation surgery is undertaken.

Selection of adjunctive means of secondary reconstruction must depend on the patient's medical condition and ability to tolerate extended procedures, the surgeon's experience and capability, and reasonable expectations for survival. For example, electing to use a free flap in such a case adds significant surgical time, morbidity, and expense. If the patient is in poor physical condition or has other, intercurrent disease that is likely to significantly shorten life expectancy, has other risk factors, such as diabetes or peripheral vascular disease, that can impact on the likelihood of successful vascular anastomosis, or if available surgical experience with distant revascularized flaps is limited, a more conservative form of reconstruction should be considered.

Although pectoralis major myocutaneous flaps can be useful in reconstructing extended supraglottic laryngectomies, they tend to be more bulky than is either necessary or useful, but they can usually be accomplished as a one-stage procedure.[6] Whereas this characteristic of myocutaneous flaps may often be advantageous, in postradiation/chemotherapy failures, it is advisable to reconstruct in two stages, incorporating a planned, dependent fistula in the first stage.

Most cases of extended supraglottic laryngectomy that require tissue augmentation can be managed with an undelayed, medially based deltopectoral flap (Bakamjian flap) (**Fig. 19.1**).[7,8] Of necessity, tubing the chest skin inward creates a dependent fistula that decompresses the critical suture line, permits excellent drainage of saliva and mucus, and can be used as a route for a postoperative feeding tube, instead of a nasogastric tube or gastrostomy. The skin is usually non–hair bearing, thin, and pliable, and the donor defect can be closed easily with a secondary split-thickness skin graft. As with any local or distant vascularized flap, one side of the critical pharyngolaryngeal closure has not been subjected to radiation and can be expected to favor prompt healing without wound breakdown. All of this is achieved at the "expense" of requiring a second-stage closure of the tubed fistula some 4 to 6 weeks later, at which point primary healing of the critical suture line has taken place and, perhaps, the patient's nutritional status has been improved by adequate tube feedings. Although this technique has been largely abandoned in favor of myocutaneous or free revascularized flaps for reconstruction of most head and neck defects, it remains very nearly ideal in this particular application.

Of course, revision surgery following failed radiotherapy/chemotherapy or partial laryngectomy can sometimes be achieved by either near-total laryngectomy (as described by Pearson[9]) or by cricohyoidopexy (as described by Laccoureye et al[10]). Whereas both of these procedures seek to preserve a useful voice and acceptable peroral deglutition after extensive salvage surgery, only the latter can avoid a permanent laryngostoma.

Near-total laryngectomy[9] results in an internal tracheoesophageal fistula that can provide an excellent voice, while maintaining enough protective valvular function that the patient is able to use peroral alimentation without significant aspiration. A permanent tracheostoma is necessary, because the laryngeal remnant is not adequate for normal respiration. It is open to question whether the voice achieved and the avoidance of the need for a prosthesis warrant a rather difficult surgical approach, but, certainly, very good results have been reported.

Cricohyoidopexy and its variants have been largely championed by Laccoureye and coworkers.[10] They have reported good functional results insofar as ability to extubate and provide adequate airway and useful voice are concerned, but aspiration can be a problem (**Fig. 19.2**). These authors have not reported specific results after persistent disease previously treated by either radiotherapy or lesser surgery, but there should be no significant reason why these techniques cannot be used, if enough tissue can be left for reconstruction and still permit wide excision of the primary lesion.

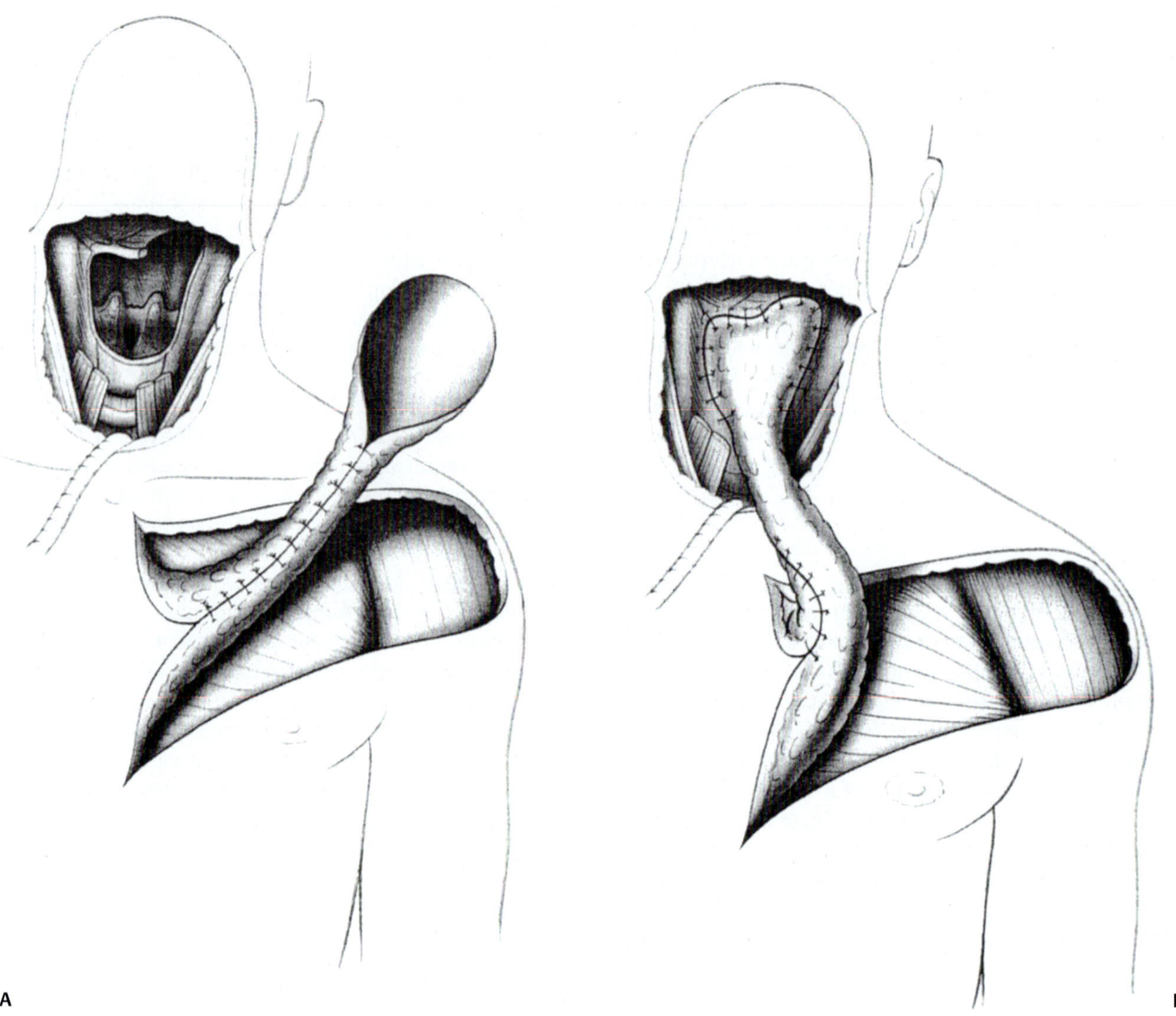

A   B

Fig. 19.1 Closure of extended supraglottic laryngectomy or partial laryngopharyngectomy by undelayed deltopectoral flap. **(A)** Note that the flap is tubed skin side in. Use of a generous apron flap for exposure facilitates this reconstruction. **(B)** Repair completed. Return of the apron flap covers most of the exposed portion of the tubed deltopectoral flap, the rest of which is skin grafted. (From Tucker HM. The Larynx. New York: Thieme Medical Publishers; 1993:Fig. 15–17. Reprinted with permission.)

Ability to Tolerate Conservation Surgery

Whenever the decision is made to attempt any type of subtotal laryngectomy in an effort to definitively control carcinoma of the larynx, certain risks of healing and eventual ability to swallow must be assumed, which would not be as likely after traditional total laryngectomy. This is especially true if the procedure is an "extended" one or if distant flaps are needed for reconstruction. The risk of these complications is increased when such procedures are elected following previous surgery or radiation/chemotherapy that has failed. Therefore, it is essential that the surgeon who attempts revision procedures evaluate the patient's general health and, in particular, his or her ability to tolerate a period of significant aspiration. Most patients in this category are able to tolerate another procedure from a cardiovascular standpoint, but many cannot safely do so because of compromised pulmonary function. A pulmonologist should evaluate such an individual's respiratory capabilities with the clear understanding that all patients aspirate significantly for at least a few weeks after subtotal laryngectomy, and that some will aspirate to some degree for the rest of their lives.[11]

The potential for prompt wound healing is also compromised following failed radiation/chemotherapy. Because salvage or revision partial laryngectomy will include resection of more tissue than is usually necessary when the same type of surgery is attempted per primum, the

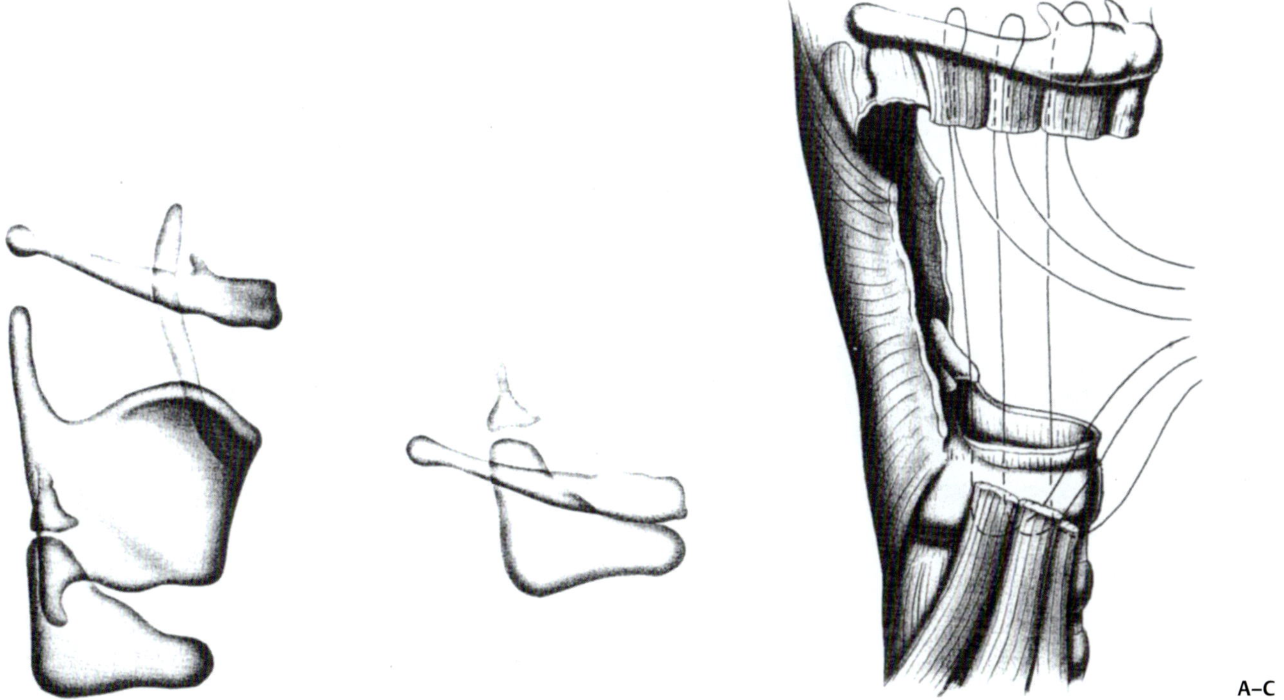

Fig. 19.2 Supracricoid partial laryngectomy. **(A)** Cricoid is approximated to the preserved hyoid bone. **(B)** View of resected larynx prior to closure. (From Tucker HM. The Larynx. New York: Thieme Medical Publishers; 1993:Fig. 15-19. Reprinted with permission.)

possibility for wound breakdown and/or fistula formation is increased. As a result, all patients undergoing revision laryngeal surgery should have adequate coverage of the carotid artery (if neck dissection is necessary), and regional flaps must be considered more frequently than is usually required following initial conservation surgery (see discussion above).

Informed Consent

The patient and his or her family should be made fully aware not only of the usual risks and benefits of conservation laryngeal surgery but also of the added risks that will be assumed in an effort to preserve airway and voice despite the failure of initial curative attempts. Only 80 to 85% of routine supraglottic laryngectomy patients are ever able to swallow without significant aspiration,[11] even after per primum attempts. It is even more likely that extended salvage procedures will result in significant numbers of patients who will have to be considered for completion laryngectomy because of an inability to maintain adequate alimentation without recurring bouts of aspiration pneumonia. If distant flap reconstruction will be needed, the patient must also weigh the relative value of conservation of voice and a tracheostoma-free airway against a generally less complicated total laryngectomy with voice restoration via tracheoesophageal puncture.

In general, these criteria are the same as those recommended for palliation attempts in patients with advanced disease who are unlikely to be cured by any means of treatment.[12]

When extended surgery is considered as a palliative procedure in hopes of at least controlling locoregional disease, the surgeon must anticipate being able to resect all gross disease. Thus, at least the possibility of curative surgery is present even in these advanced cases.

Procedure Selection and Planning

Selection of the specific surgical approach to a particular lesion will depend on the original extent and location, as well as the eventual extent of disease after chemoradiotherapy or surgery has failed.

Glottic Lesions

Most T1a and T1b lesions of the glottic larynx are cured by either radiotherapy or limited surgery. Moreover, the majority of the small number of failures can be salvaged by either partial or total laryngectomy. Perhaps because of this

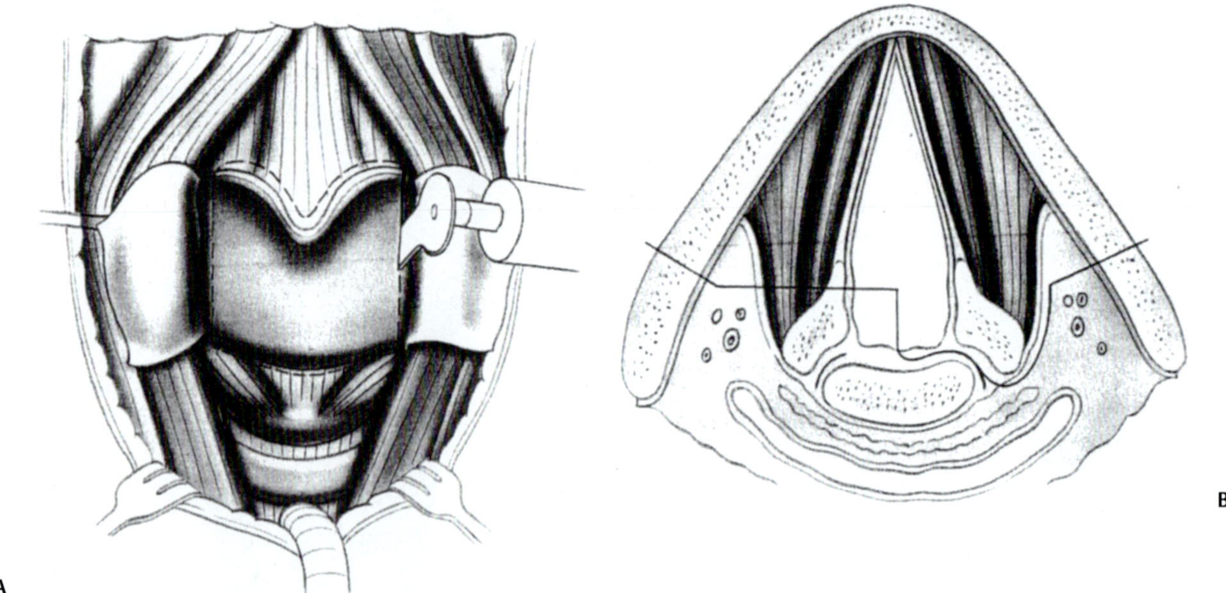

Fig. 19.3 Near-total laryngectomy. **(A)** Cartilage cuts. **(B)** Possible maximal extent of resection leaves a posterior cartilage strut bilaterally and the body of at least one arytenoid cartilage. (From Tucker HM. The Larynx. New York: Thieme Medical Publishers; 1993:Fig. 15-11. Reprinted with permission.)

"safety margin" in salvaging early failures of therapy, there has been interest of late in CO_2 and other types of laser surgery to attempt extensive endoscopic resections of lesions that might previously have been managed with radiotherapy. Early results for this technique have been promising in experienced hands,[13] but much more time will have to elapse before it can be considered a "procedure of choice." In any event, it seems likely that we will see more cases of persistent disease after this approach. Many of them should be suitable for salvage by extended vertical partial laryngectomy with epiglottic reconstruction.[14–19]

This technique permits resection of all of the glottic larynx and overlying thyroid cartilage, saving only the mobile body of one arytenoid cartilage and posterior struts of thyroid cartilage connecting the greater and lesser cornua on each side (**Figs. 19.3, 19.4**). Limited resection of the petiole of the epiglottis is also possible, especially in large male larynges, as well as resection of the anterior cricoid arch, if necessary. Better than 90% surgical cure was achieved with this technique, even in radiation failure cases.[15] Persistent glottic lesions requiring more extensive resection for salvage than outlined above are perhaps best managed by total laryngectomy, although near-total laryngectomy (as described by Pearson)[9] or cricohyoidopexy[10] may be feasible in selected cases.

Supraglottic Lesions

Supraglottic lesions that persist either in the larynx itself or, as is more often the case, in the neck can still be considered for salvage by conservation approaches. If radiotherapy for cure or with adjuvant chemotherapy has been the initial approach, any of the established techniques for supraglottic, extended supraglottic, or partial laryngopharyngectomy can be employed, providing the special precautions outlined above are followed. Many of these patients will require regional or distant flap reconstruction to optimize primary healing and to avoid severe complications. When initial subtotal surgery has failed, most cases will require total laryngectomy for salvage, although cricohyoidopexy[10] may occasionally be possible.

Subglottic and Transglottic Lesions

Fortunately, these lesions are uncommon and, in any event, generally will not qualify as "early" lesions. Total laryngectomy is almost always necessary in their management.[14] There might be an unusual case that has been managed with chemoradiation, which, when it persists, could be resected either by cricohyoidopexy[16] or resection of the cricoid and upper trachea with preservation of a functioning larynx.

Conclusion

Most of the techniques that offer the possibility of salvage or "revision" following failure either of radiotherapy/chemotherapy for cure or of limited surgical approaches have been developed in the era of conservation surgery. Whereas these were once commonly practiced by head

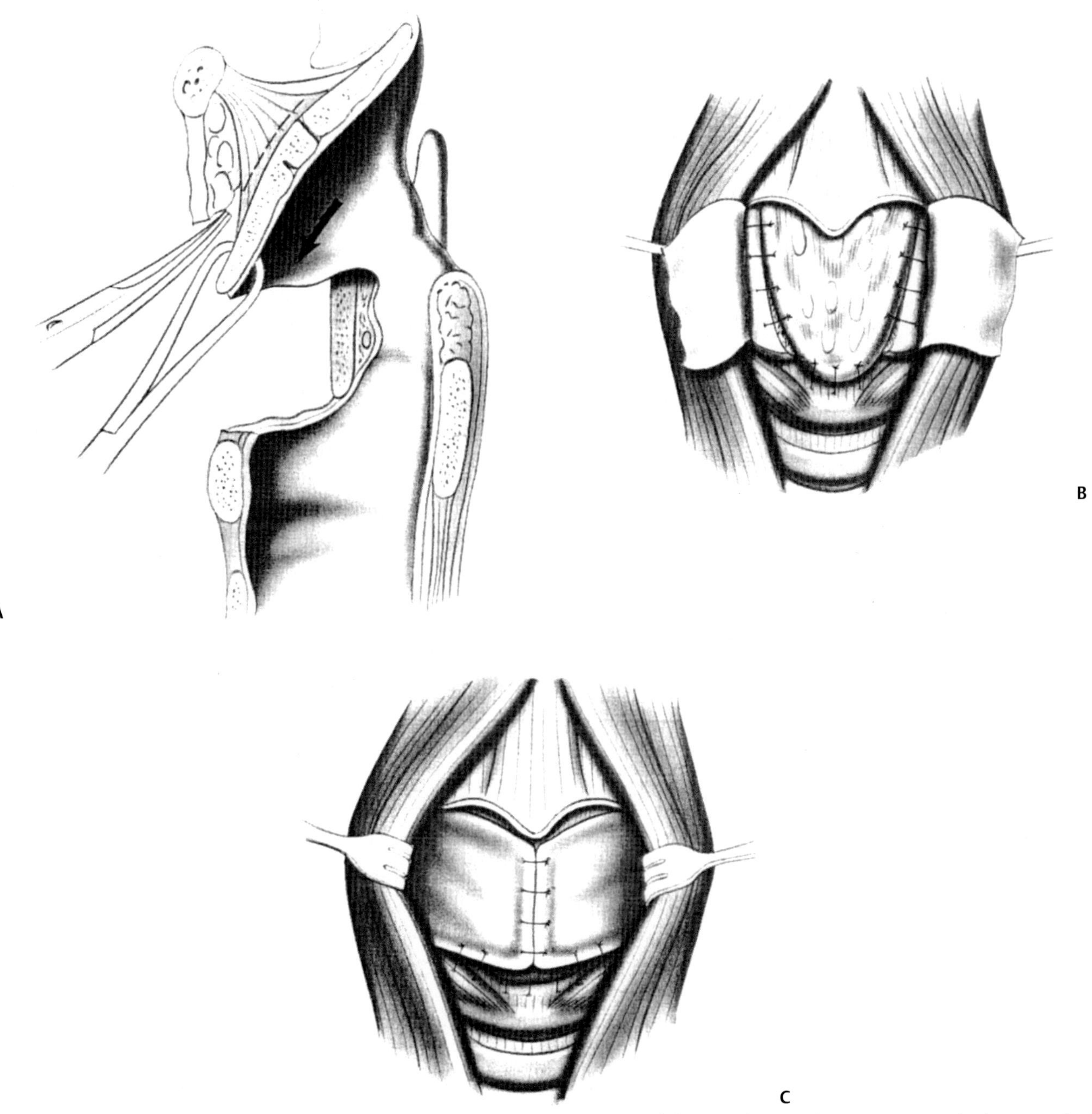

Fig. 19.4 Epiglottic reconstruction after near-total laryngectomy. **(A)** Mobilization of the epiglottis. **(B)** Epiglottis sutured to remaining cartilage struts and the cricothyroid membrane. **(C)** Perichondrial leaflets approximated. (From Tucker HM. The Larynx. New York: Thieme Medical Publishers; 1993:Fig. 15-12. Reprinted with permission.)

and neck surgeons as primary modalities for treatment, they are less often used in these days of improved radiotherapy techniques and chemotherapy. Even though results have been steadily improving with these primary treatment modalities, there are still many failures, most of which go on to total laryngectomy. The concepts outlined above may permit the surgical oncologist who has the necessary experience to salvage significant numbers of functioning larynges, avoiding permanent laryngostomas and/or gastrostomy in most salvageable cases.

References

1. Strong MS. The case for combined radiation therapy and surgery for supraglottic carcinoma. In: Snow JB, ed. Controversy in Otolaryngology. Philadelphia: WB Saunders; 1980.
2. Goldman JL, Silverstone SM. Combined preoperative irradiation and surgery for advanced carcinoma of the larynx and laryngopharynx. In: English GM, ed. Otolaryngology. Vol 5. Philadelphia: Harper & Row; 1978.
3. Fletcher GH, Goepfort H. Irradiation in management of squamous cell carcinoma of the larynx. In: English GM, ed. Otolaryngology. Vol 5. Philadelphia: Harper & Row; 1984.
4. Tucker HM. "Exploratory" surgery for advanced carcinoma of the larynx: a relatively safe approach. Ann Otol Rhinol Laryngol 1998;107:388–390.
5. Tucker HM. The Larynx. New York: Thieme Medical Publishers; 1993.
6. Fabian RL, Varvares MA. Carcinoma of the laryngopharynx and cervical esophagus. In: Fried MP. The Larynx: A Multidisciplinary Approach. St. Louis: Mosby; 1996.
7. Bakamjian VY, Long M, Rigg B. Experience with the medially based deltopectoral flap in reconstructive surgery of the head and neck. Br J Plast Surg 1971;24:174–183.
8. Wood BG, Tucker HM, Levine HL. Regional flap reconstruction during extended supraglottic laryngectomy/partial laryngopharyngectomy. Laryngoscope 1985;95:199.
9. Pearson BW. Management of the primary site: larynx and hypopharynx. In: Pillsbury HC, Goldsmith MM. Operative Challenges in Otolaryngology–Head and Neck Surgery. Chicago: Year Book Medical Publishers; 1990:358–361.
10. Laccourreye H, Laccourreye O, Weinstein G, et al. Supracricoid laryngectomy with cricohyoidopexy: a partial laryngeal procedure for selected supraglottic and transglottic carcinomas. Laryngoscope 1990;100:735–741.
11. Flores TC, Levine HL, Wood BG, Tucker HM. Factors in successful deglutition following subtotal laryngeal surgery. Ann Otol Rhinol Laryngol 1982;91:579–583.
12. Tucker HM, Rabuzzi DD, Reed GF. Massive surgery for palliation in malignancy of the head and neck. Laryngoscope 1973;83:1635–1643.
13. Eckel HE, Thumfart WF. Laser surgery for the treatment of larynx carcinomas: indications, techniques, and preliminary results. Ann Otol Rhinol Laryngol 1992;101:113–118.
14. Tucker HM, Wood BG, Levine HL, Katz R. Glottic reconstruction after near-total laryngectomy. Laryngoscope 1979;89:609–618.
15. Moreau PR. Treatment of laryngeal carcinomas by laser endoscopic microsurgery. Laryngoscope 2000;110:1000–1006.
16. Shaha AR, Shah JP. Carcinoma of the subglottic larynx. Am J Surg 1982;144:456–458.
17. Steiner W. Results of curative laser microsurgery of laryngeal carcinomas. Am J Otolaryngol 1993;14:116–121.
18. Rudert HH, Werner JA. Endoscopic resection of glottic and supraglottic carcinomas with the CO2 laser. Eur Arch Otorhinolaryngol 1995;252:146–148
19. Schechter GL. Epiglottic reconstruction and subtotal laryngectomy. Laryngoscope 1983;93:729–734.

Surgery for Recurrence after Organ Preservation Management of Advanced Squamous Cell Cancers of the Larynx

Pierre Lavertu

The pattern of care for the management of advanced laryngeal cancer has changed over the past 20 years. The traditional approach consisted of surgery followed by radiation therapy. All patients with glottic tumors and more than 70% of patients with supraglottic tumors underwent a total laryngectomy. The morbidity of a total laryngectomy, with its permanent tracheal stoma, is well recognized. Alternative therapies have been developed to preserve the laryngeal function. A major step toward the acceptance of alternative therapy came after the publication of the results from the Department of Veterans Affairs Laryngeal Cancer Study Group.[1] In many centers, organ preservation approaches, either with radiation therapy alone,[2,3] with radiation therapy combined with induction[1] or concurrent chemotherapy,[4] or with subtotal laryngectomy techniques,[5,6] are now the preferred treatment modalities for the management of advanced laryngeal cancers. When extirpative surgery is not part of the initial treatment, the risk of local recurrence is greater than after surgery. The diagnosis and treatment of tumor persistence or recurrence after radiation therapy or after chemoradiation therapy can be challenging.

In reality, the only recurrences that can be salvaged successfully are local recurrences. Approximately 30 to 50% of these can be salvaged. Patients with neck recurrences can rarely be successfully salvaged. Therefore, it has been my personal preference to perform a neck dissection, 6 to 8 weeks after completion of therapy, for all necks with less than a complete response, and for all necks stage N2 or higher on initial presentation, regardless of the response to therapy.[7] The following discussion will be centered on the diagnosis and management of laryngeal recurrences.

Diagnosis

Clinical Evaluation

The determination of tumor persistence after therapy can be difficult. Some of the changes seen after therapy can mimic signs and symptoms of tumor persistence or recurrence. Mucosal and soft tissue abnormalities are expected after therapy for advanced laryngeal cancer. Mucositis and edema are almost always seen early after therapy. These changes tend to be worse and more prolonged after chemoradiotherapy than after radiation alone. Mucositis usually disappears within the first 2 months. Cartilage exposure and/or amputation of the superior aspect of the epiglottis are not unusual, especially after chemoradiation. This is accompanied by persistent pain that is aggravated on swallowing. Concentric scarring and stenosis of the oropharynx, larynx, and hypopharynx are sometimes seen as the mucositis resolves.

Persistence of laryngeal edema after irradiation is seen in ~5% of patients.[8] After chemoradiation the incidence has not been reported, but in my opinion it is present in the majority of patients. Late occurrence of edema is often a sign of tumor recurrence, but it can also be secondary to therapy and/or radionecrosis.

The persistence of vocal cord immobility after treatment does not necessarily imply tumor persistence.[8] Late onset of vocal cord immobility is somewhat more ominous. The detection of vocal cord immobility can be sometimes difficult in patients with significant supraglottic edema.

Adequate documentation of the original location of the lesion is also useful in understanding some of the changes. Amputation of the area initially involved by the tumor is a common finding, especially at the level of the epiglottis. Residual ulceration after tumor necrosis can persist for a long time and in some patients forever.

Tumor pain that is present before therapy often disappears during therapy. Pain induced by the treatment is almost always present within the first 2 or 3 weeks of irradiation. Persistence of pain for months after therapy is not unusual. Most often this pain is associated with persistent areas of ulceration and necrosis. Late onset of pain after therapy is highly suspicious for tumor recurrence, but it can also be secondary to radionecrosis.

In conclusion, signs and symptoms observed after therapy can be significant even without tumor persistence or recurrence. Therefore, detection of tumor persistence and/or recurrence can be difficult and often delayed.

Decision tree for the evaluation and management of recurrent laryngeal cancer after chemorodiation

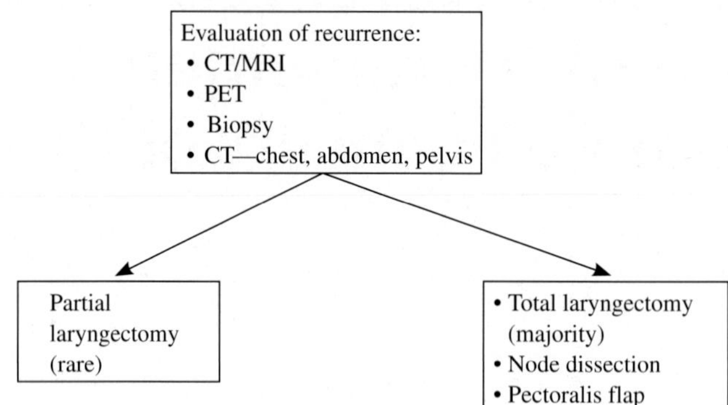

Imaging Techniques

Imaging techniques are essential for the initial diagnosis and staging of laryngeal tumors in patients treated with organ preservation therapies. These techniques can also be used for the diagnosis of tumor recurrence. Hermans et al suggested that, in ~40% of patients, the routine use of computed tomography (CT) allowed for earlier detection of recurrence than clinical examination alone.[9] However, anatomical studies such as CT and magnetic resonance imaging (MRI) are often difficult to interpret. Unless obvious changes such as tumor enhancement and/or necrosis are identified, the radiologist is often puzzled by the significant edematous changes noted after therapy.[8] Few practitioners routinely order these diagnostic tests unless tumor recurrence or persistence is suggested by clinical findings.

The recent addition of dynamic imaging techniques for the diagnosis of head and neck malignancies may be promising. Greven et al reported on 45 patients evaluated with positron emission tomography (PET) before and after irradiation.[10] They tested patients as early as 1 month after therapy and concluded that a positive scan at any time post-therapy correlated with a high likelihood of tumor recurrence. They also noted that early negative scans were not accurate for the absence of disease: 7 of 25 patients with negative scans at 1 month eventually recurred. Terhaard et al reported on 75 patients, previously treated with irradiation, with suspected recurrent disease on clinical examination.[11] PET scanning was positive in 36 of the 37 patients who eventually were proven to have recurrence. False-positive results were found in 7 of 38 patients who never recurred. The researchers concluded that a laryngoscopy and biopsy, with their inherent risk, could be avoided in patients with a negative PET. A positive PET warrants a biopsy.

Routine imaging post-treatment is rarely performed. These tests are best reserved when tumor recurrence is suspected clinically. CT and MRI scanning are the techniques of choice. More data are needed before PET is recommended for routine evaluation of possible persistent disease.

Tissue Diagnosis

Tumor recurrence needs to be proven by biopsy. It is generally accepted that biopsies obtained prior to 6 weeks after completion of therapy may not be reliable. Unless there is obvious clinical evidence of tumor growth, biopsies should not be obtained before 6 weeks after therapy. These standards have been established with irradiation. With chemoradiation, this period may be extended. Early biopsies obtained after extensive tumor necrosis can be misleading and erroneously interpreted as persistent tumor by the pathologist. Unless there is obvious tumor

growth, biopsies in necrotic areas can be deferred until 10 weeks after completion. The decision to perform a laryngeal biopsy cannot be made lightly in this patient population. The trauma associated with a biopsy can aggravate the already present edema and result in airway compromise and the need to control the airway, usually with a tracheotomy. Because of the risk of further damage to the larynx, prolonged intubation is not a recommended practice to secure the airway while the edema resolves. For this same reason, it is probably appropriate to plan definitive surgery at the time of biopsy for patients with tumor recurrence.

Other Testing

Before subjecting a patient to surgery for recurrent locoregional disease, the patient should be submitted to a thorough distant work-up. This is especially important in patients with an advanced neck stage at presentation. The work-up classically includes a CT of the chest, abdomen, and pelvis, as well as a bone scan. The place of PET scanning in the evaluation of distant disease remains to be determined but is promising.

The decision to perform a major extirpative surgery in a patient with known distant disease is beyond the scope of this discussion. However, I believe it should rarely be considered. An argument can be made to perform a palliative operation in some patients with minimal distant disease (i.e., a patient with two or three small lung lesions). This obviously needs to be thoroughly discussed with the patient.

Treatment

The best available therapy for management of tumor recurrence is surgery. In general, surgical salvage after local recurrence is possible in the majority of patients. In a large series of 386 patients with T3–T4 laryngopharyngeal tumors treated with radiation therapy, Davidson et al witnessed locoregional recurrence in 163 patients.[12] Surgical salvage was performed on 108 (66%) of these patients. Leon et al reported on 110 patients with advanced laryngeal carcinomas treated with induction chemotherapy and radiotherapy.[13] Forty-two patients had local and/or regional recurrence. Surgical salvage was possible in 28 of 42 (67%) patients. The great majority of patients in these series had surgical salvage for local recurrence. Isolated regional recurrence is often diagnosed when already unresectable and is therefore rarely amenable to surgical salvage.

Surgery for recurrence is offered to patients with resectable disease and free of distant metastases. The extent of surgery can be determined by the original T-stage, the T-stage on recurrence, and the quality of the tissues.

In patients with tumor persistence or recurrence early after therapy, with large tumor recurrence, and/or with significant laryngeal edema, although a partial laryngectomy may occasionally be possible, the operation of choice and the most often performed is a total laryngectomy with the appropriate neck dissection. The occasional patient with a small tumor persistence or recurrence should not be denied an attempt at either endoscopic removal or partial laryngectomy. Davidson et al reported on 108 patients who underwent salvage surgery after irradiation for the treatment of advanced laryngopharyngeal cancers.[12] Only 1 of the 62 patients who required a laryngectomy had a partial laryngectomy. In a similar series of patients treated with induction chemotherapy followed by irradiation, 1 of 25 patients requiring laryngeal surgery had an endoscopic resection, and 24 had a total laryngectomy.[13] Every patient undergoing an open procedure should also have some type of neck dissection, regardless of the original neck stage. Early after therapy, the extent of neck dissection should be based on the original neck staging: selective (levels 2, 3, and 4) for the N0 neck, and radical or modified radical (spinal accessory nerve [SAN] preservation) for the N+ neck. For late recurrence, the extent of neck dissection should be based on the initial staging or on the recurrent neck staging when more advanced. An ipsilateral thyroidectomy and paratracheal nodal dissection are also often performed.

The need for reconstruction with a regional or free tissue transfer is based on the extent of the mucosal deficit created. As long as the residual pharyngeal walls will approximate without undue tension and the resulting lumen will be adequate for functional deglutition, no tissue augmentation is recommended. Different closing techniques are available. The author's preference is a double-layer closure, including the mucosa and submucosa. The muscular layer is not approximated, and a unilateral pharyngeal plexus neurectomy is performed to facilitate phonation. Occasionally, when the quality of the tissue and/or closure is less than optimal, or if the overlying skin flap is of poor quality or nonexistent, the closure will be reinforced with a pectoralis myogenous flap. The skin paddle is purposely not included to minimize tissue bulk and avoid twisting of the pedicle. The exposed muscle surface is then skin grafted. The need to reinforce the pharyngeal closure is probably more frequent for surgical salvage cases compared with primary surgery cases.

Complications of Surgery

The incidence of complications from surgery performed after organ preservation therapies has been reported to be between 23 and 64%.[12] Comparisons between these different groups is difficult because of the difference in the definitions of both minor and major complications. As could be expected, the most common major complication is a pharyngocutaneous fistula. Lavertu et al[14] reported one instance of fistula in 19 patients (5%) who underwent a combination of pharyngeal and neck surgery after failure of either radiation therapy or concurrent chemoradiation in a randomized trial. Sassler et al[15] reported a fistula rate of 50% in 18 patients treated with induction chemotherapy followed by definitive radiation therapy. A review of the published information on surgical complications after organ preservation treatment resulted in the following conclusions:[16]

- Planned neck dissections have an acceptable complication rate.
- The surgical complication rate increases dramatically when the pharynx is entered via a cervical approach.
- The addition of chemotherapy to radiotherapy does not seem to increase the complication rates.
- There is a trend toward a decrease in surgical complications the longer the resection is performed from the time of completion of radiotherapy or chemoradiotherapy.
- When negative margins are achieved with surgical resection, there is a decrease in the complication rate in comparison with positive margins.
- More liberal use of vascularized flaps seems to reduce the incidence of complications.
- Patients should be maximally optimized nutritionally and metabolically. Particular attention should be paid to thyroid function and correction of hypothyroidism.

Outcome of Surgical Salvage

Approximately 60 to 70% of patients with recurrent laryngeal cancer are amenable to surgical salvage. A few authors have reported on the outcome of surgical salvage in this population. Kraus et al reported on 14 patients who had salvaged laryngectomy following failure of induction chemotherapy and irradiation.[17] Local control was achieved in 86%. Disease-specific survival in this population was 56%. The authors concluded that laryngectomy offers a reasonable outlook for cure and provides long-term palliation. Clayman et al reported on 55 patients treated with induction chemotherapy followed by radiation therapy for laryngeal and hypopharyngeal cancer.[18] Nine of 26 patients with laryngeal cancer required a laryngectomy either after induction chemotherapy or after both chemotherapy and radiation therapy. The 2-year survival rate in this group was 78%. However, with a median follow-up of 24 months, only four of these nine patients were free of disease. The researchers showed that timely surgical salvage of patients failing organ preservation therapy resulted in a survival similar to a matched group treated surgically. Davidson et al reported on 336 patients with T3–T4 laryngopharyngeal cancers randomized to either standard fractionation or hyperfractionated radiation therapy.[12] Of the 163 patients who failed these therapies, 108 (66%) underwent salvage surgery. The overall survival for the surgical salvage group was 37% at 3 years and 18% at 5 years. Survival rates were significantly correlated with the stage at recurrence. All patients with positive margins were dead at 3 years. Goodwin[19] presented the results of a meta-analysis representing 225 patients with stage III and IV recurrent laryngeal cancers. The 5-year survival rate was 36.7%. In his personal series, Goodwin showed a 58% 2-year disease-free survival rate. Recurrent stage was a significant predictor of survival. Leon et al reported a series of 110 patients with T3–T4 laryngeal cancers treated with induction chemotherapy followed by radiation therapy.[13] Of the 42 patients who recurred, 28 (67%) had salvage surgery. The 5-year survival for this cohort of patients was 57%. Weber et al presented the results of salvage laryngectomy from the Radiation Therapy Oncology Group (RTOG) 91–11 trial.[20] This study randomized 517 patients to three organ preservation regimens. Salvage laryngectomy was performed on 129 patients. The overall survival at 18 months for patients treated with induction chemotherapy followed by radiation therapy was 82.2%, 79.8% for patients treated with concurrent chemoradiation, and 86.1% for patients treated with radiation alone. The researchers concluded that locoregional control is excellent and that survival following surgical salvage was not influenced by the initial organ preservation treatment. The following conclusions can be drawn from these reviews:

- Approximately 60 to 70% of patients with locoregional recurrence will be amenable to salvage surgery.
- Survival of this cohort of patients varies from 20 to 60% and is significantly related to tumor stage on recurrence. Patients with disease limited to the primary site will do better than patients with neck disease. Patients with lower T-stage recurrence will do better than patients with higher T-stage recurrence.
- Survival is also correlated with the ability to obtain negative surgical margins. All or most patients with positive margins eventually die of the disease.
- Survival after surgical salvage is not influenced by the prior therapy.

Conclusion

The more generalized acceptance of laryngeal preservation protocols has resulted in an accepted risk of local recurrence in the range of 25 to 40%. This has not resulted in a worse survival for patients presenting with advanced laryngeal cancer. Post-treatment evaluation and management of these patients are more complex and depend on clinical and imaging expertise. Surgical salvage is more challenging and results in a higher incidence of complications, despite the more frequent use of vascularized reconstruction flaps. Patients with tumor persistence and recurrence definitely carry a worse prognosis than patients with no recurrence. However, their prognosis remains good in the absence of regional and/or distant metastases.

References

1. The Department of Veterans Affairs Laryngeal Cancer Study Group. Induction chemotherapy plus radiation compared with surgery plus radiation in patients with advanced laryngeal cancer. N Engl J Med 1991;324: 1685–1690.
2. Mendenhall WM, Parsons JT, Mancuso AA, Pameijer FJ, Stringer SP, Cassisi NJ. Definitive radiotherapy for T3 squamous cell carcinoma of the glottic larynx. J Clin Oncol 1997;15:2394–2402.
3. Parsons JT, Mendenhall WM, Stringer SP, Cassisi NJ. T4 laryngeal carcinoma: radiotherapy alone with surgery reserved for salvage. Int J Radiat Oncol Biol Phys 1998;40: 549–552.
4. Adelstein DJ, Lavertu P, Saxton JP, et al. Mature results of a phase III trial comparing concurrent chemoradiotherapy with radiation therapy alone in patients with stage III and IV squamous cell carcinoma of the head and neck. Cancer 2000;88:876–883.
5. Laccourreye O, Brasnu D, Biacabe B, Hans S, Seckin S Weinstein G. Neo-adjuvant chemotherapy and supracricoid partial laryngectomy with cricohyoidopexy for advanced endolaryngeal carcinoma classified as T3–T4: 5-year oncologic results. Head Neck 1998;20:595–599.
6. Lecanu JB, Monceaux G, Perie S, Angelard B, St-Guily JL. Conservative surgery in T3–4 pharyngolaryngeal squamous cell carcinoma: an alternative to radiation therapy and to total laryngectomy for good responders to induction chemotherapy. Laryngoscope 2000;110:412–416.
7. Lavertu P, Adelstein DJ, Saxton JP, et al. Management of the neck in a randomized trial comparing concurrent chemotherapy and radiotherapy with radiotherapy alone in resectable stage III or IV squamous cell head and neck cancer. Head Neck 1997;19:559–566.
8. O'Brien PC. Tumour recurrence or treatment sequelae following radiotherapy for larynx cancer. J Surg Oncol 1996; 63:130–135.

9. Hermans R, Pameijer FA, Mancuso AA, Parsons JT, Mendenhall WM. Laryngeal or hypopharyngeal squamous cell carcinoma: can follow-up CT after definitive radiation therapy be used to detect local failure earlier than clinical examination alone? Radiology 2000;214:683–687.

10. Greven KM, Williams DW, McGuuirt F, Harkness BA, D'Agostino RB, Keyes JW, Watson NE. Serial positron emission tomography scans following radiation therapy of patients with head and neck cancer. Head Neck 2001; 2001:942–946.

11. Terhaard CH, Bongers V, van Rijk PP, Hordijk GJ. F-18-fluor-deoxy-glucose positron-emission tomography scanning in detection of local recurrence after radiotherapy for laryngeal/pharyngeal cancer. Head Neck 2001;23: 933–941.

12. Davidson J, Keane T, Brown D, et al. Surgical salvage after radiotherapy for advanced laryngopharyngeal carcinoma. Arch Otolaryngol Head Neck Surg 1997;123:420–424.

13. Leon X, Quer M, Orus C, Lopez M, Gras JR, Vega M. Results of salvage surgery for local or regional recurrence after larynx preservation with induction chemotherapy and radiotherapy. Head Neck 2001;23:733–738.

14. Lavertu P, Bonafede JP, Adelstein DJ, et al. Comparison of surgical complications after organ preservation therapy in patients with stage III and IV squamous cell head and neck cancer. Arch Otolaryngol Head Neck Surg 1998;124: 401–406.

15. Sassler AM, Esclamado RM, Wolf GT. Surgery after organ preservation therapy: analysis of wound complications. Arch Otolaryngol Head Neck Surg 1995;121:162–165.

16. Gokhale AS, Lavertu P. Surgical salvage after chemoradiation of head and neck cancer: complications and outcome. Curr Oncol Rep 2001;3:72–76.

17. Kraus DH, Pfister DG, Harrison LB, et al. Salvage surgery for unsuccessful larynx preservation therapy. Ann Otol Rhinol Laryngol 1995;104:936–941.

18. Clayman GL, Weber RS, Guillamondegui O, et al. Laryngeal preservation for advanced laryngeal and hypopharyngeal cancers. Arch Otolaryngol Head Neck Surg 1995;121: 219–223.

19. Goodwin WJ Jr. Salvage surgery for patients with recurrent squamous cell carcinoma of the upper aerodigestive tract: when do the ends justify the means? Laryngoscope 2000;110(93 Suppl):1–18.

20. Weber RS, Berkey BA, Forastiere A, et al. Outcome of salvage total laryngectomy following organ preservation therapy: the radiation therapy oncology group trial 91–11. Paper presented at: Annual Meeting of the American Head and Neck Society; May 13, 2002; Boca Raton FL.

Revision Surgery for Paranasal Sinus Tumors

Michael K. Kim and Randal S. Weber

Cancer of the paranasal sinus remains a difficult and challenging problem, despite attempts to improve survival and quality of life over the last 2 decades. The prognosis for patients with squamous cell carcinoma of the paranasal sinus remains poor even with advancements in surgical, radiotherapeutic, and chemotherapeutic techniques.

Paranasal sinus cancer is uncommon and represents only 0.2 to 0.8% of all malignancies. Cancer of the paranasal sinus constitutes 3% of all carcinomas of the upper aerodigestive tract.[1] The majority of paranasal sinus malignancies, 50 to 80%, originate within the maxillary sinus antrum. Malignancies rarely occur within the other sinuses, and originate in the ethmoid, frontal, and sphenoid sinuses in 10%, 1%, and 1%, respectively.[2]

The cause of paranasal sinus malignancies is unknown. However, several risk factors have been associated with neoplasms of the paranasal sinus. Exposures to radium, chromium, nickel, wood, and leather have been associated with higher incidence of paranasal sinus malignancies.[3] The carcinogenic potential of tobacco, alcohol, and viruses has not been directly linked to squamous cell carcinoma of the paranasal sinus.

The destructive and devastating nature of squamous cell carcinoma of the paranasal sinus is manifested in the low overall survival rates and high local recurrence rates seen in these patients. Although the ideal curative treatment of paranasal sinus malignancies is dependent upon early diagnosis and controlling the primary tumor site, there is a limited role for salvage surgical intervention for recurrent, persistent, or progressive disease. The indications for revision surgical intervention for recurrent paranasal sinus malignancies will be reviewed.

Diagnosis

The diagnosis of paranasal sinus malignancies requires a thorough history and physical examination of the head and neck region. The priorities of any clinician who encounters a paranasal sinus neoplasm must include establishing a histologic diagnosis, determining the anatomical extent of the neoplasm, and planning an effective treatment strategy.

Typically, the signs and symptoms of early-stage paranasal sinus neoplasm are nonspecific. Initial symptoms may mimic benign paranasal sinus and nasal disorders, including nasal stuffiness, facial pain, headaches, and intermittent epistaxis.[4] The natural air-filled cavities of the paranasal sinuses allows for significant growth of the malignancy prior to producing signs and symptoms of local extension.[5] The expanding paranasal sinus neoplasm may produce sign and symptoms related to the orbit, brain, nasal cavity, oral cavity, facial soft tissues, and cranial nerves.[1,3]

Radiologic imaging provides extremely valuable information regarding the location, size, extent, and invasiveness of the paranasal sinus cancer. The imaging studies are invaluable in determining a preoperative treatment plan because they allow the surgeon to better appreciate the extent of the disease and the involvement of important structures. Although there are several imaging techniques available to the surgeon, computed tomography (CT) and magnetic resonance imaging (MRI) have been the most effective modalities for evaluating paranasal sinus cancer.

Evaluating a paranasal sinus neoplasm requires a CT scan with intravenous contrast in both the coronal and axial planes. The CT scan provides information regarding the bony architecture of the orbital apex, infratemporal fossa, pterygoids, cribriform plate, and sphenoid and ethmoid sinuses.[3,4]

When evaluating the paranasal sinus for recurrent, persistent, or progressive cancer, the information from the MRI is additive to the CT scan and provides critical information regarding the soft tissue detail of this complex anatomical region. Involvement of the infratemporal fossa, pterygopalatine fossa, periorbital tissues, peripheral nerves, brain parenchyma, carotid artery, cavernous sinus, and prevertebral fascia can be delineated with MRI scans.[3,4] The MRI provides the additional advantages of being able to distinguish tumor from retained secretions and offering image structures in multiple planes.

Obtaining the histologic diagnosis of the neoplasm is paramount to determining the treatment plan and prognosis for the patient. The majority of tumors are approachable for biopsy via the endonasal route. If, however, the tumor is contained within the maxillary sinus cavity without extension into the nasal cavity, antrostomy of the sinus may be performed. Either an inferior meatus antrostomy or a Caldwell-Luc approach may be used. It is important to obtain an adequate amount of tissue for histological, immunohistochemical, and electron microscopic analysis.[3,6]

199

Decision tree for recurrent sinonasal tumors

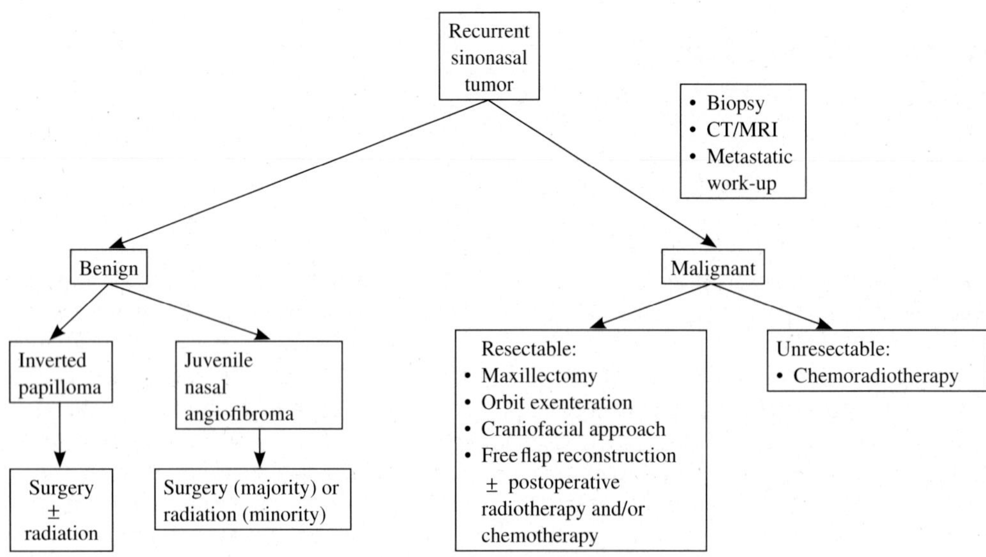

Treatment

Paranasal sinus malignancies continue to present therapeutic challenges to the head and neck surgeon. The fact remains that the majority of these malignancies are diagnosed as locally advanced disease because of the vague and nonspecific nature of symptoms in early-stage lesions. Several studies report a preponderance of patients presenting with T3 or T4 lesions.[2,4,5,7,8] The primary treatment strategies of various institutions has consisted of surgery, radiation therapy, or combination therapy.[4,6] Although considerable experience have accumulated in the treatment of paranasal sinus cancer with primary radiation therapy, only combined modality and revision surgical therapy will be discussed.[5,8]

Advanced lesions of the paranasal sinuses traditionally have been treated with combination therapy consisting of either pre- or postoperative radiation therapy and surgery. The surgical procedures consist of either partial maxillectomy, total maxillectomy, radical maxillectomy, or cranial base surgery.[4,9–11] The descriptions of the surgical techniques are beyond the scope of this chapter and are well described elsewhere. Surgery of recurrent, persistent, or progressive paranasal sinus cancers is designed to achieve the highest possible cure rates with the least anatomical and functional deformities.[4] Revision surgery is often limited to cryotherapy or laser debulking, because the primary surgical treatment usually consists of a total maxillectomy, radical maxillectomy, or cranial base surgery of a locally advanced paranasal sinus cancer.[1,4,11] The extent of revision surgery is predicated upon the respectability of the lesion. The extension of the primary, recurrent, or progressive paranasal sinus cancer into a substantial portion of the brain parenchyma, bilateral cavernous sinuses, or both optic nerves may preclude the lesion from being surgically resectable.[3,4] However, in selected cases of extensive disease, revision surgical treatment may offer the most effective form of palliation.[3,4,11]

The debate over whether radiation therapy should be given before or after surgery continues. The proponents of preoperative radiation therapy advocate giving radiation first because the blood supply to the tumor has not been altered; hence the tumor tissue is better oxygenated. Additionally, it may be more likely to achieve clear surgical margins because preoperative radiation has its greatest impact on the periphery of the tumor.[9,12] The proponents of postoperative radiation therapy maintain that radiation therapy is most effective when the tumor burden is small. Also, postoperative radiation therapy allows for more accurate assessment of the extent of disease and reduces concern with surgical wound healing, allowing for the administration of a higher total dose of radiation.[13]

Advances in the planning and delivery techniques of radiation therapy have allowed for innovative protocols for treating recurrent or persistent paranasal sinus malignancies. Further advances in intensity modulated radiation therapy (IMRT), three-dimensional conformal therapy, brachytherapy, and altered fractionation of radiation therapy have allowed for re-irradiation protocols for recurrent paranasal sinus cancers.[14] IMRT allows precise delivery of radiation beams, thus reducing associated morbidity. Although the follow-up period has been short, several studies have shown that radiation treatment with IMRT for paranasal sinus cancers is associated with lower rates of dry eye syndromes and other visual disturbances.[13,14]

Chemotherapy has several roles in the treatment of recurrent paranasal sinus cancers. As an induction agent, it may cause tumor shrinkage. In combination with radiation, it may act as a radiosensitizing agent for recurrent or metastatic disease. However, chemotherapy in several protocols has not increased survival rates.[12,15]

The higher incidence of paranasal sinus cancer in Japan has encouraged investigators there to develop alternative combined therapy. The combined treatment modality used by several institutions in Japan consists of simultaneous radiation therapy, intra-arterial chemotherapy, and conservative surgery.[16] The surgical component of the combination therapy involved frequent curettage of devitalized tissues via an antrostomy in the anterior face of the maxilla. Revision surgical treatment for recurrent or progressive paranasal sinus malignancies would also entail curettage of the tumor or a completion maxillectomy.[16] This particular combined treatment regimen has shown encouraging results for controlling paranasal sinus cancer locally and with favorable overall survival rates.[16]

Malignant adenopathy at the time of clinical presentation is uncommon with paranasal sinus malignancies, ranging from 5 to 20% in various studies.[2,8,17–19] Regional recurrence in the neck without evidence of local recurrence is also uncommon.[2,8,19] However, if there is treatment failure in the neck, surgical salvage can be successfully performed in the majority of those patients without evidence of local recurrence.[8,19,20]

Unfortunately, most cases with nodal involvement after primary treatment are also associated with local recurrence.[2,6,8,18,19]

Surgical Management of the Orbit

The surgical management of the orbit in paranasal sinus malignancies continues to be a controversial subject among head and neck surgeons. The periorbita is believed to be the defining barrier to tumor spread; however, the criteria for orbital exenteration continue to evolve.[10,21]

Orbital exenteration is typically indicated if the patient presents with preoperative ophthalmic signs and symptoms of exophthalmos, limitation of ocular motility, or decreased visual acuity. These preoperative ophthalmic findings usually correspond with tumor invading the periorbita, orbital fat, orbital muscles, and/or orbital nerves.[10,21]

The debate of removing the eye for recurrent or persistent paranasal sinus cancers ultimately centers on the ability to obtain negative margins oncologically. A further important consideration in determining the fate of the involved eye is the consideration of the effects of adjuvant therapy on the functional aspects of the orbit. Although modern techniques in radiation therapy have made significant gains in local and regional control, the morbidity associated with radiation to the orbit is significant. Several studies have demonstrated blindness in 4 to 15% of patients and brain necrosis in 15 to 21% of patients following radiation therapy for paranasal sinus malignancies.[17,22] It is of note that, with the further refinement of IMRT, the orbital complications induced by radiation may be significantly reduced.[12,14]

The histology of the paranasal sinus cancer will also determine the surgeon's ability to preserve the eye at the time of surgery. Orbital preservation is more likely with less aggressive tumors, such as low-grade esthesioneuroblastomas, low-grade adenocarcinomas, and benign tumors of the paranasal sinuses. Aggressive tumors, such as squamous cell carcinomas and high-grade adenocarcinomas of the paranasal sinuses, that encroach upon the orbital cavity will typically lead to an orbital exenteration to achieve oncologically negative margins.[1,21]

In revision paranasal sinus surgery, every patient must be prepared for the possibility of an orbital exenteration. However, the decision for orbital exenteration is often made at the time of surgery.

Reconstruction of Paranasal Sinus and Orbital Surgical Defects

The midface is a complex region anatomically, and tumor removal in this area is devastating to the patient for many reasons. Generally, limited resection of the maxilla results in minor reconstructive problems that are managed best by prosthesis.[23] Advanced tumors of the paranasal sinuses and orbital area that require ablation often result in massive defects with exposed dura, brain, and nasal and oral cavities. These large and complex defects require sophisticated reconstruction with vascularized or nonvascularized tissue and bone flaps.

The aim of reconstruction of these defects is to achieve an effective barrier between the cranial cavity and the aerodigestive tract, support the midfacial and orbital structures, and replace skin, soft tissue, and mucosal deficits. Complex three-dimensional reconstruction is necessary in

maintaining or restoring speech, deglutition, and the nasal airway, in addition to optimizing the aesthetic result for the patient. The traditional skin graft and maxillofacial prosthesis adequately reconstruct the midface for many patients. However, for larger and more extensive defects, there are problems with prosthetic retention and motion.[23]

Local pedicled flaps, cranial base flaps, and pericranial flaps with or without free bone grafts have also been used to reconstruct sino-orbital surgical defects. The application of various flaps is well described in the literature.[1,3,23]

Microvascular free tissue transfer has been used to effectively reconstruct the midface. The various free flaps available for midface reconstruction can be further categorized as fasciocutaneous, musculocutaneous, and osteocutaneous free tissue transfers. The primary fasciocutaneous tissue used for sino-orbital reconstruction is the radial forearm free flap.[24] The rectus abdominis and latissimus dorsi free flap provides a musculocutaneous component for replacing large midface defects.[25,26] Furthermore, the iliac crest, scapula, and fibula free flaps allow for free tissue transfer of bone into the midface region.[25,27,28]

Benign Tumors of the Paranasal Sinuses

Revision surgery for benign paranasal sinus tumors is not uncommon secondary to significant recurrence rates of these tumors. Both inverted papillomas and juvenile angiofibromas have significant recurrence rates.[29–31] The high recurrence rates are probably due to incomplete removal of the tumor extensions.

Inverted papillomas of the nose and paranasal sinuses are an aggressive benign neoplasm. There is an association with squamous cell carcinoma in a small percentage of patients (5–15%).[32] The primary treatment for inverted papillomas involves surgical extirpation of the tumor.

Although a medial maxillectomy via a lateral rhinotomy or midfacial degloving is an effective surgical method for resecting inverted papillomas, there is considerable discussion concerning endoscopic techniques in resecting this particular tumor.[29,32]

Revision surgery for inverted papillomas may uniquely utilize endoscopic approaches for resection of the tumor.[30,33] However, if adequate margins cannot be obtained via the endoscopic method, an aggressive open surgical procedure must be performed.

Juvenile angiofibroma presents a unique challenge to the head and neck surgeon. Advances in imaging that allow a more accurate determination of tumor location and extent, improvements in interventional angiography that permit more complete embolization of the tumor bed, and refinements in the surgical approaches that provide

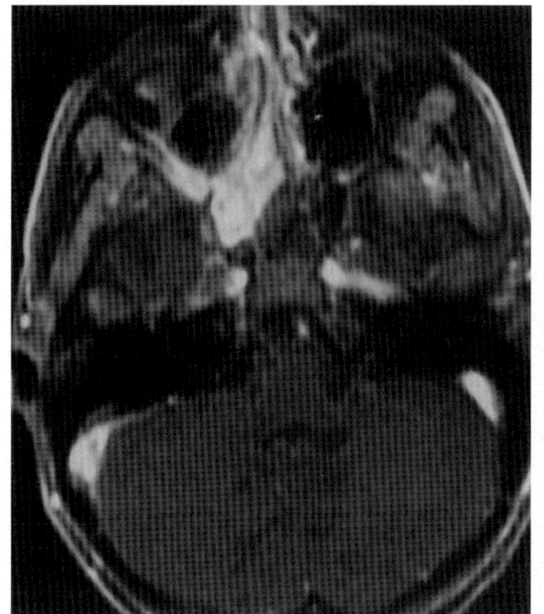

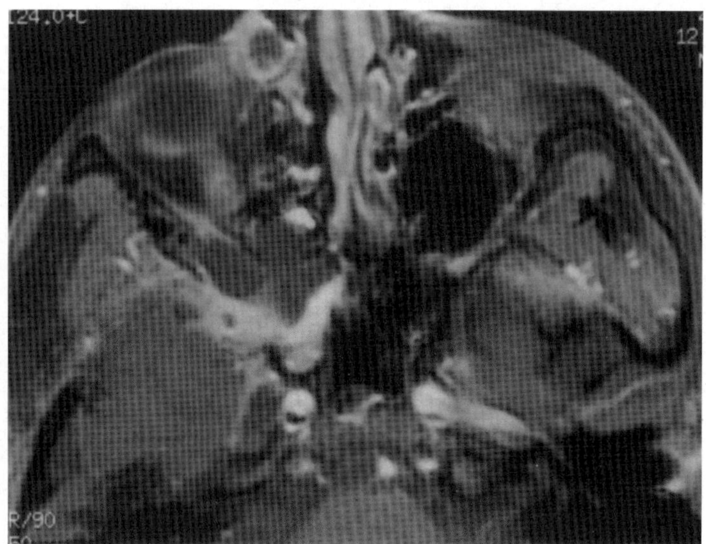

A   B

Fig. 21.1 A 14-year-old male presented with a 1-month history of right-sided nasal obstruction, epistaxis, and headaches. **(A)** Contrast-enhanced magnetic resonance imaging demonstrating angiofibroma involving the right nasal passage and pterygomaxillary fossa. **(B)** A more cephalad image demonstrating tumor in the right orbit, middle cranial fossa, and cavernous sinus.

wide exposure while minimizing morbidity have enhanced the management of this particular tumor.

Revision surgery for recurrent or persistent juvenile angiofibromas is difficult because of the anatomical location of the tumor. Although several authors have successfully shown that extensive intracranial disease can be removed with minimal morbidity and mortality through the advances in skull base surgery, cavernous sinus or brain parenchyma involvement may often prevent complete surgical removal of the juvenile angiofibroma (**Fig. 21.1**).[31]

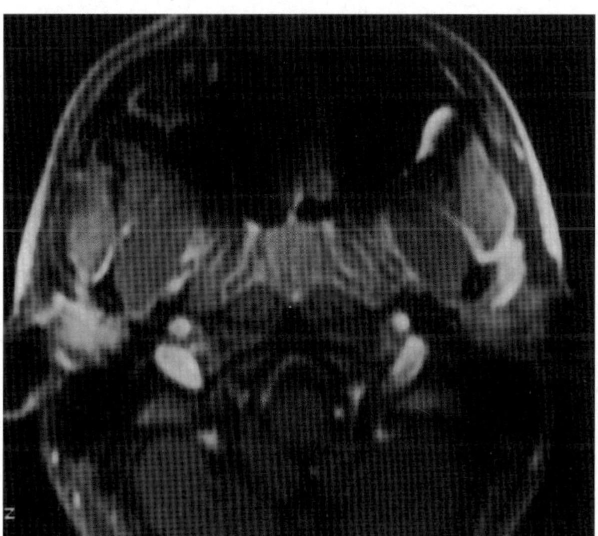

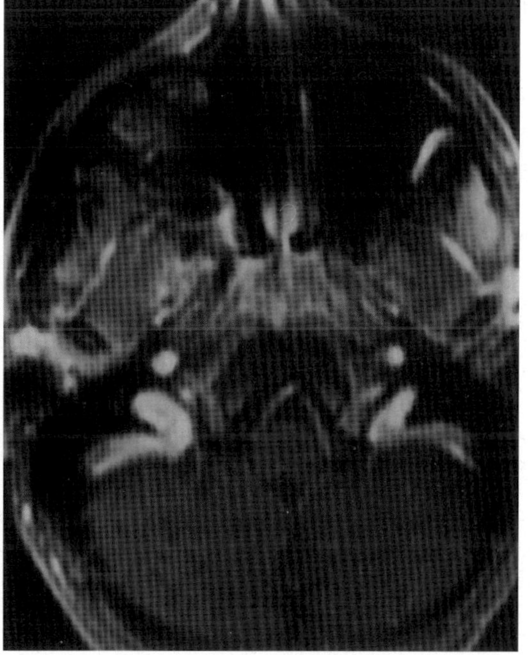

A   B

Fig. 21.2 **(A,B)** Contrast-enhanced axial magnetic resonance imaging scans 6 months after subtemporal craniectomy and transfacial resection of an angiofibroma involving the right nasal passage, sphenoid sinus, middle cranial fossa, orbit, and lateral cavernous sinus. The patient was asymptomatic, and the radiographs were interpreted as negative for disease.

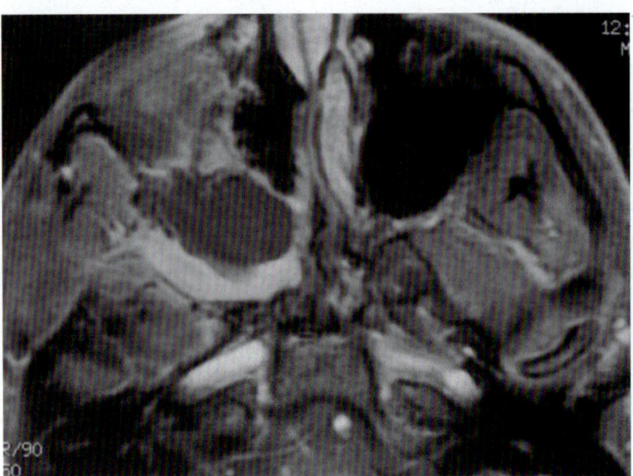

Fig. 21.3 Eighteen months following tumor resection, the patient noted fullness and discomfort in the right temporal region. An axial magnetic resonance imaging scan demonstrated recurrent tumor in the right pterygomaxillary fossa, orbit, and middle cranial fossa. Further surgical resection was not deemed feasible with acceptable morbidity, and 45 Gy of external beam radiation was administered over 5 weeks. One year following radiation, the residual angiofibroma continued to regress, and the patient remained symptom free.

The role of radiation therapy for benign paranasal sinus tumor remains controversial.[34–36] However, radiation therapy may be used for recurrent angiofibromas when extended surgical intervention might result in significant morbidity and mortality (**Figs. 21.2, 21.3**).[34,36]

Outcome

The analysis of treatment results for paranasal sinus malignancies must be viewed with caution. The conclusions drawn from many of the studies are limited by the small number of patients within the study, selection bias for certain treatment modalities, histologic heterogeneity, a lack of a standardized staging system, and the absence of prospective studies.

Local recurrence remains the major problem in the curative treatment of paranasal sinus cancers. The majority of studies present data with local recurrence rates > 50%.[4,7,8,10,37] Additionally, local recurrence remains the primary cause of treatment failures in all stages of disease.[9,10,13,19] The local control rates are considerably lower with surgical salvage of recurrent tumor.[5,11,37]

The outlook for patients with paranasal sinus malignancies remains dismal. The overall survival at 5 years ranges from 25 to 50% for most institutions.[2,5,8–10] Although several institutions in Japan have reported higher overall 5-year survival rates, at 54 to 76%, these results are not consistently being replicated elsewhere.[16,38] The overall 5-year survival for salvage surgery is, as expected, substantially lower.[5,11,36]

Distant metastasis is not common, ranging from 10 to 23%.[2,5,7,8,10,19] These rates are low and may be an underestimation, as a thorough investigation for distant disease is usually not performed, or indicated in patients with progressive incurable local disease.[8] In an autopsy study of 67 patients who died of maxillary sinus cancer, distant metastasis was found in 31% of the patients.[8,39]

Conclusion

Paranasal sinus cancer continues to present a formidable challenge to the head and neck surgeon. The refinement of radiologic imaging techniques and combined modality treatment strategies has enhanced the surgeon's ability to effectively surgically resect these cancers. Although there have been great strides made in both ablative and reconstructive cranial base surgery, a significant number of patients will fail locally.

Revision surgery for recurrent or progressive paranasal sinus malignancies presents even a greater challenge. The principles of revision paranasal sinus cancer surgery should emphasize prevention of local recurrence with development of techniques for earlier detection. The successful treatment strategy must rigorously identify the optimum treatment modality, whether it is surgery, radiation therapy, or chemotherapy alone or in combination, in a prospective manner.

References

1. Rice DH, Stanley RB. Surgical therapy of tumors of the nasal cavity, ethmoid sinus, and maxillary sinus. In: Thawley SE, Panje WR, Batsakis JG, et al, eds. Comprehensive Management of Head and Neck Tumors. 2nd ed. Philadelphia: WB Saunders; 1999:558–581.
2. Spiro JD, Soo KC, Spiro RH. Squamous carcinoma of the nasal cavity and paranasal sinuses. Am J Surg 1989;158: 328–332.
3. Stern SJ, Hanna E. Cancer of the nasal cavity and paranasal sinuses. In: Thawley SE, Panje WR, Batsakis JG, et al, eds. Comprehensive Management of Head and Neck Tumors. 2nd ed. Philadelphia: WB Saunders; 1999:205–233.
4. Sisson GA, Toriumi DM, Atiyah RA. Paranasal sinus malignancy: a comprehensive update. Laryngoscope 1989;99: 143–150.
5. Curran AJ, Gullane PJ, Waldron J, et al. Surgical salvage after failed radiation for paranasal sinus malignancy. Laryngoscope 1998;108:1618–1622.
6. Spiro JD, Spiro RH. Maxillary sinus cancer. In: Kraus DH, Levine HL, eds. Nasal Neoplasia. New York: Thieme Medical Publishers; 1997:85–102.

7. Paulino AC, Marks JE, Bricker P, et al. Results of treatment of patients with maxillary sinus carcinoma. Cancer 1998; 83:457–465.

8. Waldron JN, O'Sullivan B, Gullane PJ, et al. Carcinoma of the maxillary sinus antrum: a retrospective analysis of 110 cases. Radiother Oncol 2000;57:167–173.

9. Lee F, Ogura JH. Maxillary sinus carcinoma. Laryngoscope 1981;91:133–139.

10. Stern SJ, Goepfert H, Clayman G, et al. Squamous cell carcinoma of the maxillary sinus. Arch Otolaryngol Head Neck Surg 1993;119:964–969.

11. Janecka IP, Sen C, Sekhar L, et al. Treatment of paranasal sinus cancer with cranial base surgery: results. Laryngoscope 1994;104:553–555.

12. Claus F, De Gersen W, De Wagter C, et al. An implementation strategy for IMRT of ethmoid sinus cancer with bilateral sparing of the optic pathways. Int J Radiat Oncol Biol Phys 2001;51:318–331.

13. Jesse RH. Preoperative versus postoperative radiation in the treatment of squamous carcinoma of the paranasal sinuses. Am J Surg 1965;110:552–556.

14. Adams EJ, Nutting CM, Convery DJ, et al. Potential role of intensity modulated radiotherapy in the treatment of tumors of the maxillary sinus. Int J Radiat Oncol Biol Phys 2001;51:579–588.

15. Schuller DE, Metch B, Stein D, et al. Preoperative chemotherapy in advanced resectable head and neck cancer: final report of the Southwest Oncology Group. Laryngoscope 1988;98:1205–1211.

16. Nishino H, Miyata M, Morita M, et al. Combined therapy with conservative surgery, radiotherapy, and regional chemotherapy for maxillary sinus carcinoma. Cancer 2000;89:1925–1932.

17. Jiang GL, Ang KK, Peters LJ, et al. Maxillary sinus carcinomas: natural history and results of postoperative radiotherapy. Radiother Oncol 1991;21:193–200.

18. Jeremic B, Shibamoto Y, Milicic B, et al. Elective ipsilateral neck irradiation of patients with locally advanced maxillay sinus carcinoma. Cancer 2000;88:2246–2251.

19. Kondo M, Ogawa K, Inuyuma Y, et al. Prognostic factors influencing relapse of squamous cell carcinoma of the maxillary sinus. Cancer 1985;55:190–196.

20. Pearlman AW, Abadir R. Carcinoma of maxillary antrum: the role of preoperative irradiation. Laryngoscope 1974;84: 400–409.

21. Graamans K, Slootweg PJ. Orbital exenteration in surgery of malignant neoplasms of the paranasal sinuses: the value of preoperative computed tomography. Arch Otolaryngol Head Neck Surg 1989;115:977–980.

22. Tsujii H, Kadama T, Arimoto T, et al. The role of radiotherapy in the management of maxillary sinus carcinoma. Cancer 1986;57:2261–2266.

23. Marunick MT, Harrison R, Beumer J III. Prosthodontic rehabilitation of midfacial defects. J Prosthet Dent 1985;54: 553–560.

24. Tahara S, Susuki T. Eye socket reconstruction with free radial forearm flap. Ann Plast Surg 1989;23:112–116.

25. Coleman JJ. Microvascular approach to function and appearance of large orbital maxillary defects. Am J Surg 1989;158:337–341.

26. Shestak KC, Schusterman MA, Jones NF, et al. Immediate microvascular reconstruction of combined palatal and midfaced defects using soft tissue only. Microsurgery 1988;9:128–131.

27. Ramasastry SS, Granick MS, Futrell J. Clinical anatomy of the internal oblique muscle. J Reconstr Microsurg 1986;2: 117–122.

28. Riediger D. Restoration of masticatory function by microsurgically revascularized iliac crest bone grafts using osseous endosseous implants. Plast Reconstr Surg 1988; 81:861–877.

29. Segal K, Atar E, Mor C, et al. Inverting papilloma of the nose and paranasal sinuses. Laryngoscope 1986;96:394–398.

30. Waitz G, Wigand ME. Results of endoscopic sinus surgery for the treatment of inverted papillomas. Laryngoscope 1992;102:917–922.

31. Gullane PJ, Davidson J, O'Droyer T, et al. Juvenile angiofibroma: a review of the literature and a case series report. Laryngoscope 1992;102:928–933.

32. Benninger MS, Roberts JK, Sebek BA, et al. Inverted papilloma and associated squamous cell carcinomas. Otolaryngol Head Neck Surg 1990;103:457–461.

33. Myers EN, Petruzzelli GJ. Endoscopic sinus surgery for inverting papillomas. Laryngoscope 1993;103:711.

34. Lyons BM, Donald PJ. Intracranial juvenile angiofibroma with intradural and cavernous sinus involvement. Skull Base Surg 1992;2:87–91.

35. Jones GC, DeSanto LW, Brenner W, et al. Juvenile angiofibromas: behavior and treatment of extensive and residual tumors. Arch Otolaryngol Head Neck Surg 1986;112: 1191–1193.

36. Andrews JC, Fisch U, Valvanus A, et al. The surgical management of extensive nasopharyngeal angiofibromas with the infratemporal fossa approach. Laryngoscope 1989;99:429–437.

37. Lavertu P, Roberts JK, Kraus DH, et al. Squamous cell carcinoma of the paranasal sinuses: the Cleveland Clinic Experience 1977–1986. Laryngoscope 1989;99:1130–1136.

38. Sakai S, Hohki A, Fuchihata H, et al. Multidisciplinary treatment of maxillary sinus carcinoma. Cancer 1983;52: 1360–1364.

39. Shibuya H, Takagi M, Horivchi J, et al. Clinicopathological study of maxillary sinus carcinoma. Int J Radiat Oncol Biol Phys 1985;11:1709–1712.

Decision tree for recurrent benign parotid tumors

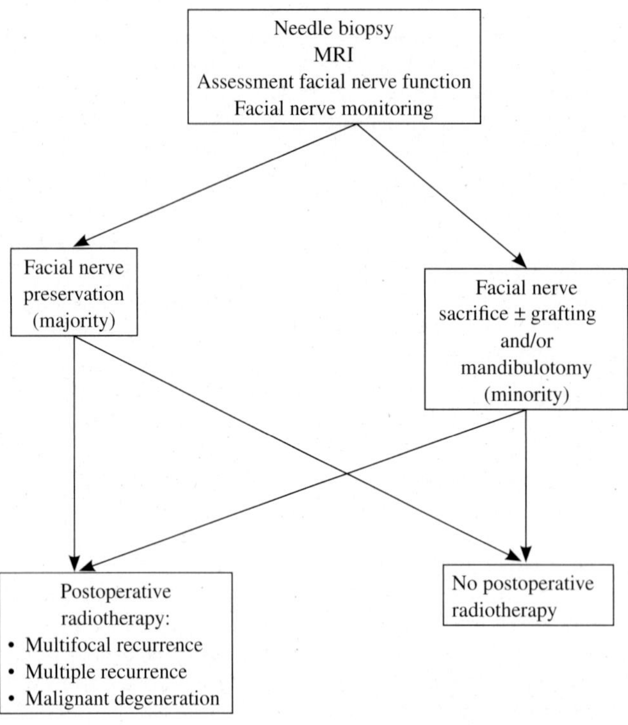

22 Parotid-Benign Disease

John F. Carew

Parotidectomy for the primary treatment of tumors of the parotid gland, in general, is a satisfying surgical procedure. These tumors are usually benign, unifocal, and freely mobile. With adequate surgical excision, including dissection and preservation of the facial nerve, the recurrence rate for these tumors is < 5%.[1–3] The cause of the recurrence may be related to surgical technique, tumor biology, or a combination of the two. Regardless of the cause of the recurrence, when tumors do recur, their surgical treatment can be tedious and technically challenging. In this chapter, the clinical characteristics of recurrent tumors of the parotid gland and their treatment will be discussed.

It should be noted that pleomorphic adenomas are by far the most common tumors to arise in the parotid gland.[4] Not surprisingly, they are also the most common benign tumor to recur. For this reason, this chapter will present comment on recurrent pleomorphic adenomas of the parotid unless specified otherwise.

Factors Predisposing to Recurrence

Many factors have been linked to the recurrence of pleomorphic adenomas of the parotid gland. The first and most well-established factor is the extent of initial surgery. There are ample data to support the contention that the enucleation or limited local excision results in a high rate of recurrence. In series published in the past, where this surgical technique was used, high rates of recurrence were seen that approached 50% in some reports.[5,6] For this reason, it is now well accepted that adequate surgical excision with at least a small cuff of normal parotid tissue surrounding the tumor should be resected at the time of primary treatment. It should be noted, however, that in many cases, at least a portion of the dissection is too close to the margin of the tumor during dissection of the facial nerve. Despite this, relatively low rates of recurrence are seen.

Occasionally, however, pleomorphic adenomas of the parotid gland may recur despite adequate primary surgical treatment. Several factors have been postulated to be related to this and include tiny microscopic extensions of the tumor beyond the pseudocapsule of the tumor, multifocality of the tumor, or rupture of the capsule of the tumor during primary surgical excision. Although these factors seem intuitively obvious, retrospective reviews by Buchman et al, Henriksson et al, and Natvig and Soberg failed to consistently reveal these as strong predictors of recurrence.[7–9] These studies, however, are limited by several factors. First, most of these studies deal with a very small number of recurrent tumors, as these tumors are uncommon and rarely recur. Additionally, they relied on operative reports for determining tumor capsule rupture. Unfortunately, operative reports do not always fully reflect the events that transpire. Surgeons may be hesitant to report capsule rupture for obvious medical and legal reasons. Despite their limitations, the reviews did not show a statistically significant increase in recurrence rate when the operative report specifically stated that the tumor capsule was ruptured.[7–9] In these reviews, the rate of recurrence when tumor capsule rupture was reported ranged from 0 to 8%. In all three studies, this is not significantly different from the recurrence rate when tumor capsule rupture was not reported. Although these studies did not show a relationship between tumor capsule rupture and recurrence, there is anecdotal evidence that this may be a source of recurrence. This evidence stems from the fact that many times when pleomorphic adenomas of the parotid recur, there are multiple tumor nodules studding the operative bed. Certainly, this pattern of recurrence is highly suggestive of tumor spillage as a possible mechanism for recurrence. Immunohistochemical studies have shown a high-level expression of integrin molecules on pleomorphic adenomas.[10] These cell surface receptors are involved in cell–cell and cell–extracellular matrix interactions. Their presence may in part account for cases where multiple tumors recur throughout the operative bed.

Although anecdotal evidence exists for tumor capsule rupture as an etiology for recurrence, more compelling evidence exists for microscopic extensions of tumor past the surgical margins. In one study, 57% of patients with microscopic extensions of tumor past the surgical margins had tumor recurrence.[7] In another, however, positive surgical margins were not shown to increase the rate of recurrence.[9] This factor, therefore, continues to remain controversial. Again, the power of these studies is limited by small sample sizes.

Finally, others have argued that this disease may be multifocal. Patient history and pathologic examples of tumor specimens rarely give evidence to support this.

From the available data, it can be concluded that recurrent tumors may be the result of either inadequate initial surgery, rupture of the capsule of the tumor with contamination of the surgical bed, or microscopic extensions of the tumor beyond its capsule. Regardless of the cause, when these tumors recur, they present a surgical challenge.

Clinical Presentation/Preoperative Evaluation

Pleomorphic adenomas of the parotid gland are relatively slow-growing tumors. For this reason, recurrences often occur decades after the primary surgery. In evaluating a patient with recurrence, several important clinical factors should be considered, including the nature of the primary surgical procedure and whether it was a formal parotidectomy or an enucleation. Treatment of patients with recurrent tumors that are the result of inadequate initial surgery tends to be more successful than treatment of patients with recurrent tumors despite adequate initial surgery.[11] Histologic characteristics of the primary tumor, with specific attention to the margins of the tumor, and accuracy of the histologic diagnosis should be obtained. Whenever possible, the original slides should be obtained and reviewed to confirm the accurate histologic diagnosis. Other critical clinical factors are the disease-free interval prior to recurrence and the rate of growth of the recurrent tumor. Additionally, the status of facial nerve function following the primary procedure is important to ascertain. If there was facial nerve weakness following the initial surgery, revision surgery will be more tedious and have a higher rate of facial nerve neuropraxia or permanent paralysis. Finally, it is important to determine if there was a history of radiation exposure or the use of therapeutic radiation in the past.

In addition to the clinical history, several aspects of the physical exam are critical to the evaluation of the patient with a recurrent tumor of the parotid. The pattern of recurrence, unifocal versus multifocal, is critical to surgical planning. Additionally, the relationship of the recurrent tumor to the overlying skin and scar tissue should be assessed. If the recurrence is immediately beneath the skin or the skin is tethered to the tumor, preparation should be made for sacrifice of the involved skin with appropriate reconstruction. The mobility of the tumor should also be assessed. The surgical incision should be inspected and kept in consideration when planning surgery for recurrent disease. In general, a modified Blair incision is most commonly used and can be extended superiorly and inferiorly to give adequate exposure when necessary for resection of recurrent disease. Finally, the function of all branches of the facial nerve should be critically examined.

Although evaluation of a patient with a primary parotid tumor may rely solely on clinical history and physical examination, in the recurrent setting it is important to obtain radiographic imaging as well as cytological evaluation. A magnetic resonance imaging (MRI) scan with attention to the parotid gland and bed is highly sensitive for soft tissue disease. Oftentimes, radiographic imaging will show minute subcutaneous nodules not appreciated on physical exam. Additionally, it gives one a sense of the extent of previous surgery based on the amount of residual parotid gland remaining. Finally, it gives critical information with regards to the third dimension or depth of the tumor and its potential relationship to the facial nerve, parapharyngeal space, and skull base.

It is often helpful to perform a fine-needle aspiration biopsy to confirm the cytologic appearance of the cells within the tumor. Occasionally, recurrent tumors following excision of pleomorphic adenomas of the parotid will display a malignant histology. This is critical information to have for preoperative planning in that a more radical and aggressive oncologic resection would be performed for a high-grade malignancy as opposed to a recurrent pleomorphic adenoma. The limitations, however, of fine-needle aspiration biopsy and cytologic evaluation must be understood. A fine-needle biopsy suggesting a recurrent pleomorphic adenoma does not guarantee that final histology will not show evidence of a malignant histology. The treatment of recurrent pleomorphic adenoma that degenerates into a malignancy is beyond the scope of this chapter, but such a malignancy requires a more aggressive surgical approach and a lower threshold for sacrifice of the facial nerve.

Surgical Technique

The extent of surgery required to adequately reset a recurrent pleomorphic adenoma of the parotid gland depends in large part on the nature of the recurrence. Occasionally, one may see a unifocal recurrence just beneath the skin and sufficiently distant from the facial nerve that can be excised through a simple local excision. These cases, however, are relatively rare, and this technique should be reserved for a very select cohort of patients. For unifocal recurrences, the surgical technique is similar to that for primary parotid tumors, although less parotid tissue will be encountered, and the dissection of the facial nerve will be tedious. Surgical excision of the unifocal recurrence begins with entering the surgical bed using the previously made incision. Care must be taken in making this incision because the recurrence can often be just beneath the scar. Additionally, the facial nerve may be relatively superficial because the superficial lobe of the parotid is no longer separated from the skin. In revision surgery, the skin flap raised tends to be thinner than in primary surgery because of the potential superficial location of the tumor and facial nerve. In males, the base of the hair follicles can be used as a guide to raising the flap in a relatively superficial plane. In females, one must rely on meticulous dissection, with frequent checks of the flap thickness. Once the flap has been raised, the facial nerve should be identified. The initial attempt to identify the facial nerve can be made using the standard landmarks of the posterior belly of the digastric, tragal pointer, and mastoid tip. If this region is heavily scarred, distal branches of the facial nerve can be identified and traced retrograde. As with any nerve dissection, it is critical to meticulously dissect directly on the nerve. Oftentimes extensive fibrosis and strands of fibrous tissue will cover the nerve and can be confused for minuscule branches coming off the nerve. The meticulous dissection and the use of a nerve simulator may aid in distinguishing between strands of fibrous tissue and facial nerve branches. With careful and meticulous dissection, however, the vast majority of unique focal recurrent pleomorphic adenomas of the parotid can be resected with preservation of the facial nerve. It is exceedingly rare to have to resect the facial nerve to get adequate tumor resection. If a recurrent tumor completely encases a single branch, this can be sacrificed and grafted. The functional aesthetic defect from this is reasonably acceptable. If, however, the main trunk of the facial nerve is encased with benign recurrent tumor, every effort should be made to preserve the nerve because of the significant aesthetic morbidity of sacrificing the main trunk, even if it is reconstructed.

In multifocal and more advanced disease, more aggressive surgical approaches and more tedious dissection are often required. If multiple subcutaneous nodules are seen beneath a scar, the scar tissue should be excised. Again, if a modified Blair incision had been used for the primary case, it is used for the excision of the recurrence. As noted above, the skin flaps are raised in a superficial plane to protect the facial nerve and the recurrent tumor. When there is evidence of recurrence in surgical scar, oftentimes these tumors can be seen in the relatively superficial subcutaneous tissue. Every effort should be made to appreciate these preoperatively and take adequate precautions to ensure adequate resection while maintaining the skin flap intact. Once the skin flaps have been raised, the facial nerve should be identified. An initial attempt should be made at the usual landmarks of the tragal pointer and posterior belly of the digastric. Again, however, if heavy scarring is encountered here, peripheral branches can be traced from distally to proximally. Although it is rarely necessary to perform a mastoidectomy to identify the proximal facial nerve, this maneuver can be considered in recurrent cases when there is massive recurrence, extensive multifocal tumors, or extremely dense scar tissue.

Once the facial nerve has been identified, meticulous dissection should be performed along its branches. As previously described, a facial nerve simulator can be used to distinguish between twigs of fibrous tissue coming off the nerve and true branches. Using the aforementioned methods, in general, most recurrent tumors, even when multifocal, can be safely resected while preserving the facial nerve.[11]

Although the facial nerve integrity can be maintained in the vast majority of these cases, the rate of temporary nerve dysfunction following surgery for recurrent tumors is much higher than in primary cases. Because of this, one should carefully counsel the patient preoperatively that he or she may have temporary weakness of the face but that this usually will resolve with time. Additionally, technologies are now available that allow monitoring of the facial nerve, which can help to identify it and minimize traumatic injury. Whereas in the primary setting, facial nerve identification and a traumatic dissection are relatively straightforward, in the recurrent setting, they can be very tedious. Certainly, routine use of a facial nerve monitor for primary parotid tumors is not necessary and has not been shown to improve outcome with regard to facial nerve function.[12] In the setting of recurrent parotid tumors, however, it may serve as a useful adjunct to meticulous anatomical dissection. Some authors have reported it to be very useful for this purpose.[13] As always, technology can never replace surgical experience, judgment, and meticulous dissection.

The vast majority of primary parotid tumors, as well as recurrences, occur in the superficial lobe of the parotid gland. Occasionally, however, recurrent tumors may arise in the deep lobe. Again, proper clinical examination and radiographic imaging are critical to preoperative planning. Similar issues as described above apply to the treatment of recurrent parotid tumors in the deep lobe. In addition, further surgical exposure may be required for the resection of recurrent deep lobe parotid tumors. Although the vast majority of primary deep lobe parotid tumors can be resected through a transcervical route, a small fraction of recurrent deep lobe parotid tumors may require a mandibulotomy to obtain adequate access for tumor resection. One should be prepared in the setting of a recurrent deep lobe parotid tumor to perform a mandibulotomy to ensure complete tumor removal. A mandibulotomy, however, is still required in only a minority of cases even in the recurrent setting.

Adjuvant treatment in the form of postoperative radiation therapy should be considered in cases of multifocal recurrence or second or third recurrences, or if the surgeon is at all concerned with the adequacy of tumor resection.[11,14,15] Although gross tumor should never be left behind, there is a level of surgical satisfaction appreciated following tumor resection that should be taken into account when deciding

Table 22.1   Local Control Rates after Surgical Treatment of Recurrent Pleomorphic Adenomas of the Parotid Gland

Author	Years	N	Local Control (%)	Follow-up (years)
Carew et al[11]	1984–1993 (9 years)	31	94	7.3*
Renehan et al[14]	1952–1992 (40 years)	114	85	14.0*
Phillips and Olsen[20]	1965–1985 (20 years)	126	68	14.5**
Samson et al[21]	1979–1988 (9 years)	21	81	2.0–11.0
Myssiorek et al[18]	1950–1983 (33 years)	27	37	12.0**
Niparko et al[19]	1935–1975 (40 years)	48	53	16.1**
Maran et al[16]	1967–1982 (15 years)	19	89.5	0.2–16.0
Fee et al[17]	1955–1973 (18 years)	26	65	Minimum 3 years

* Median length of follow-up.

** Mean length of follow-up.

if adjuvant radiation therapy is indicated. Certainly, there is a reasonable amount of data suggesting that in patients at high risk for further recurrence, postoperative radiation therapy decreases the rate of recurrence.[11,14,15]

Results

As mentioned earlier, parotid tumors are fairly slow growing, and their recurrence can occur decades after initial treatment. For this reason, the local control rate after treatment of recurrent pleomorphic adenomas is difficult to estimate and highly dependent on the length of follow-up. Recent reports indicate that local control varies from 37 to 94% (**Table 22.1**).[11,14,16–21] As would be expected, the studies with longer follow-up usually have higher rates of recurrence. The median time to failure in the treatment of recurrent pleomorphic adenomas was similar to the time to recurrence noted after initial surgery: 6.0 to 9.9 years.[19,20] In one report, none of the patients followed for less than 10 years had recurrence, whereas 43% of patients followed more than 10 years recurred.[20]

Several factors have been related to local control rates in the treatment of recurrent pleomorphic adenomas of the parotid. As expected, multifocal recurrences treated with surgery alone in one series had a much higher local failure rate (43%) compared with patients treated for unifocal disease (15%).[14] In another series, the extent of surgery for the primary tumor prior to the recurrence was related to local control rates for the treatment of the recurrence. Patients who recurred after an initial formal parotidectomy had a much higher local failure rate (37%) relative to patients who were treated for a recurrence after a limited excision (0%, $p < .01$).[11] The location of the recurrence deep to the facial nerve was also associated with a trend toward poorer local control. Patients with recurrences deep to the nerve had control rates of 67% at 7 years compared with 89% at 7 years for those with recurrence that was lateral to the nerve.[11] This is not surprising given the difficulty in resecting deep lobe tumors in a previously operated parotid bed.

The last factor that appeared to improve local control was the use of postoperative radiation therapy (PORT) in select cases. In one series, the use of adjuvant PORT improved local control rates in the cohort of patients with multinodular recurrences from 57 to 96% ($p < .01$).[14] In another series, the 10-year local control rate was 100% in patients who received adjuvant PORT compared with 71% in those patients who did not receive PORT.[11] This difference, however, was not statistically significant ($p < .28$) but may be related to the sample size and power of this study. In another study, the tumor was controlled in 18 of 20 patients (90%) whose recurrence was treated with excision and PORT, with follow-up ranging from 10 to 26 years.[15] The recurrence in these patients, however, followed a limited initial operation, a setting in which a more favorable prognosis can be anticipated. Although this issue is unlikely to be resolved by a randomized clinical trial, the evidence suggests that adjuvant PORT after surgery may benefit selected patients with ominous clinical and pathological presentations.

Conclusion

As with many recurrent disease processes, the adequate initial treatment of a tumor can avoid recurrence that often results in a much more tedious and technically challenging operation. Once a parotid tumor does recur, however, its successful treatment is facilitated by adequate preoperative clinical, radiographic, and cytologic evaluation. Adequate surgical resection can often be achieved through an unhurried and meticulous dissection with careful localization and preservation of the facial nerve. Finally, despite adequate surgical excision, a cohort of patients can be considered to be at significant risk for recurrence. Specifically, these are patients with recurrence after an initial adequate formal parotidectomy and those with extensive multinodular disease. These patients may benefit from adjuvant radiation therapy.

References

1. Leverstein H, van der Wal JE, Tiwari RM, van der Waal I, Snow GB. Surgical management of 246 previously untreated pleomorphic adenomas of the parotid gland. Br J Surg 1997;84:399–403.
2. Foote FW Jr, Frazell EL. Tumors of the major salivary gland. Cancer 1953;6:1065–1133.
3. Woods JE, Chong GC, Beahrs OH. Experience with 1,360 primary parotid tumors. Am J Surg 1975;130:460–462.
4. Conley J, Clairmont AA. Facial nerve in recurrent benign pleomorphic adenoma. Arch Otolaryngol 1979;105:247–251.
5. Maimaris CV, Ball MJ. Treatment of parotid gland tumours by conservative parotidectomy. Br J Surg 1986;73:897.
6. Krolls SO, Boyers RC. Mixed tumors of salivary glands: long-term follow-up. Cancer 1972;30:276–281
7. Buchman C, Stringer SP, Mendenhall WM, Parsons JT, Jordan JR, Cassisi NJ. Pleomorphic adenoma: effect of tumor spill and inadequate resection on tumor recurrence. Laryngoscope 1994;104:1231–1234.
8. Henriksson G, Westrin KM, Carlsoo B, Silfversward C. Recurrent primary pleomorphic adenomas of salivary gland origin: intrasurgical rupture, histopathologic features, and pseudopodia. Cancer 1998;82:617–620.
9. Natvig K, Soberg R. Relationship of intraoperative rupture of pleomorphic adenomas to recurrence: an 11–25 year follow-up study. Head Neck 1994;16:213–217.
10. Steiner MG, Kuhel WI, Carew JF, et al. Characterization of novel cell lines from pleomorphic adenomas of the parotid gland established in a collagen gel system. Laryngoscope 1997;107:654–660.
11. Carew JF, Spiro RH, Singh B, Shah JP. Treatment of recurrent pleomorphic adenomas of the parotid gland. Otolaryngol Head Neck Surg 1999;121:539–542.
12. Witt RL. Facial nerve monitoring in parotid surgery: the standard of care? Otolaryngol Head Neck Surg 1998;119:468–470.
13. Wolf SR, Schneider W, Suchy B, Eichhorn B. Intraoperative facial nerve monitoring in parotid surgery. HNO 1995;43:294–298.
14. Renehan A, Gleave EN, McGurk M. An analysis of the treatment of 114 patients with recurrent pleomorphic adenomas of the parotid gland. Am J Surg 1996;172:710–714.
15. Dawson AK. Radiation therapy in recurrent pleomorphic adenoma of the parotid. Int J Radiat Oncol Biol Phys 1989;16:819–821.
16. Maran AG, Mackenzie IJ, Stanley RE. Recurrent pleomorphic adenomas of the parotid gland. Arch Otolaryngol 1984;110:167–171.
17. Fee WE Jr, Goffinet DR, Calcaterra TC. Recurrent mixed tumors of the parotid gland—results of surgical therapy. Laryngoscope 1978;88:265–273.
18. Myssiorek D, Ruah CB, Hybels RL. Recurrent pleomorphic adenomas of the parotid gland. Head Neck 1990;12:332–336.
19. Niparko JK, Beauchamp ML, Krause CJ, Baker SR, Work WP. Surgical treatment of recurrent pleomorphic adenoma of the parotid gland. Arch Otolaryngol Head Neck Surg 1986;112:1180–1184.
20. Phillips PP, Olsen KD. Recurrent pleomorphic adenoma of the parotid gland: report of 126 cases and a review of the literature. Ann Otol Rhinol Laryngol 1995;104:100–104.
21. Samson MJ, Metson R, Wang CC, Montgomery WW. Preservation of the facial nerve in the management of recurrent pleomorphic adenoma. Laryngoscope 1991;101:1060–1062.

Decision tree for recurrent malignant parotid neoplasams

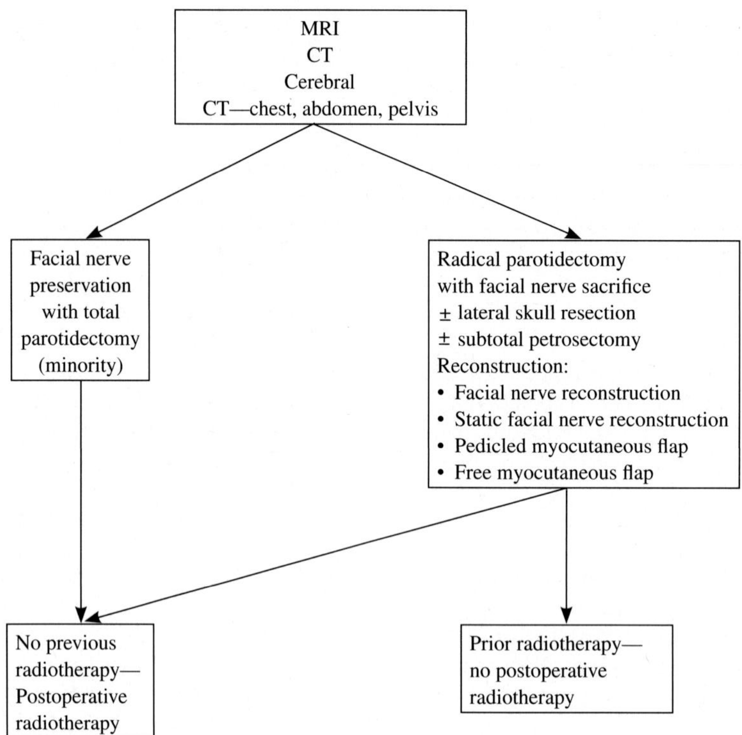

23 Recurrent Malignancy of the Parotid Gland

John P. Leonetti

The surgical management of primary malignant parotid tumors can range from a superficial parotidectomy to advanced lateral skull base resection for transcranial disease.[1] The ability to obtain locoregional control of malignant parotid neoplasms is related to the tumor-nodes-metastasis (TNM) stage, histologic grade, facial nerve involvement, and intraoperatively defined tumor extension of local neurovascular, muscular, and bony structures.[2] Despite meticulous preoperative planning, afgggressive tumor ablation, and postoperative radiotherapy, the risk of local or regional malignant parotid tumor recurrence can be as high as 50%.[3] The purpose of this chapter is to outline diagnostic and treatment options for patients with locally recurrent malignancies of the parotid gland.

Diagnosis

Follow-up Surveillance

Early detection of parotid gland tumor recurrence may affect the overall outcome in many patients. A clinical evaluation is performed on all patients with malignant disease every 3 months for 2 years and every 6 months for 3 years. A chest x-ray is obtained annually, along with a contrast-enhanced magnetic resonance imaging (MRI) scan of the parotid and neck regions.

Clinical Evaluation

A complete head and neck examination is performed, including bimanual parotid palpation, cranial nerve assessment, and microscopic otoscopy. Referred otalgia may be due to tumor invasion of the auriculotemporal branch of the trigeminal nerve, the tympanic branch of the glossopharyngeal verve, or the auricular branch of the vagus nerve.[4] A new-onset voice change or swallowing difficulty may signify lower cranial nerve tumor invasion of the jugular foramen.[5] Hearing loss may be due to tumor occlusion of the eustachian tube with resultant middle ear effusion or external auditory canal tumor involvement. Diploplia and headache suggest skull base erosion and abducens neuropathy due to petrous apex and carotid canal tumor extension.[6]

The most common presentation of locally recurrent parotid malignancy is the presence of a mass in the operated bed or a diffuse fullness between the angle of the mandible and the mastoid tip.[7] Facial paresis or paralysis in a patient with a history of parotid malignancy must be assumed to be caused by tumor recurrence with or without a clinically apparent mass.[8]

Generalized fatigue, lethargy, weight loss, or peripheral bone pain are potential symptoms of metastatic disease.

Radiographic Assessment

MRI is ideal for evaluating soft tissue, intracranial, and perineural tumor recurrence.[9] Contrast-enhanced computed tomography (CT) is helpful in the identification of temporal bone, cervical spine, petrous apex, or clival bone erosion.[10] Cerebral angiography and venography are used in patients with suspected jugular foramen tumor invasion.[11] Collateral venous return must be demonstrated if recurrent tumor resection requires jugular bulb obliteration or ligation. Failure to identify inadequate collateral venous return could result in life-threatening venous infarction.

All patients with locally recurrent parotid malignancy must undergo a metastatic evaluation, which, at a minimum, should include a CT scan of the head, chest, and abdomen and a total body bone scan. Clinical or radiographic evidence of metastatic disease will eliminate aggressive local surgical management as a treatment option.

Treatment

General

Most patients with malignant parotid tumors will receive postoperative radiotherapy as part of the initial treatment planning. If radiotherapy was not employed, it may be used as the only treatment or following salvage surgery for recurrent disease.

Surgical Approach

Total parotidectomy with facial nerve preservation can be used in the rare situation of a localized, solitary recurrent mass with normal preoperative facial nerve function. Radical parotidectomy is used in patients with multifocal tumor recurrence and/or preoperative facial twitching, paresis, or paralysis.

Lateral skull base procedures can be used for large or deep-seated recurrent lesions to obtain tumor-free margins near the external auditory canal, jugular foramen, carotid canal, or the floor of the middle cranial fossa.[12] Variations of the subtotal petrosectomy can thus be used to accomplish tumor removal through lateral skull base access based on preoperative radiographic assessment of tumor extent.

Defect Reconstruction

Primary wound closure is used following parotidectomy with facial nerve preservation or in patients who are not candidates for neural repair. Larger lateral skull base defects can be reconstructed with pedicled trapezius, latissimus dorsi, or temporalis muscle flaps. Microvascular free flap reconstruction using the serratus, gracilis, or rectus abdominis muscles can provide facial contour and movement if the proximal facial nerve can be anastomosed to the donor muscle motor nerve.[13]

Dynamic facial nerve repair is dependent upon the degree of surgical resection and may include primary nerve anastomosis, interposition greater auricular or sural nerve grafting, cross-facial anastomosis, or a hypoglossal-facial repair.[14]

Static procedures utilized after facial nerve resection include fascial or Gore-Tex slings, gingivobuccal prosthetic devices, and occuloplastic procedures such as eyelid gold weights, springs, and lower eyelid tightening techniques.[15]

Results

Despite early diagnosis and accurate radiographic mapping, recurrent malignancy of the parotid gland is often associated with a grave and fatal outcome. Calearo et al saw an overall recurrence rate of 23% in a group of 167 patients with malignant parotid tumors, with significant variation according to the tumor histology.[2] In a review of 22 patients with adenoid cystic carcinoma operated by Spafford et al, 5 (23%) patients developed locally recurrent disease.[16] Three of these patients died of the recurrence despite additional salvage surgery. Malata et al documented a 27% recurrence rate in 51 patients who underwent surgical excision of a variety of malignant parotid tumors.[17] All 14 patients in this series died within 23 months of their surgery with local disease (3 patients), metastatic disease (6 patients), and unrelated (5 patients) causes for the demise. Leverstein et al published a series of 65 patients who underwent surgical treatment for parotid epithelial malignancy.[18] Twelve of 65 (18%) developed locoregional recurrent disease. Eleven of 12 died of their recurrent tumor despite attempted salvage surgery ± radiotherapy. Twenty-five of 97 patients developed local parotid tumor recurrence in the Magnano et al. series.[19] As of their 1999 publication, 4 patients were without disease, but 21 of 25 patients (84%) were either alive with or dead of their disease, despite salvage treatment of the tumor recurrence.

Conclusion

Early detection of recurrent parotid malignancies may be possible through diligent clinical and radiographic surveillance. The surgical resection of recurrent parotid malignancies may range from completion total parotidectomy to advanced, combined lateral skull base techniques. Future reviews will demonstrate if such advanced ablative surgery will impact the overall outcome in this select patient population.

References

1. Pedersen D, Overgaard J, Sogaard H. Malignant parotid tumors in 110 consecutive patients: treatment results and prognosis. Laryngoscope 1992;102:1064–1069.
2. Calearo C, Storch O, Pastore A, Polli G. Parotid gland carcinoma: analysis of prognostic factors. Ann Otol Rhinol Laryngol 1998;107:969–973.
3. Laskawi R, Rodel R, Zirk A, Arglebe C. Retrospective analysis of 35 patients with acinic cell carcinoma of the parotid gland. J Oral Maxillofac Surg 1998;56:440–443.
4. Byrne MN, Spector JG. Parotid masses, evaluation, analysis, and current management. Laryngoscope 1988;98:99–105.
5. Leonetti JP, Smith PG, Grubb RL. The perioperative management of the petrous carotid artery in contemporary surgery of the skull base. Otolaryngol Head Neck Surg 1990;103:46–51.
6. Leonetti JP, Smith PG, Linthicum FH. The petrous carotid artery: anatomic relationships in skull base surgery. Otolaryngol Head Neck Surg 1990;102:3–12.
7. Theriault C, Fitzpatrick PJ. Malignant parotid tumors: prognostic factors and optimum treatment. Am J Clin Oncol 1986;9:510–516.
8. Woods JE. The facial nerve in parotid malignancy. Am J Surg 1983;146:493–496.

9. Horowitz SW, Leonetti JP, Azar-Kia B, et al. CT and MR of the temporal bone and parotid regions for malignancy. AJNR Am J Neuroradiol 1994;15:755–762.

10. Som PM, Biller HF. High grade malignancies of the parotid gland: identification with MR imaging. Radiology 1989;173:823–826.

11. Fisch U, Feagan P, Valvanis A. The infratemporal fossa approach for the lateral skull base. Otolaryngol Clin North Am 1984;17(3):513–552.

12. Leonetti JP, Smith PG, Anand VK, Kletzker GR, Hartman JM. Management of advanced parotid neoplasms. Otolaryngol Head Neck Surg 1993;108:270–276.

13. Izquierdo R, Leonetti JP, Origitano TC, et al. Refinements using free tissue transfer for complex cranial base reconstruction. Plast Reconstr Surg 1993;92:567–574.

14. Anand VK, Al-Mefty O, Leonetti JP. Complications of skull base surgery and how to avoid them. Instructional Course AAO-HNS 1993;6:323–359.

15. Leonetti JP, Scannichio LS, Kelly TF. Prosthetic restoration of the paralyzed face. Otolaryngol Head Neck Surg 1993;108:201–203.

16. Spafford PD, Mintz DR, Hay J. Acinic cell carcinoma of the parotid gland: review and management. J Otolaryngol 1991;20:262–266.

17. Malata CM, Camiller IG, McLean NR, et al. Malignant tumors of the parotid gland. Br J Plast Surg 1997;50:600–608.

18. Leverstein H, Van Der Wal JE, Triwari RM, et al. Malignant epithelial parotid gland tumors: analysis and results in 65 untreated patients. Br J Surg 1998;85:1267–1272.

19. Magnano M, Fernando C, Cravero L, et al. Treatment of malignant neoplasms of the parotid gland. Otolaryngol Head Neck Surg 1999;121:627–632.

Decision tree for recurrent nasopharynx cancer

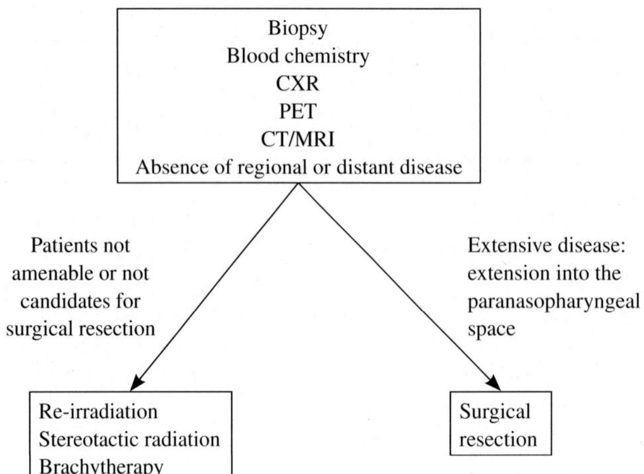

Recurrent Nasopharyngeal Carcinoma

William I. Wei and Anthony P. W. Yuen

Nasopharyngeal carcinoma (NPC) is a nonlymphomatous, squamous cell carcinoma that originates from the epithelial cells lining the pharyngeal recess located medial to the medial crura of the eustachian tube. This malignant disease is common in southern China, especially among Cantonese speakers. The incidence is around 25 cases per 100,000 population.[1] NPC is radiosensitive; therefore, external radiotherapy is the primary treatment modality. As there is a high propensity for NPC to metastasize to cervical lymph nodes, the neck is always included in the irradiation field even when there is no clinical positive neck node. The nasopharynx and upper neck nodes are usually treated in one target volume, using two lateral opposing facial fields and one anterior facial field delivering a total of 60 to 70 Gy. In recent years, concurrent chemoradiation with cisplatinum (cisplatin), followed by three courses of adjuvant chemotherapy using cisplatinum and fluorouracil, has significantly improved both the 3-year progression-free survival and the 3-year overall survival.[2] The overall 5-year survival is stage dependent and ranges from 70 to 80% for stage I disease and 20 to 30% for stage IV disease.[3,4] In some patients, however, despite radical therapy with chemotherapy and radiation, the primary tumor persists or recurs. When the disease is localized in the nasopharynx, and in the absence of regional or distant metastasis, salvage therapy may be possible.

Assessment of Tumor

Salvage therapy is performed only after accurate assessment of the recurrent tumor. The choice of salvage treatment also depends on the findings of the assessment.

A metastatic work-up should be performed to ensure that the tumor is localized in the nasopharynx. The work-up should include a clinical examination, tests on blood biochemistry, such as liver and renal function tests, a chest x-ray, and, when indicated, a positron emission tomography of the body.

Assessment of a local tumor in the nasopharynx should be performed by an endoscopic examination to visualize its mucosal extent. Computed tomography is useful to evaluate the extent of bone erosion, especially at the skull base. Magnetic resonance imaging should also be performed to assess the three-dimensional extension of the tumor in the nasopharynx.

Options of Salvage Therapy

Re-irradiation

For re-irradiation to be effective, a radiotherapeutic dose of 60 Gy or more is required.[5] Although the reported 5-year disease-free survival rate with re-irradiation ranges from 18.7 to 50%, the associated morbidities are significant. Trismus and the effects of cranial nerve damage can be incapacitating. Complications related to neuroendocrine damage and poor nonverbal memory recall have been reported.[6] In a large retrospective review of treatment results after local recurrence, it was shown that successful local salvage was achieved in 32% of patients who received re-irradiation. The cumulative incidence of late post-re-irradiation sequelae was 24%, and the treatment mortality was 1.8%.[7]

To avoid the high incidence of complication resulting from re-irradiation brachytherapy, surgical resection and stereotactic radiosurgery can be considered for patients with relatively small and localized tumors.

Stereotactic Radiotherapy

Stereotactic radiotherapy for the management of recurrent NPC can achieve a local tumor control rate of 10 to 60%. However, only a small number of patients have been treated this way, and long-term follow-up data are not available.[8] In the future, 3-D conformal radiotherapy, stereotactic radiotherapy, and intensity modulated radiotherapy may permit larger recurrent tumors to be treated with high conformity. This would allow dose escalation, better local control, and fewer complications.

Brachytherapy

When the recurrent cancer in the nasopharynx is small ($<$ 2 cm diameter) and does not involve underlying bony structures, brachytherapy with split palate implantation of radioactive gold grains (Au^{198}) can achieve a good local tumor control rate.[9] This technique involves splitting the palate under general anesthesia. The mucoperiosteum over the hard palate is then retracted to expose the tumor in the nasopharynx. This allows radioactive gold grains to be inserted accurately into the tumor under direct vision. The palatal wound is then closed in layers.[10]

From 1988 to 1999, brachytherapy was performed in our hospital for 106 patients with small tumor localized in the nasopharynx. All patients were followed up for between 8 months and 8 years (median 4.5 years) after having been discharged. The 5-year actuarial local tumor control rate for recurrent tumor was 65%. Although palatal fistula was the major morbidity (20%), its incidence could be reduced by more precise closure of the palatal wound. The results achieved with brachytherapy using gold grain implantation support its use for patients with small recurrent tumors in the nasopharynx. When the expertise required for gold grain implantation is unavailable, treatment with afterloading intubation brachytherapy may prove a suitable alternative. A retrospective study of 61 patients with local recurrent NPC was performed. High-dose intracavitary brachytherapy gave an actuarial 3-year local relapse-free survival rate of 45%.[11] This treatment is therefore effective when the brachytherapy source can be placed close to the tumor in the nasopharynx to achieve a good dosimetry.

Surgical Resection

Brachytherapy is unsuitable for recurrent NPCs that are extensive or have extended into the paranasopharyngeal space. The location of the tumor, such as over the crura of the eustachian tube or on the posterior nasal septum, also precludes the accurate insertion of the gold grains. Therefore, for these patients, surgical resection is an alternative salvage option. Step serial sectioning studies of specimens obtained following nasopharyngectomy for recurrent NPC after radiotherapy have shown that the disease was usually extensive. Over 90% of the 19 specimens studied showed (1) submucosal extension beyond the tumor edge of up to 2 cm (median 1 cm) and (2) malignant cells in close association with the eustachian tube cartilage.[12] Adequate exposure of the recurrent NPC is necessary for an oncological resection to be performed. As the nasopharynx is located in the center of the head, it is difficult to obtain an adequate exposure for a curative resection. Although the inferior approach through the palate exposes the tumor to allow insertion of radioactive gold grains, it does not allow resection of a larger tumor with adequate margins. This is particularly true when the tumor has extended laterally into the paranasopharyngeal space. All approaches to the nasopharynx reported in the literature have their own particular indications and limitations. The choice of approach for each patient depends on the location, size, and extent of the recurrent tumor in the nasopharynx.[13] Because most recurrent cancer in the nasopharynx after radiotherapy is located at the lateral wall, we have developed an anterolateral approach for resection of these tumors.[14,15] The facial and palatal incisions are similar to those employed for

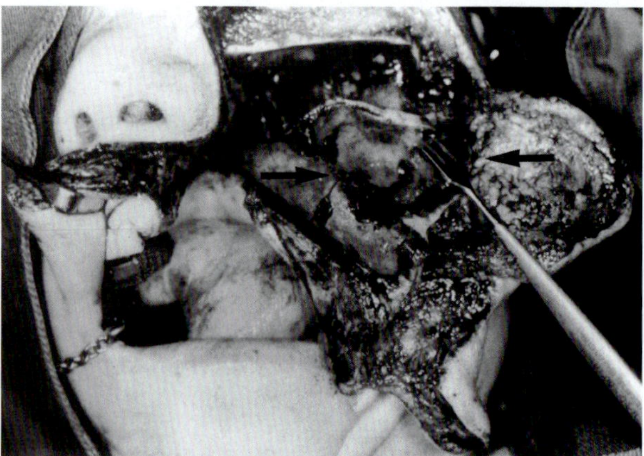

Fig. 24.1 The maxilla (*arrows*) attached to the anterior cheek flap is swung laterally to expose the nasopharynx for tumor extirpation.

maxillectomy. The anterior cheek flap is left attached to the anterior wall of the maxilla. After appropriate osteotomies, the osteocutaneous complex consisting of the maxilla and the anterior cheek flap can be turned laterally to offer a wide exposure of the nasopharynx and its vicinity, the paranasopharyngeal area (**Fig. 24.1**). Tumors in this region can be resected with an adequate margin under direct vision. After the resection, the maxilla that is attached to the anterior cheek flap can be returned to its original position and fixed with miniplates to the facial skeleton. When this approach was initially employed for the surgical salvage of postradiotherapy recurrent cancer in the nasopharynx, the 5-year actuarial local disease control rate was 52%, and the 5-year actuarial disease-free survival rate was 43%.[15] Between February 1989 and September 1999, this approach was employed as surgical salvage for 71 patients with recurrent primary nasopharyngeal cancer after radiotherapy. Fifty-four patients (47 males and 7 females; ages between 27 and 76 years, median 52 years) received curative resections as negative resection margins were achieved. All 71 patients survived and were discharged home. The follow-up period for those who had curative resection ranged from 6 to 125 months (median 38 months). The 5-year actuarial local cancer control rate was 62%, and the 5-year actuarial survival rate was 49%.[16]

Morbidity associated with the operation included trismus of different severity resulting from further dissection of the radiated pterygoid muscles at the time of surgery. The trismus, however, usually improved with passive stretching. Palatal fistula developed in 14 patients (19.7%). The fistula was closed in one patient, while the remaining patients were managed with a dental plate. All patients could take a normal diet, and there was no functional disability. With the modification of the palatal incision, the problem of palatal fistula has been eliminated.[17] Two patients developed facial sinus, which healed after removal of the plate and screws.

The improved salvage results compared with our early reports were achieved through careful patient selection, early detection of recurrence after external radiotherapy, and modification of surgical techniques. Removal of the pterygoid plates and the attached muscle increased the exposure of the nasopharynx for complete tumor extirpation. The posterior part of the nasal septum, rostrum, and superior surface of the soft palate were routinely included with the resection of tumor. Besides increasing the resection margin, removal of these structures enhanced the exposure of the whole nasopharynx. The anterior wall of the sphenoid sinus was removed to increase both the deep resection margin and drainage of the sinus. Parts of the prevertebral muscle and anterior portion of the clivus could also be removed to gain additional clearance. The internal carotid artery could be exposed and any bleeding secured under direct vision. Facial scarring of the patients had become almost invisible 12 months after the operation, and the associated morbidity was low.

Choice of Salvage Therapy

Salvage therapy for recurrent NPC with a curative intent is performed only when there is no evidence of regional or distant metastasis. The choice of therapy depends on evaluation of the extensiveness of the tumor using endoscopy or imaging studies (**Fig. 24.2**). For recurrent nasopharyngeal carcinomas that are located within accessible sites in the nasopharynx, brachytherapy with gold grain implantation offers a good local tumor control rate with minimal morbidity. However, this modality is effective only for NPCs that are < 2 cm in diameter and exhibit no bony erosion. Nasopharyngectomy via the anterolateral approach is appropriate for circumstances that include a tumor infiltration of >1 cm, location of a tumor that is not amenable to gold grain implantation, and when the tumor has extended to the paranasopharyngeal tissue. This technique offers a reasonable chance of eradicating the disease with an acceptable morbidity. However, when the skull base bone or the clivus has been infiltrated by tumor or when the tumor has encroached onto the internal carotid artery, then a successful curative resection is remote.

When an unsuitable medical status precludes a patient from undergoing surgery or where microscopic residual tumors exist after nasopharyngectomy, then stereotactic therapy is applicable. Its efficacy is decreased for tumors that have extended inferiorly. Therefore, the value of stereotactic therapy as a salvage procedure remains to be confirmed. Further external radiotherapy may control the recurrent nasopharyngeal carcinoma when other options are not applicable. The eradication of recurrent tumor with this option is, however, frequently associated with significant morbidities, especially on long-term follow-up.

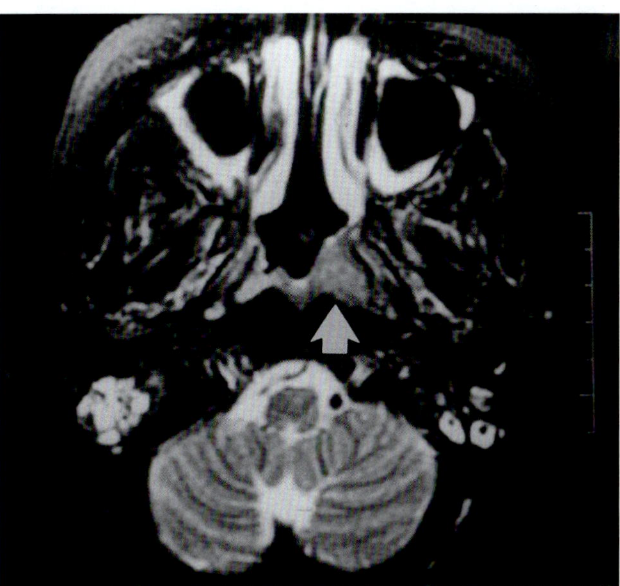

Fig. 24.2 Magnetic resonance imaging showing tumor (*arrow*) extending to the paranasopharyngeal space, too thick for gold grain implantation but amenable to surgical resection.

References

1. Parkin DM, Ferlay J, Raymond L, Young J. Cancer incidence in five continents. I Arc 1997;143:814,815.
2. Al-Sarraf M, LeBlanc M, Giri PG, et al. Chemoradiotherapy versus radiotherapy in patients with advanced nasopharyngeal cancer: phase III randomized intergroup study 0099. J Clin Oncol 1998;16:1310–1317.
3. Chao KS, Low DA, Perez CA, Purdy JA. Intensity-modulated radiation therapy in head and neck cancers: the Mallinckrodt experience. Int J Cancer 2000;90:92–103.
4. Wei WI, Sham JST. Nasopharyngeal carcinoma. Lancet 2005;365:2041–2054.
5. Wang CC. Re-irradiation of recurrent nasopharyngeal carcinoma—treatment techniques and results. Int J Radiat Oncol Biol Phys 1987;13:953–956.
6. Woo E, Lam K, Yu YL, Ma J, Wang C, Yeung RT. Temporal lobe and hypothalamic-pituitary dysfunctions after radiotherapy for nasopharyngeal carcinoma: a distinct clinical syndrome. J Neurol Neurosurg Psychiatry 1988;51:1302–1307.
7. Lee AW, Law SC, Foo W, et al. Retrospective analysis of patients with nasopharyngeal carcinoma treated during 1976–1985: survival after local recurrence. Int J Radiat Oncol Biol Phys 1993;26:773–782.
8. Chua DT, Sham JST, Hung KN, et al. Stereotactic radiosurgery as a salvage treatment for locally persistent and recurrent nasopharyngeal carcinoma. Head Neck 1999;21:620–626.
9. Kwong DLW, Wei WI, Cheng ACK, et al. Long term results of radioactive gold grain implantation for the treatment

of persistent and recurrent nasopharyngeal carcinoma. Cancer 2001;91:1105–1113.

10. Wei WI, Sham JST, Choy D, Ho CM, Lam KH. Split-palate approach for gold grain implantation in nasopharyngeal carcinoma. Arch Otolaryngol Head Neck Surg 1990;116:578–582.

11. Leung TW, Tung SY, Wong VY, et al. High dose rate intracavitary brachytherapy in the treatment of nasopharyngeal carcinoma. Acta Oncol 1996;35:43–47.

12. Wei WI. Carcinoma of the nasopharynx. Otolaryngol Head Neck Surg 1998;12:119–132.

13. Wei WI, Lam KH, Sham JST. New approach to the nasopharynx: the maxillary swing approach. Head Neck 1991;13:200–207.

14. Wei WI, Ho CM, Yuen PW, Fung CF, Sham JST, Lam KH. Maxillary swing approach for resection of tumors in and around the nasopharynx. Arch Otolaryngol Head Neck Surg 1995;121:638–642.

15. Wei WI. Salvage surgery for recurrent primary nasopharyngeal carcinoma. Crit Rev Oncol Hematol 2000;33:91–98.

16. Wei WI. Nasopharyngeal cancer: current status of management. Arch Otolaryngol Head Neck Surg 2001;127:766–769.

17. Ng RWM, Wei WI. Elimination of palatal fistula after the maxillary swing procedure. Head Neck 2005;27:608–612.

25 Revision Neck Dissection

Paul A. Kedeshian

Revision surgery for cervical metastatic disease presents a difficult therapeutic challenge whose scope and potential for success depend on the extent of prior therapy. In general, revision surgery is complicated by the fact that there is usually more extensive and poorly defined disease in a debilitated patient, leading to increased technical challenges, surgical morbidity, and postoperative complications. For the purposes of this discussion, recurrent metastatic disease arising from primary squamous carcinomas of the head and neck will be considered. However, some of the principles that are elaborated may be extended to nonsquamous pathologies or to cervical metastases from infraclavicular primary sites.

Work-up

All patients with recurrent cervical metastases must have a thorough head and neck physical examination (including endoscopy of the upper aerodigestive tract). At the time of this evaluation, the primary site must be carefully investigated to rule out a recurrence, and the aerodigestive tract in general must be investigated to exclude a second primary neoplasm. The physical examination of patients with recurrent neck disease must focus specifically on the location and size of the metastasis. Additionally, the physical characteristics of the metastasis, including fixation to local structures (suggestive of direct invasion), cephalocaudad mobility overlying the carotid sheath, tethering or erosion of the overlying skin, and paresis or paralysis of cranial nerves, must be determined. The location and orientation of any prior skin incisions should also be noted. Biopsy via fine-needle aspiration (FNA) should be performed whenever possible to broadly characterize the tumor mass and potentially separate a metastatic recurrence from other pathologies.

Patients should also undergo a metastatic work-up, including chest radiographs followed by a chest computed tomography (CT) scan if any abnormalities are detected on plain radiographs. Additional imaging should include magnetic resonance imaging (MRI) with gadolinium encompassing both the initial primary site and the neck. (The soft tissue resolution provided by MRI in the setting of prior treatment, with the obliteration of tissue planes, far exceeds that of CT.) In particular, the relationship of the neck disease to the carotid artery (encasement, abutment, and invasion) needs to be visualized and the metastases investigated for any features that might suggest unresectability (see below).

Determining the resectability of cervical metastases as they relate to the carotid arterial system should include an assessment of both the anatomical and functional status of the carotid artery. Magnetic resonance angiography (MRA) and/or conventional angiography are quite valuable for the determination of arterial compression, displacement, stenosis, and flow as well as the patency of contralateral flow through the circle of Willis. This information can then be supplemented by the functional data obtained from balloon occlusion and subsequent single photon emission computed tomography (SPECT) scanning. With these data, a better sense of the likelihood of carotid resection can be ascertained and, if the carotid needs to be resected, the potential consequences better anticipated.

Finally, whole-body positron emission tomography (PET) scan imaging is frequently beneficial in the evaluation of recurrent disease, particularly when MRI findings are equivocal, a tissue confirmation of tumor recurrence is not available, or systemic metastases are suspected.

The extent and nature of the neck disease prior to a patient's initial treatment are of critical importance (particularly when the prior treatment was rendered by a different surgeon). In particular, information regarding the size and location of the initial metastatic disease is vital. Moreover, the nature and the timing of prior therapy (to separate disease recurrence from persistence) must be ascertained. Any available surgical pathology reports should be reviewed with a particular emphasis on (1) the size and number of involved lymph nodes, (2) the presence or absence of extracapsular disease, and (3) the inclusion of any nonlymphatic structures (submandibular gland, sternomastoid muscle, and skin) within the pathologic specimen. Additionally, any prior operative reports should be obtained and carefully reviewed and, when possible, the prior treating physicians directly contacted. If radiotherapy has been employed, treatment doses, sources (including the use of nonphoton sources), ports, fractionation, and treatment duration need to be investigated. The occurrence of any significant breaks in treatment should be determined as well as reports of any chemotherapeutics administered and whether they were delivered sequentially or concomitantly.

Decision tree for recurrent neck cancer

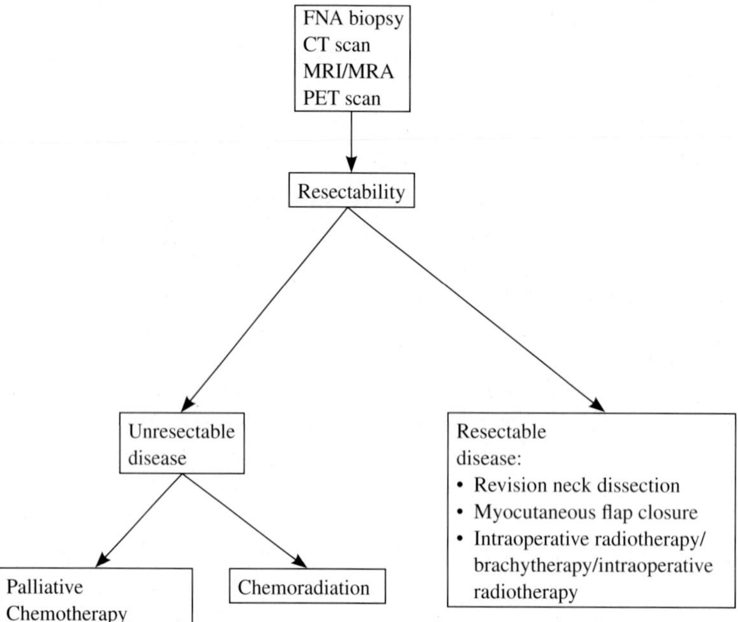

Contraindications to Surgery

Features that suggest unresectability include

1. Carotid encasement/invasion/occlusion
2. Dermal lymphatic invasion/dermal metastases
3. Invasion of deep neck musculature/fixation to deep neck/brachial plexus invasion
4. Base of skull invasion/extension/erosion

Recurrence after Radiotherapy

When cervical metastatic disease recurs following radiotherapy, the extent of the pretreatment neck disease and the technical details of the radiotherapy are essential to ascertain. These details must include specifics as to the doses and regions of the neck irradiated because radiotherapy doses to sites of known N[+] disease that are <63 Gy are likely inadequate to fully sterilize metastatic squamous cell carcinoma.[1] Although excellent cure rates are reported for primary radiotherapy in the treatment of N1 disease,[2] the results are not as promising if radiotherapy is the sole treatment modality for either N2 or N3 disease (except in the case of metastases from nasopharynx primaries).[3] Moreover, combined modality treatment is of greater effectiveness for nodal disease that demonstrates aggressive histopathologic features, such as extracapsular spread (ECS).

The extent of surgical resection necessary if a cervical recurrence presents following radiotherapy is usually dictated by the location of the recurrence. A type 1 neck dissection is usually sufficient to adequately encompass the metastatic disease. However, the dissection may need to be extended to include the spinal accessory nerve (radical neck dissection) or occasionally broadened in anatomical extent to include sacrifice of the marginal nerve, vagus nerve, mandibular periosteum, skin, or other structures (extended neck dissection). The neck dissection incisions used to resect recurrent metastatic disease following radiotherapy can usually be reapproximated primarily (with a low incidence of wound complications) if the integrity of the overlying skin can be maintained. However, regional myocutaneous free flap coverage must be considered when a portion of "contaminated" skin needs to be resected, concern over carotid artery exposure exists, a tension-free primary closure cannot be obtained, or brachytherapy or intraoperative radiotherapy is to be employed.

The specific scenario of cervical recurrence after open neck biopsy and subsequent radiotherapy deserves mention at this juncture. When sufficient radiotherapy doses are employed (63 Gy or greater), ample data as to the curability of these patients (without the need for neck dissection)

exist.[4] However, if this approach is to be employed, important patient selection criteria that must be adhered to include (1) the open biopsy needs to have been excisional (with no gross tumor thought to be remaining), (2) a solitary node was excised, (3) the node's maximal diameter is <3 cm, and (4) the node was lacking evidence of ECS.[4]

A brief mention should be made of patients with recurrent neck disease following organ preservation therapy (chemotherapy and radiotherapy delivered either concurrently or sequentially). Although a complete clinical response for N[+] disease following the completion of chemo- and/or radiotherapy may be observed (and many advocate that the neck can be carefully observed in this situation), the probability of recurrent neck metastasis (particularly for advanced N2 or N3 neck disease) is not negligible.[5,6] Additionally, if a complete clinical response is not achieved for N[+] disease following chemotherapy and/or radiotherapy (regardless of N stage), surgical salvage may not be feasible.[5] In many of these cases, therefore, a PET scan obtained following the completion of nonsurgical treatment may provide a rationale for neck dissection by detecting active tumor *prior to* the clinical or radiographic detection of recurrent or residual disease.

Recurrence after Supraomohyoid Neck Dissection

Recurrent neck disease following supraomohyoid neck dissection (SOHND) or type II, whether followed by radiotherapy or not, presents a much more formidable surgical challenge than recurrence following radiotherapy alone. In particular, SOHND involves the comprehensive resection of fatty and lymphatic tissue from levels 1 to 3. Consequently, if recurrent metastatic disease occurs anywhere within these nodal levels, it may be adherent to the great vessels, thereby making complete gross tumor resection unlikely. However, in situations where the recurrent disease is present in either level 4 or 5 (not routinely dissected during SOHND), the potential for complete resectability may be greater, although the risks of chyle fistula and accessory nerve sacrifice are high.

When recurrence after SOHND occurs and the recurrence is thought to be resectable, the patient and the treating surgeon must recognize the likely palliative nature of any revision surgery. Therefore, the adjunctive use of either brachytherapy or intraoperative radiotherapy (IORT) should be addressed in an effort to increase the chances of cure, as both of these modalities have been reported to yield satisfactory results.[7,8] Whether IORT or brachytherapy is employed, the need for myocutaneous flap coverage in these cases is mandatory. In the specific case of metastatic disease affixed to the carotid artery, the likely palliative nature of any revision surgery for cervical metastases must be appreciated. Unless preoperative anatomical and functional studies suggest that the carotid artery potentially may need to be resected and that its resection would not likely result in major cerebrovascular compromise, the benefit of carotid artery resection is questionable and its morbidity potentially catastrophic.[9] In these circumstances, brachytherapy has shown some success; therefore, iodine 125 implants and myocutaneous flap coverage may be a lower risk alternative to consider.[10]

Recurrence after Type 1 Neck Dissection/Radical Neck Dissection

Secondary to the extensive dissection of tissue planes adjacent to critical neurovascular structures, as well as the resection of the sternomastoid muscle, when cervical metastatic disease occurs after either a type 1 neck dissection or radical neck dissection, the likelihood that the disease can be completely resected is essentially nil. Such a clinical situation should be universally regarded as incurable; therefore, any palliative surgical interventions (as well as their morbidity and complications, see below) need to be carefully balanced against the morbidity of unrestrained tumor growth and tumor-related symptoms (pain, skin ulceration, cranial neuropathies, etc.).

Complications of Surgery

Complications of recurrent neck surgery include

1. Chyle fistula
2. Wound breakdown/carotid exposure/carotid rupture
3. Cranial neuropathies
4. Vascular injury/cerebrovascular accident

References

1. Peters LJ, Goepfert H, Ang KK, et al. Evaluation of the dose for postoperative radiation therapy of head and neck cancer: first report of a prospective randomized trial. Int J Radiat Oncol Biol Phys 1993;26:3–11.
2. Mendenhall WM, Million, RR, Cassisi NJ. Squamous cell carcinoma of the head and neck treated with radiation therapy: the role of neck dissection for clinically positive neck nodes. Int J Radiat Oncol Biol Phys 1986;12(5):733–740.
3. Million RR, Cassisi NJ. General principles for treatment of cancers in the head and neck: selection of treatment for the primary site and for the neck. In: Million RR, Cassisi NJ, eds. Management of Head and Neck Cancer: A Multidisciplinary Approach. Philadelphia: JB Lippincott;1984;43–62.
4. Mack Y, Parsons JT, Mendenhall WM. Squamous cell carcinoma of the head and neck: management after excisional biopsy of a solitary metastatic neck node. Int J Radiat Oncol Biol Phys 1993;25:619–622.
5. Armstrong J, Pfister D, Strong E, et al. The management of the clinically positive neck as part of a larynx preservation approach. Int J Radiat Oncol Biol Phys 1993;26:759–765.
6. Wolf GT, Fisher SG. Effectiveness of salvage neck dissection for advanced regional metastases when induction chemotherapy and radiation are used for organ preservation. Laryngoscope 1992;102:934–939.
7. Zelefsky MJ, Zimberg SH, Raben A, et al. Brachytherapy for locally advanced and recurrent lymph node metastases. J Brachytherapy Int 1998;14:123–131.
8. Freeman SB, Hamaker RC, Rate WR, et al. Management of advanced cervical metastasis using intraoperative radiotherapy. Laryngoscope 1995;105:575–578.
9. Brennan JA, Jafek BW. Elective carotid artery resection for advanced squamous cell carcinoma of the neck. Laryngoscope 1994;104:259–263.
10. Paryani SB, Goffinet DR, Fee WE Jr, et al. Iodine 125 suture implants in the management of advanced tumors in the neck attached to the carotid artery. J Clin Oncol 1985;3(6):809–812.

26 Zenker Diverticulum

Richard L. Scher

Hyphopharyngeal diverticula, to which Zenker's name has been inextricably linked, were initially described by Ludlow in 1769.[1] A clear understanding of the pathogenesis of Zenker (or Zenker's) diverticulum (ZD) has been lacking, but most theories have focused on the structural or physiologic abnormality of the cricopharyngeal muscle and its relationship to pharyngeal and esophageal function to explain diverticular development.[2] Several creative surgical approaches have been used to treat patients with ZD, including diverticulectomy,[3] diverticulopexy,[4,5] diverticular invagination,[6,7] cricopharyngeal myotomy,[8] and endoscopic diverticulotomy.[9] Each of these techniques has had proponents who have reported the efficacy of their particular approach while offering evidence of low morbidity. The selection of appropriate surgical treatment has been facilitated by a clearer understanding of the pathogenesis of ZD and a continuing concern for perioperative complications in patients who are often elderly, debilitated, or have significant associated medical illnesses. Unfortunately, not as much attention has been directed to the reporting of recurrence rates following various methods of treatment for ZD, although most surgeons now advocate including some method of dealing with the cricopharyngeus muscle to produce effective relief of symptoms and minimize recurrence.[8,10,11]

Clinical Features

Esophageal diverticula are classified based on anatomical location (pharyngoesophageal, midesophageal, or epiphrenic) and mechanism of formation (pulsion or traction). Of the various types of esophageal diverticula, Zenker, or pharyngoesophageal, diverticulum is the most common symptomatic esophageal form, with an annual incidence of 2 per 100,000 people per year.[12] Men are affected 2 to 3 times more often than women, with peak incidence in the 7th and 8th decades of life. For those referred for an examination of the upper gastrointestinal tract, the incidence can reach as high as 1 in 1000.[13,14] ZD is a pulsion-type diverticulum consisting of mucosal and submucosal membranes herniating through Killian dehiscence, an area of potential anatomical weakness located between the inferior constrictor and the cricopharyngeus muscles, first described in 1907 by Killian.[15]

The predominant symptom in patients with ZD is dysphagia. Other symptoms include regurgitation of food, belching, noisy deglutition, halitosis, choking, coughing, hoarseness, globus sensation, weight loss, aspiration, and pneumonia. There are often few physical findings, but these may include emaciation and only rarely Boyce sign, a swelling in the neck that gurgles on palpation.[16]

In those patients who have been treated for ZD, persistent or recurrent symptoms are usually similar in type to the symptoms seen before surgery, but the degree of severity may differ. Careful attention should be directed to the historical features of the patient's complaints to ascertain whether the symptoms are similar to and as severe as those present before treatment. Other causes for the symptoms, such as gastroesophageal reflux, esophageal dysmotility, hiatal hernia, neuromuscular dysfunction, and xerostomia, not uncommonly seen in conjunction with ZD, should be kept in mind, evaluated, and treated, if possible.

In all cases, diagnosis is made by barium contrast radiography of the pharynx and esophagus to confirm the presence, size, and position of the diverticulum. Endoscopic confirmation of the diverticulum should only be undertaken as part of the definitive surgical therapy, as it is otherwise unnecessary and potentially dangerous. Given the extremely low incidence of carcinoma occurring in the diverticulum, endoscopic evaluation should be done only when sufficient symptomatology and abnormality on barium esophagram exist to raise suspicion of malignancy.[17]

The radiographic findings of recurrent ZD depend on the surgical procedure used for initial treatment. Those patients treated with an endoscopic diverticulotomy approach will routinely demonstrate a diverticular remnant on the barium study (**Fig. 26.1**).[18,19] The hallmark of recurrent ZD in this setting is retention of barium in the remnant after repeated swallowing, combined with persisting or recurring symptoms. Similar radiographic features, along with possible enlargement of the diverticulum, may be present in those patients treated by means other than diverticulectomy or endoscopic diverticulotomy. Those patients treated initially by diverticulectomy will demonstrate the presence of a diverticulum on barium studies, although symptoms as severe as before the initial treatment may be present even though the recurrent ZD may be smaller than the original. Radiographic signs of distal pharyngeal or proximal esophageal narrowing should

225

Decision tree for treatment of recurrent Zenker's diverticulum

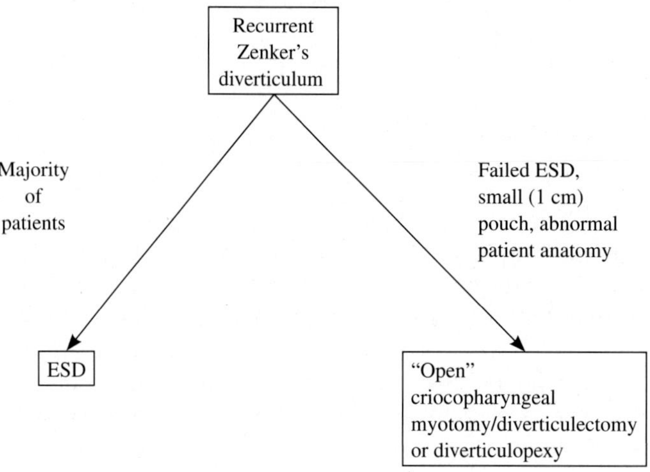

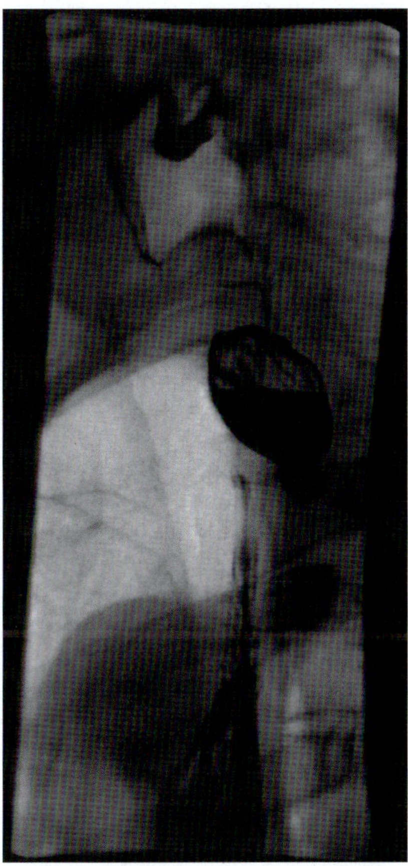

Fig. 26.1 Lateral view, barium esophagram demonstrating a recurrent Zenker diverticulum after prior endoscopic staple diverticulostomy. Barium retention is noted in the diverticulum after multiple swallows.

also be looked for in those patients previously treated by diverticulectomy, or in whom initial surgery may have been complicated by fistula and associated infection.

Pathogenesis and Rationale for Treatment Selection

Although it was widely accepted that ZD was an acquired pulsion diverticulum, there was and still remains considerable controversy on the mechanism of formation. Ludlow[1] gave the first anatomical description of a pulsion diverticulum of the hypopharynx in 1769, but it was not until 1878 that the basic pathophysiology was described by Zenker and von Ziemssen.[20] In 1816 Bell[21] proposed inappropriate coordination of the inferior constrictor muscle against a closed cricopharyngeus muscle as an etiology for ZD. The endoscopic observations of Jackson and Shallow[22] reported in 1926 provided clinical evidence suggesting that the cricopharyngeus muscle was responsible for development of ZD. Ever since, variations on this mechanistic theme

behind the formation of ZD have been proposed, including studies supportive of premature cricopharyngeal relaxation, delayed cricopharyngeal relaxation, and cricopharyngeal spasm as the responsible factors in the genesis of the diverticulum.[22] Regardless of the theory, the cricopharyngeus muscle was most commonly believed to be the culprit responsible for the formation of ZD. This led to the concept of including cricopharyngeal myotomy in the surgical management of ZD, either as a primary procedure or in conjunction with diverticular resection or suspension.[3,8,13,14]

Even with this generally accepted concept as to causation, no such agreement was present regarding the appropriate means of treatment for patients with ZD. Proponents could be found supporting cricopharyngeal myotomy alone,[8] diverticulectomy or diverticulopexy alone,[4] or a combined approach of myotomy together with diverticular resection or suspension.[3,5] Despite refinements in surgical techniques, no approach proved clearly superior to the others in treatment outcome. All of these techniques were reported to provide symptomatic relief in ~80 to 90% of patients, although with serious complication rates of up to 30% and mortality as high as 3%.[3,9,14,23] In most cases, no direct comparisons were made by prospectively studying one treatment method against another, and long-term analysis of results was often lacking. Furthermore, none of the techniques proved to be superior to the others at preventing recurrence of the ZD, with recurrence rates reported to range from 0 to 20%.[3,9,14,23]

These results made it difficult to determine whether the addition of cricopharyngeal myotomy would prevent recurrence or improve symptom outcome. As a result, efforts were directed at trying to minimize the immediate morbidities associated with surgical treatment, while still incorporating management of the cricopharyngeus muscle into the overall treatment scheme. One of the first such efforts was made in 1917 by Mosher,[9] who first described endoscopic esophagodiverticulostomy using a knife to divide the common wall. This technique proved successful at relieving symptoms, but it was abandoned after the seventh patient died from mediastinitis. Sieffert[24] in 1937 reintroduced the endoscopic technique, but it was Dohlman and Mattson[25] who popularized the procedure. In 1960 they presented the results of endoscopic management of ZD in a series of 100 patients without treatment-related deaths or serious complications, with 93% of patients reporting relief of symptoms.

However, because of concern related to the "sutureless" division of the common wall between the diverticulum and the esophagus, with the potential for pneumothorax, bleeding, or mediastinitis, endoscopic management of ZD did not gain truly wide acceptance. Various refinements in endoscopic technique have been introduced in an attempt to alleviate these concerns and eliminate the severe complications Mosher[9] initially experienced. Dohlman and Mattsson[25] used diathermic coagulation to divide the common wall in 1958. More recent modifications to this method included the use of the microscope and carbon dioxide (CO_2) laser described by van Overbeek et al[26] in 1984 and potassium titanyl phosphate (KTP)/532 laser in 1992 by Kuhn and Bent.[27] Gastroenterologists Ishioka et al[28] in Brazil and Mulder et al[29] in the Netherlands simultaneously introduced flexible endoscopic incision using electrocautery in 1995. Yet even these refinements in endoscopic technique were associated with rates of mediastinitis as high as 8 to 10%.

To address this concern, a modification of the endoscopic technique was described in 1993 by Martin-Hirsch and Newbegin[30] in England and Collard et al[31] in Belgium, who simultaneously introduced the endoscopic stapling technique of performing an esophagodiverticulostomy for ZD. This technique was refined and introduced to the United States in 1996 by Scher and Richtsmeier[32] as endoscopic staple esophagodiverticulostomy (ESED). Several advantages have been shown for the stapling technique compared with endoscopic approaches using laser or electrocautery or the open surgical techniques, including greatly reduced risks of perforation, mediastinitis, and laryngeal nerve injury, more rapid return to oral diet, and shorter operative times and hospital stays.[32–34] When compared with other treatment approaches, endoscopic staple diverticulostomy (ESD) has been shown to have at least equal effectiveness at providing symptom resolution.[33,34] These features have proven especially attractive in patients who are often elderly and may have coexistent significant medical illness. The results reported for ESD now support the use of this technique as the treatment of choice for all patients with ZD.

Recurrent Zenker Diverticulum

Although treatment for ZD has evolved to provide predictably effective and safe treatment by the ESD technique, recurrent ZD may occur following this or any other treatment. Rates of recurrence from 0 to 20% have been reported regardless of technique.[11,13,14,26,33,34] As stated, although the altered function of the cricopharyngeus muscle has received the greatest focus, and failure to adequately perform cricopharyngeal myotomy has been proposed by most surgeons as the primary reason for recurrence, neither this factor nor any others have consistently proved to be clearly associated with recurrence of symptoms from ZD following treatment. Factors such as gastroesophageal reflux and esophageal or pharyngeal dysmotility are often present in patients with ZD, and failure to address these disorders may lead to continued complaints of difficulty swallowing.[12]

In those patients shown to have dysphagia from recurrent ZD, the best management should clearly aim to produce resolution of symptoms while minimizing potential for recurrence in the safest manner possible. Few reports have looked specifically at treatment of recurrent ZD.[10,11,35,36] Skinner and Zuckerbraun[11] demonstrated that cricopharyngeal myotomy alone was a relatively safe and effective means of dealing with recurrence after previous diverticulectomy or cricopharyngeal myotomy. In eight patients with recurrent ZD treated with cricopharyngeal myotomy (seven patients) or myotomy and diverticulectomy (one patient), these authors found that all patients had good (minor symptoms persisted) or excellent (complete relief of symptoms) outcomes after treatment. Only one patient had a complication, this being a persistent salivary fistula in the patient treated with diverticulectomy. Huang and colleagues[36] also reported a series of 31 patients with recurrent ZD treated with diverticulectomy alone (15 patients), diverticulectomy with cricopharyngeal myotomy (12 patients), or myotomy alone (4 patients). In this series, 96% of the patients had good to excellent results, but there was a 35% morbidity and 3% mortality associated with treatment.

More recent reports have described the use of ESD as treatment for recurrent ZD.[10,35] Koay et al[35] successfully used ESD to treat three patients with ZD recurring after prior diverticulectomy (one patient) or ESD (two patients). Scher[10] has also used ESD to treat recurrent ZD. In a series of 18 patients, 9 were treated by prior ESD and 9 by external approaches (4 by diverticulectomy and myotomy, 3 by diverticulectomy alone, and 2 by diverticulopexy and myotomy). Sixteen patients were treated successfully with improvement or complete relief of symptoms. In two patients ESD was not possible because of the small diverticulum size (1 cm). In all others, the ESD procedure was found to be technically identical to that used as the initial treatment of patients with ZD. The only complication noted in this series was postoperative fever due to atelectasis, occurring in one patient. The overall average hospital stay was less than 1 day (range 0–2 days), with all patients resuming oral diet by the first day after surgery.

Surgical Technique

Endoscopic Approach

As demonstrated by recent clinical experience, the efficacy and safety profile of ESD makes it the preferred method for treatment of recurrent ZD.[10,33,37,38] All patients with recurrent ZD are felt to be acceptable candidates for an attempt at revision by ESD except those patients with evidence on barium esophagram of a very small recurrent

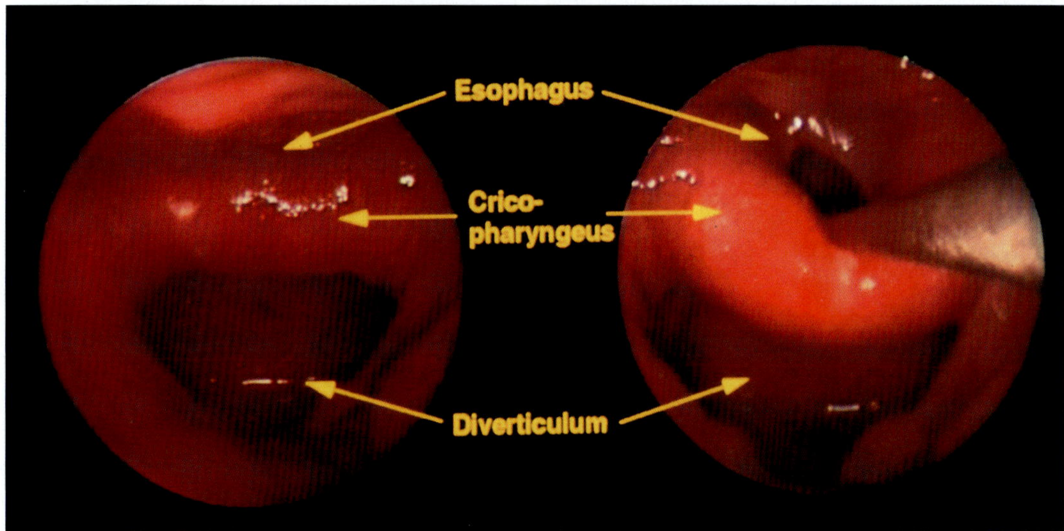

Fig. 26.2 Endoscopic view of Zenker diverticulum prior to performing endoscopic staple diverticulostomy.

diverticulum (1 cm) treated previously by external approach with a definite or likely cricopharyngeal myotomy. The scarring from prior treatment and the small diverticulum size make retraction of the common wall into the endostapler blades unlikely to be technically feasible. Depending on symptom severity, these patients should be counseled to undergo either continued observation and treatment with dietary modification or a revision external cricopharyngeal myotomy. All other patients are good candidates for revision by ESD, providing no other factors exist that would preclude successful endoscopic exposure of the diverticulum.

The procedure is performed with the patient under general endotracheal anesthesia with muscle relaxants. Following induction of anesthesia and oral endotracheal intubation, the patient is positioned as for routine rigid laryngoscopy. The Weerda bivalved laryngoscope (Karl Storz, Culver City, California) is used for the procedure. This laryngoscope allows adjustment of the angulation and aperture size of the proximal and distal openings. The laryngoscope is inserted posterior to the larynx after thorough evaluation of the upper aerodigestive tract. The distal ends of the instrument are adjusted to expose the esophageal lumen and the diverticulum, without inserting the blades of the laryngoscope into the pouch or esophageal introitus. The common wall between the esophagus and diverticulum, formed by the cricopharyngeus muscle and overlying mucosa, is positioned between the laryngoscope blades. Telescopic visualization (0 or 30 degrees) connected to a video camera is used for all observations and manipulations (**Fig. 26.2**).

Revision of a prior esophagodiverticulostomy or creation of a new opening in those patients treated initially by diverticulectomy or diverticulopexy with or without cricopharyngeal myotomy proceeds identically to ESD performed as primary treatment for ZD[32,33] (**Fig. 26.3**). The Endo-GIA 30 endosurgical stapler (US Surgical Corp., Norwalk, Connecticut) is used to create the diverticulostomy. The Endo-GIA 30 stapler is a trigger-activated device that allows simultaneous stapling and sectioning of tissue. The instrument has a distal replaceable cartridge that contains three rows of staples on each side of a midline retractable knife blade. The two anvils of the cartridge are placed around the tissue to be stapled and divided; by activating the trigger mechanism, the knife is advanced through the tissue at the same time the staples are placed. The stapler easily fits through the lumen of the Weerda laryngoscope without obstructing the surgeon's telescopic view.

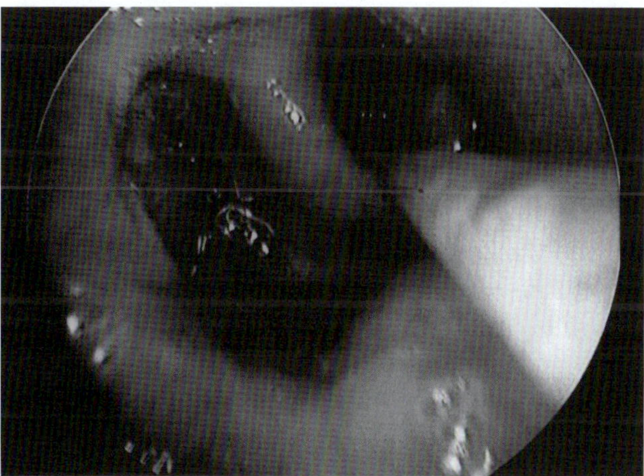

Fig. 26.3 Endoscopic view of recurrent Zenker diverticulum after prior diverticulectomy. Staples used for resection of diverticulum at first operation are still present in the anterior wall of the recurrent diverticulum. A well-formed common wall is present.

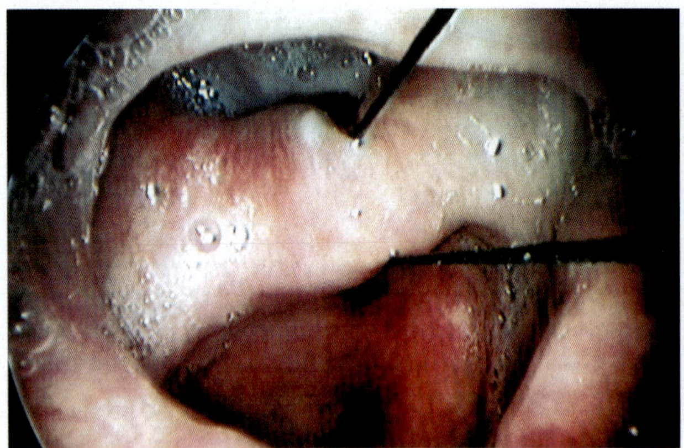

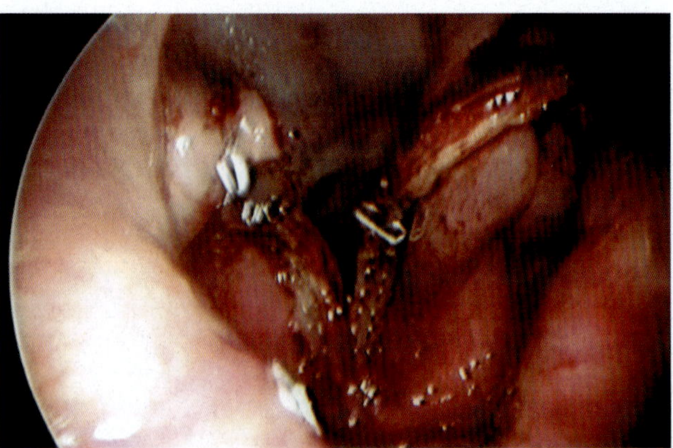

Fig. 26.4 Endoscopic view of Zenker diverticulum during endoscopic staple diverticulostomy. **(A)** Retraction suture in place in common wall (diverticulum posterior) to assist in providing traction during placement of endosurgical stapler. **(B)** Diverticulostomy performed (staples present) with retraction suture still in position.

Prior to insertion of the endosurgical stapler, placement of retraction sutures through the lateral edges of the common wall on each side of the proposed diverticulostomy helps to maintain traction while positioning the Endo-GIA 30 stapler (**Fig. 26.4**). This helps to more effectively position the common wall into the stapler blades before making the diverticulostomy, especially in recurrent diverticula that are small (< 2 cm). The retraction sutures are placed using the Endostitch autosuture device (US Surgical Corp.) with a 2–0 silk suture. Once the diverticulostomy is completed, the retraction sutures are cut and removed, with care taken not to leave a portion of the suture that may have been incorporated in the line of staples.

After placement of the retraction sutures, the stapler is positioned around the common wall with one blade in the esophagus and the other in the diverticulum. Placement of the stapler blade containing the staple cartridge into the esophageal lumen usually allows a more complete division of the common wall. The stapler blades are closed while confirming their position with the telescope. The endostapler is then activated, dividing and stapling the common wall to create a diverticulostomy (**Fig. 26.4**). If further division of the common wall is felt necessary in a larger diverticulum, the staple cartridge can be replaced and the diverticulostomy extended distally from the apex of the first cut.

After completing the diverticulostomy, the retraction sutures are removed, the diverticulum, esophagus, and pharynx are thoroughly examined with the telescopes, and then the laryngoscope is removed. The patient is observed in the postanesthesia care unit and either discharged the day of surgery if medically indicated or observed in the hospital. If no signs of morbidity exist (fever, chest or back pain, subcutaneous crepitance, hemoptysis, tachycardia), a clear liquid diet is started on the day of surgery, with resumption of regular diet as tolerated starting on the first postoperative day. No antibiotics are given, and no naso- or orogastric tube is placed. Antireflux medication (proton-pump inhibitor) is prescribed for all patients and continued for 2 months after surgery. Other than postoperative office evaluation and examination, no studies are performed unless concern for morbidity or recurrence of symptoms develops.

Limitations of Endoscopic Staple Diverticulostomy

Though few in number, there are limitations to the endoscopic stapling technique. Exposure of the diverticulum may be difficult or impossible due to factors associated with patient anatomy, such as kyphosis, large cervical osteophytes, small oropharyngeal opening, or severe retrognathia. Also, in patients with a small ZD, an insufficient diverticulostomy may be performed even though placement of retraction sutures improves the exposure and positioning of the common wall into the stapler blades. Even with retraction sutures, retraction of the common wall may not be possible in patients with recurrent small ZD following prior external approaches secondary to scarring. Collard et al[31] proposed sawing off the distal part of the Endo-GIA 30 stapler anvil to allow the common wall to be divided to the bottom of the diverticulum. However, besides introducing avoidable risks to the procedure by potentially affecting the integrity of the staple closure, this modification has proven unnecessary.[32,33]

Lastly, though the pouch can be inspected thoroughly and biopsies obtained, a complete specimen is not available for pathologic assessment, as is the case following diverticulectomy. This may prevent the discovery of carcinoma in the pouch. Fortunately, carcinoma in a diverticulum is extremely rare, found in $< 0.5\%$,[17,30] though in one review of 50 excised ZD, an unusually high percentage (8%) was reported to contain squamous cell carcinoma or carcinoma in situ.[39] Along with intraoperative assessment, possible malignancy may be suggested when there is a sudden increase in symptom severity of progressive dysphagia, pain, hemoptysis, or more marked regurgitation of food. Barium swallow may also suggest a malignancy when it reveals a loss of smooth contour within the pouch interior and a persistent filling defect.[39] In these situations, ESD is contraindicated, and open excision of the diverticulum is recommended.

Complications unique to ESD are rare and described in case reports. Esophageal perforation was reported secondary to possible technical failure of the endostapler or excessive width of the common wall.[40] However, Richtsmeier and Monzon[41] brought to light that differences do exist between stapler cartridges and discovered that one particular type (TR45B 3.5 mm cartridge for Endopath ETS Flex45 Endoscopic Articulation Linear Cutter stapler, Ethicon Endo-Surgery Inc., Cincinnati, Ohio) was more prone to leaks at the incisional apex at lower intraluminal pressures. In another case, persistent foreign body sensation and odynophagia were reported 2 months after ESD due to retention of staples.[42] Removal of the staples resulted in symptomatic relief. Similarly, a retained silk retention suture was shown to be the etiology of recurrent ZD in one patient.[38] Removal of any loose, exposed staples and foreign debris intraoperatively after activating the stapler can prevent these complications. Finally, a fatal case of mediastinitis due to delayed perforation on postoperative day 2 has also been reported.[43] In this case report, no mention was made whether the pouch and diverticulostomy were examined carefully for perforation, a practice that needs to be performed after every procedure.

In reports by Scher and colleagues,[10,33,38] there has no mortality after ESD, either when used for initial treatment of ZD or for recurrences. Morbidity was minimal, with a rate of serious complications of only 1.4% in all patients, and none in the 18 patients treated for recurrent ZD. Postoperative fever was found in 4.2% of all treated patients and shown to be secondary to atelectasis in all patients except one. This patient had persistent aspiration pneumonia from the ZD that worsened after surgery, with eventual resolution and prevention of subsequent aspiration. Dental damage was found in 7%. Significant complications of perforation and transient true vocal cord paralysis occurred in only one patient each. The perforation was detected in the one patient during ESD and repaired intraoperatively, with no postoperative fever and complete resolution of preoperative symptoms.[38] The other patient had transient true vocal cord paralysis secondary to pressure on the posterior larynx by the laryngoscope that resolved completely 2 weeks after surgery.

Comparing morbidity reported for other endoscopic techniques, complication rates averaged 2.35% for cautery, 6% for CO_2 laser, and 2.36% for ESD.[25,28,29,31,33,44–47] Only 6 deaths have been reported in the endoscopic literature from a total of 1468 patients (0.4% mortality). Of these patients, 389 underwent ESD, with a mortality rate of 0.5%.

External Approach

An external approach is indicated for patients with recurrent ZD when ESD is not technically feasible either because the pouch is too small (1 cm) or patient anatomy does not allow endoscopic exposure of the ZD. In all patients, an attempt at ESD is reasonable, but patients in the categories noted above should be advised and prepared preoperatively for a probable external approach.

All patients treated by external approach should have as complete a cricopharyngeal myotomy performed as possible. Whether to include diverticulectomy or diverticulopexy depends on the individual patient's overall health, size of the diverticulum, and findings at the time of operation. The primary objective should be effective relief of symptoms and prevention of future morbidity, while minimizing the risks associated with treatment. For smaller pouches and in more frail individuals, myotomy is often all that is necessary. Larger pouches should be resected in combination with myotomy, unless significant fibrosis or adhesions prevent adequate mobilization or exposure of the pouch.

The surgical procedure is performed under general anesthesia. Intravenous cefazolin and clindamycin are given. Prior to making the incision, endoscopy is performed to pack the pouch with gauze and to place an esophageal dilator (~40 French size). This facilitates identification of the diverticulum and the esophagus during the external approach. A transverse incision is made in the left neck at approximately the level of the cricoid cartilage. Subplatysmal skin flaps are raised in a caudal and cephalad direction to expose the underlying sternocleidomastoid muscle. The fascia over the medial aspect of the sternocleidomastoid muscle is incised and the muscle retracted laterally to expose the carotid sheath and omohyoid muscle. The omohyoid muscle may be either retracted or divided to expose the contents of the carotid sheath. Dissection is continued medial to the carotid artery and internal jugular vein, and the middle thyroid vein is ligated and divided. The vessels are retracted laterally, and care is taken to identify and preserve the recurrent laryngeal nerve.

The dissection proceeds in a posterior direction into the retropharyngeal space. The pharynx and esophagus are exposed and rotated medially to allow visualization of their posterolateral surfaces and identification of the diverticulum. The diverticulum should be mobilized from surrounding fascia or fibrous attachments by careful dissection. The cricopharyngeus muscle is identified, and a myotomy is performed for as long a segment as is safely possible. The external muscular fibers are divided vertically to expose the submucosa, but no attempt is made to resect any of this muscle. If the diverticulum is to be resected, the neck of the diverticulum is identified and the line of transection noted so as to maintain adequate esophageal lumen diameter. This is done with the esophageal dilator in place. Any packing that is present in the diverticulum is removed, and then an Endo-GIA or Endo-TA stapler is placed across the neck of the diverticulum. The stapler is activated and the pouch resected. No additional second layer of closure is required. The wound is closed in routine fashion.

A nasogastric tube is not routinely placed. If one is felt to be necessary, it should be placed under direct endoscopic visualization prior to performing the myotomy and diverticulectomy to avoid the potential for inadvertent perforation of the esophagus by the tube. Patients are allowed to take clear liquid diet beginning on the day after surgery, and advanced to soft diet as tolerated, provided there is no evidence of complication. No radiographic studies are performed prior to initiating feeding, unless there is evidence of perioperative morbidity

External approaches to treat ZD have long been associated with significant morbidity, but reliable data regarding complications after treatment of recurrence are lacking. Though morbidity is partly due to technical factors, the majority of patients are elderly, and many have numerous medical problems. Engel and Panje[48] summarized the results of surgical complications observed from transcervical approaches reported in large series published in the English literature since 1985 and compiled rates of fistula (6.3%), recurrent nerve palsy (3.6%), pneumomediastinum (0.8%), mediastinitis (3.1%), and mortality (2.0%) in 245 patients. Payne[3] reported a morbidity rate of 7.9%, mortality rate of 1.2%, and recurrence rate of 3.6% in 888 patients. Mortality rates of 1 to 2% were also found in the 1996–1997 report from the National Confidential Enquiry into Perioperative Deaths in head and neck surgery.[49] These results should be kept in mind when considering and performing myotomy with or without diverticulectomy for recurrent ZD.

Conclusion

Recent experience with ESD has demonstrated it to be an excellent approach for treatment of recurrent ZD, with excellent symptom resolution and low morbidity and mortality. Unlike the endoscopic approaches using CO_2 laser and cautery, ESD provides a "sutured" closure of the diverticulostomy edges with staples, minimizing the chance for salivary leakage and bleeding. Additionally, ESD does not emit thermal energy, eliminating possible damage to underlying structures such as the recurrent laryngeal nerve. ESD for recurrent ZD is technically identical to the procedure when used for initial treatment, with no greater morbidity or mortality. Given the mainly elderly population who often had multiple medical problems along with ZD, ESD offers an excellent alternative to open surgical procedures that require longer operative times and hospital stays and are associated with higher rates of morbidity and mortality. In rare situations, external approaches with myotomy, with or without diverticulectomy, may be necessary to treat recurrent ZD and should be considered as needed.

However, endoscopic staple diverticulostomy is a safer and better alternative to standard transcervical approaches to treating Zenker diverticulum and should be considered the treatment of choice for patients with ZD and for those with recurrences.

References

1. Ludlow A. A case of obstructed deglutition, from a preternatural dilatation of, and bag formed in, the pharynx. Med Observ Inq 1769;3:85–101.
2. McConnel FMS, Hood D, Jackson K, O'Connor A. Analysis of intrabolus forces in patients with Zenker's diverticulum. Laryngoscope 1994;104:571–581.
3. Payne WS. The treatment of pharyngoesophageal diverticulum: the simple and complex. Hepatogastroenterology 1992;39:109–114.
4. Laccourreye O, Menard M, Cauchois R,. Esophageal diverticulum: diverticulopexy versus diverticulectomy. Laryngoscope 1994;104:889–892.
5. Konowitz PM, Biller HF. Diverticulopexy and cricopharyngeal myotomy: treatment for the high-risk patient with a pharyngoesophageal (Zenker's) diverticulum. Otolaryngol Head Neck Surg 1989;100:146–153.
6. Morton RP, Bartley JRF. Inversion of Zenker's diverticulum: the preferred option. Head Neck 1993;15:253–256.
7. Johnson JT, Weissman J. Diverticular imbrication and myotomy for Zenker's. Laryngoscope 1992;102:1377–1378.
8. Schmit PJ, Zuckerbraun L. Treatment of Zenker's diverticulum by cricopharyngeus myotomy under local anesthesia. Am Surg 1992;58:710–716.
9. Mosher HP. Webs and pouches of the esophagus: their diagnosis and treatment. Surg Gynecol Obstet 1917;25:175–187.
10. Scher RL. Endoscopic staple diverticulostomy for recurrent Zenker's diverticulum. Laryngoscope 2003;113:63–67.
11. Skinner KA, Zuckerbraun L. Recurrent Zenker's diverticulum: treatment with crycopharyngeal myotomy. Am Surg 1998;64:192–195.

12. Feussner H, Siewert JR. Zenker's diverticulum and reflux. Hepatogastroenterology 1992;39:100–104.
13. Jamieson GG, Duranceau AC, Payne WS. Pharyngo-oesophageal diverticulum. In: Jamieson GG, ed. Surgery of the Esophagus. London: Churchill Livingstone; 1988; 435–443.
14. Gregoire J, Duranceau A. Surgical management of Zenker's diverticulum. Hepatogastroenterology 1992;39:132–138.
15. Killian G. Uber den Mund der speiserohre. Z Ohrenheilkd Krankheiten Luftwege 1908;55:1–41.
16. Siddiq MA, Sood S, Strachan D. Pharyngeal pouch (Zenker's diverticulum). Postgrad Med J 2001;77:506–511.
17. Huang BS, Unni KK, Payne WS. Long-term survival following diverticulectomy for cancer in pharyngoesophageal (Zenker's) diverticulum. Ann Thorac Surg 1984;38: 207–210.
18. Hadley JM, Ridley N, Djazaeri B, Glover G. The radiological appearances after the endoscopic crico-pharyngeal myotomy: Dohlman's procedure. Clin Radiol 1997;52:613–615.
19. Ong CC, Elton PG, Mitchell D. Pharyngeal pouch endoscopic stapling—are post-operative barium swallow radiographs of any value? J Laryngol Otol 1999;113: 233–236.
20. Zenker FA, von Ziemssen H. Dilatations of the esophagus. Cyclopedia Pract Med 1878;3:46–48.
21. Bell C. Surgical Observations. London: Longmans, Greene; 1816:64–70.
22. Jackson C, Shallow TA. Diverticula of the oesophagus, pulsion, traction, malignant and congenital. Ann Surg 1926;83:1–19.
23. Payne WS, King RM. Pharyngoesophageal (Zenker's) diverticulum. Surg Clin North Am 1983;63:815–824.
24. Sieffert A. Operation endoscopique d'un gros diverticule de pulsion. Bronchoscop Oesophageoscop Gastroscop 1937;3:232–234.
25. Dohlman G, Mattsson O. The endoscopic operation for hypopharyngeal diverticula. AMA Arch Otolaryngol 1960;71:744–752.
26. van Overbeek JJ, Hoeksema PE, Edens ET. Microendoscopic surgery of the hypopharyngeal diverticulum using electrocoagulation or carbon dioxide laser. Ann Otol Rhinol Laryngol 1984;93:34–36.
27. Kuhn FA, Bent JP. Zenker's diverticulotomy using the KTP/532 laser. Laryngoscope 1992;102:946–950.
28. Ishioka S, Sakai P, Maluf Filho F, Melo JM. Endoscopic incision of Zenker's diverticula. Endoscopy 1995;27:433–437.
29. Mulder CJ, den Hartog G, Robijn RJ, Thies JE. Flexible endoscopic treatment of Zenker's diverticulum: a new approach. Endoscopy 1995;27:438–442.
30. Martin-Hirsch DP, Newbegin CJ. Autosuture GIA gun: a new application in the treatment of hypopharyngeal diverticula. J Laryngol Otol 1993;107:723–725.
31. Collard JM, Otte JB, Kestens PJ. Endoscopic stapling technique of esophagodiverticulostomy for Zenker's diverticulum. Ann Thorac Surg 1993;56:573–576.
32. Scher RL, Richtsmeier WJ. Endoscopic staple-assisted esophagodiverticulostomy for Zenker's diverticulum. Laryngoscope 1996;106:951–956.
33. Cook RD, Huang PC, Richstmeier WJ, Scher RL. Endoscopic staple-assisted esophagodiverticulostomy: an excellent treatment of choice for Zenker's diverticulum. Laryngoscope 2000;110:2020–2025.
34. Wouters B, van Overbeek JJ. Endoscopic treatment of the hypopharyngeal (Zenker's) diverticulum. Hepatogastroenterology 1992;39:105–108
35. Koay CB, Commins D, Bates GJ. The role of endoscopic stapling diverticulotomy in recurrent pharyngeal pouch. J Laryngol Otol 1998;112:954–955.
36. Huang B, Payne WS, Cameron AJ. Surgical management for recurrent pharyngoesophageal (Zenker's) diverticulum. Ann Thorac Surg 1984;37:189–191.
37. Ardran GM, Kemp FH. The radiography of the lower lateral food channels. J Laryngol Otol 1961;75:358–370.
38. Scher RL, Richtsmeier WJ. Long-term experience with endoscopic staple-assisted esophagodiverticulostomy for Zenker's diverticulum. Laryngoscope 1998;108: 200–205.
39. Bradley PJ, Kochaar A, Quraishi MS. Pharyngeal pouch carcinoma: real or imaginary risks? Ann Otol Rhinol Laryngol 1999;108:1027–1032.
40. Hilton M, Brightwell AP. Oesophageal perforation during stapling of a pharyngeal pouch: adverse clinical incident report. J Laryngol Otol 2000;114:549–550
41. Richtsmeier WJ, Monzon JR. Postendoscopic Zenker esophagodiverticulostomy leaks associated with a specific stapler cartridge. Arch Otolaryngol Head Neck Surg 2002;128:137–140
42. Arunachalam PS, Cameron DS. Persistent foreign body sensation and pharyngeal pain due to retention of staples: an interesting sequela of endoscopic stapling procedure. J Laryngol Otol 2001;115:425–427.
43. Nix PA. Delayed oesophageal perforation following endoscopic stapling of a pharyngeal pouch. J Laryngol Otol 2001;115:668.
44. Wayman DM, Byl FM, Adour KK. Endoscopic diverticulotomy for the treatment of Zenker's diverticulum. Otolaryngol Head Neck Surg 1991;104:448–452.
45. Von Doersten PG, Byl FM. Endoscopic Zenker's diverticulotomy (Dohlman procedure): forty cases reviewed. Otolaryngol Head Neck Surg 1997;116:209–212.
46. Narne S, Cutrone C, Bonavina L, Chella B, Peracchia A. Endoscopic diverticulotomy for the treatment of Zenker's diverticulum: results in 102 patients with staple-assisted endoscopy. Ann Otol Rhinol Laryngol 1999; 108:810–815.
47. van Overbeek JJ. Meditation on the pathogenesis of hypopharyngeal (Zenker's) diverticulum and a report of endoscopic treatment in 545 patients. Ann Otol Rhinol Laryngol 1994;103:178–185.
48. Engel JJ, Panje WR. Endoscopic laser Zenker's diverticulotomy. Gastrointest Endosc 1995;42:368–370.
49. Resouly A. Pharyngeal pouch surgery: the report of the National Confidential Enquiry into Perioperative Deaths. Royal College of Surg Eng 1996;7:32.

Decision tree for revision free flap surgery

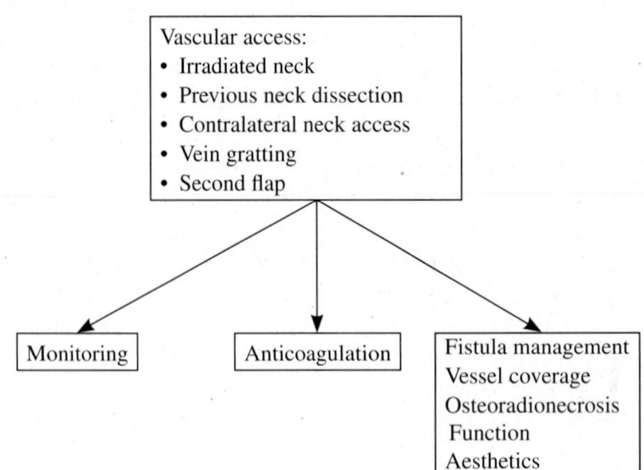

27 Free Flap Reconstruction

Dimitrios P. Mastorakos and Joseph J. Disa

Major head and neck extirpative surgery is frequently followed by plastic surgery reconstructive procedures in an attempt to restore function, cover a vital structure, or improve cosmesis. This need becomes ever more pressing after a secondary procedure, even if during the first procedure no such need was appreciated.[1–3] This makes reoperative head and neck surgery a formidable undertaking that demands coordination between the ablative and reconstructive teams. A multidisciplinary approach is crucial to the successful completion of such an undertaking. This chapter examines the reasons for free flap reconstruction, the timing and purposes of such surgery, the technical issues involved, and specific problems associated with it.

Reasons for Reconstruction

The return of a patient to the operating room (OR) after a head and neck procedure is usually due to recurrence of the original pathology or a complication of the previous treatment modalities.[2,3] A recurrence usually involves the suture lines around the previous resection or the tissues neighboring the previous reconstruction. It is associated with increasing induration or mass effect of the tissues near the previous pathology. As a result of a possible infiltration of previous reconstruction,[4] by the time the resection is completed, the new defect is usually larger than the old one, while at the same time the previous reconstruction is, for the most part, resected.

A complication in this setting is usually the result of either radiation therapy[5,6] or the development of a fistula.[7] The changes associated with radiation therapy usually involve all the tissues exposed to it, including bone and blood vessels.[8,9] This makes issues such as coverage of hardware and identification and dissection of recipient vessels for microanastomoses very challenging. Equally challenging from a different standpoint can be the management of a fistula. It is usually the result of a flap or a suture line failure and can result in probably the most feared of complications, namely, the carotid artery blowout.[10] In such a situation, addressing the problem becomes rather pressing.[7]

Timing of Surgery

Because reoperative head and neck surgery is never a trivial undertaking, the timing of such a procedure can be very critical. Depending on the reason for the return to the OR, this can be done emergently, urgently, or at a later date. Emergency surgery is usually associated with massive bleeding or airway obstruction. The role of the reconstructive surgeon in this setting is to ensure coverage of sensitive structures, with living and well-vascularized tissue, once the bleeding or airway obstruction has been relieved.[11] This includes the revision of previous reconstructive solutions once hemostasis has been assured. Preventing such complications with reliable coverage of all vascular structures beforehand, prompt drainage of collections, and securing of a stable airway is always easier than salvage surgery in an emergency setting. Urgent management is usually associated with hardware or sensitive structure exposure, such as bone, vessels, or meninges. The approach here should be one of proactive management, trying to minimize the extent of damage caused. Lastly, late approaches are usually associated with radiation-induced changes, exposure of heavily irradiated or even necrotic tissue, or aesthetic shortcomings of the previous surgery outcome.

Purposes of Reoperation

The rationale behind returning to the OR for reoperative head and neck surgery is damage control, another attempt at curing the patient, palliation, or functional/cosmetic improvement. Keeping in mind the purposes of the surgery can be crucial because this could dictate the extent of resection, the sophistication of the reconstruction, and the length to which one is prepared to go to accomplish it.

Condition of the Patient

Evaluating the general medical condition of the patient is paramount before embarking on a lengthy and complicated reoperative endeavor.[12] Issues such as nutrition, tobacco or alcohol or even drug abuse, and history of chemotherapy or radiation, as well as the Acute Physiology and Chronic Health Evaluation (APACHE) II score,[13] are extremely important when assessing the patient preoperatively. Virtually all patients have long histories of alcohol and/or tobacco abuse. A large number of them will be debilitated because of malnutrition secondary to the disease itself, other treatment modalities, or long-standing poor health.[14] Pulmonary and cardiovascular assessment is always critical, as it was before the first procedure. Aspiration pneumonia, adult respiratory distress syndrome (ARDS), prolonged respiratory insufficiency or intensive care stay, stroke, and myocardial infarction are well-known complications after such surgeries. Actually, many would argue that even before the first procedure, one should evaluate the ability of a patient to go through reoperation.[15] A negative answer should steer the reconstructive surgeon away from complex and lengthy reconstruction toward an expeditious and reliable procedure. It appears, therefore, that a reoperative approach is one of potentially significant morbidity and mortality, and this should be made clear to the patient beforehand.

One should always take into consideration the patient's priorities and wishes.[10] Oftentimes what the physician considers important will not coincide with the patient's views. A better cosmetic outcome, for instance, might not be worth a prolonged stay in the hospital. Therefore, getting to know the patient's views and needs and describing the functional, aesthetic, and structural defects anticipated can be very helpful in providing the best possible solution to the patient's problem.

Approaching Reoperative Free Flap Surgery

When faced with a reoperative head and neck surgery, one should first try to visualize the defect present once the ablative surgeon has completed his or her part. The extent of soft tissue deficit, the bony structures missing, the neurovascular structures resected or ligated, and the functional deficit are all issues to be taken into consideration. To do that, one should be able to communicate fully and reliably with the ablative team preoperatively but also during the surgery itself, assessing or even modifying the defect while it is created. Preoperative imaging and a physical examination will help a great deal by allowing a fairly accurate estimate of the anticipated defect.

The next step is to take an inventory of all the possible reconstructive options available once the resection is completed. To that end, one should take into consideration the possible vascular and neural structures affected by the surgery, as this could determine the strength of particular surgical options. Local, regional, and distant flaps, simple and composite tissue reconstructions, single- or multiple-stage procedures, use of bone/nerve/vein/skin grafts, even the use of medical prosthetics, are all options to be considered. This decision process must also take into consideration the condition of the patient, and whether it would or would not allow some of these options.[14,16] Additionally, local conditions are crucial. By now most patients will have already been irradiated, and many of the locally present landmarks and planes will have been obscured. This raises the degree of difficulty associated with the dissection and makes the presence/condition of the structures dissected rather unpredictable.

Technical Issues

In the reoperative setting, one will obviously come across the stigmata of previous surgery, such as scar tissue, obscured tissue and fascial planes, and displaced and distorted anatomical relationships. Some of the native vessels would have been ligated or used during the earlier procedure. This setting, coupled with the fewer vessels available to the reconstructive surgeon, makes dissecting a reoperative neck and establishing recipient vessels for microvascular anastomoses formidable undertakings. Fine instruments, atraumatic blunt and sharp dissection, and a concerted effort to get out of the zone of injury are all ways to approach this challenge. The full extent of the reconstructive ladder, including classic and reliable options such as the deltopectoral or the forehead flap, all the way to free flaps and composite tissue transfers, should be considered.[17–19] The option best suited to the patient's needs should be the one chosen, and age alone should not be considered a contraindication to free flap reconstruction.[16]

When microvascular tissue transfer is the procedure of choice, careful attention must be given to the perioperative management of the patient. Due to the long operative time and the complexity of the procedure, a multidisciplinary approach is warranted. Anesthesia, medicine, cardiology, intensive care, infectious diseases, nursing, and respiratory and physical therapy are all disciplines needed to come together to assist in getting the patient through the perioperative period.[13] Careful positioning during surgery, prevention of hypothermia, invasive cardiovascular monitoring of patients with compromised cardiac or pulmonary function, and optimization of the fluid status become significant issues.

The Irradiated Neck

Particular attention is due to the irradiated neck. Aside from the inherent difficulty of redissecting a previously dissected neck due to scar tissue adhesions, the added fibrosis and friability of radiated tissue make the environment even more hostile.[9] The vessels are usually incorporated in thick scar tissue, completely obscuring the anatomical planes.[5] Judicious use of blunt dissection with fine-tipped instruments can be very helpful. In addition, particular attention should be given to the quality of the soft tissue and skin covering the vital neck structures. Any doubt of viability should prompt resurfacing with fresh, well-vascularized, and healthy soft tissue and skin.

Vascular Access

Obtaining vascular access should always be the first step toward a complex reconstruction in the neck.[20] Unless good quality vascular access has been established, one should avoid raising any kind of flap as a free tissue transfer. In addition, a fallback option of a local flap should always be in place, if possible, should the securing of a vascular access prove impossible. Helpful points include the following:

1. Going for major vessels with well-known and fairly constant anatomy (external carotid, lingual artery, common facial artery, superficial temporal artery) preferably outside the zone of injury/ radiation
2. Minimal threshold before going to the opposite side or using the external carotid artery in an end-to-side fashion if the ipsilateral vascular access proves impossible
3. Avoiding vein grafts, if possible, and using flaps with long vascular leashes
4. Unless a perfect match to the donor vessels is found, preferring the internal jugular vein (IJV) with its optimal sump flow characteristics to any other vein of the area for vascular outflow
5. The reconstructive team, given their precise concept of the characteristics and quality needed for a successful reconstruction, should ideally perform the vascular access dissection.

Second Flap

Once vascular access is obtained, attention should be turned to raising and transferring an appropriate flap. This is the time to accurately assess the defect created as well as the characteristics required from the flap to be used. On occasion only a combination of flaps can provide the optimal characteristics of structural rigidity and surface conformity. For example, a free fibula would provide the best structural characteristics but only mediocre surface coverage, whereas a radial forearm free flap would provide the best coverage with thin, pliable, well-

vascularized skin but a bone that is only marginally adequate.[21] This is the time to think of a combination of flaps. This becomes a daunting task, especially taking into account the difficulties mentioned regarding vascular access. Attaching both flaps to the same recipient vessels or piggybacking the second flap on the first is always an option to be considered, keeping in mind that one may end up overtaxing the vascular access vessels. In general, separate vascular access should be provided for each flap if at all possible.

Once the free flap is inset and the vessels are functioning properly after the microvascular anastomosis, one has to assess the quality of the soft tissue. As mentioned, the already scarred and most probably irradiated soft tissue envelope may prove inadequate (due to intraoperative swelling or débridement) or unsuitable to be used. This is often the case when using a jejunum free flap for a hypopharyngeal reconstruction. One should not compromise the result of the whole of the reconstruction by covering it with poor, scarred, irradiated skin under tension. This is the time to use a second flap, such as the deltopectoral or the pectoralis major pedicled flap, or a second free flap if an adequate local flap is unavailable[1] (**Figs. 27.1–27.7**).

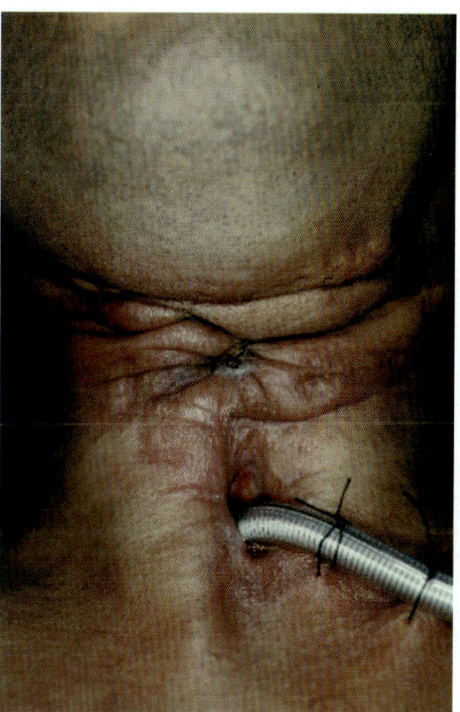

Fig. 27.1 Recurrent hypopharyngeal malignancy in setting of prior irradiation. Note skin involvement.

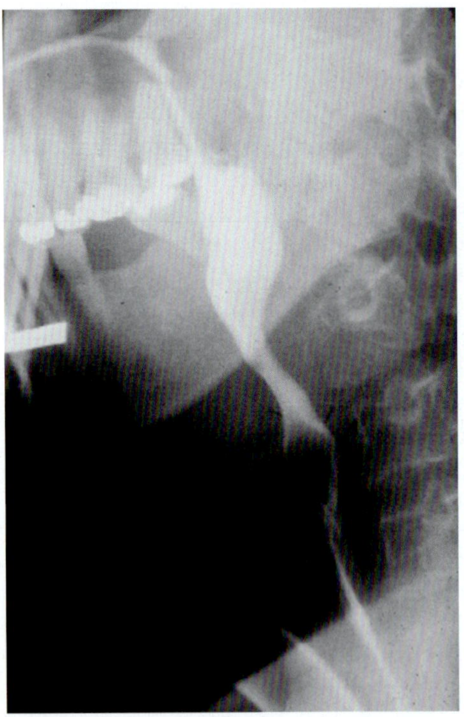

Fig. 27.2 Barium study showing recurrent malignancy.

Postoperative Care

Flap Monitoring and Anticoagulation

Once a reoperative reconstructive surgery is completed, our attention turns to the safe postoperative course of the patient. Because the head and neck region harbors a multitude of valuable and sensitive structures (brain, eye, vessels, nerves, trachea, esophagus), it becomes critical to

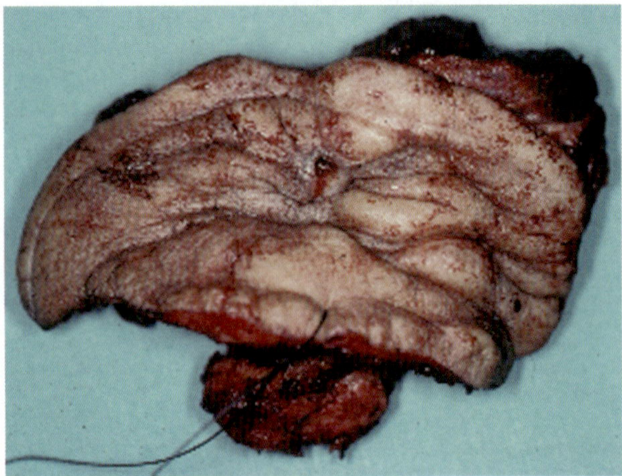

Fig. 27.3 Surgical specimen.

follow the condition of the flap and to know immediately when a flap is failing in order to take appropriate measures. This is the reason for careful monitoring of the free tissue transfer. Many different modalities have been used, including capillary refill, pinprick bleed, handheld Doppler probes, implantable Doppler probes, laser Doppler, surface temperature probes, and fluorescein. In our hands the handheld Doppler, coupled with experienced nursing and clinical follow-up, provides the best outcome in terms of early diagnosis of flap failure.[22]

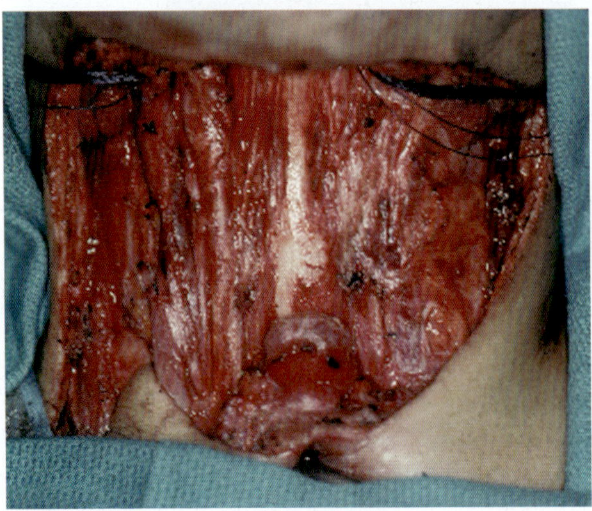

Fig. 27.4 Defect of hypopharynx and skin after resection.

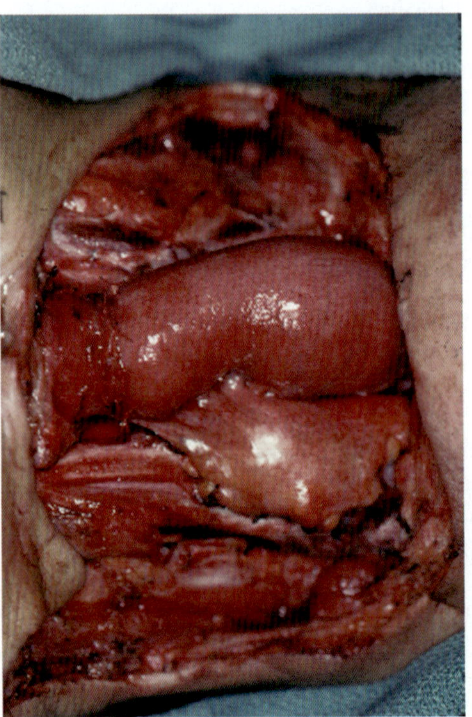

Fig. 27.5 Reconstruction with jejunum free flap.

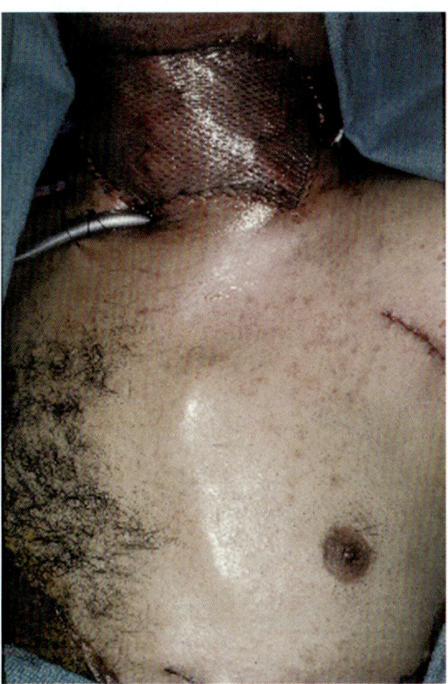

Fig. 27.6 Free jejunum covered with pectoralis major flap and split-thickness skin graft. Immediate postoperative appearance.

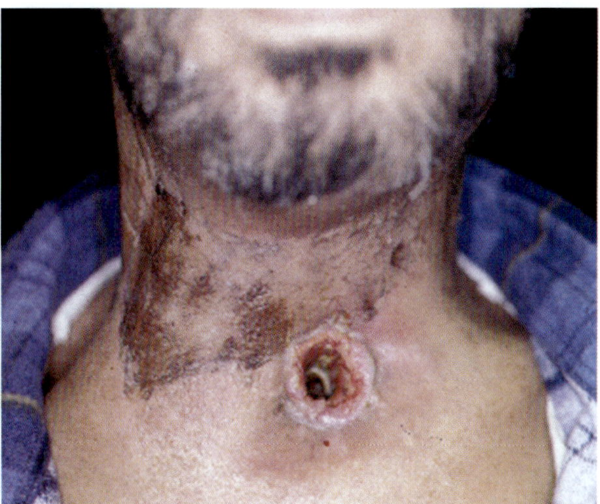

Fig. 27.7 Late postoperative appearance.

Regarding the use of anticoagulation, this is an area of wide variability. Many modalities have been used, including full anticoagulation with heparin. We are currently limiting our approach to 325 mg of aspirin by mouth, or more often via tube, daily for 5 days. This provides an improved environment near the microanastomosis while this is being repopulated by endothelium; at the same time, the complications associated with full anticoagulation (heparin) or volume overload (dextran) are minimized.

Emergency Returns to the Operating Room

At the completion of a reoperative procedure involving a free flap, one should outline a plan of action should this flap fail. After having described the multiple difficulties of reoperative free flap surgery, it becomes obvious that the degree of difficulty increases with each subsequent trip to the OR. This is why the plan of action should be decided by the head of the reconstructive team at the completion of the reconstructive effort, given the availability of all the intraoperative information regarding alternatives and fallback options. If the decision is one of pursuing the salvage of the flap to the fullest, then one should return to the OR at the first sign of a compromised flap. Then and there, under the microscope is the best time and optimal conditions to tackle such issues. Given that the majority of such mishaps occur during the first 6 hours following surgery, the best defense against them is to accept nothing less than a perfect flap at the conclusion of the surgery, and to keep a high level of vigilance post-op, especially during those first 6 hours. If the flap appears to become compromised, prompt return to the OR will provide the best opportunity for salvage, as the vast majority of causes are related to errors in technique or vascular compromise from extrinsic compression.[23]

Addressing Specific Problems

Fistula

Fistula constitutes one of the major complications after reconstructive head and neck surgery. The incidence after myocutaneous flap reconstruction can vary from 13 to 29%; with free flap reconstruction, from 0 to 15%.[24] Factors considered to increase the rate of fistulas include radiation, malnutrition, large defects, closure under tension, ischemic wound edges, and infection.[7,25]

One of the key aspects of reconstructing the oropharyngeal area is providing a watertight seal between the mucosa left in situ and the epithelial surface (epidermis or mucosa) brought in with the free tissue transfer. The absence of such a seal, especially coupled with one or more of the above factors, provides the setting for a collection between tissue planes. This is the first step toward infection and subsequently fistulization. This problem can be minimized by carefully approximating the epithelial linings and attempting to stop the progression of the above-mentioned sequence by prompt, effective, and complete drainage of the possible collections.

These principles dictate, to a certain extent, the management of a fistula. Once a collection is noted, this is drained adequately, taking care not to jeopardize the microvascular anastomoses. Packing is started in an attempt to provide for good granulation tissue. Biopsy may be considered, to rule out a possible recurrence or positive margin. If the fistula is small enough and is surrounded by well-vascularized tissue, conservative measures will usually suffice to control and heal the fistula.

If the fistula is large or if it exposes a vital structure (brain, carotid artery), especially if it is surrounded by indurated, irradiated tissue, then the case is made for a return to the OR for débridement and vascularized tissue resurfacing.[26] This, of course, is the time to consider the patient's overall medical condition and ability to tolerate another procedure, in conjunction with the availability of local and regional tissue for reconstruction. Antibiotics are usually helpful only until all collections are fully drained and the cellulitis is under control. After that débridement will be much more helpful in removing dead or ischemic tissues.

A special word of caution is warranted for a failed jejunal flap used for hypopharyngeal reconstruction. In that case, prompt return to the OR and débridement is warranted, as this can be a life-threatening complication. Once the area is fully débrided and clean, one has to proceed with either exteriorization of the proximal and distal segments of the cervical esophagus/pharynx or perform a second pharyngoesophageal reconstruction using locoregional (pectoralis major) or distant (jejunum, radial forearm) tissue transfer. The latter will usually provide a better long-term outcome, assuming the patient's condition can tolerate it (**Figs. 27.8–27.21**).

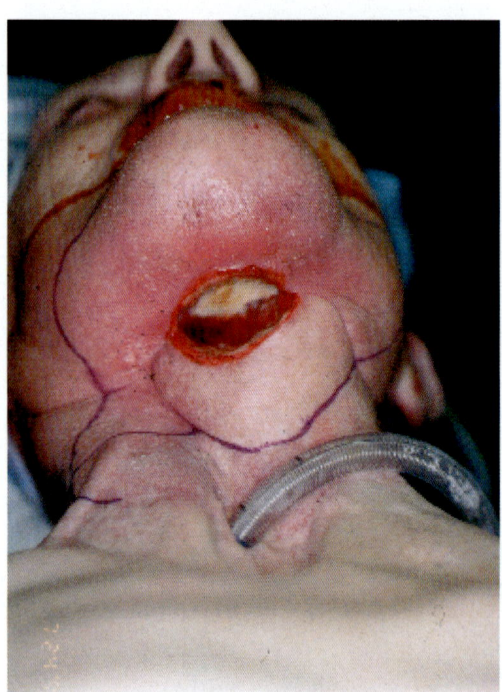

Fig. 27.9 Planned resection is outlined in pen.

Carotid Artery Blowout

Carotid artery exposure and subsequent possible rupture is one of the most feared complications associated with head and neck surgery. As mentioned above, this will usually complicate large resections, especially in the setting of a leak between tissue planes, formation of a fistula, or tumor recurrence.[27,28] The mortality rate is reported to be between 10 and 50%[5,11,29] once the blowout occurs.

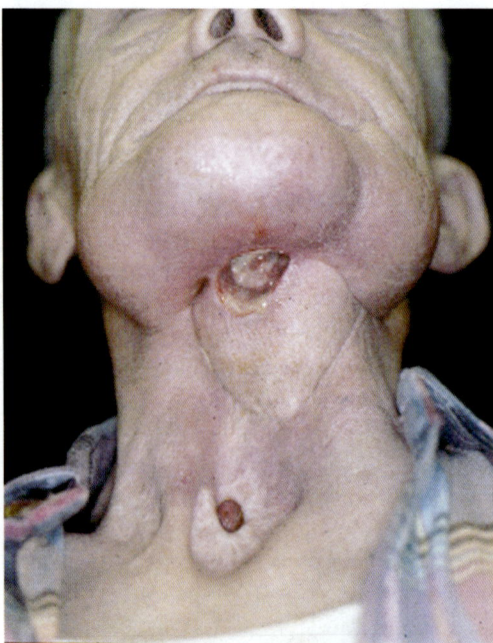

Fig. 27.8 Patient with recurrent floor of mouth malignancy. He has developed a tumor fistula recurrence at the site of a previous pectoralis major flap reconstruction.

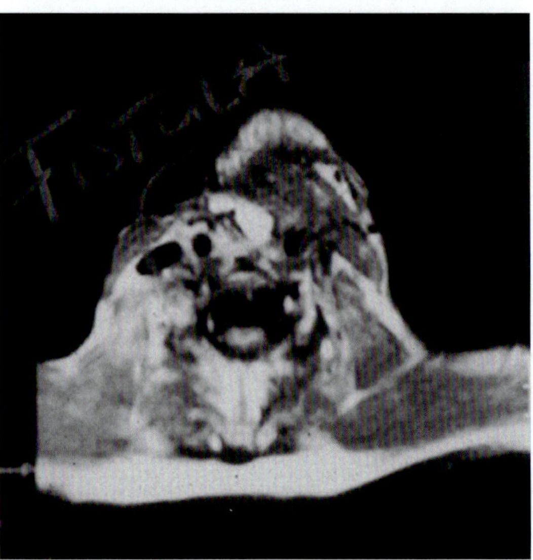

Fig. 27.10 Computed tomography scan demonstrating tumor fistula.

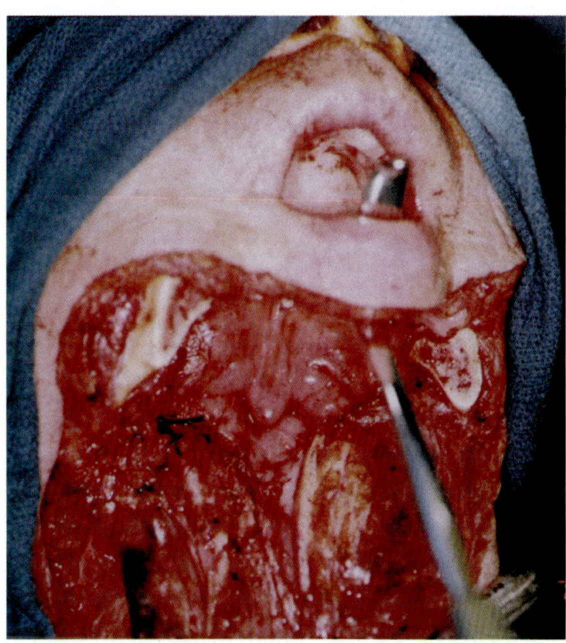

Fig. 27.11 Surgical defect. Anterior mandible, floor of mouth, anterior hypopharynx, tongue, and cutaneous cover have all been resected.

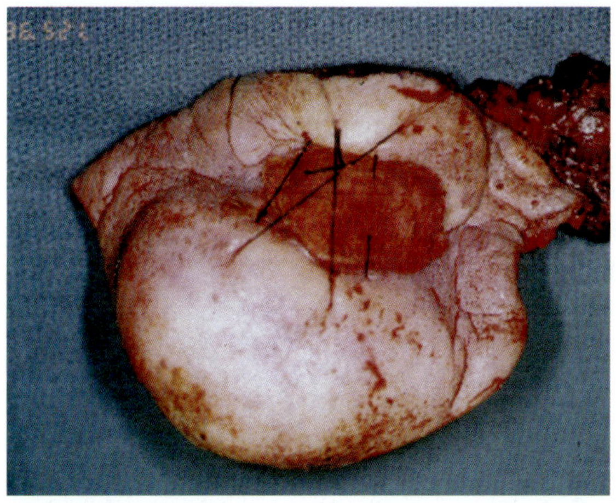

Fig. 27.13 Surgical specimen, inferior view.

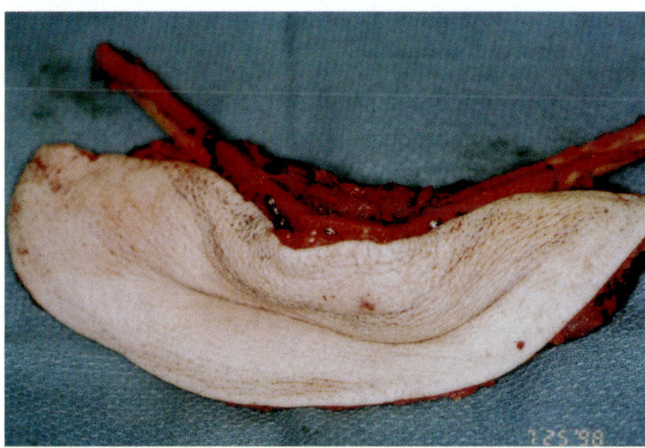

Fig. 27.15 Fibula free flap shaped to restore mandible. Large skin island will be used for external skin coverage.

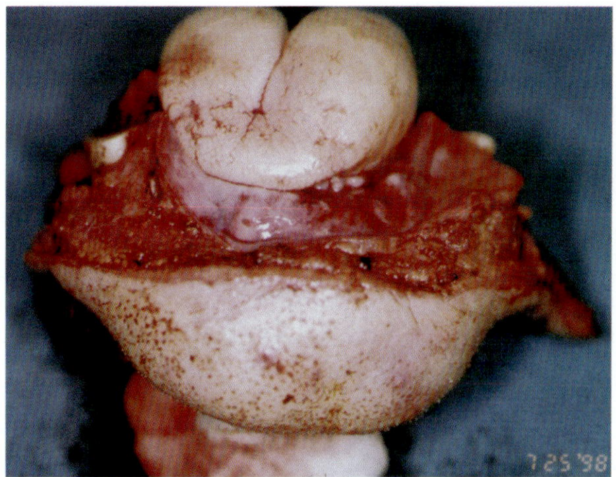

Fig. 27.12 Surgical specimen, anterior view.

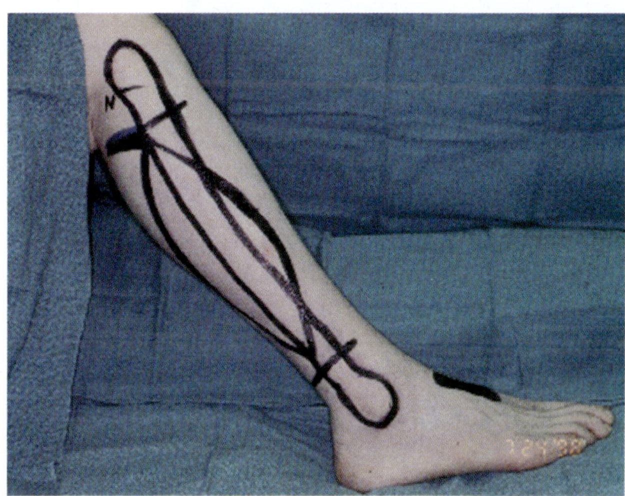

Fig. 27.14 Mandible reconstruction planned with fibula free flap.

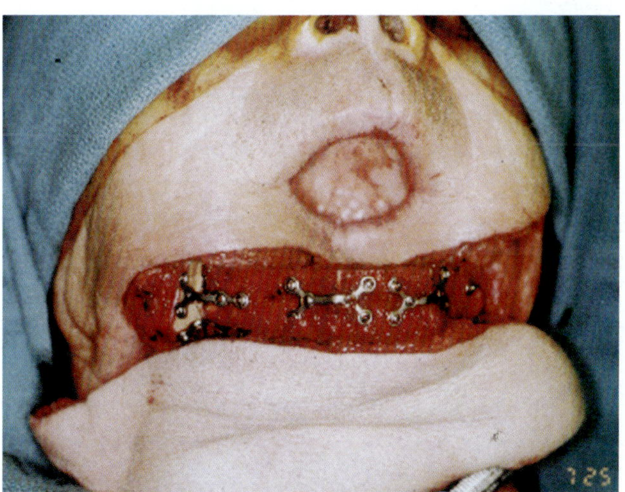

Fig. 27.16 Fibula free flap rigidly fixed in place.

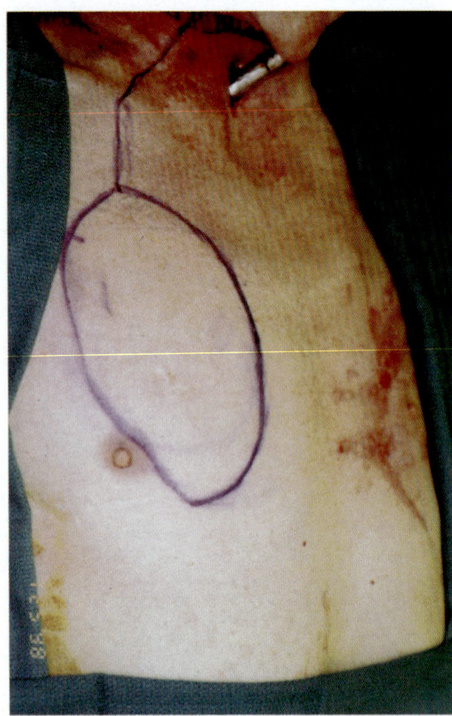

Fig. 27.17 Pectoralis major myocutaneous flap planned to repair floor of mouth, tongue, and anterior hypopharynx defect.

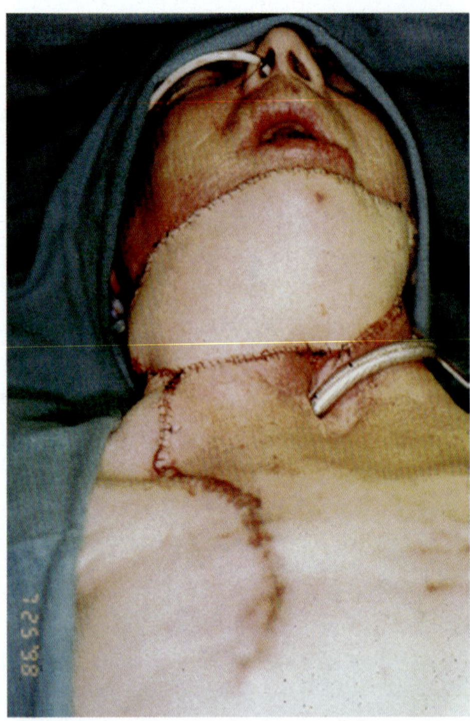

Fig. 27.19 Intraoperative view. Large skin island externally is from fibula free flap.

The true incidence of carotid blowout, however, is not clearly known.[26]

Several flaps and grafts have been used for the prevention of this complication, including dermal grafts, muscle flaps, and fascia lata grafts.[30] Some have advocated choosing an incision that provides additional vessel coverage.[31]

It appears that the best treatment of carotid artery blowout is its prevention, by coverage with well-vascularized tissue, prompt drainage of collections and hematomas, and minimal unnecessary dissection, especially in the setting of previous radiation. Careful attention to nutrition in this already compromised patient population will also be very effective in preventing vascular complications.[30] The low incidence of complications associated with free flap coverage could well be the result

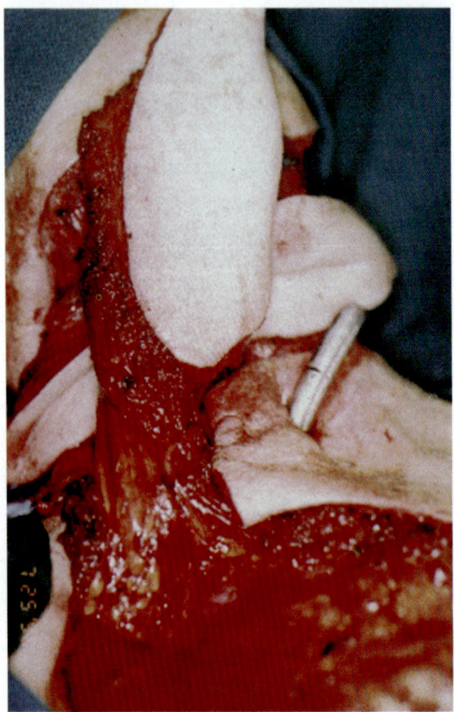

Fig. 27.18 Pectoralis flap being elevated.

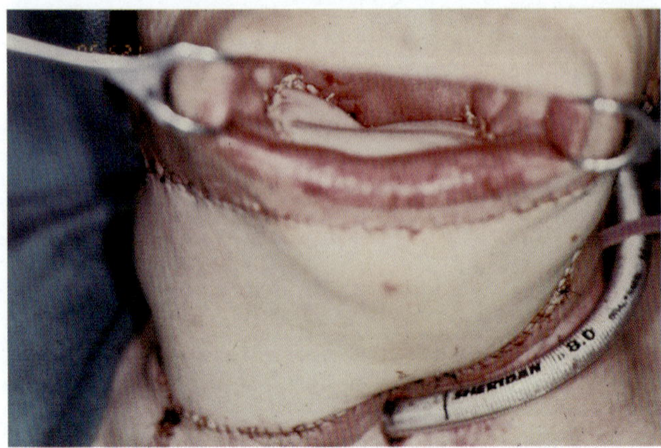

Fig. 27.20 Intraoperative view. Pectoralis major flap inset intraorally.

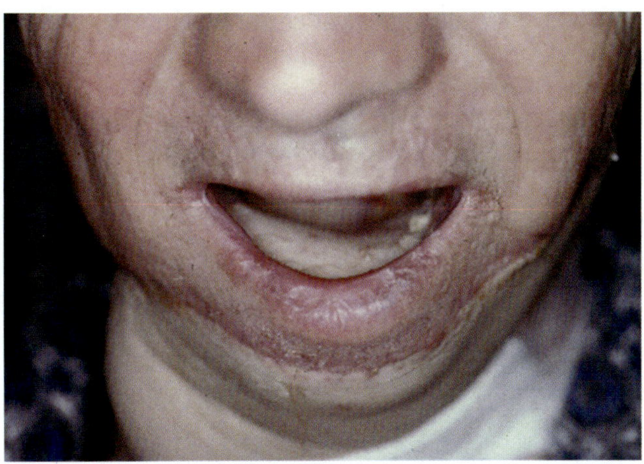

Fig. 27.21 Late postoperative appearance. All wounds have healed well.

of the better blood supply of the free tissue transfers compared with pedicled flaps.[24]

Once it has occurred, carotid blowout constitutes a surgical emergency. The patient is taken to the OR; pressure is applied to control the bleeding, and the neck is explored. One may choose to use a shunt in the carotid system, but the two vessel ends are rarely adequate for repair or reanastomosis. Generally, ligation of the vessels and tissue débridement are performed. Once control of the wound has been obtained, the area can be resurfaced, either immediately or in a delayed fashion when the wound is suitable. Several reports on recurrent carotid rupture mention the use of endovascular and radiological techniques in the management of this problem.[32]

Osteoradionecrosis

Osteoradionecrosis (ORN), or the collective changes caused by radiation therapy on bone, is in itself a significant source of morbidity, especially once the dose delivered is > 6000 cGy. Because head and neck tumors are often treated with radiation, it is common to see the full spectrum of ORN, including sequestration of bone, pathologic fractures, fistulization, and soft tissue loss.[33,34] The pathophysiology of ORN includes the tissue hypoxia associated with the progressive microvascular changes of radiation together with the scarring that results. In soft tissue this will most often result in an indurated, brawny discoloration with multiple telangiectasias. On bone that receives significant loads, such as the mandible, this problem can easily translate into bone loss or fracture, especially after a trivial trauma, such as a tooth extraction.[35] The amount of trauma required to show signs of ORN appears to decrease as the dose of radiation increases.

Hyperbaric oxygen has been very promising in counteracting the effects of ischemia associated with ORN.[36] This modality can be used either prophylactically, trying to increase the oxygen content of the tissue during the time of injury (i.e., tooth extraction), or therapeutically once the signs of ORN develop. Once all conservative modalities have been exhausted, the next step is wide débridement of involved tissues and reconstruction with well-perfused tissue in the form of a pedicled or free flap.[37,38]

Hardware Exposure and Nonunion

Hardware in the form of plates and screws used for rigid fixation is invaluable in providing a stable construct able to withstand the tremendous pressures that can be produced by the masseteric musculature. Complications after free flap reconstruction can include exposure of hardware and nonunion of bone. Both can be produced by ischemia of the bone or the soft tissue envelope. Ischemia should be avoided by minimizing periosteal stripping and ensuring well-vascularized soft tissue cover of hardware. In addition, a watertight closure between the oropharynx and the hardware will minimize the risk of chronic contamination. The use of miniplates appears to combine minimal stripping of the periosteum while maximizing construct rigidity, especially if they are placed along two perpendicular planes.[39] Creating bone-to-bone contact and rigid fixation between two well-vascularized bones seems to be the best possible setting for complete and prompt bony union.

In the setting of poor wound healing and hardware exposure, with or without fistulization, consideration must be given to conservative management with aggressive local wound care. If the surrounding tissue is healthy, secondary healing can occur without a second flap. If the conservative management fails and the decision is to operate, then poorly placed or loose hardware has to be removed, ischemic tissues need débridement, and infection needs to be controlled. To maximize the chance for union, the bone should be adequately reduced and rigidly fixed. Cancellous bone grafting should be considered, and well-vascularized soft tissue should isolate the hardware from the oropharyngeal flora.[40]

Aesthetics

To successfully rehabilitate a patient after head and neck tumor ablation, the final aesthetic outcome has to be taken into consideration. The first concern is the control of the tumor and optimizing functional recovery. However, if these efforts are not followed by appropriate concern about the aesthetic outcome, the patient will have great difficulty coming to terms with the new reality faced after surgery.

These issues become more complex still if we consider reoperative surgery. As outlined above, the tissues available and the choices present will be limited, and previous treatment will have left scars and an indurated, possibly fibrosed soft tissue envelope, which will only add to the difficulty of the aesthetic reconstruction of the patient. Sometimes while correcting a different problem aesthetics can be improved as well (i.e., when closing a fistula). Most of the time, however, the first procedure will be the time to optimize aesthetic outcome. Appropriate color match for the skin choice, proper design of bone length and shape, accurate assessment of the soft tissue defect and volume deficit, and accurate replacement will all set the stage for an aesthetically optimal reconstruction.

When deciding to reoperate with the sole purpose of improving aesthetics, there are several options. Flap debulking, sharply or with suction-assisted lipectomy, serial excision, dermal or fat grafting to improve contour, delayed insetting, and serial excision or the principle of the disappearing flap are all options to improve the final result.

The pedicle of a free flap is always an area of concern. The safest course of action is to try and leave it intact, especially when the flap is lying in a radiated, scarred bed, where revascularization from the periphery is unreliable. If it appears that the pedicle would be placed at risk, staging the contouring of the flap and possibly delaying it to give time for the flap to become vascularized is warranted.

Finally, one should consider the option of prosthetic reconstruction. The advances in the area of materials and coloring are such that it is not rare to find the best reconstruction being accomplished by a prosthetic rather than a surgical method. The reconstructive team should always be cognizant of their limitations, and if the result is expected to be suboptimal, they should not hesitate to cooperate with the prosthetics specialist, even intraoperatively, to provide the best possible platform for a prosthetic reconstruction. Such an approach could be the best suited for the patient, providing an aesthetic reconstruction with minimal pain and morbidity and expediting the return of the patient to society.

Conclusion

Head and neck reoperative surgery is a formidable undertaking best handled in a multidisciplinary approach by experienced surgeons. The best defense against the need for reoperation is, as always, careful assessment and planning as well as execution of the first operation and careful utilization of the other treatment modalities available. Prompt attention to complications is warranted, because some could be life threatening or significantly compromise the patient's quality of life. Lastly, respect of the patient's wishes and factoring into the decision-making process the patient's condition and life expectancy appear integral to tailoring the treatment, including the reconstruction options, to each individual patient.

References

1. Blackwell KE, Buchbinder D, Biller HF, Urken ML. Reconstruction of massive defects in the head and neck: the role of simultaneous distant and regional flaps. Head Neck 1997;19:620–628.
2. Bradford CR, Esclamado RM, Carroll WR, Sullivan MJ. Analysis of recurrence, complications, and functional results with free jejunal flaps. Head Neck 1994;16:149–154.
3. Haas I, Hauser U, Ganzer U. The dilemma of follow-up in head and neck cancer patients. Eur Arch Otorhinolaryngol 2001;258:177–183.
4. Ellison DE, Hoover LA, Ward PH. Tumor recurrence within myocutaneous flaps. Ann Otol Rhinol Laryngol 1987;96:26–28.
5. McCready RA, Hyde GL, Bivins BA, Mattingly SS, Griffen WO Jr. Radiation-induced arterial injuries. Surgery 1983;93:306–312.
6. Cheng SW, Wu LL, Ting AC, Lau H, Lam LK, Wei WI. Irradiation-induced extracranial carotid stenosis in patients with head and neck malignancies. Am J Surg 1999;178:323–328.
7. Sanders EM, Davis KR, Whelan CS, Deckers PJ. Threatened carotid artery rupture: a complication of radical neck surgery. J Surg Oncol 1986;33:190–193.
8. Larson DL, Kroll S, Jaffe N, Serure A, Goepfert H. Long-term effects of radiotherapy in childhood and adolescence. Am J Surg 1990;160:348–351.
9. Deutsch M, Kroll SS, Ainsle N, Wang B. Influence of radiation on late complications in patients with free fibular flaps for mandibular reconstruction. Ann Plast Surg 1999;42:662–664.
10. Baxter WF. Survival after unplanned carotid rupture. Laryngoscope 1979;89:385–392.
11. Coleman JJ III. Treatment of the ruptured or exposed carotid artery: a rational approach. South Med J 1985;78:262–267.
12. Fogarty BJ, Khan K, Ashall G, Leonard AG. Complications of long operations: a prospective study of morbidity associated with prolonged operative time (>6 h). Br J Plast Surg 1999;52:33–36.
13. De Melo GM, Ribeiro KC, Kowalski LP, Deheinzelin D. Risk factors for postoperative complications in oral cancer and their prognostic implications. Arch Otolaryngol Head Neck Surg 2001;127:828–833.
14. Bhattacharyya N, Fried MP. Benchmarks for mortality, morbidity, and length of stay for head and neck surgical procedures. Arch Otolaryngol Head Neck Surg 2001;127:127–132.

15. Chen AY, Matson LK, Roberts D, Goepfert H. The significance of comorbidity in advanced laryngeal cancer. Head Neck 2001;23:566–572.

16. Bridger AG, O'Brien CJ, Lee KK. Advanced patient age should not preclude the use of free-flap reconstruction for head and neck cancer. Am J Surg 1994;168:425–428.

17. Boeckx W, Fossion E, Guelinckx P, Demey R, Dewilde R. Free flaps in head and neck surgery. Acta Chir Belg 1982;82:219–229.

18. Blackwell KE. Unsurpassed reliability of free flaps for head and neck reconstruction. Arch Otolaryngol Head Neck Surg 1999;125:295–299.

19. Disa JJ, Hu QY, Hidalgo DA. Retrospective review of 400 consecutive free flap reconstructions for oncologic surgical defects. Ann Surg Oncol 1997;4:663–669.

20. Blackwell KE, Brown MT, Gonzalez D. Overcoming the learning curve in microvascular head and neck reconstruction. Arch Otolaryngol Head Neck Surg 1997;123:1332–1335.

21. Cordeiro PG, Hidalgo DA. Conceptual considerations in mandibular reconstruction. Clin Plast Surg 1995;22:61–69.

22. Disa JJ, Cordeiro PG, Hidalgo DA. Efficacy of conventional monitoring techniques in free tissue transfer: an 11-year experience in 750 consecutive cases. Plast Reconstr Surg 1999;104:97–101.

23. Hidalgo DA, Jones CS. The role of emergent exploration in free-tissue transfer: a review of 150 consecutive cases. Plast Reconstr Surg 1990;86:492–498.

24. O'Brien CJ, Lee KK, Stern HS, et al. Evaluation of 250 free-flap reconstructions after resection of tumours of the head and neck. Aust N Z J Surg 1998;68:698–701.

25. Lundgren J, Olofsson J. Pharyngocutaneous fistulae following total laryngectomy. Clin Otolaryngol 1979;4:13–23.

26. Rees R, Cary A, Shack RB, Harris PF. Pharyngocutaneous fistulas in advanced cancer: closure with musculocutaneous or muscle flaps. Am J Surg 1987;154:381–383.

27. Heller KS, Strong EW. Carotid arterial hemorrhage after radical head and neck surgery. Am J Surg 1979;138:607–610.

28. Mika H, Bumb P, Gunther R. Rupture, emergency ligature and elective ligature of the carotid artery. Laryngol Rhinol Otol (Stuttg) 1982;61:634–638.

29. Porto DP, Adams GL, Foster C. Emergency management of carotid artery rupture. Am J Otolaryngol 1986;7:213–217.

30. Shumrick DA. Carotid artery rupture. Laryngoscope 1973;83:1051–1061.

31. Kambic V, Sirca A. H incision—method of choice for radical neck dissection. J Laryngol Otol 1977;91:383–390.

32. Chaloupka JC, Roth TC, Putman CM, et al. Recurrent carotid blowout syndrome: diagnostic and therapeutic challenges in a newly recognized subgroup of patients. AJNR Am J Neuroradiol 1999;20:1069–1077.

33. Murray CG, Herson J, Daly TE, Zimmerman S. Radiation necrosis of the mandible: a 10 year study, I: Factors influencing the onset of necrosis. Int J Radiat Oncol Biol Phys 1980;6:543–548.

34. Murray CG, Herson J, Daly TE, Zimmerman S. Radiation necrosis of the mandible: a 10 year study, II: Dental factors; onset, duration and management of necrosis. Int J Radiat Oncol Biol Phys 1980;6:549–553.

35. Marx RE, Johnson RP, Kline SN. Prevention of osteoradionecrosis: a randomized prospective clinical trial of hyperbaric oxygen versus penicillin. J Am Dent Assoc 1985;111:49–54.

36. Hao SP, Chen HC, Wei FC, Chen CY, Yeh AR, Su JL. Systematic management of osteoradionecrosis in the head and neck. Laryngoscope 1999;109:1324–1327.

37. Shaha AR, Cordeiro PG, Hidalgo DA, et al. Resection and immediate microvascular reconstruction in the management of osteoradionecrosis of the mandible. Head Neck 1997;19:406–411.

38. Citardi MJ, Chaloupka JC, Son YH, Ariyan S, Sasaki CT. Management of carotid artery rupture by monitored endovascular therapeutic occlusion (1988–1994). Laryngoscope 1995;105:1086–1092.

39. Hidalgo DA. Titanium miniplate fixation in free flap mandible reconstruction. Ann Plast Surg 1989;23:498–507.

40. Boyd JB, Mulholland RS, Davidson J, et al. The free flap and plate in oromandibular reconstruction: long-term review and indications. Plast Reconstr Surg 1995;95:1018–1028.

Decision tree for recurrent hypopharynx cancer

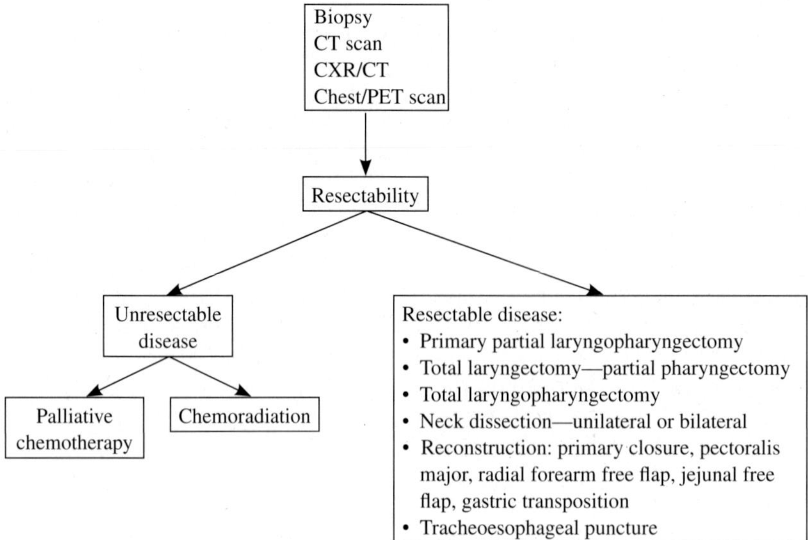

Hypopharyngeal Cancer

Peter E. Andersen and Douglas Reh

Primary malignant tumors of the hypopharynx are uncommon, representing only a small fraction of the total cancers diagnosed in the United States. The American Cancer Society (ACS) estimated 8600 new diagnoses of cancer of the pharynx in the United States in 2002, with 2100 deaths from pharyngeal cancer in that same period.[1] Because the ACS figures include cases of nasopharyngeal and oropharyngeal as well as hypopharyngeal cancers, these figures are an upper limit of the magnitude of the problem, and actual incidence is, of course, less. Hypopharyngeal cancer is closely associated with laryngeal cancer in terms of its anatomical location as well as its risk factors. These include principally tobacco and alcohol use. Although many different types of malignant tumors can arise within the anatomical boundaries of the hypopharynx, the vast majority of hypopharyngeal cancers are squamous carcinoma. This discussion will focus solely on this histologic type.

The pyriform sinus is the most common site of malignancy in the hypopharynx, followed by the posterior pharyngeal wall and postcricoid region. The most common presenting symptoms in a patient with hypopharyngeal cancer include the presence of a neck mass, throat pain, ipsilateral otalgia, dysphagia, and hoarseness.[2] Because of the rich lymphatics in this region, there is early spread of the disease to regional lymph nodes. An estimated two thirds of patients have palpable lymph node metastasis on initial evaluation, and almost half of the clinically N_0 patients will be found to have occult cervical lymph node metastasis if elective neck dissection is performed.[3] Because of the propensity for regional nodal metastasis, high stage at presentation is common, with ~80% of patients presenting with stage III or IV disease.[4] The most common sites of nodal metastasis are to the jugular chain of nodes,[3] although the retropharyngeal, paratracheal, parapharyngeal, and paraesophageal nodes may also be involved. Survival rates in patients with hypopharyngeal cancers tend to be poor. The disease-free 5-year survival rate has been estimated at 56% in patients with pyriform sinus cancer and 30% in those with cancer of the posterior wall of the hypopharynx.[5]

Initial treatment for hypopharyngeal cancer is beyond the scope of the current discussion; however, it should be noted that multiple methods often are employed to treat hypopharyngeal cancer. Hypopharyngeal cancers have a high risk of recurrence after initial therapy. This has been attributed to the high rate of submucosal extension, including extension into the thyroid cartilage and surrounding tissue. Small-stage lesions or lesions that occur in patients who are unsuitable for more aggressive treatment are often treated with radiotherapy alone. Radiotherapy alone has been reported by Stoeckli et al to have a recurrence rate as high as 59%.[6] Commonly, patients with cancer of the hypopharynx are treated with combined therapy, either surgical resection followed by radiation therapy or combinations of chemotherapy and radiation therapy given sequentially or simultaneously. Most patients with hypopharyngeal cancer undergo some combination of surgical resection, reconstruction, and radiotherapy/chemotherapy. Conservation surgery may be indicated for T1 and T2 cancers in which the pyriform sinus is solely involved above the apical region. This includes partial laryngopharyngectomy. Supracricoid and hemicricoid laryngopharyngectomy have also been described. These patients also have an extremely high incidence of neck disease; consequently, planned neck dissections are an important part of their surgery.[7]

Evaluation and Work-up of Patients with Recurrent Hypopharyngeal Cancer

Because of the high rates of recurrence in patients treated for hypopharyngeal cancer, salvage surgery and treatment have become an increasingly important aspect in the management of these patients. The remainder of our discussion will focus on the evaluation, work-up, and treatment of patients with recurrent hypopharyngeal cancer.

The aforementioned high recurrence rates necessitate careful follow-up after initial treatment. Consequently, patients are usually monitored very closely through serial examinations. The presenting symptoms in patients with recurrence are essentially the same as those of patients with new-onset hypopharyngeal cancer. The presence of a neck mass is the most common complaint and may be accompanied by throat pain, ipsilateral otalgia, dysphagia, odynophagia, and hoarseness. These and other symptoms should be monitored in patients who are being followed after their initial treatment for hypopharyngeal cancer.

Patients being referred for suspicion of a recurrence need a full and detailed history and physical examination.

The history should focus on a careful analysis of the patient's symptoms. These can be useful in determining the location and extent of the tumor and the patient's functional status. The past medical history should focus on the location and size of the original tumor, as well as the extent of any neck disease. The consulting head and neck surgeon must know the initial treatment course. These are principally either surgery, radiation, combination surgery and radiation, or concurrent versus sequential chemo- and radiation therapy. If the patient underwent surgical resection of the initial tumor, it is important to obtain the operative note to get details regarding the approach, findings at the time of surgery (including extent of the tumor), and techniques used in the tumor's excision. Treatment of any neck disease is also important. This will be essential in determining the treatment options for this patient's recurrence. If the patient underwent radiation therapy, it is also important to obtain the details of the radiation therapy. This includes overall dose, port size, and the time to failure after completion of the therapy. Obviously, these details will be most easily obtainable from the records of the previous treatment rather than from the patient. Those patients who have had a recurrence within a year of their primary radiotherapy are much less likely to be able to be radiated for their recurrence. If the patient underwent chemotherapy, it is important to establish which chemotherapeutic regimens were used. This will be important, not only in determining what can be used for the treatment of the recurrence

but also in establishing any comorbidities that may have been caused by the initial therapy. These include renal impairment caused by cisplatin or peripheral neuropathy caused by both cisplatin and docetaxel.

Careful attention should be paid to understanding the patient's other underlying comorbid conditions. Diseases such as diabetes, coronary artery disease, chronic obstructive pulmonary disease (COPD), and liver disease can significantly impact a patient's outcome in terms of the existing cancer, as well as the patient's response and morbidity to treatment. This information will help in determining ideal treatment options. A careful review of the patient's medications is also important. Certain medications, such as steroids, can significantly impact a patient's outcome, especially in terms of his or her recovery from surgery. Establishing overall performance status for a patient is another important component of the medical history. This includes an understanding of the patient's daily functional status, social support, and overall health. It determines the level of medical and social care that the patient will need, both during and after treatment (**Table 28.1**).[8] Overall nutritional status is another essential piece of information. If a surgery is being planned, the patient's nutritional status must be ascertained and any steps must be taken to maximize their overall nutrition prior to surgery and/or any other form of treatment for the cancer.

A detailed review of systems should also be performed as part of the consultation. This may help to establish

Table 28.1 Karnofsky Performance Status Scale

Definitions	Rating (%)	Criteria
Able to carry on normal activity and to work; no special care needed	100	Normal no complaints; no evidence of disease
	90	Able to carry on normal activity; minor signs or symptoms of disease
	80	Normal activity with effort; some signs or symptoms of disease
Unable to work; able to live at home and care for most personal needs; varying amount of assistance needed	70	Cares for self; unable to carry on normal activity or to do active work
	60	Requires occasional assistance, but is able to care for most of his personal needs
	50	Requires considerable assistance and frequent medical care
Unable to care for self; requires equivalent of institutional or hospital care; disease may be progressing rapidly	40	Disabled; requires special care and assistance
	30	Severely disabled; hospital admission is indicated although death not imminent
	20	Very sick; hospital admission necessary; active supportive treatment necessary
	10	Moribund; fatal processes progressing rapidly
	0	Dead

symptoms consistent with distant metastasis, which will affect treatment decisions.

During physical examination, careful attention must be given to the examination of the neck because of the significant incidence of regional metastasis in patients with recurrent hypopharyngeal cancer. Focus should be on levels 2, 3, and 4,[4] as well as the contralateral neck. Flexible laryngoscopy should be performed by an experienced endoscopist. Attention should be paid to establishing the size and location of the tumor, as well as involvement of contiguous anatomical structures, such as invasion of the tumor into the larynx. The head and neck surgeon must understand the involvement of the vocal cords and assess any fixation. This is especially important in planning surgical treatment, as vocal cord fixation will necessitate a total laryngectomy.

Laboratory examination should be directed by findings on history and physical examination. When appropriate, liver and renal function work-ups should be performed. Hematologic abnormalities must be ruled out, especially in those patients who have received chemotherapy. Prealbumin can be obtained to establish nutritional status.[9] Hypercalcemia is suggestive of distant metastasis.

The rates of neck metastasis are 69 to 72% (pyriform sinus and posterior hypopharynx, respectively); distant metastasis rates approach 17% in patients presenting with hypopharyngeal cancer.[5] These rates can be assumed to be the same or higher in patients with recurrence. Consequently, imaging modalities are helpful in ruling out regional and distant metastasis. A computed tomography (CT) scan of the neck with contrast is warranted in all patients with recurrence, as it is fairly sensitive in determining regional spread. The 5-year survival in patients who undergo salvage surgery hypopharyngeal recurrence remains a dismal 20%.[6] We do not perform radical head and neck surgery on patients with inoperable disease or distant metastases. Therefore, the work-up must also rule out pulmonary metastasis or second primary. Chest x-ray has been shown to be less sensitive than CT (21%) but extremely specific (99%) for the diagnosis of pulmonary tumor. We advocate a screening chest x-ray followed by a chest CT only if the x-ray is negative. This allows a cost-effective yet sensitive method of ruling out pulmonary involvement.[10]

Positron emission tomography (PET) scan has remained controversial in terms of its sensitivity and specificity in diagnosing both occult head and neck metastasis and pulmonary tumors (metastasis or primary). Stoeckli et al's study suggests poor sensitivity (25%) in patients with N0 necks and oropharyngeal and oral cavity cancer.[11] Teknos et al looked at 12 patients with stage III or IV head and neck cancer. Three patients had positive findings of mediastinal tumor not detected by chest x-ray or CT.[12] Wax et al found high sensitivity (100%) for PET scan in the detection of synchronous lung lesions in their study.[13] However, PET scan does provide a complete survey of the entire body and therefore is a very efficient means of assessing the entire patient; it therefore has become a standard part of our workup.

Surgical Therapy

Because the majority of patients with cancer of the hypopharynx receive combination therapy as their initial therapy, options for treatment of recurrent disease are more limited than those for patients with cancer of other head and neck sites. Therefore, the major decisions regarding surgical treatment of recurrent cancer of the hypopharynx center not around choices for the extirpative surgical procedure but rather around the decision whether or not to proceed with surgical therapy at all, and if so, around reconstructive options. For the vast majority of patients, the extirpative procedure required will be that of total laryngectomy with partial or total pharyngectomy. It may be possible in a very small percentage of patients of high-performance status with small recurrent tumors to perform a less than total laryngectomy; this should be considered the exception to the rule and should only be undertaken by surgeons highly experienced in such procedures. The need for total laryngectomy in treatment of cancer of the hypopharynx is sometimes confusing. In cases where the primary tumor extends into the larynx, such as direct mucosal spread or fixation of the hemilarynx, the need for total laryngectomy is obvious. However, even in cases where the larynx is not directly involved, laryngectomy is required because postsurgical deglutition will be so disordered that the risk of severe aspiration requires the separation of the airway and foodway. The remaining portion of this discussion will focus on patients undergoing some form of laryngopharyngectomy.

The extent of pharyngeal wall resection required will vary according to the size and location of the primary tumor. Carcinoma of the hypopharynx is prone to spread submucosally through the submucosal lymphatics of the hypopharynx. Therefore, the actual extent of the tumor may be larger than what is evident on clinical examination. In general, we believe that 2 cm of normal-appearing mucosa should be excised around the obvious lesion. Cancers of the pyriform sinus where the primary tumor is located solely within the pyriform sinus can generally be excised with enough remaining pharyngeal mucosa to consider primary closure of the pharyngotomy. However, when the tumor extends from the pyriform sinus to another location in the hypopharynx, such as the posterior wall, the surgical defect will be too large to allow primary closure, and some form of reconstruction will be required. Tumors originating on the posterior pharyngeal wall or postcricoid area will require total pharyngectomy with appropriate reconstruction. Although it is often technically possible to perform primary closure of the pharyngeal defect in patients with tumors located within the pyriform sinus, the surgeon should recognize that if attempted in patients who have been previously treated with radiation therapy or chemotherapy and radiation, there is an extremely high incidence of postoperative pharyngocutaneous fistula. Thus, although reconstruction is not absolutely required in these cases, it should be considered if only for the fact that doing so greatly reduces the incidence of pharyngocutaneous fistula.

Reconstructive options are varied in these patients and will depend both on the physical status of the patient and on the resources available to the surgeon. Every attempt should be made to accomplish the reconstruction in as few steps as possible. The treating surgeon should recognize that the median survival time in patients with recurrent cancer of the hypopharynx is distressingly low; therefore, elaborate multistage reconstructions that require prolonged periods of time are unacceptable, as the goal of the procedure should be to rehabilitate the patient as soon as possible.

Perhaps the simplest reconstructive technique in these patients is the pectoralis musculocutaneous flap. The reliability, proximity to the primary site, ease of elevation, and minimal donor site morbidity make this an acceptable choice for pharyngeal reconstruction. However, the skin paddle of this flap is not freely mobile relative to its vascular pedicle; also, the skin paddle is less reliable in females with large breasts and the flap is bulky, making reconstruction of circumferential pharyngeal defects difficult. Our choice for reconstruction of less than circumferential pharyngeal defects is the radial forearm free tissue transfer (RFFTT). This flap is hardy and has a long vascular pedicle, allowing reach to recipient vessels virtually anywhere in the neck. The skin is pliable and makes an excellent patch for a partial pharyngectomy defect. Investigators have reported good results with reconstruction of circumferential pharyngeal defects with the RFFTT. Our experience has been that this is an acceptable technique of reconstruction but that our patients with visceral reconstructions of such defects tend to have better swallowing results.

For those patients undergoing total laryngectomy with total pharyngectomy, reconstructive options depend on the amount of cervical esophagus remaining in the neck for anastomosis. When enough esophagus remains to allow safe anastomosis to the visceral flap, our reconstructive method of choice is the jejunal free flap (JFF). This flap provides an excellent match in caliber to the native esophagus and replaces mucosal tissue with similar mucosal tissue. Disadvantages to this flap include the morbidity of laparotomy and jejunectomy, the tendency toward excessive mucus secretion of the transferred jejunal segment, and dysphagia due to peristalsis of the jejunal

segment. This flap is also technically more difficult to perform than the RFFTT. In situations where tumor resection requires cervical esophagectomy, there may not be enough esophagus remaining in the neck to safely perform the lower anastomosis. In those cases the surgeon may consider performing a blunt transhiatal esophagectomy and gastric transposition and pharyngogastric anastomosis.

Microvascular reconstruction has been shown to be effective in patients who are heavily pretreated; however, a special circumstance exists in patients who lack vessels in the neck suitable for microvascular anastomosis. In these cases microvascular techniques must be abandoned in favor of older techniques of reconstruction, such as the pectoralis major musculocutaneous flap, gastric transposition, or colonic transposition. In patients felt to be at extremely high risk for wound healing complications, the surgeon may consider the construction of a planned pharyngostome to be closed at a secondary procedure later.

As with any procedure involving total laryngectomy, restoration of speech is vital. In most cases immediate tracheoesophageal puncture (TEP) is possible and has been shown not to significantly increase postoperative complications. We believe that the benefit to the patient by early restoration of speech outweighs the very small possibility of increased postoperative complications; however, we will not place a TEP through an area of reconstructed pharynx.

Conclusion

Recurrences following treatment for hypopharyngeal cancers are frequent due to the early spread of disease at the time of the primary diagnosis, the submucosal spread potential, and the presence of nodal neck disease. The usual symptoms of recurrence include throat pain, otalgia, dysphagia, and hoarseness. The surgeon taking care of the primary disease should be diligent in close follow-up with periodic laryngoscopies and CT scan evaluation of the neck and lungs if any questionable recurrence arises. Distant metastasis should be considered in addition to nodal disease that is high at the recurrent presentation and with most recurrences of hypopharyngeal cancer. Because most of the patients with primary disease have already undergone some form of surgery with radiation and chemotherapy, the decision for care of the recurrence is complex and depends on the patient's nutritional, social, and emotional status. Surgery is a difficult option, with laryngopharyngectomy being the most common salvage procedure with completion neck dissections, if necessary. Reconstruction flaps are usually required to prevent pharyngocutaneous fistula. Hypopharyngeal cancers are uncommon, and recurrence rates are high, offering many challenges to the treating surgeon.

References

1. American Cancer Society. Cancer Facts and Figures. Atlanta: Author; 2002:4.
2. Marks JE, Smith PG, Sessions DG. Pharyngeal wall cancer: a reappraisal after comparison of treatment methods. Arch Otolaryngol 1985;111:79–85.
3. Shah JP. Patterns of cervical lymph node metastasis from squamous carcinomas of the upper aerodigestive tract. Am J Surg 1990;160:405–409.
4. Shah JP. Head and Neck Surgery. 2nd ed. New York: Mosby-Wolfe; 1996:236.
5. Spector JG, Sessions D, Haughey B, et al. Delayed regional metastases, distant metastases and second primary malignancies in squamous cell carcinomas of the larynx and hypopharynx. Laryngoscope 2001;111:1079–1087.
6. Stoeckli SJ, Pawlik A, Lipp M, Huber A, Schmid S. Salvage surgery after failure of nonsurgical therapy for carcinoma of the larynx and hypopharynx. Arch Otolaryngol Head Neck Surg 2000;126:1473–1477.
7. Weinstein GS. Supracricoid laryngectomy with cricohyoidepiglottopexy. Otolaryngol Head Neck Surg 1994;111(5):684–685.
8. O'Toole DM, Golden AM. Evaluating cancer patients for rehabilitation potential. West J Med 1991;155:384–387.
9. Bernstein L, Pleban W. Prealbumin in nutrition evaluation. Nutrition 1996;12(4):255–259.
10. Houghton DJ. Role of chest CT scanning in the management of patients presenting with head and neck cancer. Head Neck 1998;20:614–618.
11. Stoeckli SJ, Steinert H, Pfaltz M, Schmid S. Is there a role for positron emission tomography with 18f-fluorodeoxyglucose in the initial staging of nodal negative oral and oropharyngeal squamous cell carcinoma? Head Neck 2002;24:345–349.
12. Teknos TN, Rosenthal EL, Lee D, Taylor R, Marn CS. Positron emission tomography in the evaluation of stage III and IV head and neck cancer. Head Neck 2001;23:1056–1060.
13. Wax MK, Myers LL, Gabalski EC, Husain S, Gona JM, Nabi H. Positron emission tomography in the evaluation of synchronous lung lesions in patients with untreated head and neck cancer. Arch Otolaryngol Head Neck Surg 2002;128:703–707.

Decision tree for revision surgery for non-melanoma skin cancer

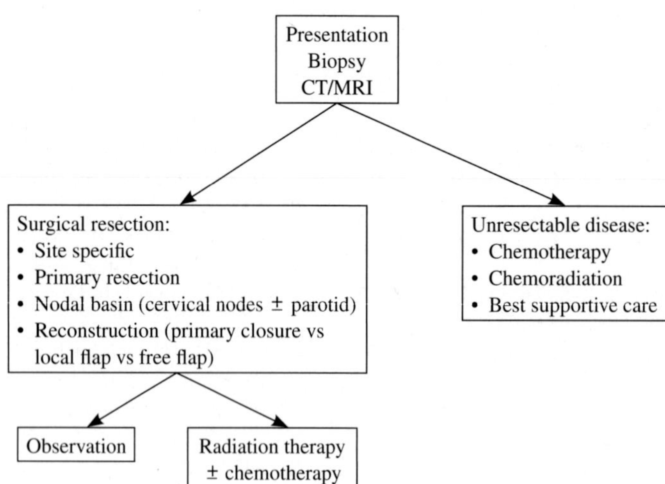

Revision Surgery for Non-melanoma Skin Cancer

Brian A. Moore and James L. Netterville

Non-melanoma skin cancer (NMSC), comprising primarily squamous cell carcinoma (SCC) and basal cell carcinoma (BCC), has emerged as a global health problem of epidemic proportions. Epidemiologic surveys have estimated that 1.3 million cases are diagnosed each year in the United States, with 2.75 million new cases worldwide. Unlike other forms of cancer, the incidence is expected to rise at alarming rates over the next 30 years.[1,2] The economic impact of this disease is burgeoning as well, with over $425 million spent per year on the diagnosis and treatment of NMSC within the Medicare population of the United States.[3] The recognized association between these lesions and sun exposure dictates that cutaneous SCC and BCC typically arise on sun-exposed areas of the body, with > 80% of the lesions appearing on the head and neck.

Despite the frequency with which cutaneous malignancies arise on the head and neck, the majority of lesions are evaluated and treated by our colleagues in dermatology or even primary care. However, more advanced lesions, such as recurrent, deeply invasive, and metastatic lesions, remain the purview of the head and neck surgeon. We will discuss our management of these aggressive skin malignancies, describing our pretreatment assessment, the principles employed in treating the various subsites in the head and neck, and an overview of the current controversies such as indications for parotidectomy, neck dissection, and temporal bone resection. Also, we will describe available adjuvant or alternative therapies, including chemotherapy, radiation, and re-irradiation. Due to the broad scope of cutaneous SCC and BCC, we will limit our description to non-melanoma skin cancer. In our opinion, cutaneous melanoma represents a different biologic entity with unique pathophysiology and behavior whose management merits separate discussion.

Aggressive Non-melanoma Skin Cancer

The majority of cutaneous SCC and BCC cases arise on sun-exposed areas of the body, accounting for the disproportionate incidence of these lesions on the head and neck. Exposure to ultraviolet radiation, particularly ultraviolet B (UVB) light, has been identified as the primary risk factor for developing NMSC. Once present, a typical NMSC may be treated with any number of techniques, including electrodissection and curettage, cryotherapy, simple excision, topical agents, and even radiotherapy. Cure rates from all of these modalities are comparable, ranging from 90 to 98% across numerous studies. The widespread availability of Mohs micrographic surgery, a technique in which horizontal frozen section analysis is performed in an attempt to achieve total margin control, has improved cure rates for NMSC to ~99%.[4] Nevertheless, a subset of NMSC exists that defies these accepted modalities and demands more aggressive therapy.

Lai and colleagues have described the features of aggressive NMSC, in terms of their propensity to recur, invade, and metastasize.[5] Recurrent tumors, lesions > 2 cm in maximum dimension on initial evaluation, and those exhibiting rapid growth or regional metastases are commonly considered aggressive NMSC. Poorly differentiated or spindle cell SCC, as well as morpheaform and basosquamous forms of BCC, constitute more virulent histopathologic variants.[5] Finally, lesions located in the central "H zone" of the face or at sites of embryonic fusion planes, such as the glabella, nasal root, and melolabial sulcus, have been noted to exhibit more aggressive behavior, with deep invasion occurring prior to extensive surface expansion.[6,7]

Lesions that fit many of these characteristics are more likely to recur following initial treatment, and these are the lesions with which the head and neck surgeon will be faced. With recurrence also comes the issue of advanced disease, metastases, and invasion into adjacent structures, such as the orbit and temporal bone. Thorough patient evaluation and critical decision making with regard to parotidectomy, neck dissection, temporal bone resection, and the use of adjuvant therapies will maximize the ultimate result in terms of local and regional disease control and survival.

Patient Evaluation

Historical Points

Patients with recurrent NMSC who present to a head and neck surgeon have usually been referred by a dermatologist, plastic surgeon, otolaryngologist, or other practitioner. Nevertheless, as with all conditions, a thorough

253

Table 29.1   Risk Factors for Non-melanoma Skin Cancer

Ultraviolet Radiation B Exposure

Patient Characteristics

– Light skin color

– Inability to tan, easily burns

– Light eye color

Precursor Lesions

– Bowen disease

– Actinic keratoses

Immunosuppression

Syndromes

– Xeroderma pigmentosum

– Nevoid basal cell syndrome

– Albinism

– Epidermodysplastic verruciformis

– Epidermolysis bullosa dystrophica

Ionizing Radiation

Polycyclic aromatic hydrocarbons

history and physical examination are the cornerstone of patient evaluation, although radiographic images provide invaluable data for treatment planning. The risk factors for NMSC are widely known and are summarized in **Table 29.1.** Key features in the history include the extent and severity of previous sun exposure, exposure to ionizing radiation, and immunosuppression from infectious, neoplastic, or iatrogenic causes, as in the case of organ transplant patients. Patients should be queried about the duration of the lesion in question, the rapidity with which it has grown, the presence of subjective facial weakness or asymmetry, and the detection of any locoregional pain or paresthesias.

A detailed dermatologic history is mandatory, focusing on the location and previous management of all prior lesions on the head and neck, including premalignant conditions such as actinic keratoses. If possible, medical records, operative notes, and pathology reports should be reviewed for previous treatment of the lesion(s) in question. The pathology reports in particular provide key information regarding the status of surgical margins, depth of invasion, and the presence of perineural invasion—this information may be augmented by having the dermatopathologist review the actual slides or tissue blocks from the outside facility.

Physical Examination

In addition to performing a complete head and neck examination, attention should be focused on the lesion of concern, its relationships to surrounding structures, and the lymph node basins that provide first and second echelon drainage for the anatomical subsite of the head and neck. Careful assessment of the lesion and its mobility relative to adjacent structures is important. Non-melanoma skin malignancies may directly invade the cartilage of the external auditory canal and the bone of the craniofacial skeleton, including the mandible, midface, orbital rim, and calvarium. Preservation of the skin's innate mobility over the underlying bony and cartilaginous framework suggests that these structures are not involved. The external auditory canals and tympanic membranes merit scrutiny under the operating microscope in the setting of an auricular or preauricular primary, as sleeve resection of the external auditory canal and lateral temporal bone resection may be determined based on the visible invasion of the lesion toward or into the middle ear. For periorbital lesions, the eye should be assessed for proptosis, chemosis, extraocular mobility, and visual acuity, as any impairment of ocular appearance or function may suggest gross invasion into the orbital cavity or perineural spread along the infraorbital nerve (V2) or the supraorbital and supratrochlear nerves (V1).

Palpation of the neck, including the parotid gland, may determine whether a parotidectomy or neck dissection will be undertaken. Lymph node metastases in NMSC are more common in SCC, occurring with an incidence of 0.5 to 16%.[8] BCC metastases do occur, but the incidence is negligible. The nodal basins most commonly involved by NMSC depend on the location of the primary lesion, as depicted in **Fig. 29.1.** Lesions of the ear, lateral cheek, and periorbital and temporal regions commonly drain to lymph nodes within the parotid gland, whereas occipital, upper jugular, perifacial, and submandibular lymph nodes provide common avenues for most other sites in the head and neck. When the parotid gland is involved by metastatic NMSC, up to 26% of patients will have clinical involvement of the cervical lymphatics, with ~33% of patients with clinically negative necks exhibiting pathologic nodal involvement.[9] The lymphatics accompanying the external jugular vein are also important sites of metastasis in NMSC. The cervical lymphatics on the contralateral side should also be examined, as lesions of the midface and lip exhibit a propensity for bilateral metastases.

Cranial nerves must also be examined, with particular emphasis on the branches of CN V and VII that innervate the area of the primary lesion, as these nerves are commonly involved by perineural tumor spread.[10] Perineural tumor invasion represents a form of direct tumor extension, rather than a metastatic focus of disease. Aberrant sensation or subtle facial weakness may be detected on close evaluation, although these are commonly late findings.

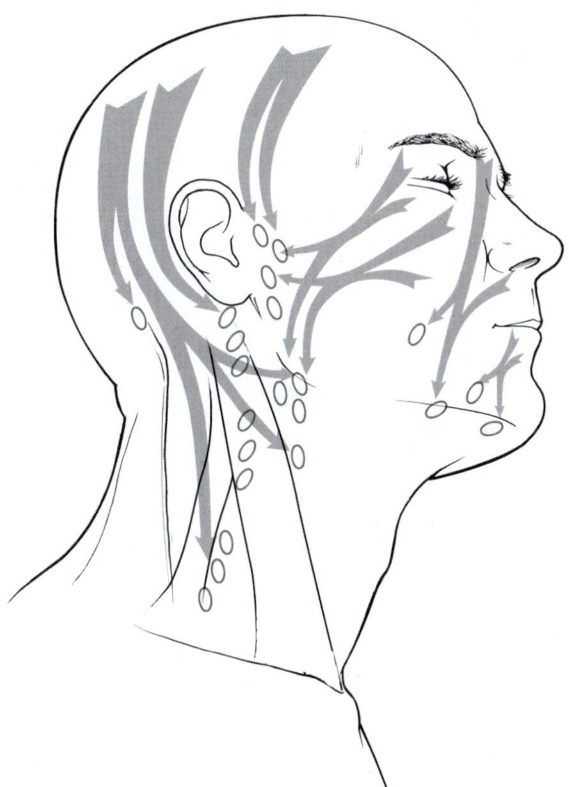

Fig. 29.1 Lymphatic drainage pathways of the skin of the head and neck. Lymph nodes within the parotid bed, the perifacial nodes, and those in levels II and III provide the most common avenues for lymphatic metastases. Anterior lesions involving the lip and midface may exhibit bilateral drainage. Lymph nodes along the external jugular vein also provide a common avenue for metastasis. Note that posterior scalp lesions may spread directly to level V along the spinal course of accessory nerve.

Imaging

We regard imaging as imperative in the preoperative assessment of the aggressive NMSC patient. Although physical examination can provide important information regarding the location of the lesion, its fixation to underlying structures, and motor or sensory nerve malfunction, imaging provides the key data that determine the operative plan. Computed tomography (CT) scanning is the most common modality employed, as it details the extent of soft tissue involvement, bony destruction, spread into the middle ear and temporal bone, orbital extension, and the presence of parotid or cervical lymphatic metastases. By depicting widening of neural foramina or the pterygomaxillary fissure, it can reveal subclinical perineural invasion.[10]

Magnetic resonance imaging (MRI) is used selectively, depending on the location of the lesion and the clinical findings. For deeply invasive scalp lesions, MRI can demonstrate the relationship of the tumor to the dura and vascular structures such as the sagittal sinus. MRI is invaluable in the evaluation of perineural invasion because the affected nerve may be subtly thickened along its proximal course to the skull base. Because deeply invasive lesions may spread to the skull base or sinonasal cavities, MRI is also useful in the differentiation of tumor from secretions. Finally, patients routinely undergo standard chest plain films to screen for pulmonary metastases.

Surgical Management

The goal of treating recurrent NMSC is achieving locoregional control and minimizing distant metastasis, with the ultimate aim of improving patient survival. Although Mohs micrographic surgery has demonstrated great effectiveness for controlling local disease in small recurrences, it is usually inadequate for the aggressive NMSC with which the head and neck surgeon is faced. Nevertheless, we employ the fundamental principles of Mohs surgery during tumor resection: excision of all tumor with a negative three-dimensional margin and preservation, if possible, of key structures such as the eye. The hallmark of our surgical philosophy is to anticipate the aggressiveness of the lesion and perform oncologically sound anatomical dissections of the primary lesion, with management of contiguous structures and metastatic sites driven by preoperative assessment and intraoperative findings.

We do not follow a concrete dictum on surgical margins, although 1 cm margins are the minimum employed for recurrent BCC. Morpheaform BCCs and SCCs generally are resected with initial margins of 1.5 to 2.0 cm. Margins are assessed circumferentially and on the deep surface via frozen section analysis until negative margins are achieved. For the deep margin, we seek to clear the margin one layer beyond the last grossly involved structure. Elimination of gross perineural invasion provides another cornerstone of our ablative philosophy, often necessitating lateral temporal bone resection, maxillectomy, and even orbital exenteration.

Microscopic perineural invasion, in the absence of preoperative symptoms, is resected to the skull base or until the nerve margin is negative, although the possibility of skip lesions mandates the use of adjuvant radiotherapy. Aggressive treatment of perineural invasion with surgical resection to a negative margin (if possible) and postoperative radiation therapy is important, given the association between perineural spread and local recurrence, metastasis, and mortality.[11]

The surgical management of aggressive NMSC does not end with extirpation of the tumor, as reconstruction of the defect should focus on both surveillance and the cosmetic and functional outcomes. We regard reconstruction as another component of the comprehensive care of the head and neck cancer patient. These principles comprise the foundations of our management of NMSC, but each anatomical subsite presents its own unique challenges and considerations.

Scalp

Resection of recurrent NMSC on the scalp provides the clearest example of our management principles. Wide local excision with margins of 1 to 2 cm is the initial step; the challenge arises in determining the depth of resection. If the tumor does not extend beyond the skin or subcutaneous tissues, the pericranium is left in place, as it provides an excellent recipient bed for a split-thickness skin graft. However, if tumor involves the musculoaponeurotic system, the pericranium is sent as a margin and the calvarium is drilled down to the marrow space to accommodate a skin graft. Often the skin graft is delayed until the exposed marrow generates a healthy bed of granulation tissue. This will allow the defect to be more level with the native scalp, providing a more acceptable cosmetic appearance. When the pericranium is positive, but the underlying skull appears normal, then drilling away the outer cortex down to the marrow space will usually clear the margin. However, if the tumor has eroded the outer cortex, then a craniotomy is performed in conjunction with our neurosurgical colleagues, and we will routinely send samples from the surrounding bone marrow for frozen section analysis. If dura is grossly involved, it too is resected (**Fig. 29.2**). The same applies to the brain parenchyma, although invasion into important vascular structures such as the sagittal sinus has been a relative contraindication for continued dissection, provided that the patient is a candidate for postoperative radiation therapy.

More than other head and neck sites, the scalp is amenable to more conservative reconstructive techniques. If pericranium or diploë remains at the base of a wound, the defect may be allowed to heal by secondary intention or covered with a split-thickness skin graft. The poor tissue laxity of the scalp makes primary closure often unsatisfactory, if not impossible. Larger defects, particularly in patients who have previously been irradiated, may require the transposition of vascularized tissue in the form of pedicled flaps or free tissue transfer. Lateral defects may be reconstructed with a pedicled latissimus dorsi flap or an extended island trapezius flap.[12] Free flap reconstructive options include the scapular and parascapular systems, latissimus dorsi, radial forearm, anterolateral thigh, and rectus abdominis flaps.

Ear

For auricular NMSC, we again resect all gross disease with at least one tissue layer of clearance. The potential for subclinical extension and horizontal growth along the dermis and perichondrium, as well as the possibility of deep invasion along embryologic fusion planes, supports aggressive resection in the periauricular region.[13]

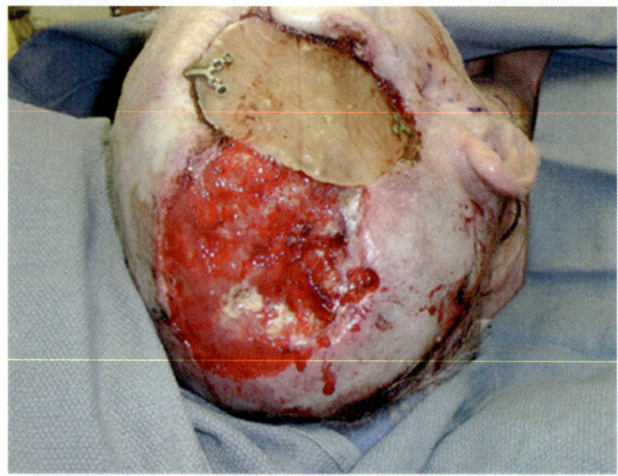

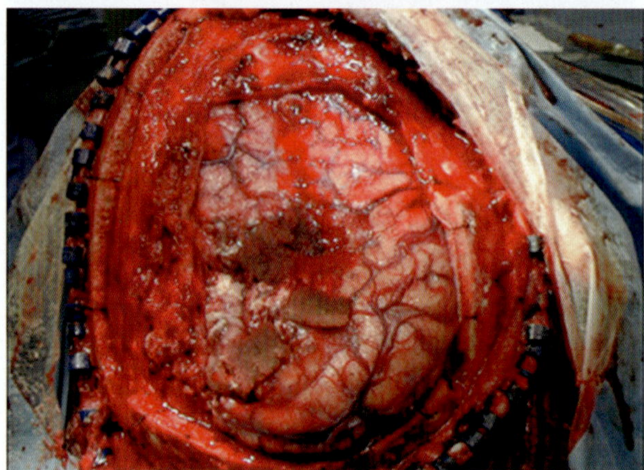

Fig. 29.2 Recurrent basal cell carcinoma of the scalp with invasion through the calvarium into the brain parenchyma. The patient had previously required a craniectomy and cranioplasty for the index lesion 5 years earlier.

The tight apposition of the skin to the perichondrium of the auricle demands that perichondrium be resected in continuity with the lesion. We commonly then resect the underlying cartilage, if it is grossly negative, as a margin and preserve the deeper perichondrium. When the cartilage is clinically involved, we resect that portion of the auricle with a margin of 1 to 2 cm, depending on tumor histology.

Involvement of the tragus and anterior cartilaginous ear canal is carefully assessed, as tumor can spread into the parotid and even into the glenoid fossa through the fissures of Santorini. Again, all gross disease is resected with a wide margin, even if it requires dissection medially toward the middle ear; anteriorly into the parotid, temperomandibular joint, and infratemporal fossa; posteriorly toward the mastoid; and superiorly toward the skull base. In general, we adhere to the indications for temporal bone resection promulgated by Gal and colleagues.[13] Lesions with extension into the external auditory canal that do not extend beyond the bony-cartilaginous junction

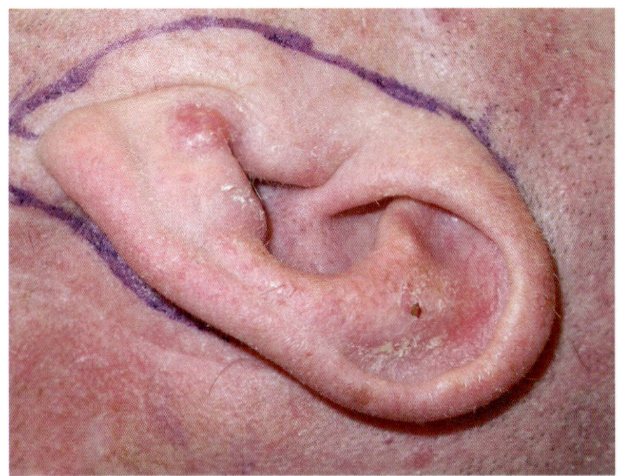

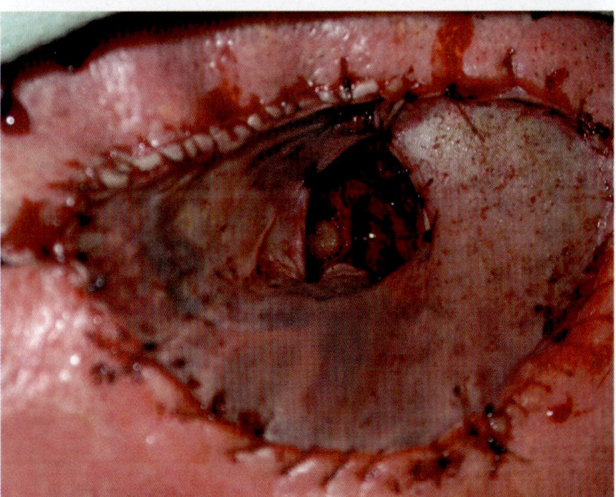

Fig. 29.3 Infiltrative basal cell carcinoma of the auricle. The tumor extended proximally into the cartilaginous external auditory canal. A lateral temporal bone resection was performed, with split-thickness skin grafting of the defect in anticipation of prosthesis placement. (Photos courtesy of Gary Clayman, DMD, MD)

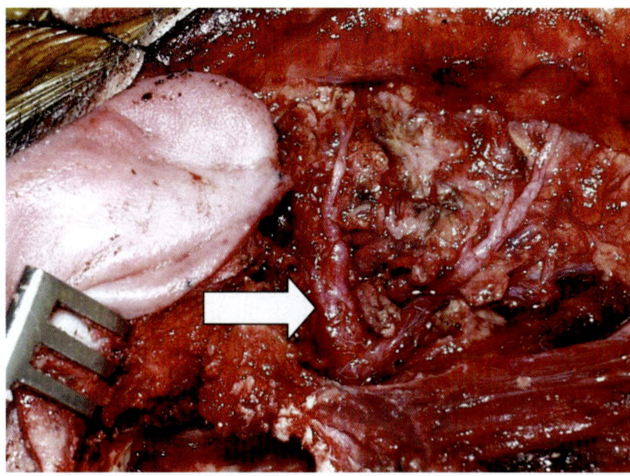

Fig. 29.4 Gross involvement of the facial nerve by cutaneous squamous cell carcinoma. The arrowhead points to thickening and discoloration of the trunk and initial divisions.

are treated with a sleeve resection (**Fig. 29.3**). Extension into the bony canal requires lateral temporal bone resection, and gross involvement of the middle ear space or mastoid merits subtotal temporal bone resection.[12]

Parotidectomy is performed for auricular NMSC if there is clinical, radiographic, or intraoperative evidence of direct extension or lymphatic metastases. Total parotidectomy is the procedure of choice, with preservation of the facial nerve if it appears grossly normal or had normal preoperative function. When the nerve is clinically positive, usually manifest as marked swelling and discoloration, it is resected with a proximal negative margin achieved via lateral or subtotal temporal bone resection, if possible (**Fig. 29.4**). Primary nerve grafting using the medial antebrachial cutaneous nerve or sural nerve is then performed if the proximal, histologically negative nerve stump is in the tympanic or vertical segments.

Reconstruction of auricular and lateral temporal defects follows the principles of the reconstructive ladder, as in all subsites. Most wounds are too large for primary closure, or too extensive and cosmetically important for healing by secondary intention. Full-thickness skin grafts may be used with excellent cosmetic result for aggressive auricular lesions that do not invade into cartilage. For more extensive lesions, the preservation of a small remnant of the superior helix, if oncologically safe, is gratefully accepted by patients who wear eyeglasses. Other reconstructive options for lateral temporal and temporal bone defects include the temporalis system of flaps, pedicled flaps such as the latissimus dorsi, trapezius, and pectoralis flaps, cervicofacial rotation flap, and free tissue transfer.

Orbit

Management of NMSC around the eye remains a challenging issue. In general, periorbital NMSCs that do not invade the maxilla, sinonasal cavities, and bony orbital rim, or that do not exhibit clinical or radiographic evidence of perineural invasion, may be amenable to Mohs surgical excision. The supraorbital and supratrochlear nerves are sampled if they are adjacent to the lesion, and they may be freed from their foramina and dissected within the periorbita to achieve negative margins if they are initially positive in the supraorbital region. When the infraorbital nerve is involved with gross perineural invasion, the orbital floor can be resected to clear the nerve of macroscopic disease. Deep penetration in the medial canthal region and glabella may necessitate external ethmoidectomy or anterior skull base dissection to remove all gross disease. Our indications for orbital exenteration include tumor extension into the orbital apex, entry into the periorbital fat, impairment of extraocular movement, and in situations where microscopic disease will inevitably remain and radiation will be required. Although in these cases, the eye could theoretically be saved, it may ultimately lose function and become a source of chronic pain if it is left in situ.

Myriad techniques are available for periorbital and orbital reconstruction, but this topic is beyond the scope of this chapter. In our experience, orbital exenteration defects may be effectively handled in two ways: obliterating the defect with a free flap, such as a rectus abdominis, or lining the orbital cavity with vascularized tissue, such as a superficial temperoparietal fascia flap (**Fig. 29.5**), followed by placement of an ocular prosthesis. We attempt to save the eyelids if doing so does not

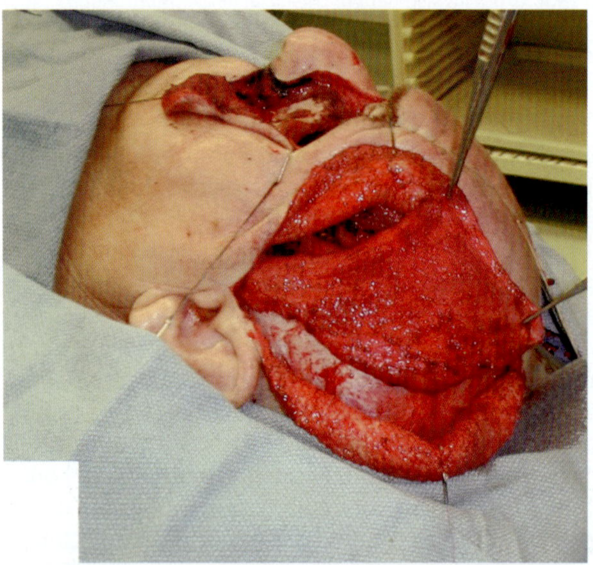

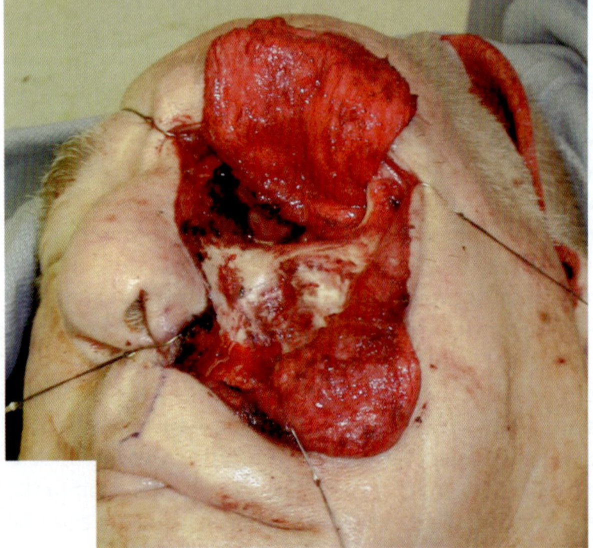

Fig. 29.5 Elevation and rotation of a superficial temperoparietal fascia flap based on the superficial temporal vessels for an orbitectomy defect.

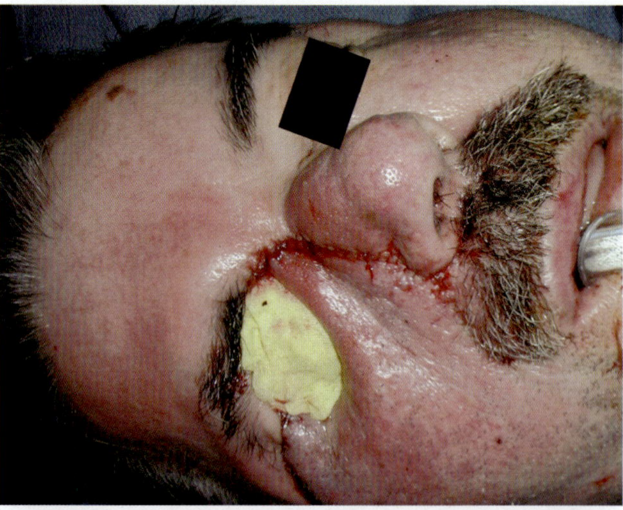

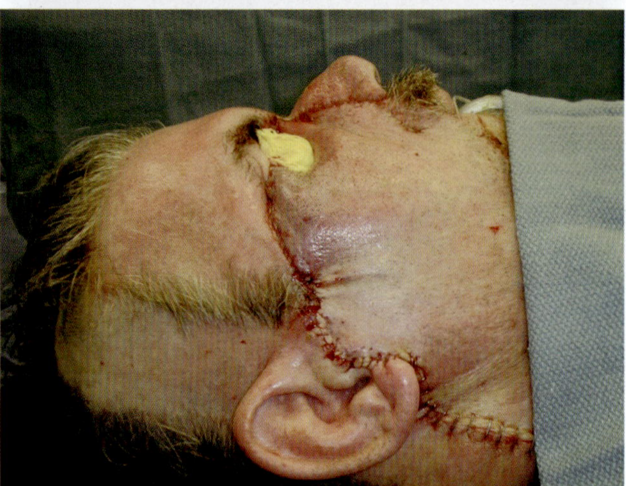

Fig. 29.6 A cervicofacial flap has been employed to close a defect of the medial canthus and lateral nasal wall arising during wide local excision and orbital exenteration. This flap provides excellent color and texture match for defects of the infraorbital region, cheek, and periauricular region.

violate the margins of resection. For lower eyelid and medial canthal defects, elevation and rotation of a cervicofacial flap can provide an excellent tissue match in terms of color and texture (**Fig. 29.6**).

Cheek and Midface

Aggressive NMSCs of the cheek, lip, and midface are managed in a similar fashion to the areas previously described. Incisions are fashioned in accordance with the relaxed skin tension lines or with the local flap design in mind without compromising the oncologic principles. Circumferential frozen section control of margins is accomplished, and the depth of resection depends on the degree of tumor invasion. If necessary, through-and-through defects are created to eliminate gross disease. Tumors overlying the maxilla and mandible may require resection of the periosteum, and tumors affixed to the periosteum may necessitate a medial maxillectomy or marginal mandibulectomy as an additional margin of safety. Again, close scrutiny is given to major sensory and motor nerves in these regions, and evidence of perineural spread is aggressively sought.

Although split- and full-thickness skin grafts may be readily employed for reconstruction of the resultant surgical defects, the pliability of the tissues in these subsites allows some to be closed primarily and the majority to be closed with simple rotational flaps of various design, including rhomboid, bilobed, and melolabial flaps. A cervicofacial rotation flap may also be used to close defects of the cheek, as the anterior incision of the cervicofacial or cervicothoracic flap may be placed at any point in the neck or chest to create the optimum flap for lateral defects (**Fig. 29.7**). Once again, a thorough defect analysis should be performed and the optimum technique chosen by moving up the reconstructive ladder.

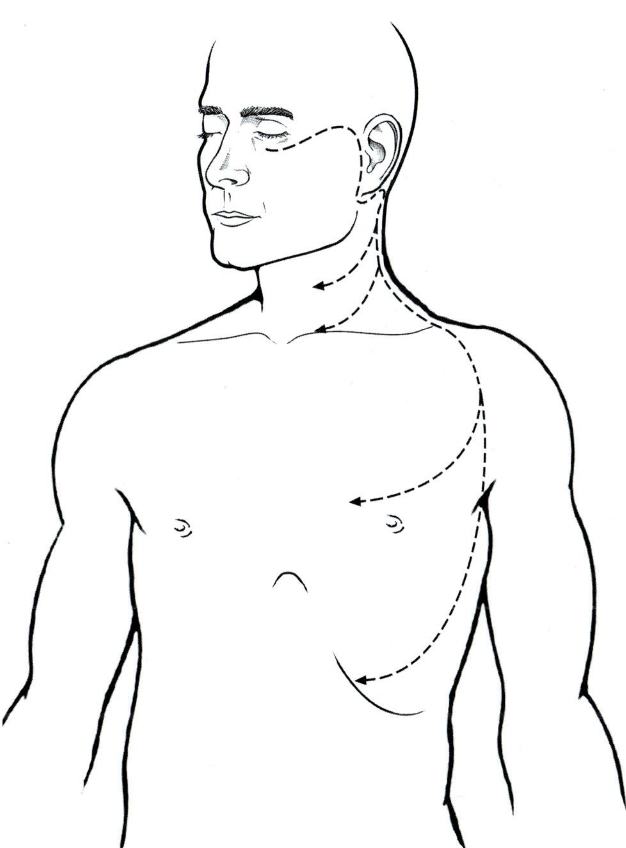

Fig. 29.7 The cervicofacial and cervicothoracic flaps constitute a flexible system of reconstruction of lateral and infraorbital defects, as the inferior limb may be extended as necessary to allow for adequate tissue rotation.

Metastatic Disease

As previously stated, lymph node metastases occur in 0.5 to 16.0% of cutaneous SSC, and they are less common in BCC. Lymphatic drainage pathways in the head and neck are well established for cutaneous malignancies, and these patterns indicate which sites and cervical levels are at risk for a particular lesion. Because the intraparotid lymph nodes provide the first echelon of drainage for the temperoparietal scalp, periorbital region, ear, and cheek, patients with aggressive NMSC often present with palpable parotid masses. In fact, a history of an antecedent skin malignancy should be elicited from any patient presenting with a parotid mass. Previous investigations have demonstrated that the majority of the parotid lymph nodes are located lateral to the retromandibular vein, indicating that they can be lateral or medial to the branches of the facial nerve.[14] Aggressive NMSC may also involve the parotid gland by direct invasion or via perineural infiltration along a branch of the facial nerve or auriculotemporal nerve.

Metastatic disease in the parotid gland has been associated with diminished locoregional control attributed to a higher likelihood of extracapsular spread and resultant positive margins, as well as with cervical metastases.[5,15] Up to 26% of patients with clinically evident parotid metastases have palpable cervical adenopathy, and at least one third of patients with clinically negative necks may have pathologic evidence of disease in the setting of parotid metastases.[9] However, no direct association between parotid metastases and survival has been elucidated. Nevertheless, cervical metastases are an independent risk factor for diminished survival, with advanced neck stage indicating a worse prognosis.[15]

Based on these data, our indications for parotidectomy in NMSC include the following: invasion of the parotid capsule by an overlying NMSC, extension of an auricular lesion into the parotid parenchyma, evidence of perineural invasion along a branch of CN V or VII, and clinical or radiographic evidence of enlarged intraparotid lymph nodes. Although tumors > 2 cm in maximum dimension and depth of invasion > 4 mm have been shown to be associated with cervical lymphatic metastases, we do not routinely proceed with elective parotidectomy, preferring instead to monitor the gland closely for evidence of delayed metastases.[16]

When the decision has been made to proceed with parotidectomy, we perform at least a subtotal parotidectomy, excavating all glandular and lymphatic tissue lateral to the retromandibular vein. Unless the facial nerve is grossly involved with tumor or is paralyzed preoperatively, we make every attempt to preserve it, even sharply dissecting tumor from the nerve sheath. If the nerve is clinically or grossly involved, we will then extend the operation proximally along the course of the nerve as required to achieve a negative neural margin. Minor microscopic disease at the geniculate ganglion may be left behind, as postoperative radiation therapy is given to all patients with perineural invasion, with the ports adjusted to accommodate the projected path of the nerve to the brainstem. After the completion of a standard course of external beam radiation, a boost of stereotactic radiation is often directed at the proximal stump of the positive nerve root.

When the parotid is clinically or radiographically involved with metastatic NMSC, we will perform a selective neck dissection of at-risk cervical zones. For lesions of the lateral face and temperoparietal scalp, our practice is to perform a selective neck dissection of levels II to IV, along with the anterior and superior aspects of level V. Due to the potential for metastases along the external jugular chain, we routinely resect this vessel and its accompanying lymphatics. For lesions of the midface and lips, which are less likely to spread first to the parotid gland, we will perform a selective neck dissection of levels I to III, often dissecting both necks and ensuring that the perifacial nodes are removed.[17] In the setting of obvious nodal metastases, our practice is to perform a comprehensive neck dissection of all levels, preserving, if possible, the internal jugular vein and spinal accessory nerve. The selection of a modified radical neck dissection or radical neck dissection is predicated on obvious invasion of these important structures, and these procedures are infrequently performed.

Neoadjuvant/Adjuvant Therapy

Although external beam radiation therapy remains a reasonable alternative as primary therapy for aggressive NMSCs, we primarily employ it as an adjuvant modality. For early lesions, particularly BCC, radiation therapy has been touted as a means of achieving comparable cure rates to surgical methods in cosmetically important areas.[18] Previous work has demonstrated the efficacy of radiation therapy in controlling primary and recurrent T2 and T3 lesions, as well as stage III lesions in patients who refuse surgery or who are deemed to be poor operative candidates. However, radiation therapy alone has been shown to be inadequate for managing T4 lesions, with 5-year local control rates improving from 50 to 80%.[19] Furthermore, the cosmetic advantage of radiotherapy has not been supported by randomized studies, and there exists the possibility of inducing a delayed soft tissue sarcoma in the radiation field.[20]

Our primary indications for radiation therapy include the following: perineural spread, perivascular invasion, involvement of deep structures such as cartilage and bone, multiple positive lymph nodes, and the presence of extracapsular spread. Histologic subtypes such as spindle cell variants of SCC and the morpheaform or basosquamous forms of BCC are also more likely to be irradiated.

In certain situations, re-irradiation of NMSC may be employed. Patients who have been previously treated with radiotherapy and who recur in the treatment area may readily undergo excision of the involved area, particularly if the initial treatment employed superficially penetrating electrons. If re-excision is not planned, then re-irradiation may also be performed, although with a higher risk of local complications. Data from a small series of patients indicate that the optimum salvage result may be achieved if the accumulated biologic effective dose (BED) is <110 Gy at the skin surface.[21]

Similarly, the use of chemotherapy in NMSC is in its nascence. Preoperative treatment with cisplatin and bleomycin appears promising based on a limited case series, but significant randomized, controlled studies are lacking.[22] We have anecdotal evidence to support neoadjuvant therapy with carboplatin and taxol in extremely aggressive, metastatic NMSC. The most common scenario in which we employ neoadjuvant chemotherapy involves a rapidly progressing parotid mass in a patient with a past history of locoregional NMSC. These patients do not fare well with surgery as a first-line modality, and their response to any form of therapy may be assessed with two or three cycles of carboplatin and taxol. Patients who progress are then treated on a palliative basis, but those who exhibit a complete response then receive concomitant chemotherapy and radiation with surgical salvage, provided they have not been previously irradiated. Patients who have a partial response to chemotherapy are then taken to surgery as outlined in previous sections. We have seen some promising results in this treatment paradigm, although the data have not yet been published (B. Murphy, personal communication, June 2003).

Conclusion

Non-melanoma skin cancer is a worldwide health problem whose incidence is expected to increase, with a concomitant rise in directed expenditures. Although numerous techniques are effective in treating early or primary lesions, an aggressive form of NMSC exists that demands aggressive surgical management, often in conjunction with radiotherapy and chemotherapy. We have described our philosophy and practices in dealing with these aggressive cases of NMSC.

Following a thorough history and physical examination that includes cranial nerve assessment, we prefer to image these patients with CT scanning as a primary modality, reserving MRI for those cases in which there is a concern for perineural infiltration. After widely excising the lesion(s) in question, we then are prepared to proceed with parotidectomy, neck dissection, orbital exenteration, and temporal bone resection, as previously described. We regard reconstruction as an integral component of the comprehensive care of the NMSC patient and let the defect determine the reconstructive technique without sacrificing the oncologic safety of the procedure. We commonly employ adjuvant radiotherapy to maximize local and regional control rates, and we believe that neoadjuvant and adjuvant chemotherapy has an evolving role in the management of aggressive and recurrent NMSC.

References

1. Miller DL, Weinstock MA. Nonmelanoma skin cancer in the United States: incidence. J Am Acad Dermatol 1994; 30:774–778.
2. Armstrong BK, Kricker A. Skin cancer. Dermatol Clin 1995;13:583–594.
3. Chen JG, Fleischer AB, Smith ED, et al. Cost of nonmelanoma skin cancer treatment in the United States. Dermatol Surg 2001;27:1035–1038.
4. Hruza GJ. Mohs micrographic surgery local recurrences. J Dermatol Surg Oncol 1994;20:573–577.
5. Lai SY, Weinstein GS, Chalian AA, Rosenthal DI, Weber RS. Parotidectomy in the treatment of aggressive cutaneous malignancies. Arch Otolaryngol Head Neck Surg 2002; 128:521–526.
6. Panje WR, Ceilley RI. The influence of embryology of the mid-face on the spread of epithelial malignancies. Laryngoscope 1979;89:1914–1920.
7. Baker SR, Swanson NA, Grekin RC. An interdisciplinary approach to the management of basal cell carcinoma of the head and neck. J Dermatol Surg Oncol 1987;13: 1095–1106.
8. Tavin E, Persky M. Metastatic cutaneous squamous cell carcinoma of the head and neck region. Laryngoscope 1996;106:156–158.
9. O'Brien CJ, McNeil EB, McMahon JD, Pathak I, Lauer CS. Incidence of cervical node involvement in metastatic cutaneous malignancy involving the parotid gland. Head Neck 2001;23:744–748.
10. Mendenhall WM, Amdur RJ, Williams LS, Mancuso AA, Stringer SP, Mendenhall NP. Carcinoma of the skin of the head and neck with perineural invasion. Head Neck 2002;24:78–83.
11. Goepfert H, Dichtel WJ, Medina JE, Lindberg RD, Luna MD. Perineural invasion of squamous cell carcinoma of the head and neck. Am J Surg 1984;148:542–547.
12. Netterville JL, Panje WR, Maves MD. The trapezius myocutaneous flap: dependability and limitations. Arch Otolaryngol Head Neck Surg 1987;113:271–281.
13. Gal TJ, Futran ND, Bartels LJ, Klotch DW. Auricular carcinoma with temporal bone invasion: outcome analysis. Otolaryngol Head Neck Surg 1999;121:62–65.
14. Jackson GL, Ballantyne AL. Role of parotidectomy for skin cancer of the head and neck. Am J Surg 1981;142: 464–469.
15. O'Brien CJ, McNeil EB, McMahon JD, Pathak I, Lauer CS, Jackson MA. Significance of clinical stage, extent of surgery, and pathologic findings in metastatic cutaneous squamous cell carcinoma of the parotid gland. Head Neck 2002;24:417–422.
16. Kraus DH, Carew JF, Harrison LB. Regional lymph node metastasis from cutaneous squamous cell carcinoma. Arch Otolaryngol Head Neck Surg 1998;124:582–587.
17. Netterville JL, Sinard RJ, Bryant GL, Burkey BB. Delayed regional metastasis from midfacial squamous carcinomas. Head Neck 1998;20:328–333.
18. Wilder RB, Kittelson JM, Shimm DS. Basal cell carcinoma treated with radiation therapy. Cancer 1991;68:2134–2137.
19. Mendenhall WM, Parsons JT, Mendenhall NP, Million RR. T2–T4 carcinoma of the skin of the head and neck treated with radical irradiation. Int J Radiat Oncol Biol Phys 1987;13:975–981.
20. Avril MF, Auperin A, Margulis A, et al. Basal cell carcinoma of the face: surgery or radiotherapy? Results of a randomized study. Br J Cancer 1997;76:100–106.
21. Chao CK, Gerber RM, Perez CA. Reirradiation of recurrent skin cancer of the face: a successful salvage modality. Cancer 1995;75:2351–2355.
22. Denic S. Preoperative treatment of advanced skin carcinoma with cisplatin and bleomycin. Am J Clin Oncol 1999;22:32–34.

IV
Facial Plastic Surgery

Decision tree for revision nasal tip surgery

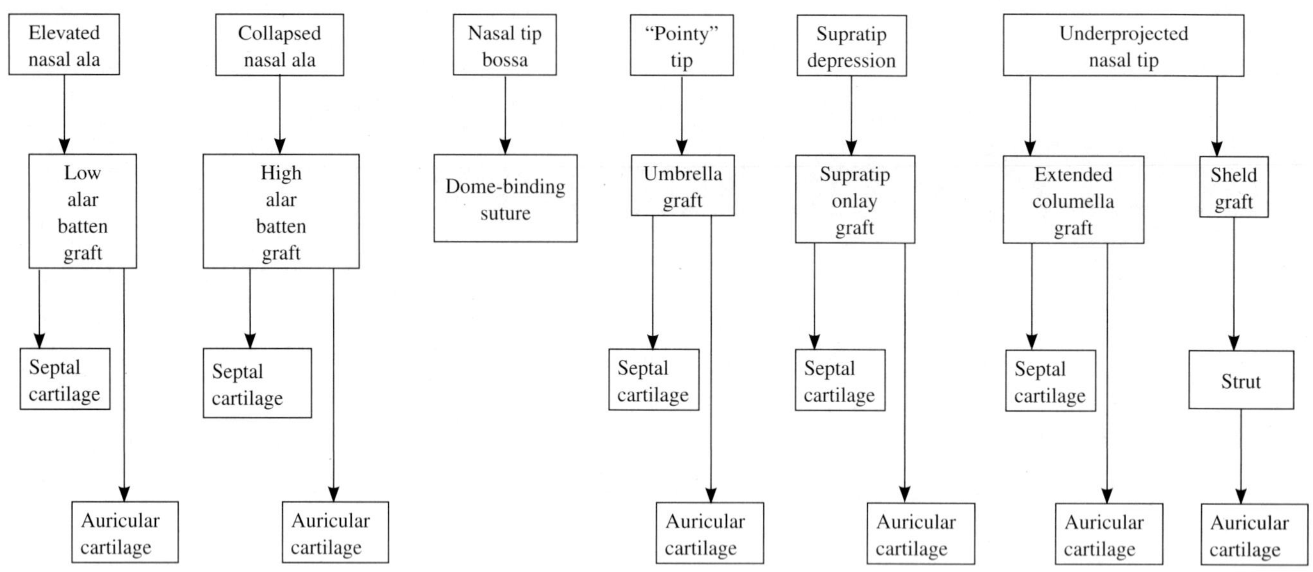

Revision Surgery of the Nasal Tip

Norman J. Pastorek and Frank P. Fechner

Most aesthetic problems following rhinoplasty involve the lower one third of the nose. The ability to adequately and consistently refine the nasal tip remains the holy grail of the rhinoplasty surgeon. Fortunately, most postrhinoplasty tip problems are minor; some, however, can be daunting. Most postrhinoplasty deformities can be repaired with a fairly reliable degree of aesthetic resolution. It is impossible to assure perfection in any case. The most challenging aspect of revision surgery of the nasal tip may be the surgeon's ability to balance the patient's expectations with the reality of what is possible.

Postoperative aesthetic problems in the nasal tip result from an inappropriate preoperative evaluation and diagnosis, an inappropriate operative procedure, or both. Each case where the postoperative result is not adequate should represent a valuable learning experience for the surgeon. In each of these less than desirable cases, the preoperative photos should be examined, the operative plan should be reevaluated, and the operative procedure should be reconsidered. Where did the judgmental error occur? This question must be answered. When the surgeon is dealing with his or her own results, the reevaluation provides a humbling but very important enlightening experience in the quest for consistently good results in rhinoplasty. It is much more difficult, though, when the patient has come for secondary surgery with the primary procedure done elsewhere.

When a patient who has had a primary rhinoplasty comes to the same surgeon for a secondary procedure, it is usually because the patient has faith in the primary surgeon and trusts that he or she can adequately adjust the aesthetic concerns. It is important that the surgeon acknowledge the problem with which the patient is concerned. It is the beginning point for any reasonable conversation about secondary surgery. There is a strong tendency for the surgeon's ego to deny that any problem exists. A comment such as "I don't see any problem" or "It looks fine to me" instantly destroys the patient's confidence in the surgeon. After all, if the surgeon cannot see the problem, how could he or she fix it? The patient's next thought would be, "Maybe I shouldn't have come here in the first place." It is always best to acknowledge the problem (unless there really is no problem) and deal with it from that point. It is much better to say, "I see what you're talking about. It's very minor; I think we should leave it alone." If the problem, however, is significant, the patient should be told to wait for an appropriate time, and a secondary procedure will be done. If the problem is significant and it is beyond the surgeon's ability to correct, the case should be referred.

When the patient has had surgery elsewhere a long time ago, there is a different set of psychological circumstances. Patients who have had their initial rhinoplasty years ago have usually adjusted to the aesthetic problems, and although they have never been happy with the results, they tend not to be hostile. In many cases financial or family circumstances have had a priority in their life. The initial surgeon may no longer be available. Referring such patients back is not an option. These patients usually are realistic about what can be achieved with secondary surgery. With this group of patients, it is unwise to change their appearance too much, especially relative to overall nasal size and retroussé. Many older patients have the small noses that routinely resulted from operations done in the 1960s and 1970s. They have assimilated the small size into their self-image. The secondary procedure should be designed to bring symmetry and harmony to the nose without significantly enlarging it. These patients will not tell you they do not want the nose larger. Unhappiness about the new, larger nose will be expressed following the secondary procedure.

Patients who are seeking secondary rhinoplasty following a recent procedure (1–3 years) represent yet another set of psychological circumstances. Invariably, such a patient has made a decision not to return to the initial surgeon for a secondary procedure. It has been written many times that the primary surgeon should never be admonished about the result. This advice is still true. It accomplishes nothing in helping the patient; Instead, it rekindles any hostility the patient may have. The condemnation of another surgeon always results in some repercussion. It is best to state truthfully that you were not present at the initial surgery and could not possibly know the details of the surgery or the exact reasons that led to the current appearance. You should indicate that you have to examine and evaluate the nose and formulate a plan for secondary rhinoplasty.

Not all patients who come for consultation for secondary rhinoplasty are psychologically fit for surgery. The patient who immediately tells the surgeon that he or she expects perfection from the procedure is not a candidate. The patient who belittles the first surgeon and praises you as wonderful is not a candidate. The patient who brings in photos and diagrams may just be trying to be complete in his or her explanation. A long consultation may be necessary to explain the process and make sure the patient is realistic. If you feel that you have made your case carefully, thoughtfully, and completely, that should be the end of any detailed explanation. When this patient, just before surgery, sends a letter or package of further diagrams and notes detailing minutia, you should cancel the case. These patients are probably obsessive-compulsive, and their nose is the focus of their lives. You cannot make them happy. Patients who you consider less than "normal" in their manner of dress and personal appearance or hygiene also should be suspect. Finally, any patient who makes you feel uncomfortable should be considered inappropriate.

There are certain patients who are not physically suited for surgery. For example, a patient with exquisitely thin skin may not be suitable for any further manipulation of the tip skin and may not be a candidate for grafting. Conversely, a patient with extremely thick skin may also present a problem for revision surgery. Invariably, such a patient had thick skin when he or she presented to the original surgeon. In an attempt to modify the tip contours, most or all of the lower lateral cartilages (LLCs) were removed, leaving the patient with an even worse looking nose. Most of these patients can be helped by nasal tip grafts, but it is the expectations of these patients that may be a problem. These patients always seem to bring photos of models with small, highly refined noses as their ideal. Surgery should proceed only after the patient truly understands the limitations of revision surgery. Multiple nasal tip procedures in some patients have created a subcutaneous scar tissue density that resists expansion of grafts. Some patients complain more about the dense erythema of the nose following multiple rhinoplasties than about the configuration of the nose. Although newer technologies such as laser and intense pulsed light treatments may be of help, these patients should know that the erythema may worsen. Finally, any medical condition that would preclude other elective procedures would also preclude revision nasal surgery.

Most postoperative tip problems result from misjudgments about the preoperative condition of LLCs and a failure to appreciate the significance of thick skin. The most common complaints following rhinoplasty are tip asymmetries (including bossae), poor projection, pollybeak, and tip ptosis. These nasal tip deformities have in common the lack of structural support of the LLCs following surgical intervention. It is almost certain that these patients had LLCs that were relatively nonsupporting before surgery. The second most common complaint is related to alar retraction, alar convexity/concavity, or hanging columella. In the case where tip asymmetries or poor projection has occurred, the surgeon either did not appreciate the relative weakness of the LLCs or did not adapt the rhinoplasty procedure to compensate for the weakness. Where increasing lower lateral strength was imperative, it was instead weakened. In the case of alar retraction, the surgical procedure involved an over-resection of the lateral ala of the LLC or a failure to recognize mild alar retraction preoperatively. The ala retracted superiorly as scar tissue contracted in response to the removed lateral ala cartilage. The hanging columella usually results from over-resection of the ala or a failure to identify a potential for the columella to appear redundant following surgery.

The Elevated Nasal Ala: The Alar Graft

Most ala deformities following rhinoplasty are a combined elevation of the alar rim into an arch with a smaller radius preoperatively and a flattening or concavity of the normal alar arch. This deformity is caused by removal of too much of the vertical height of the lateral crus of the LLC. If at least 6 mm of vertical height of cartilage is left at the conclusion of the rhinoplasty, the appearance of the ala usually is adequate. Almost all alar arch elevation is secondary to overexcision of the lower lateral alar cartilage.

The alar arch can be restored with either septal or auricular cymba concha cartilage grafting. It can be done as an independent procedure or can be part of a more extensive nasal tip reconstruction. The cartilage graft must be placed at a position that is near the alar margin to cause the desired effect. A cartilage graft placed in the normal anatomical position will not lower the alar margin once scar retraction has occurred. A pocket is created by entering the ala through the original surgical incision. The dissection is carried downward toward the alar margin. The ideal end point is 1 mm above the free margin of the ala. The graft need not extend laterally into the alar base when only the arch of the ala is of concern. The graft size in the 22 × 6 mm range is usually adequate. In most cases the alar skin lining is not deficient, and a composite skin–cartilage graft is not necessary. It is rare for the original surgeon to have removed alar skin lining. Once the scar tissue bed between the skin and the alar lining is dissected, the alar lining adequacy becomes evident. If, preoperatively, the alar margin is noted to be not only elevated but also rolled inward, there may be a possibility that alar skin lining may have to be replaced. The most desirable graft in such circumstances would be a cymba concha cartilage graft lined with attached cymba conchal skin. It is important that the graft be fairly straight or slightly curved. If too much effort is used to make the

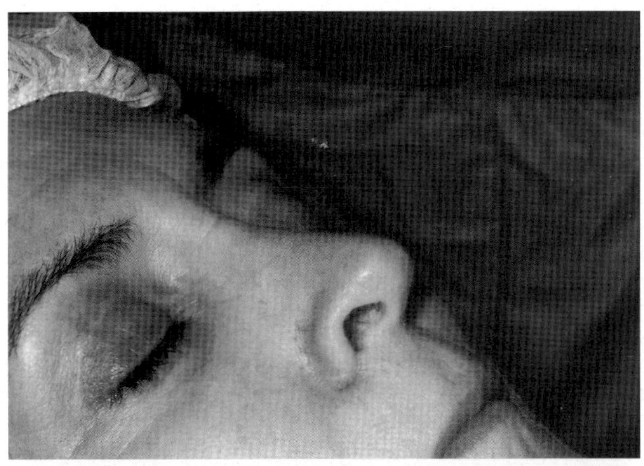

A

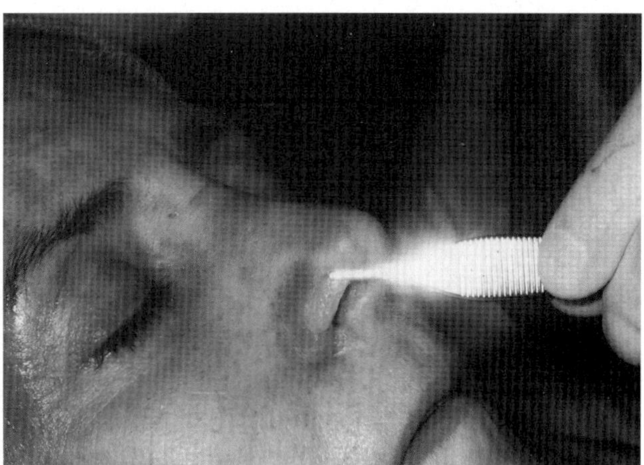

B

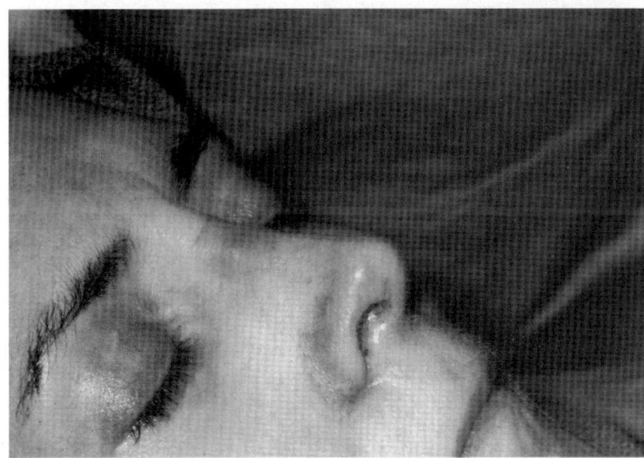

C

Fig. 30.1 **(A)** Postoperative rhinoplasty patient with marked elevation of the right alar margin secondary to overexcision of the lower lateral cartilage. **(B)** Surgical photo indicating the shape and size of the alar batten graft to support the right ala. The graft must be thick enough to be effective, but thin enough so as not cause distortion of the ala. The graft must be placed in a pocket to within 1 mm of the alar margin to effectively lower the rim position. **(C)** Immediate postoperative showing the effect of the alar batten graft placement.

graft curve so that it mimics the curve of the nasal ala, it will curve even more when it is placed in the alar pocket. This can produce an undesirable flaring of the nostril. The cartilage graft will maintain its position if the pocket is the same size as the graft. The alar skin is closed with 4–0 chromic suture (**Figs. 30.1, 30.2**). If a composite graft is used, the alar skin is sutured to the composite graft skin with 4–0 chromic sutures.

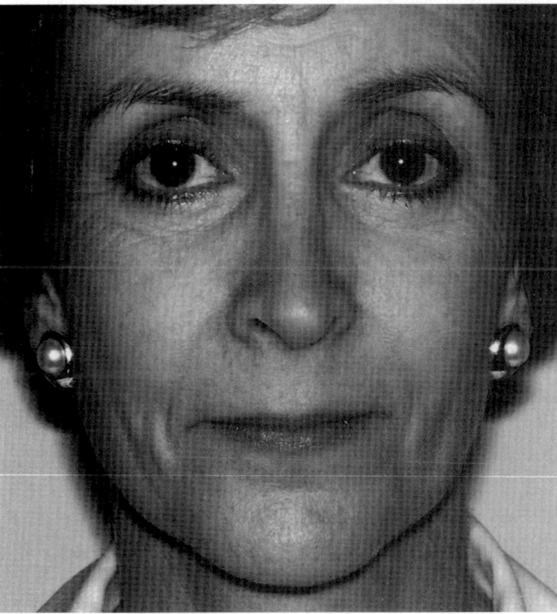

A

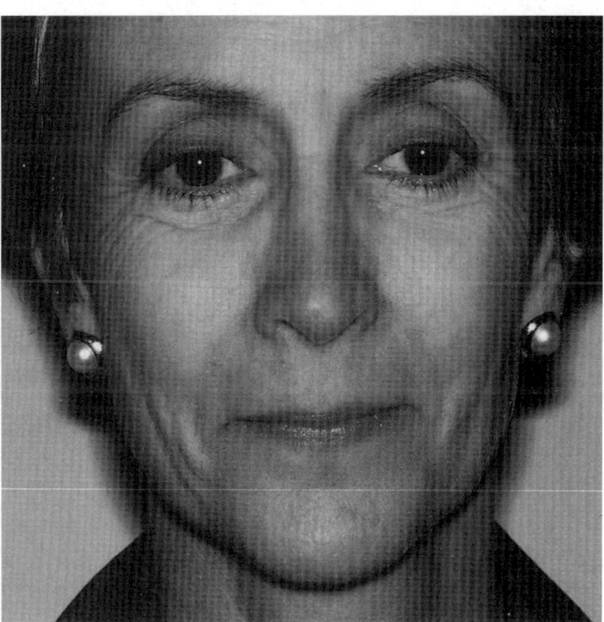

B

Fig. 30.2 **(A)** Preoperative frontal view of elevated right alar margin secondary to overexcision of the lower lateral cartilage. **(B)** Postoperative frontal view following alar batten grafting.

The Collapsed Ala: The Alar Batten Graft

The collapsed ala is a result of the same postoperative contraction that cause the elevated ala but more severe because the airway is compromised. The graft that is used to reverse the concavity is wider and longer and placed at a slightly higher level. This graft is usually thicker and stronger than the alar graft. Besides elevating the concavity at the alar groove region, it must resist the negative pressure of respiration. The graft also must extend to and just beneath the pyriform aperture for support. These grafts can be formed from either septal or auricular cartilage. They can be used as independent grafts to alleviate respiratory obstruction or as part of a nasal tip reconstruction (**Figs. 30.3, 30.4, and 30.5**).

Nasal Tip Bossa: The Dome-Binding Suture

One of the most common complaints of patients seeking secondary surgery is the formation of bossae, either unilateral or bilateral. The patient describes the slow, progressive development of "knobs" or "bumps" in the nasal tip. These bossae are often accompanied by a central tip depression. The cause is related to excision of LLC. The reason for bossa formation after rhinoplasty is always overexcision of the LLC. The remaining LLC could not sustain the central position of the domes. As scar contraction occurs laterally to fill the void created by excision of the LLC, the dome (or domes) is pulled laterally. This lateral dislocation of the dome causes a bossa to occur. There is usually the history of a subtle beginning and progressive worsening until a permanent lateral position is noted. The LLCs following cephalic excision lost their integrity to maintain a central and forward position. The lateral positioning of the domes may be associated with a slight loss of projection. If overprojection was one facet of the preoperative aesthetic problem, then this loss of projection may be welcomed. Simple excision or shave of the bossa via a marginal incision may reduce the bossa, but this usually contributes to an overall roundness of the nasal tip. It is much more functional to approach and mobilize the LLC via intracartilaginous and marginal incisions. The LLC can be examined. It is always a learning experience to see what the previous surgeon has done and relate that surgery to the outcome. Repositioning the lateralized domes into their original midline and contiguous position is

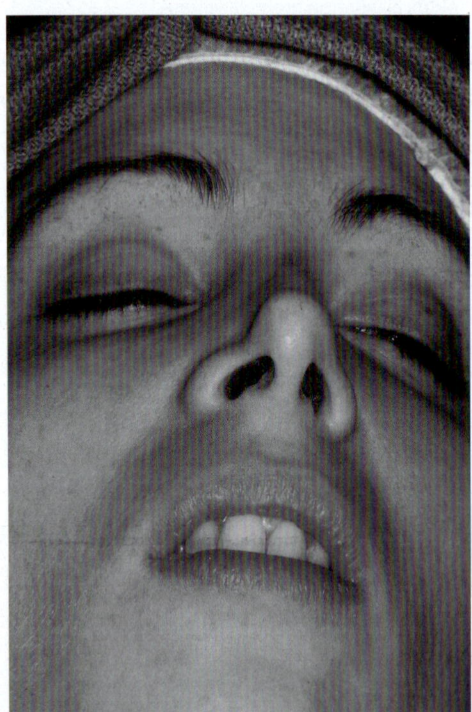
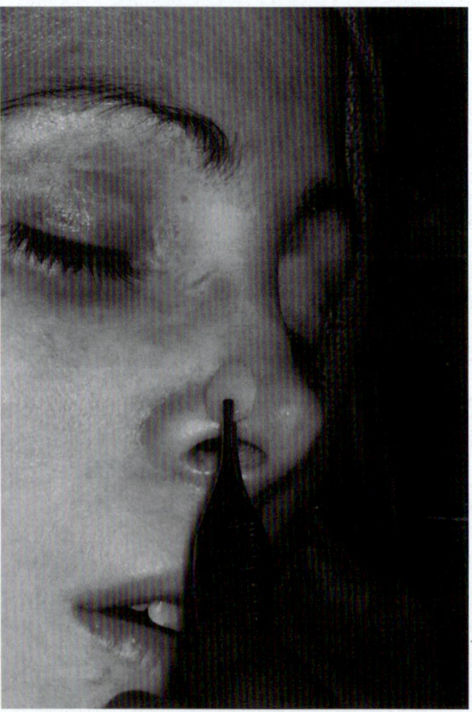

A

B

Fig. 30.3 **(A)** Preoperative surgical view of alar retraction and elevation following overexcision of the lower lateral cartilage and upper lateral cartilage (ULC) on the right. The ala is both collapsed and retracted. **(B)** Operative view showing the size and shape of a septal cartilage graft designed to elevate the collapsed lateral ala and fill the depression caused by excision of the ULC. The graft must extend to within 1 mm of the alar margin to achieve a downward repositioning of the alar margin.

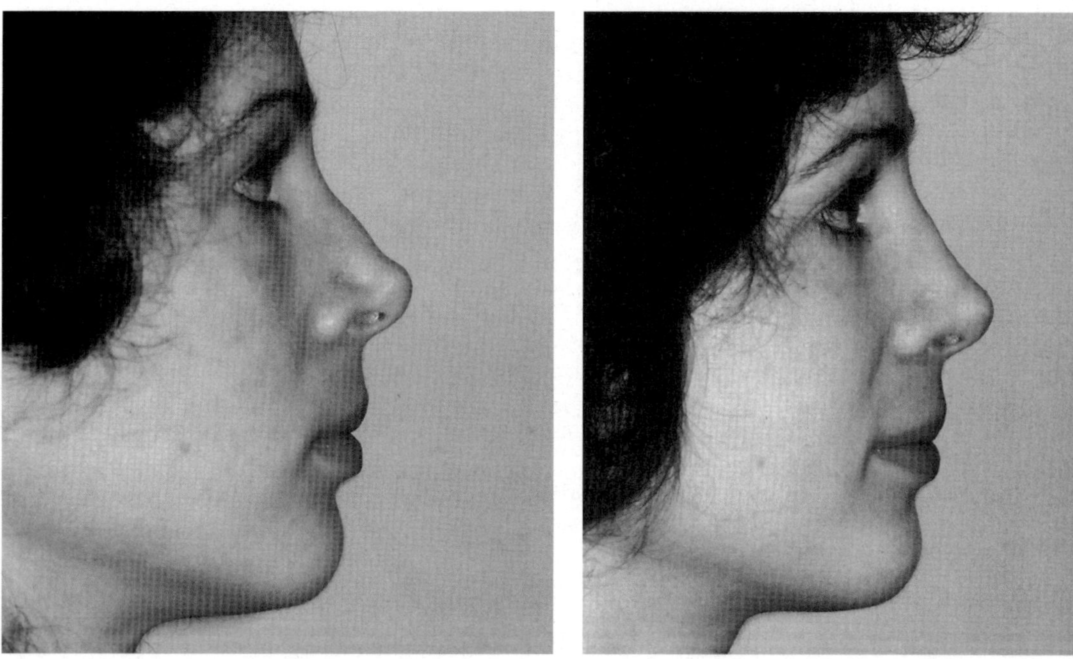

Fig. 30.4 (A) Pre- and **(B)** postoperative lateral view of a patient with an elevated and collapsed right ala.

much more effective in giving the nasal tip its normal triangular shape (rather than unnatural rounded appearance). This is most easily done by using a dome-binding suture. This is a permanent mattress suture with the knot buried between the domes. Suturing the domes at the initial procedure could have prevented the occurrence of a bossa.

The suture gives remarkable support to the entire nasal tip, narrowing it horizontally and projecting it forward. The reason the domes lateralize following rhinoplasty is that the inherent strength of the LLC was lacking. This is an identifiable feature preoperatively. LLC weakness is one of the most important preoperative features to be

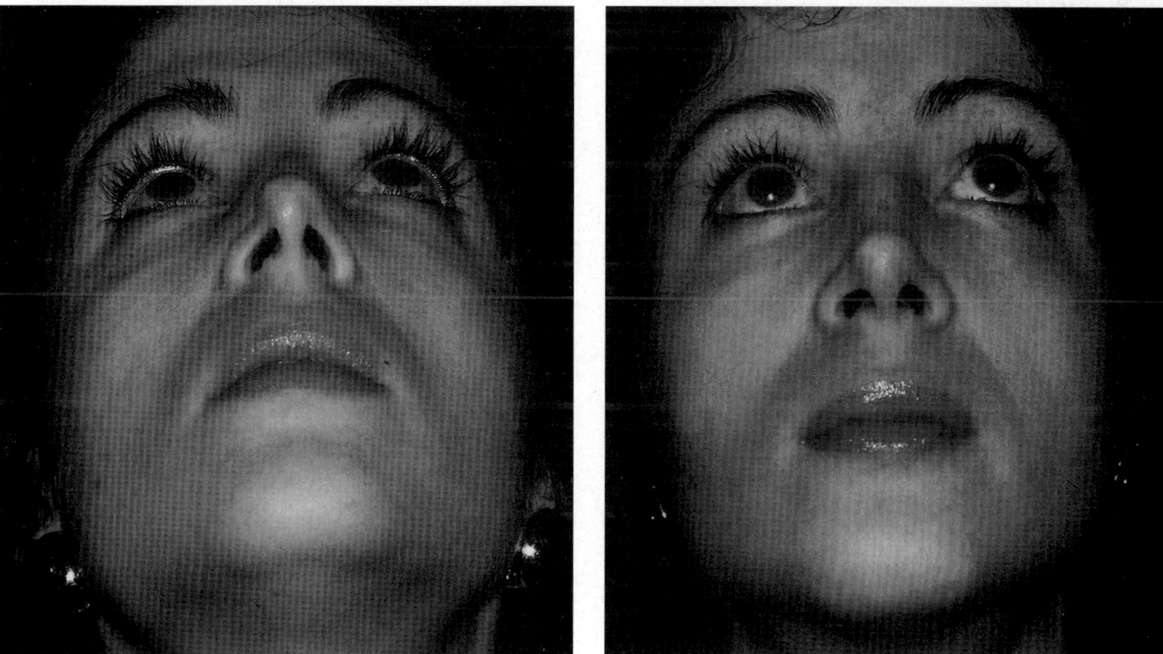

Fig. 30.5 (A) Pre- and **(B)** postoperative submental views of a patient with an elevated and collapsed right ala.

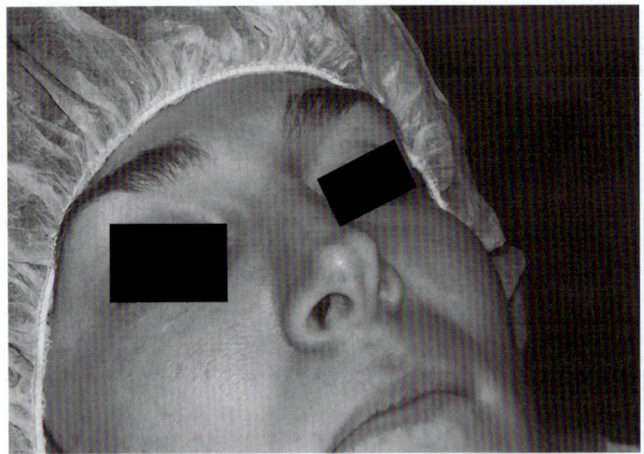

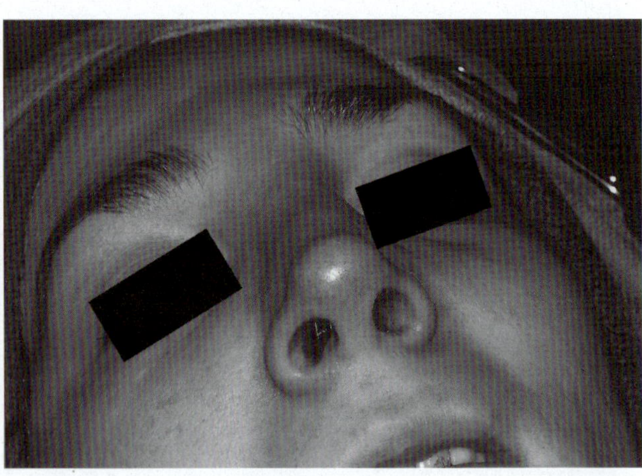

Fig. 30.6 **(A)** Preoperative surgeon's view of a patient with separated domes. The bifidity with central clefting occurs in patients with weak LLC who have had an intracartilaginous approach to the primary rhinoplasty. As the domes drift laterally, they produce the appearance seen in this patient. **(B)** The immediate postoperative view of the patient in **(A)** following delivery of the LLC remnants and application of the dome-binding suture. The bifidity and clefting are eliminated.

determined before surgery (**Figs. 30.6, 30.7**). The weakest LLCs are commonly associated with thick skin in an inverse proportion. When the lateral crura of the LLC were very weak preoperatively, often the medial crura were very weak as well. In these cases a strut must be placed at secondary surgery to support the LCC even though a dome-binding suture has been used to bring the domes forward and centrally into unity.

The Umbrella Graft

Occasionally, the problem with the nasal tip is the patient's perception of sharpness or a complaint that the tip is "too pointy." This can occur following a rhinoplasty where the dome division was performed but the gap between the projecting central crura and the cut lateral crura is great. This results in a sharp, pointed, triangular-shaped tip. In

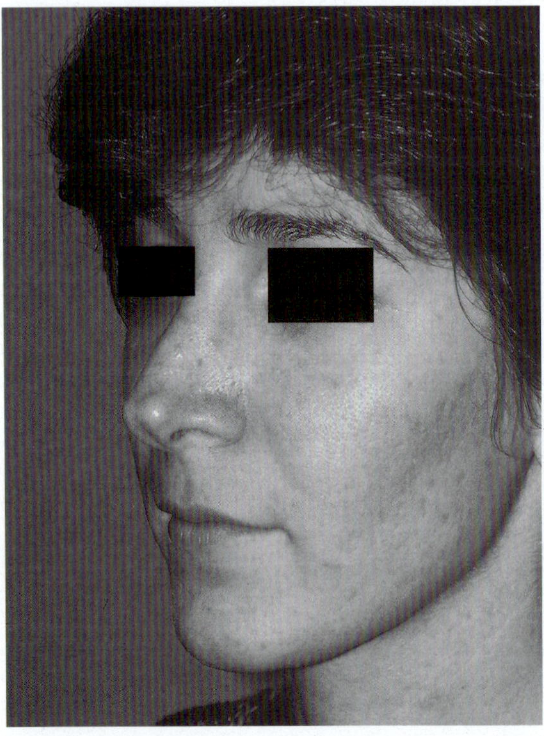

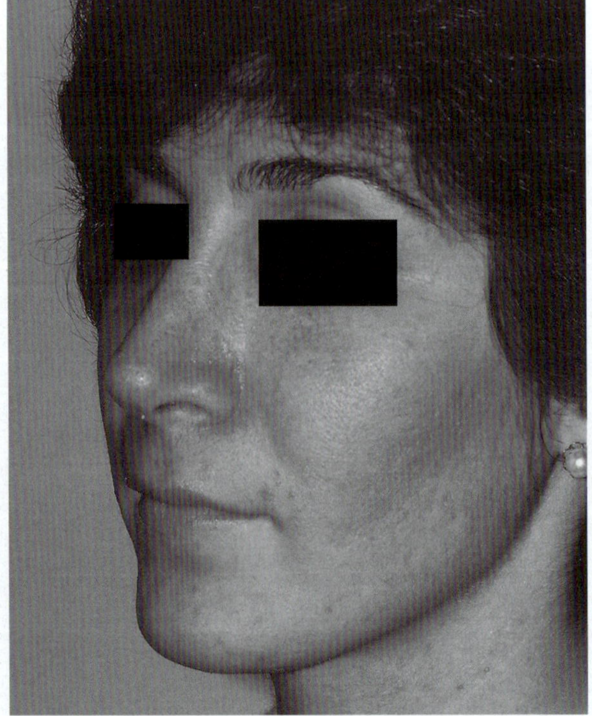

Fig. 30.7 **(A)** Pre- and **(B)** postoperative views of the patient with postrhinoplasty dome separation corrected by the dome-binding suture.

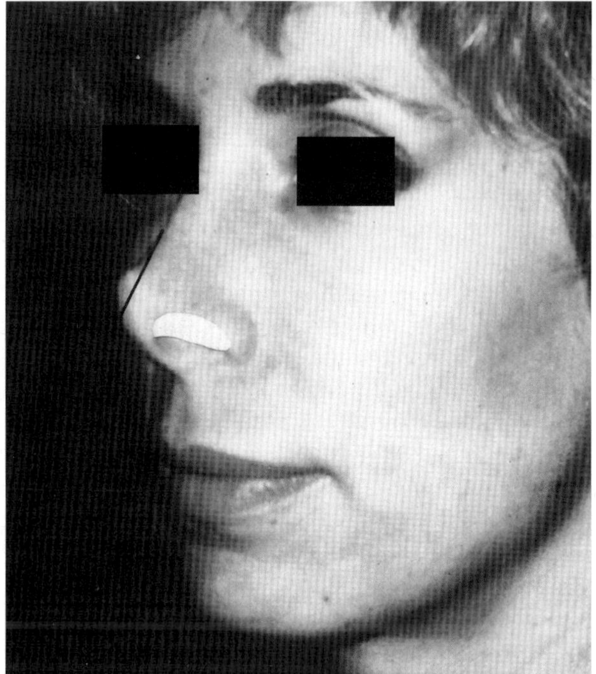

A

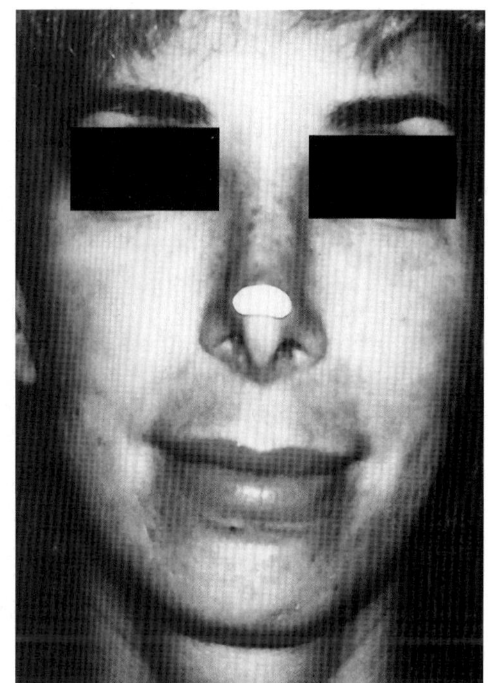

B

Fig. 30.8 (A) Oblique and **(B)** frontal views of a patient who had a dome-splitting-type rhinoplasty performed years earlier. This has resulted in a major tip overprojection. The excision of the lateral ala of the lower lateral cartilage (LLC) has produced marked elevation of the alar margins. The oval-shaped opacity indicates the position of the umbrella graft used to smooth the tip following amputation of the overprojecting medial crura of the LLC. The straight line on the oblique view indicates the level of excision of the projecting medial crura. The opacity over the ala indicates the position of the alar batten graft.

most cases, the resolution requires a delivery approach, with amputation of the offending projecting dome element. To maintain the projection and create tip width, an umbrella graft often is the answer. This graft is ovoid in shape and extends over the tip. It is essential that the edges be shaved sharply to prevent the edges from showing through the tip skin (**Figs. 30.8, 30.9**). The graft must be slightly curved to follow the natural curve of the nasal tip.

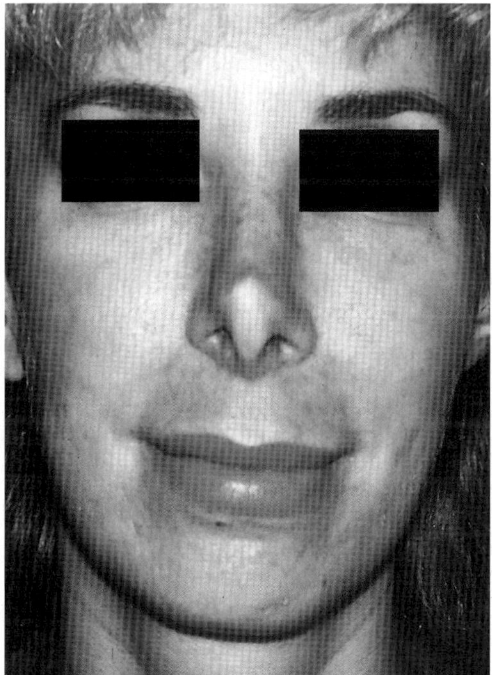

A

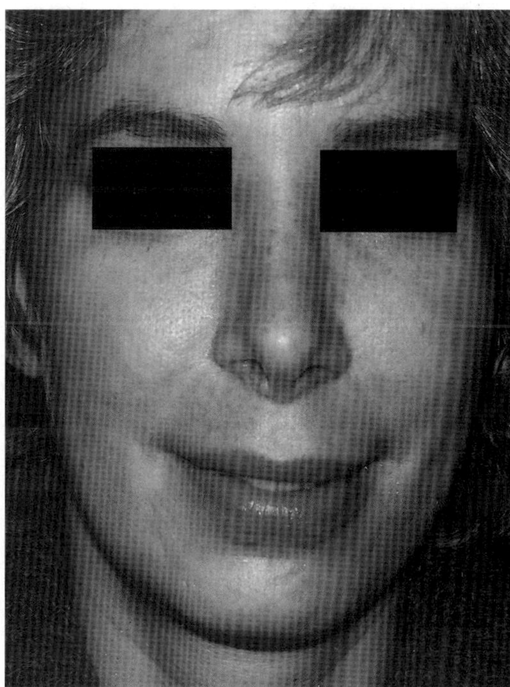

B

Fig. 30.9 (A) Pre- and **(B)** postoperative frontal views of a patient following umbrella grafting of the nasal tip.

The Supratip Onlay Graft

A unilateral concavity immediately above the supratip can result from a deviation of the septal angle of the cartilaginous septum. This deformity can occur as a tip deformity when the LLCs themselves are in good position. The deformity can be corrected if the nasal septum can be straightened to plum midline. If the skin is thin and the deviated dorsal septal angle is all that remains of the nasal septum, it may be impossible to correct this deformity by straightening the septum alone. Partial-thickness incisions on a deviated septum concave surface can be used to move the cartilage in an opposite direction. However, when the deviated cartilage strut is the only support of the nasal supratip, this technique may cause the midnose to collapse. In such cases, an exact-fitting supratip graft can fill the area and give symmetry to the supratip (**Fig. 30.10**).

The Extended Columella Tip Graft

On of the most common postoperative rhinoplasty deformities is a total loss of tip projection. This occurs when the initial surgeon failed to appreciate the inherent weakness of the LLC. The roundness or fullness of the nasal tip in these cases was often approached as needing significant reduction of the LLC. The expectation was that the tip skin would drape over the reduced LLC, producing a more attractive nasal tip. When the LLCs are small, thin, weak, soft, and easily compressible, there is no chance they will retain their quality of projection when they are reduced in size. In these cases, some projection mechanism must be used to cause the tip to either lie at the level of the dorsal line or project forward of the dorsal line. The original surgeon could have prevented the loss of projection by limiting the amount of LLC excision and/or using a columellar strut, a dome-binding suture, a premaxillary graft, or a tip graft to maintain or improve tip projection. Once the problem has occurred, however, usually one or more tip-projecting techniques must be used to move the tip forward and overcome the scar forces that resulted from the initial rhinoplasty. The extended columellar tip graft was developed to both strengthen and stiffen the columella and provide shape and extension to the lobule and sublobule in a single cartilage graft placed endonasally. The graft is best fashioned from the nasal septum but can be formed from the cavum concha also.

This graft is usually placed at the conclusion of the reconstructive procedure. The need for this graft is determined at the time of the preoperative assessment. When the domes of the LLC are retropositioned to such a degree that neither dome binding nor strut placement can produce enough projection, the extended columella tip graft

should be considered. The graft is usually 2.5 to 3.0 cm in length. It is shaped into a long isosceles triangle. The short length of the triangle, which gives form and shape to the nasal tip, is usually ~10 to 12 mm in length. It is important that the edges of the graft be beveled around the entire graft. This is especially true along the edge that lies beneath the domes. The bevel on the surface that is in contact with the skin will turn up slightly, allowing for a soft appearance at the tip. Failure to bevel the edges will result in the graft showing through the skin.

The graft is self-retentive because of the pocket in which it is placed. At the conclusion of the rhinoplasty, all mucosal and septal sutures are placed except at the margin incision on the right (if the surgeon is right-handed). Using a curved Stevens scissors, a pocket is made by blunt dissection, via the marginal incision, beneath the skin of the lobule. The pocket is carefully extended over the feet of the LLC down to the columella–lip junction. It is important that the marginal incision not be extended down onto the columella. It is the long, narrow pocket in the precrural space that will give the graft stability and maintain its central position. Prior to making the pocket, the distance from the columella–lip junction to the leading edge of the domes is made. Two to three millimeters are added for desired extent of the projection. The graft is then prepared once the measurement is determined from the new proposed tip position to the columella–lip junction. The amount of available cartilage will determine how long the pocket will be. The graft must extend at least halfway down into the columella to achieve stability. To place the graft, grasp it with a Brown-Adson forceps and push through the marginal incision onto the lower nasal dorsum, then push it carefully inferiorly into the precrural pocket. At times, adjustments must be made to either widen the precrural columellar pocket or narrow the long dimension of the graft for a proper fit. The surgeon must be mindful that the narrower the graft is, the less projection power it will exert. Also, the narrower the graft, the more risk there is that the graft can fracture. Once the graft is in position, the amount of projection is easily seen. It is better that the tip seem overly projected at this point. There is always some settling of the projection postoperatively. Usually a single chromic suture is needed at the region of the nasal isthmus and another at the area of the junction of the columella and the nares to stabilize and centralize the graft. When the graft is in position, the skin of the nasal tip is gently massaged of edema so the position and projection potential of the graft can be appreciated. It is not a problem to be able to see the outline of the graft at this point. Once the vasoconstriction from the local anesthesia abates, the outline of the graft will no longer be seen. During bandaging of the nose, it may be necessary to place a small Telfa bolster just above the anterior margin of the tip graft to help

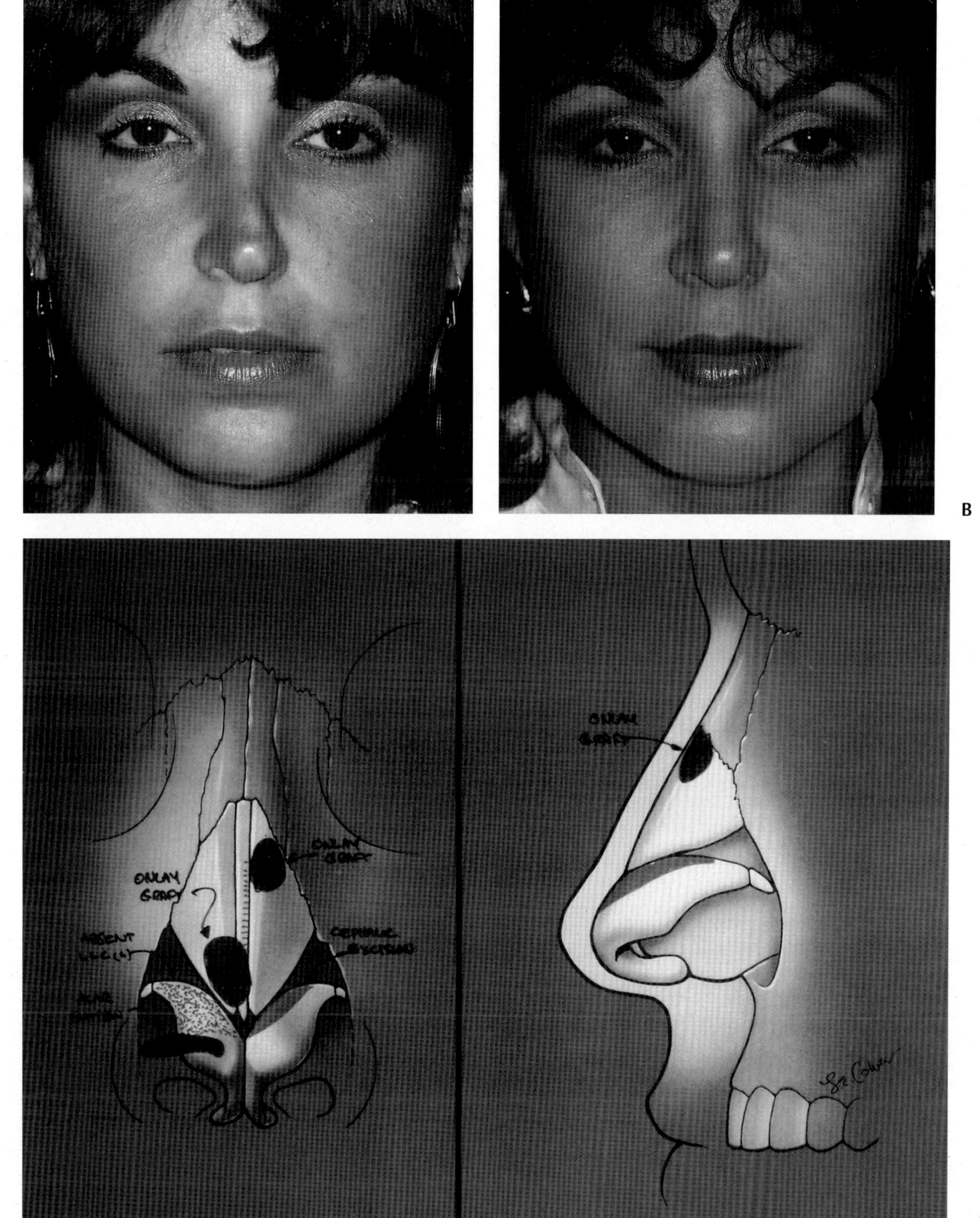

Fig. 30.10 **(A)** Pre- and **(B)** postoperative frontal views of a patient with an acute deviation of the nasal septum at the nasal septal angle. Straightening of the septum and use of a supratip onlay graft produce the normal appearance seen in the postoperative view. **(C)** The surgical diagram indicates the area of supratip onlay grafting. The patient also required onlay grafting and alar batten grafting on the right.

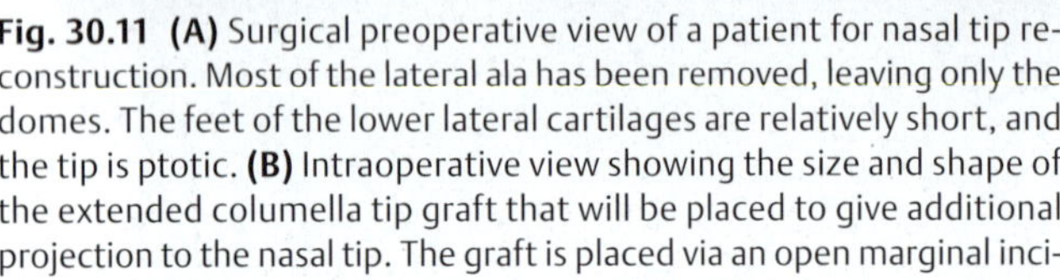

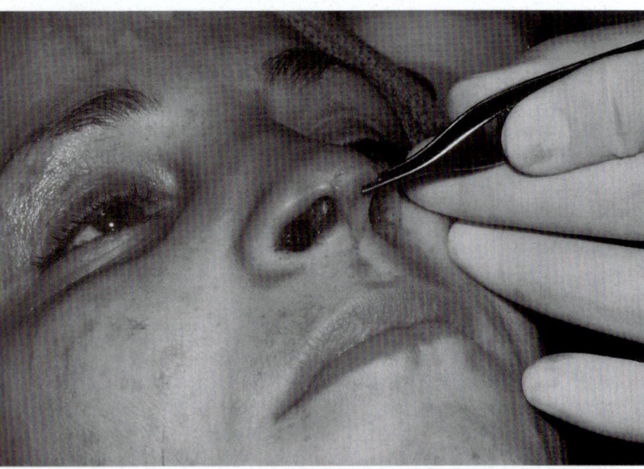

B

Fig. 30.11 (A) Surgical preoperative view of a patient for nasal tip reconstruction. Most of the lateral ala has been removed, leaving only the domes. The feet of the lower lateral cartilages are relatively short, and the tip is ptotic. **(B)** Intraoperative view showing the size and shape of the extended columella tip graft that will be placed to give additional projection to the nasal tip. The graft is placed via an open marginal incision on the right side. All other incisions are closed prior to the placement of the graft. A pocket is dissected in the precrural space down toward the premaxilla. The graft is pushed through the marginal incision onto the nasal dorsum while holding it with a Brown-Adson forceps. The graft is then slowly pulled down into the dissected precrural space. The right marginal incision is then closed with multiple chromic sutures.

stabilize the graft during initial healing (**Figs. 30.11, 30.12, and 30.13**).

The Shield Graft

Occasionally, a projection tip graft is needed, but the cartilage specimens that are available (septal and/or auricular) are not long enough to produce an extended tip columellar graft that is self-stabilized in the precrural space. A shorter triangle of cartilage can be stabilized in the tip by using a suture anchor between the base of the graft and the base of the columella. Any remaining dome remnants are sutured with a dome-binding suture, as described above. This is important even if there is only a small remnant remaining. The sutured domes give a posterior support to the shield graft. Once the rhinoplasty is completed, all mucosal incisions are sutured with the exception of the right marginal incision. The right marginal incision is used to place the graft the last maneuver of the procedure. The graft is as wide as possible at the nasal tip and as long as possible where it will fit into the precrural pocket. A pocket is made via the right marginal incision into the precrural space. The size should just fit the graft. If the graft is placed without an anchor, it is likely to ride up toward the tip. To

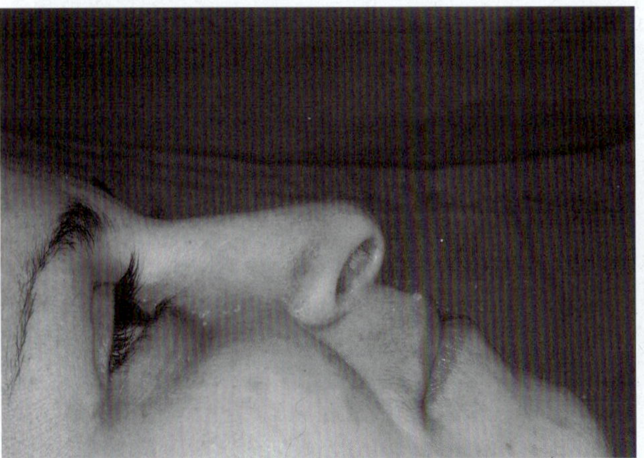

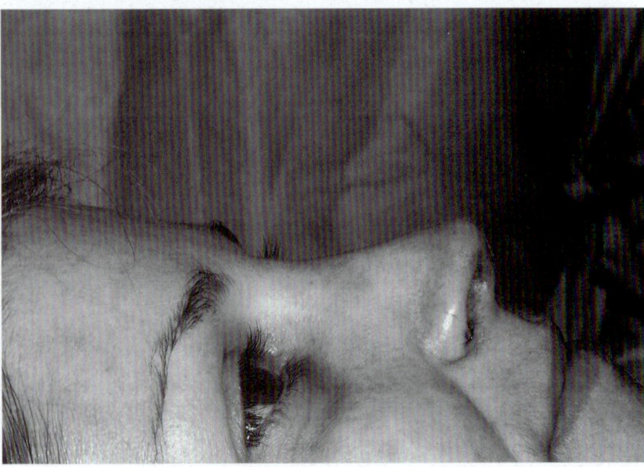

B

Fig. 30.12 (A,B) Intraoperative views of the patient just prior to the procedure and following columellar strut, dome-binding suture, and extended columella tip graft.

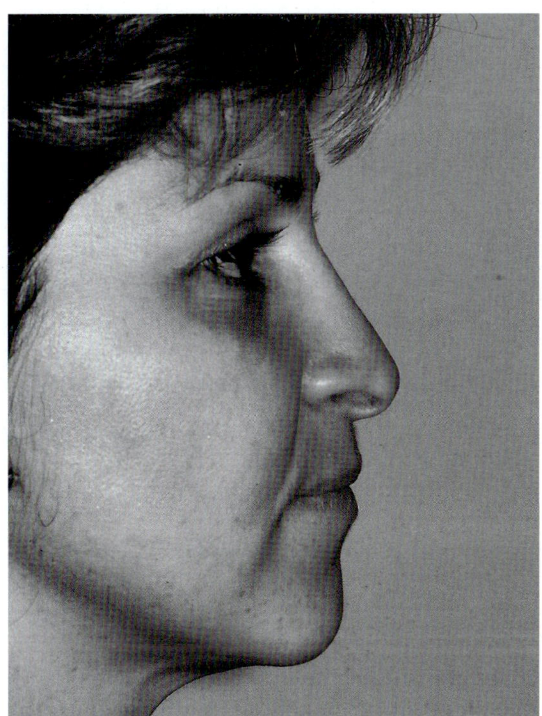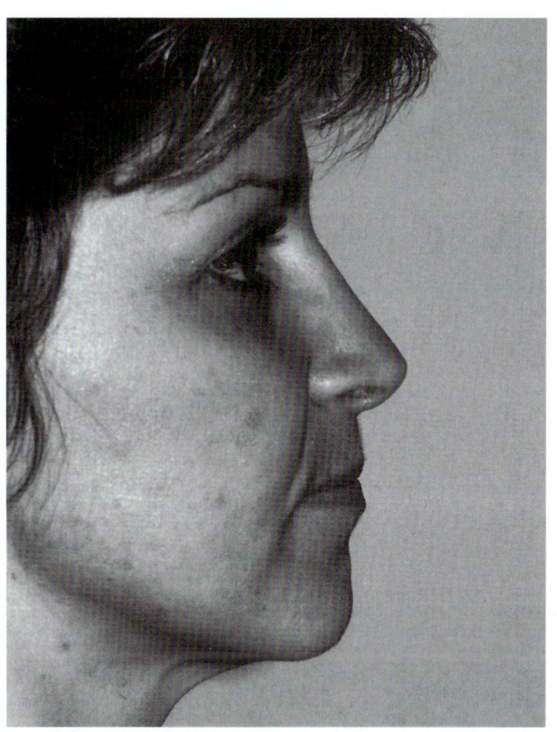

A

B

Fig. 30.13 (A) Preoperative and **(B)** 1-year postoperative lateral views following nasal tip reconstruction.

anchor the graft, a double-armed straight needle 4–0 Prolene is used. One needle is placed through the base of the graft. It is pulled through until the needles are held together as a unit. The needles are placed together as a unit into the precrural pocket, then pushed down along the center of the columella to exit at the columella base. The needles are then pulled to allow the graft to move toward and into the pretrial pocket. Once the graft is in good position, slight tension is placed on the suture so that it is securely in place. Care is taken not to put too much tension on the graft, or the suture may pull through the cartilage. A small square of Telfa (4 × 4 mm) is cut as a bolster. The needles are pushed through the Telfa, and a knot is tied to fit snuggly. This anchor will hold the graft in position. The suture can remain until the splint is removed. The remaining right marginal incision is then closed with 4–0 chromic suture (**Figs. 30.14, 30.15, and 30.16**).

Postoperative Management

The postoperative management following one or more of these grafts is similar to the management of any primary or secondary rhinoplasty case. Antibiotics are used universally. The authors prefer to use a small Telfa wick in both nares until the morning following surgery. The patient is instructed to remove the wicks with a tweezers. A cortisone–antibiotic ointment is used sparingly for several days in each nostril. A paper tape and Aquaplast splint is applied following the procedure and is removed on the 6th postoperative day.

Complications

Complications are no different than any found in the postoperative course following primary and secondary rhinoplasty. Bleeding is always a significant problem following rhinoplasty if packing is required. It is always best if the surgeon who has done the reconstruction sees the patient concerning the bleeding rather than another surgeon who does not have a vested interest in the case. Someone who is interested only in stopping the bleeding may not be as gentle with a recently operated nose. Infection should always be preventable. Liberal use of Betadine is advised for surgical prep, both on the exposed skin surface and in the nares. It is imperative that no permanent suture comes into contact with the teeth. Operative and postoperative antibiotics are advisable in secondary rhinoplasty when grafts are used.

The advantage of the endonasal approach with the grafts described above is that contour on the external nose can immediately be appreciated. The most significant

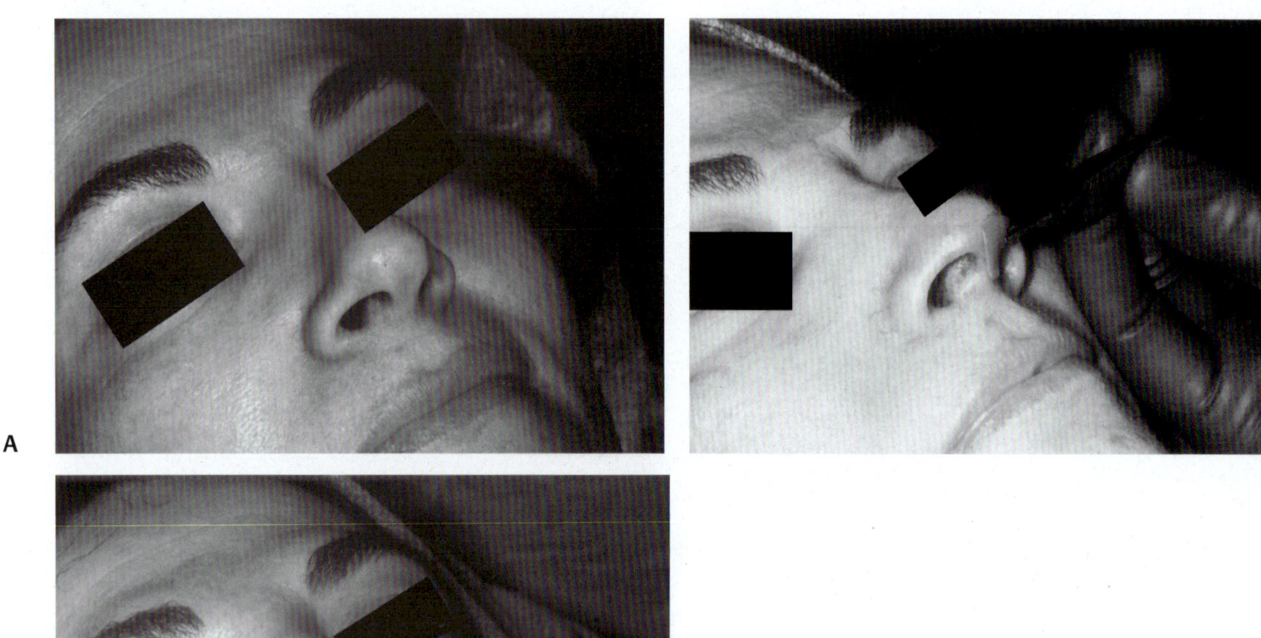

Fig. 30.14 (A) Preoperative view of a patient for nasal tip reconstruction. The patient has lost support of the nasal tip secondary to excision of most of the lower lateral cartilage (LLC). The LLC remnants are weak and nonsupportive, producing a pollybeak deformity. **(B)** Intraoperative view of the size and shape of the auricular cartilage graft to be placed to augment the nasal tip. Septal cartilage was not available because of previous septoplasty. **(C)** Once the tip graft is in position, the needles are pushed through a small bolster of Telfa and tied. This suture remains in position for 4 days.

problem with any of these grafts is the visual aesthetics of misplaced grafts, grafts that are too big or too small, and the perceptible edge of grafts that have not been shaved razor thin. All of these problems can be prevented with focused attention on the detail of graft planning and implantation.

Conclusion

These various grafts and sutures have been used successfully in many hundreds of endonasal revision rhinoplasties involving repair of the nasal tip. Success in revision rhinoplasty requires careful analysis and close attention to the

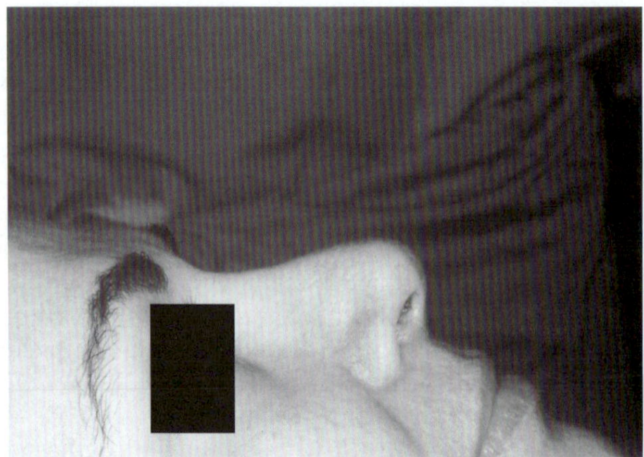

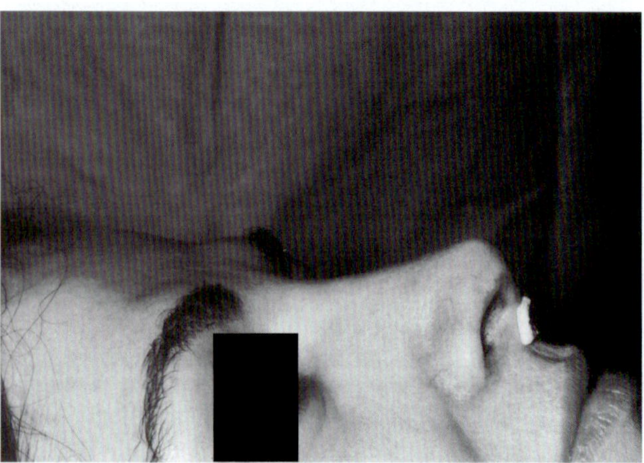

Fig. 30.15 (A) Immediate pre- and **(B)** postoperative lateral views of the patient following placement of the short tip graft.

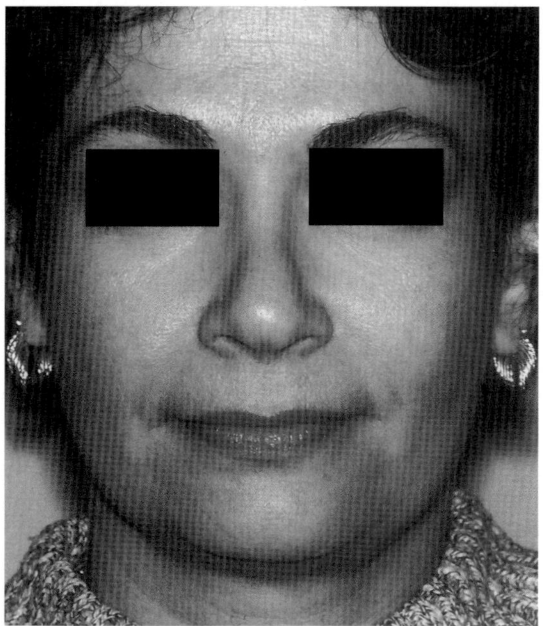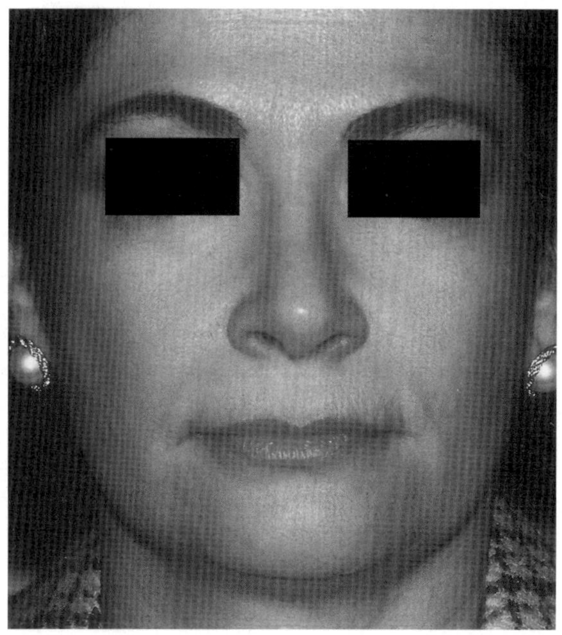

A

B

Fig. 30.16 **(A)** Preoperative and **(B)** 1-year postoperative frontal views following a short tip graft placement to restore projection and form to the nasal tip following primary rhinoplasty.

details of camouflage and projection of the nasal tip. The endonasal approach requires the surgeon to evaluate the deficiencies in the nasal tip prior to surgery. The surgeon must be able to explore the possible need for one or several of the grafts described above and visualize their placement and the effect they will have on restoring the nasal tip to normal. Skin thickness, the amount of remaining cartilage, support characteristics of the remaining cartilage, the position of the remaining cartilage, the type and amount of scarring, the condition of the nasal septum, the presence or absence of the cartilaginous nasal septum, and the availability of auricular cartilage all must be firmly appreciated and be a part of the surgical plan to restore the nasal tip to normal.

Suggested Reading

Gunter JP, Rohrich RJ. Correction of the pinched nasal tip with alar spreader grafts. Plast Reconstr Surg 1992;90(5): 821–829.

Johnson CM, Toriumi DM. Open Structure Rhinoplasty. Philadelphia: WB Saunders; 1998.

Kim DW, Toriumi DM. Nasal analysis for secondary rhinoplasty. Facial Plast Surg Clin North Am 2003;11(3):399–419.

Peck GC Jr, Michelson L, Segal J, Peck GC. An 18-year experience with the umbrella graft in rhinoplasty. Plast Reconstr Surg 1998;102(6):2158–2165.

Rohrich RJ, Raniere J Jr, Ha RY. The alar contour graft: correction and prevention of alar rim deformities in rhinoplasty. Plast Reconstr Surg 2002;109(7):2495–2505.

Sheen JH. Tip graft: a 20-year retrospective. Plast Reconstr Surg 1993;91(1):48–63.

Tardy ME Jr. Rhinoplasty: The Art and the Science. Philadelphia: WB Saunders; 1997.

Toriumi DM, Josen J, Weinberger M, Tardy ME Jr. Use of alar batten grafts for correction of nasal valve collapse. Arch Otolaryngol Head Neck Surg 1997;123(8):802–808.

Decision tree for revision rhinoplasty

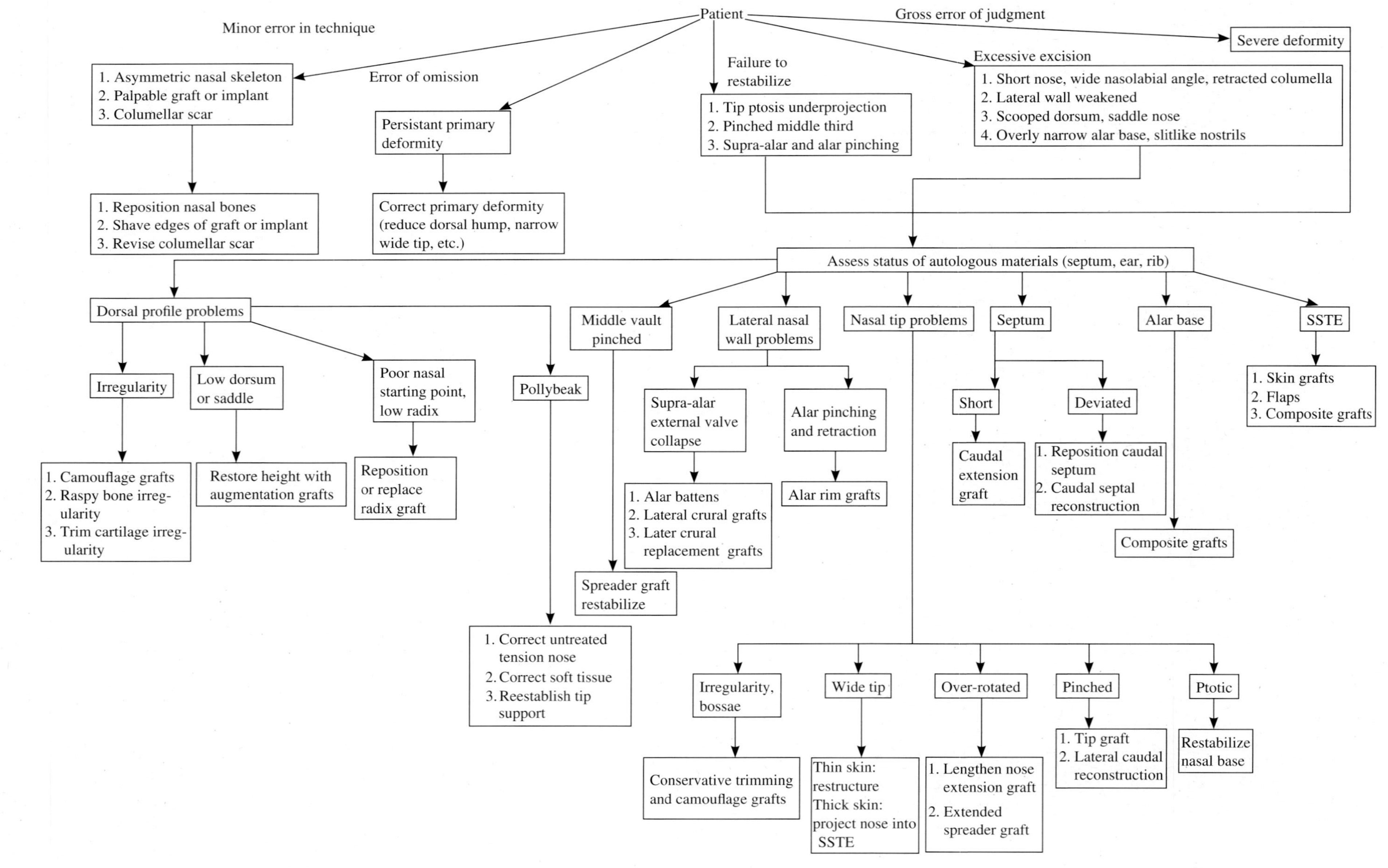

Secondary External Rhinoplasty

David W. Kim, Benjamin A. Bassichis, and Dean M. Toriumi

Surgery of the nose poses numerous unique challenges. There is incredible heterogeneity in nasal anatomy and form. The nose is a prominent three-dimensional structure, in which form is determined by material (bone and cartilage) that is awkward to reshape. Disruption of the nasal structure may lead to weakening and undesired alterations in appearance, particularly in the face of relentless postoperative scar contracture. For these reasons, primary rhinoplasty frequently results in a suboptimal outcome, with a need for revision surgery in an estimated 8 to 15% of cases.[1] Revision rhinoplasty creates additional difficulties. Following primary surgery, the nasal anatomy is altered and highly variable. This compromised baseline means that traditional techniques may be of limited usefulness. Treatment must become based on diagnosing and understanding the problems caused by the previous operations and selecting the correct techniques to address them. Thus, in many ways, the study of secondary rhinoplasty is the study of the complications of primary rhinoplasty.

Patient Interview

It is imperative that the surgeon obtains as much information as possible concerning the problems that led to the patient's visit. The typical individual seeking revision surgery is often more knowledgeable, demanding, and emotional than primary rhinoplasty patients. The patient must understand that the greater the degree of baseline damage, the more limited the possibilities for improvement. Therefore, it is critical that the surgeon instill realistic outcome expectations in these patients. Surgery should not be performed unless common expectations are reached between patient and surgeon.

During the initial consultation, old operative notes and rhinoplasty worksheets may provide useful information. However, they may be incomplete or erroneous regarding grafting material, implants, and previous surgical maneuvers. Pre- and postoperative photographs may help in determining the nature and time course of the given problems. Photographs can also reveal which problems resulted from surgery and which predated the primary surgery. These original images are valuable, as many patients may have had variant nasal anatomy that set up a predisposition to a specific postrhinoplasty deformity.

The physician should list and prioritize patient complaints and gauge how reasonable and achievable these requests are. Functional airway problems that result from anatomical disturbances are surgically correctable. Cosmetic problems should be discussed in detail with the aid of photographs and computer imaging. Each aesthetic complaint should be discussed with regard to possible etiology and prospects for repair.

Physical Examination

Cosmetic nasal analysis of the secondary nose begins with a global assessment of the deformities. Often one or two areas of deformity may be immediately noticeable to the physician. These may include an asymmetric tip, dorsal irregularities, or a narrowed base. It is important to prioritize these deformities during surgery, as surgery on each subunit of the nose affects the appearance of the others. The surgeon must modify a given structure based on the status of adjacent structures. Knowing that one aspect of the nose is particularly problematic allows the surgeon to focus on it and modify the rest of the nose around those corrections.

Analysis should continue with a systematic assessment of each view of the nose. Although analysis of the patient is done in the office setting, quality preoperative photographs allow for more detailed study at a later time. On the frontal view, symmetry and width should be assessed in each of the vertical thirds of the nose. An irregular brow-tip aesthetic line should prompt the surgeon to determine the anatomical cause. Middle vault collapse may be manifest as pinching in the middle third of the nose or as an inverted-V deformity. Previously over-resected lower lateral cartilages (LLCs) may lead to supra-alar pinching and alar retraction (revealed as excessive nostril show). Common iatrogenic tip deformities include pinching, bossae, and asymmetry.

The base view also provides information about the shape and size of the columella, alar base, nostrils, and lobule. Excessively narrowed or asymmetric nostrils, malposition of alar insertion, and the presence of visible scars are signs of complications from alar base reduction. Other stigmata of previous surgery on the base view include alar pinching, tip irregularities, alar notching or pinching, and persistent caudal septal deviation.

On the lateral view, the dorsum is assessed for a smooth profile, nasal starting point, and presence of a supratip break. An over-resected dorsum may lead to a convex appearance in the presence of a projecting tip. A low dorsum will also lead to an appearance of excessive width on the frontal view. A pollybeak may be present as the result of relative supratip excess (soft tissue or cartilaginous) or deficiency in tip projection. In the lower third, the overall projection and rotation of the nasal tip must be assessed. Using Goode's method, the nasal tip projection as defined from the alar crease to the tip-defining point should be just over half (0.55) the length of the nose.[2,3] The ideal length should be based on a nasal starting point near the superior palpebral fold and a tip-defining point determined by the ideal degree of tip rotation. One measure of rotation is the nasolabial angle, which in men should be between 90 and 95 degrees and in women between 95 and 105 degrees. In cases of relative tissue excess or deficiency at the premaxilla, this angle may not reflect the degree of rotation at the tip and infratip lobule. In these cases, use of the columellar facial angle may be more appropriate.[4] This is the angle formed by the intersection of the columella and a vertical reference line perpendicular to the Frankfort horizontal line. A common secondary deformity occurs after excessive caudal septal resection and cephalic trim of the LLCs. In such cases, the nose is foreshortened, the nasolabial angle overly obtuse, and the ala retracted. In other cases in which the nasal base was previously inadequately supported, the tip may become ptotic, resulting in a long nose with an acute nasolabial angle. Both lateral views should be compared, as deformities may differ from side to side.[5]

The surgeon must note the thickness and sebaceous quality of the nasal skin–soft tissue envelope (SSTE). Particularly in thick-skinned individuals, previous reduction of the underlying skeletal framework may cause significant scarring in the dead space. This can cause the SSTE to be exceptionally thick and inelastic. Further structural reduction should be avoided in these patients so that subsequent additional scar formation may be prevented. In such cases, one should augment the relative deficiency of the underlying structural framework to project into the thick soft tissue envelope. An advantage of such thick SSTE is that irregularities of the underlying nasal skeleton and grafts are camouflaged.

The SSTE may have been overly thinned, damaged, or devascularized during prior surgery. The presence of acquired cutaneous telangiectasias, purple or blue discoloration of the nasal skin with cold temperature, and visible irregularities are signs of such a condition. In these patients, the dissection of the SSTE of the underlying structural framework must be precise and deliberate, as extensive soft tissue elevation will increase the risk of ischemia and wound breakdown. Although patients with thin skin may not have injury to the SSTE, it is important to remember that there is added risk of contour irregularities becoming visible or palpable. Care must therefore be taken to ensure that all existing bony and cartilaginous structures, grafts, and implants are precisely positioned and smoothly contoured. The benefit of thin skin is that general contour changes made at the time of surgery will translate into similar final contours postoperatively, requiring less of a compromise on what one would consider an ideal aesthetic outcome.[6]

It is crucial to obtain an assessment of the patient's nasal airflow, which should be undertaken prior to and after decongestion of the nasal mucosa. The surgeon must note the external stigmata of an obstructed nose or one that is prone to develop postoperative problems. These characteristics include thin SSTE, a narrow or collapsed middle vault, short nasal bones, supra-alar pinching, a prominent supra-alar crease, narrow nostrils, and thin lateral nasal walls. Intranasal exam may reveal a narrow internal valve angle, internal recurvature of the lateral crura, dynamic lateral wall collapse, septal deviation, inferior turbinate hypertrophy, mucosal synechiae, or shortage of lining from prior excision. Assessment of dynamic function should be performed by observing the lateral wall of the nose with inhalation. Obvious collapse indicates lateral wall weakness. Significant improvement of breathing by supporting the lateral wall with a small instrument may predict airway improvement with placement of a supporting graft to the lateral wall. All of these factors must be considered in formulating a surgical plan that will restore or preserve a functional airway.

Palpation of the nose is important to determine the shape, position, and strength of the nasal structure. Dorsal irregularities may not be visible beneath a thick SSTE and may require digital palpation to be detected. An attempt should be made to trace the LLCs to assess position and stability. The resistance and recoil of the nasal tip to digital pressure will provide information of tip support. Finally, palpation of the caudal nasal septum will help to determine the position and integrity of the caudal septal strut.[7]

General Considerations

Patients who seek revision rhinoplasty may come with any number of problems. Small asymmetries, malposition, and irregularities may occur as the result of errors of omission or technique. These problems are generally straightforward and easily corrected. Significant asymmetries, functional obstruction, and gross deformities are more likely to result from errors of judgment. In such cases, the primary surgeon may have been overly aggressive in excisional or reductive maneuvers or failed to resupport destabilized structures. These problems may not become apparent for years and may therefore escape the awareness of the original surgeon.

There are several categories of complications, each of which results from different types of surgical errors. Identification, diagnosis, and correction of these problems depend on a thorough understanding of the surgical pitfalls and postoperative processes. The various groups of complications are listed in **Table 31.1.**

A common problem is one of subtle asymmetry or malposition of structures, grafts, or implants secondary to technical errors. In thin-skinned patients, imprecise graft placement or uneven excision of cartilage may lead to cosmetic imperfections. Asymmetric skeletal modifications can lead to nasal pyramid imperfections. These complications are typically minor and are readily correctable. An exception to this is the case of alloplastic implants that become infected and have begun to extrude. Though such a problem can be easily corrected by removing the implant, if left untreated, the infection can become serious and lead to permanent damage to the nose. Additionally, these implants may lead to a contractile process of the skin envelope, making it difficult to re-expand the area of desired augmentation. Failure to reapproximate the columellar incision exactly and appropriately can result in a visible scar. Even after an appropriate and technically sound operation, the forces of scar contracture, mechanical trauma, and edema may result in an imperfect outcome.

Errors of omission result in variable degrees of postoperative problems, depending on the severity and nature of the original problem. This type of error, often committed by an inexperienced or overly conservative surgeon, may be evident in preoperative photographs. Common examples include the twisted nose, asymmetric middle vault, and various tip deformities. These problems are readily corrected with the proper techniques.

A third class of error involves failure to resupport destabilized structures. Many maneuvers in primary rhinoplasty require disassembling the various support structures of the nose. Left unsupported, these destabilized areas become more susceptible to the forces of scar contracture, gravity, and facial mimetic function. The most common problems of this type include failure to stabilize the nasal tip at the base after compromising tip support mechanisms, failure to resupport the upper lateral cartilages onto the dorsal nasal septum after cartilaginous hump removal, and failure to support the lateral nasal wall in patients with a lateral wall deficiency. Correction of such problems usually requires structural grafting techniques to restore strength to the nasal framework.

A more problematic type of error is one of excessive reduction and excision. Excessive caudal septal resection, lateral crural cephalic trim, dorsal hump reduction, alar cartilage division, and alar base reduction may result in an assortment of cosmetic and functional sequelae. The type and severity of deformity resulting from over-reduction of the underlying nasal structure partially depend on the quality of the SSTE. Many of these problems are challenging to repair, as there is a deficiency of tissue that may not be able to be replaced. This is particularly true when a portion of the internal lining of the nose has been excised.

Table 31.1 Complications and Errors

Class of Surgical Error	Common Examples	Resulting Deformities
Minor error of technique	• Asymmetric skeletal modification (e.g., osteotomies, dome sutures) • Malpositioned graft • Malpositioned implant • Poor closure of columellar incision	• Asymmetric nasal skeletal • Palpable or visible graft • Palpable or visible implant (possible infection) • Columellar scar
Error of omission	• Various	• Persistent primary deformity
Failure to restabilize	• Failure to stabilize nasal base • Failure to stabilize middle vault • Failure to stabilize lateral wall	• Tip ptosis and underprojection • Pinched middle third, collapse of ULC, inverted V, internal valve obstruction. • Supra-alar and alar pinching, dynamic external valve obstruction
Excessive excision	• Caudal septum • Cephalic trim of LLC • Dorsal hump reduction • Alar cartilage division • Alar base reduction	• Short nose, wide nasolabial angle, retracted columella • Lateral wall weakness, supra-alar and alar pinching, alar retraction • Scooped dorsum, saddle deformity, bony open roof, middle vault collapse • Palpable or visible graft • Overly narrow alar base, narrow slitlike nostrils
Gross error of judgment	• Various	• Possible severe deformity

LLC, lower lateral cartilage; ULC, upper lateral cartilage.

The final category of error represents deformities stemming from gross errors of judgment. Although the problems outlined above may result from the poor execution of a reasonable surgical strategy, this last class of deformity usually results from a fundamentally flawed plan. These problems may be catastrophic and may not be possible to correct. These mistakes may stem from faulty analysis, disregard for basic principles of rhinoplasty, or use of improper techniques. The inexperienced but aggressive surgeon is most likely to commit such an error. These problems are varied and tend to cause a highly unnatural appearance. Some of the most difficult cases involve situations in which large areas of soft tissue have been excised or violated (**Fig. 31.1**).

Grafting Material

Inspection of potential sources of autogenous grafting material will aid in surgical planning. Palpation of the nasal septum and conchal cartilage aids in determining the amount of remaining cartilage available. At a minimum, a 1.0 to 1.5 cm dorsal-septal strut must remain for support of the nasal bridge and tip. The cartilage incisions should not extend into the peripheral vertical component of the concha or into the eminentia corresponding to the root of the helix to avoid distorting the shape of the ear. If there is a clear shortage of septal and auricular cartilage, the possibility of costal cartilage harvesting should be considered.[5]

Specific Deformities

The common problems requiring revision surgery are outlined according to determinants of preoperative analysis. For any given deformity, the thickness of the SSTE will determine the likelihood of its being detected and diagnosed prior to surgery.

Nasal Septum

Caudal Septum Deviation

Persistent caudal septal deviation is one of the most common causes of a significant postoperative deviated tip and nasal airway obstruction. Intranasal examination should focus on the shape of the caudal septal margin. It may be tilted, C-shaped, fractured, or dislocated from the nasal spine. The nasal spine itself and the posterior septal angle must be examined for position and symmetry. The remainder of the septum must also be thoroughly visualized to check for persistent bony spurs or cartilaginous deviation obstructing the airway. The strength and caudal-cephalic position of the caudal margin must be assessed to determine the ideal method of correction. A severely weakened or retracted septum may require reconstruction with a large caudal extension graft. A strong, severely deviated caudal septum may need to be removed and replaced with a straight segment of cartilage.

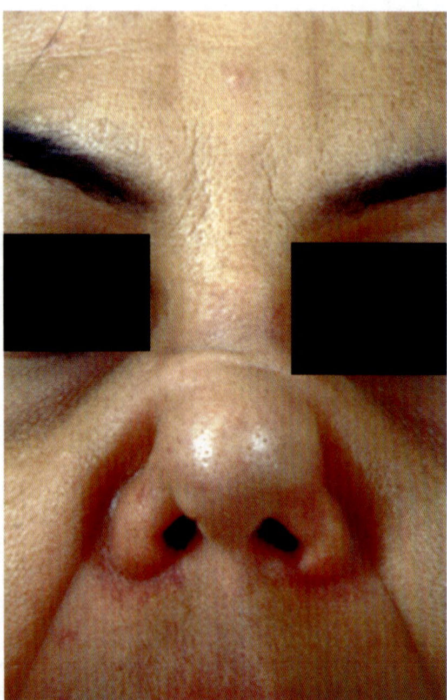
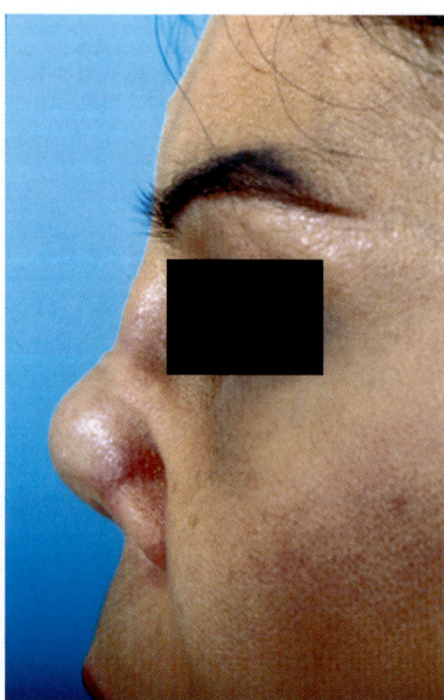

Fig. 31.1 (A,B) Patient with a severe deformity resulting from previous over-reductive rhinoplasty and a destructive infection of an alloplastic implant.

Caudal Septal Excision (Short Nose)

Excessive caudal septal excision may result in rotation of the tip and a foreshortened nose. With the entire tip tripod cephalically rotated, the nasolabial angle is widened and the columella retracted. Careful analysis of the nasal base, tip projection and rotation, and palpation of the caudal margin of the septum is critical. The internal vestibular lining should be inspected for previous resection, as redundancy of skin and mucosa would ensue following septal truncation.

Correction requires restoring septal length with a caudal extension graft and fixating the tip cartilages onto the new caudal margin. Minor deformities may be addressed with plumping grafts at the premaxilla for posterior caudal septal deficiency or columellar onlay grafts. If there is a shortage of vestibular lining, an assessment must be made whether or not the compromised SSTE will tolerate expansion with such grafts. If not, a composite graft must be considered.

Lateral Nasal Wall

Weak, unsupported lateral nasal walls may lead to a variety of postrhinoplasty problems. Destabilization of the lateral wall due to aggressive cephalic trim of the lower lateral crura or division or resection of the alar cartilages may lead to this problem. In addition, a failure to correct preexisting lateral wall weakness and supra-alar pinching, failure to support the alar lobule and margin in patients with inherently weak cartilage, and failure to address cephalically positioned lateral crura may lead to lateral wall problems.

Supra-alar and External Valve Collapse

Exaggeration of the supralobular crease may represent an inherent deficiency of cartilage and support of the lateral wall of the nose. This is exaggerated in individuals with narrow, projecting noses. This deformity can also develop as the result of scar contracture on the tissue void caused by previous excision of lower lateral crura. Aggressive cephalic trim and interruption of the lateral crus will decrease support of the lateral wall and contribute to eventual collapse, which is best detected on frontal and oblique views. Inspiration may lead to further dynamic collapse of the weakened external valve. Intranasal inspection may reveal fixed or dynamic inspiratory medialization of the alar lobule. Improvement of breathing achieved by supporting the lateral wall with a narrow instrument such as a cotton tip applicator or cerumen loop confirms this diagnosis. A standard Cottle maneuver is not sufficiently specific or localizing as a test for insufficiency

of the lateral wall. The degree of collapse may vary in severity and will require appropriately sized alar batten grafts for correction.[8,9] These grafts are curved cartilaginous supports placed into the area of maximal lateral wall weakness. Through the external approach, the grafts are placed into tight pockets that overlap and extend lateral to the lateral crura. The curvature of the graft should be oriented to lateralize the supra-alar area with the concave surface medial. The lateral aspect of the graft is usually caudal to the lateral crura, depending on the area of maximal pinching. In severe cases, the grafts may extend to the pyriform aperture to add support. In cases in which lateral recurvature of the native lateral crura impinges on the nostril width, the lateral crura may be sutured to the alar batten grafts for lateral stabilization. Internal vestibular stents may be placed in the postoperative period to prevent postoperative medialization of the lateral wall. These stents may be constructed with pliable plastic stents or segments cut from a standard nasopharyngeal tube (nasal trumpet) and may be maintained in the nasal vestibules while the patient sleeps for a period of 3 to 12 weeks, depending on the severity of the initial problem.[10–12]

Alar Pinching and Retraction

Excisional techniques of the lateral crura may cause weakness and contracture at the nostril margin. Cephalic retraction may cause alar retraction and excessive columellar show (unless the columella itself is also retracted). The alar margin may be notched at the apex in cases where the internal vestibular skin has become scarred from a poorly healed incision. On the lateral view, there should ideally be a columellar show of 2 to 4 mm. A distance exceeding this range suggests the presence of either a retracted ala or a hanging columella. An imaginary line through the long axis of the nostril on the lateral view serves as a marker to help in differentiating these possibilities. Normally, the top and bottom of the nostril should be equidistant to this line. If the distance of the top of the nostril to this line significantly exceeds the distance from the bottom of the nostril to the line, alar retraction is present. The converse is true for a hanging columella. This comparison may be applied in cases of decreased columellar show to differentiate between a hooded ala and a retracted columella (**Fig. 31.2**).[13]

Contracture from previous reduction of the LLC may also be evident on the base view. Particularly in cases in which the LLC are weak or cephalically positioned, excisional techniques may lead to destabilization of an inherently weak alar margin and visible alar pinching. This can also occur if the tip cartilages have been previously narrowed excessively using vertical dome division, lateral crural flap, or excessive tightening

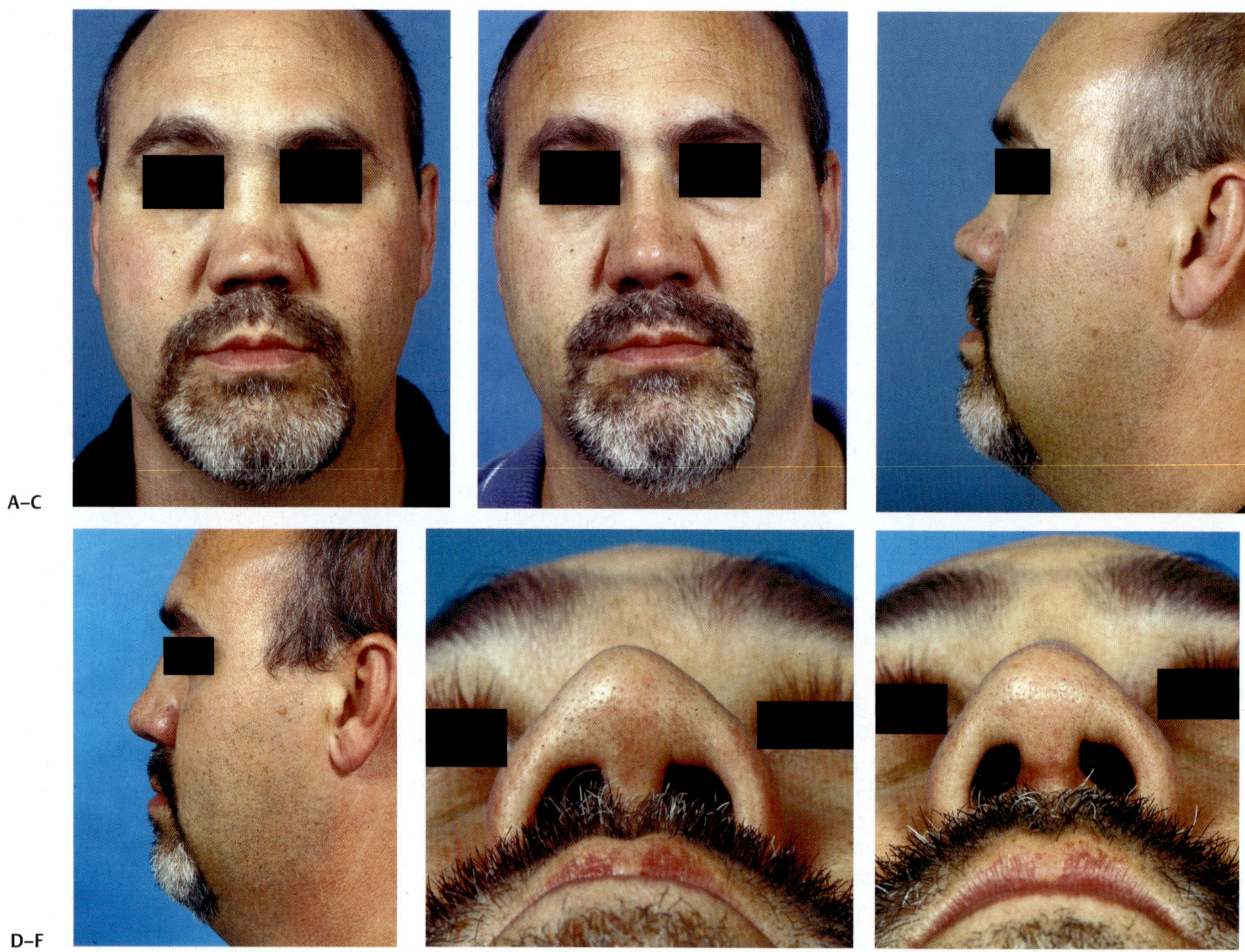

Fig. 31.2 Patient with severe alar retraction from a previous aggressive cephalic trim. Note the excessive columellar show on the lateral and oblique views and the prominence of the nostrils and infratip lobule on the frontal view. Correction required placement of alar rim grafts and internal composite grafts to the vestibular alar margin. Preoperative **(A,C,E)** and postoperative **(B,D,F)** frontal, lateral, oblique, and basal views.

of dome sutures. The nostrils may be thin and slitlike and become more prone to collapse with inspiration.

Cephalically positioned LLCs provide less support for the alar margin. Any maneuver that narrows the tip may lead to alar margin weakness in individuals with cephalic LLCs. This orientation may be detected prior to surgery by palpation of the tip and supratip areas. When curved and prominent, this anatomical variation will manifest as a parenthesis deformity on the frontal view, in which the tip is seemingly enclosed between two curved parentheses (corresponding to the caudal borders of the alar cartilages). If the SSTE is thick and the cartilages are flat, this variation may go undetected until surgery.

Placement of alar rim grafts may restore support and create a more triangular nasal base. These grafts are long, narrow cartilaginous grafts that are placed into precise pockets along the alar rim just caudal to the marginal incision. They measure 2 to 3 mm in thickness and width and 5 to 8 mm in length. Softer material, such as cartilage harvested from the ear or from cephalic trim of the LLC, is preferable. The medial aspect of these grafts may be gently bruised to aid in camouflage. They may be stabilized to the surrounding soft tissue or to the lateral aspect of a shield graft with 6.0 polydioxanone (PDS II) suture. These grafts will improve upon the concave or "knock-kneed" appearance of the rim on the base view and create a more triangular appearance on the basal view. Alternatively, cephalically positioned lateral crura may be dissected free from the underlying vestibular mucosa and repositioned into a more caudal position. If these LLCs are overly arched, this repositioning may be combined with a lateral crural strut graft and intradomal sutures. This strong, stiff graft, usually obtained from the septum, allows the lateral crura to take on a straighter orientation, allowing for triangularity of the nasal base. Severe cases of alar retraction may require the use of composite grafts of ear cartilage and skin placed into the marginal incisions to reposition the alar margins more caudally.

Nasal Tip

Some of the most noticeable deformities in secondary rhinoplasty occur in the nasal tip. Correction requires modulating tip position and shape, then maintaining the modifications against the forces of scar contracture. Tip deformities in secondary rhinoplasty patients come in all forms and may result from any of the classes of surgical errors described above. The external rhinoplasty approach in revision of the nasal tip best facilitates the correction of these deformities.

Irregularities and Bossae

Asymmetry of the tip may result from problems of unequal excision, suture modification, or grafting. Subtle discrepancies may not become evident for several months until edema resolves and scar contracture occurs. Bossae may form as the result of knuckling or angulation of the LLC and tip grafts as the SSTE contracts. Patients with thin skin and strong cartilage are particularly susceptible to this problem. These irregularities may result from the buckling of weakened or reduced alar cartilage under contractile forces or may result simply from insufficiently contoured edges of cartilage or grafts under thin skin. Conservative cartilage trimming, revising suture modification of the domal cartilage, and/or onlay camouflaging may correct such problems (**Fig. 31.3**).[5,7,9] In cases of severe structural compromise, the entire tip structure may need to be reconstructed (see below).

Persistently Wide or Bulbous Tip

A persistently wide tip after primary rhinoplasty may be due to the failure of the surgeon to account for a thick, inelastic SSTE when modifying the dome region. In these patients, performing dome-binding sutures alone may improve the shape of the alar cartilages themselves, but this

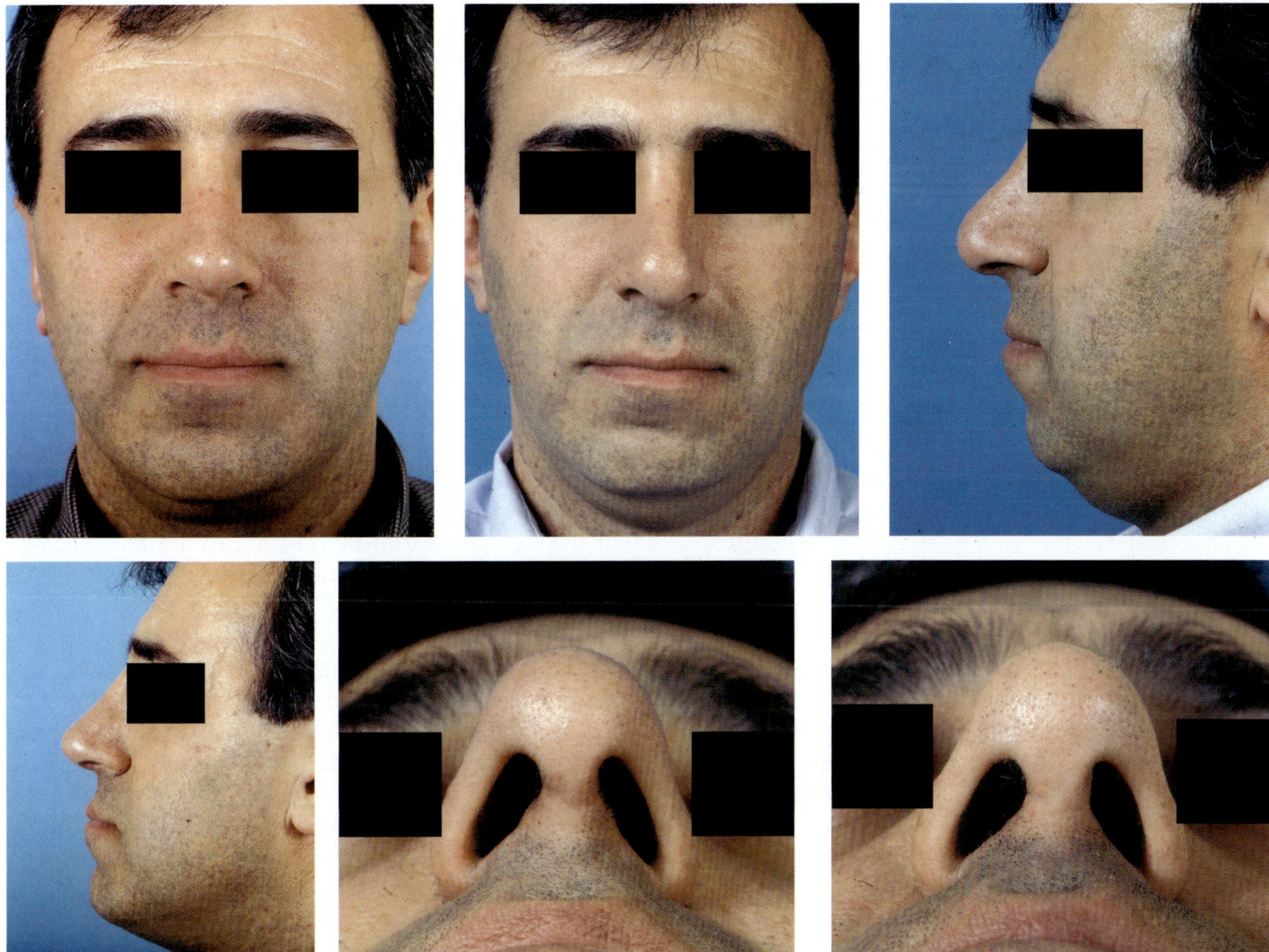

Fig. 31.3 Patient with nasal tip bossae. Preoperative (**A,C,E**) and postoperative (**B,D,F**) views.

change will not necessarily transmit through the thick SSTE. Failure to project the tip into the skin envelope and effectively stretch it to conform to the underlying tip shape will lead to this problem. Study of the overall projection and rotation of the tip, the nasolabial angle, and nasal length should be performed to determine how best to project the tip and restore optimal tip shape. A shield-shaped tip graft may be sutured to the intermediate and medial crura to provide the desired augmentation to the infratip lobule and tip. Although the nasal base remains unchanged, the leading edge of the shield graft may project beyond the domes by as much as 8 mm. A buttress or cap graft may be placed cephalad to the leading edge of the graft to support the graft and camouflage the transition to the supratip. Lateral crural grafts are placed on the existing lateral crura and sutured to the lateral edge of the shield graft when the tip graft projects > 3 mm above the existing domes. These also provide additional support and camouflage to the shield graft. Lateral crural grafts also bolster lateral alar support in cases in which the native lateral crura have been weakened or removed.

Another common error of omission leading to a persistently wide tip is the failure to straighten convex lateral crura. Domal narrowing will not result in a defined triangular tip appearance if the lateral walls of the triangle are curving outward. Unless the curvature is straightened with suture technique or lateral crural struts, persistent tip width will be present. These problems may be detected through the study of the base view of the nose. If lateral crural struts will be needed, strong segments of cartilage are required to overcome the curvature of the existing alar cartilage. These grafts are placed between the undersurface of the lateral crura and the vestibular skin that should be carefully elevated. The caudal attachment of the lateral crus and skin should remain intact to prevent caudal migration of the graft. The graft should extend from just lateral to the domes to the lateral aspect of the lateral crura. The lateral crural strut graft may be stabilized with a full-thickness chromic suture, but it should be finally secured to the lower lateral crura with a 5–0 clear nylon suture.

Pinched Tip

The pinched nasal tip results from excessive narrowing of the domes from excisional techniques, dome division, and/or excessive transdomal sutures. The narrowness of the tip may be further complicated by lateral wall collapse and alar pinching. This unnatural appearance is a clear sign of prior surgery. The normal width of the tip is created by the inherent curvature of the individual domes as well as the normal divergence of the interdomal angle. This divergence creates a natural infratip lobule width, which should be evident from both the base view as well as the frontal view. Restoring a natural tip appearance may require reconstruction of the tip with a shield graft (**Fig. 31.4**).[5]

Ptotic Tip

Maintaining tip position after rhinoplasty depends on restoring any tip support mechanisms that are weak or have been surgically violated. Separation of the LLCs from the upper lateral cartilages, freeing the medial crura from the caudal septum, and excising or weakening the LLCs are common maneuvers in primary rhinoplasty that compromise major tip support mechanisms. Stabilizing the tip tripod framework at the nasal base can help to prevent the eventual ptosis of the unsupported tip and subsequent elongation of the nose. Methods of base stabilization include suture stabilization of the medial crura onto a long caudal septum, a caudal extension graft, a columellar strut, or an extended columellar strut.[6] Failure to take such measures may lead to gradual loss of tip support, a hanging tip and infratip lobule, an overly acute nasolabial angle, and an underprojected, long nose. In addition to the obvious appearance on the lateral view, poor tip strength and recoil on palpation confirm the diagnosis. By using one of the base-stabilizing techniques, the tip position and support may be restored.

Dorsal Profile

Dorsal Irregularity

Most commonly, this problem arises after contour irregularities are created along the dorsum. Osseous hump reduction and osteotomies may lead to palpable or visible edges of bone. In the bony vault, these deformities must be smoothed or camouflaged to prevent an undesirable outcome. An open roof deformity may follow bony hump removal with osteotomies that inadequately medialize the nasal bones. In the middle third of the nose, the dorsal aspect of the upper lateral cartilage (ULC), septal cartilage, and spreader grafts (if present) must be stabilized in a horizontal and coplanar orientation. If not, an irregularity due to asymmetric collapse or migration of the ULC relative to the dorsal septum may become evident. These problems may be detected by close inspection and palpation of the nasal dorsum.

Treatment requires smoothing or camouflaging any irregularities and restabilizing the middle vault structures. Persistent osseous deformities may be addressed by remobilizing the nasal bones through previous osteotomy lines. Often digital manipulation is sufficient to reposition the bones into a symmetric midline position. Alternatively, an osteotome may be used to perform the osteotomies. The leading edge of the instrument will tend to follow the path of the previous osseous cuts. Therefore, if the prior osteotomies were poorly placed, extra caution should be exercised to redirect the revision osteotomies in the proper orientation. Subtle bony deformities may be addressed with simple rasping. In cases where the

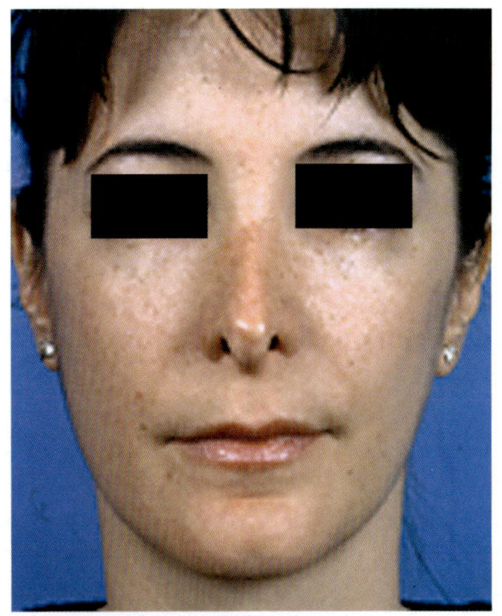
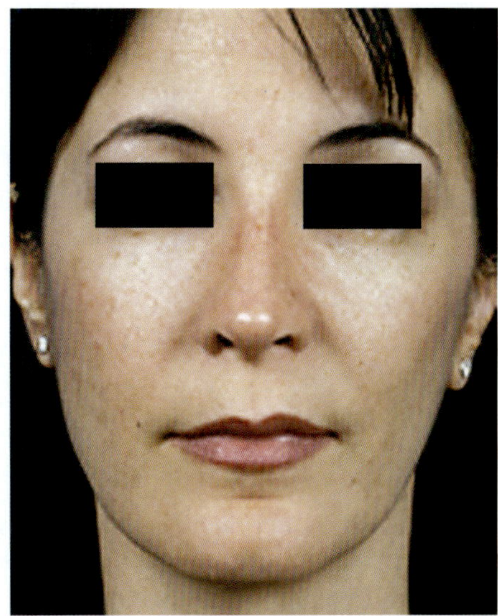
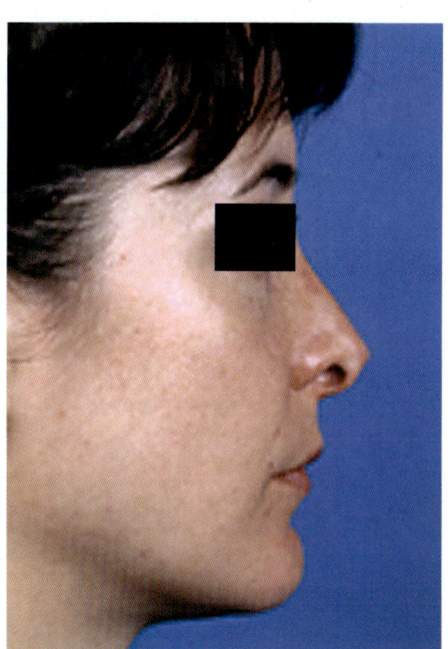

A–C

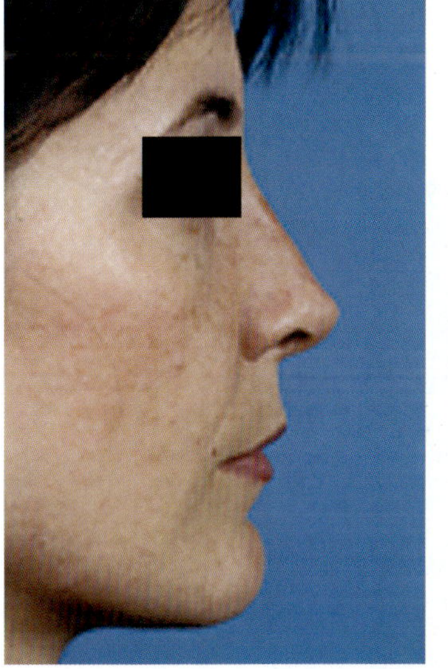
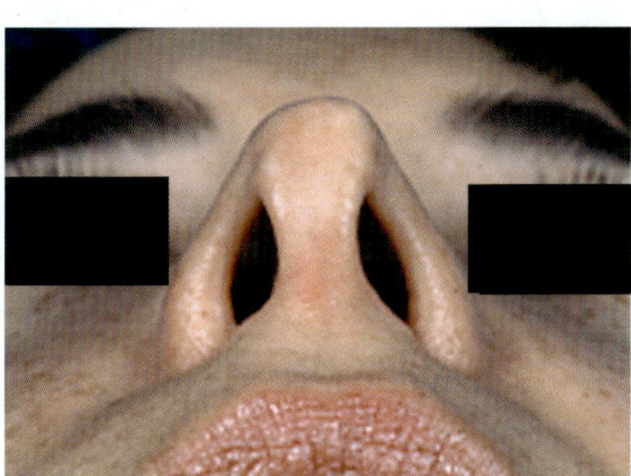
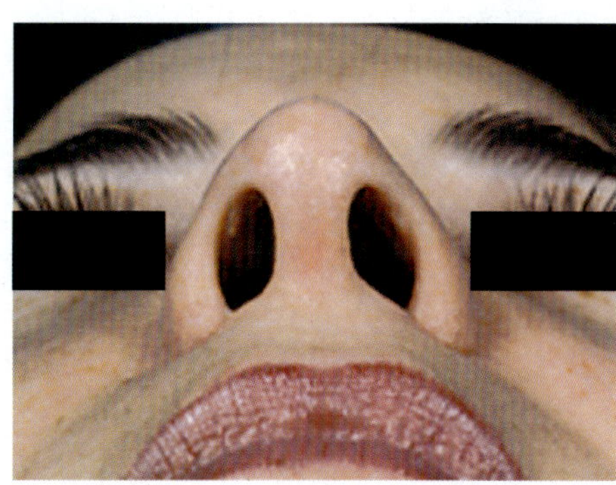

D–F

Fig. 31.4 Patient with previous reduction rhinoplasty. Excessive caudal septal trim, cephalic trim, and dome narrowing have created a short nose with alar retraction and pinching and an overly narrow tip. Treatment required a caudal extension graft, alar batten grafts, alar rim grafts, and tip reconstruction with a shield graft. Preoperative **(A,C)** and postoperative **(B,D)** frontal, lateral, and basal views. **(E)** Overly narrowed, cephalically displaced lower lateral crura.

cartilaginous dorsum is slightly decreased, onlay grafting may be used to correct irregularities. Small irregularities may be excised to restore a smooth contour.

Low Dorsum/Saddle Deformity

More dramatic dorsal abnormalities may result from the creation of improper height at the upper or middle third. An inexperienced surgeon may fail to recognize that dorsal alignment can be improved by elevating a low radix rather than by reducing a relative convexity at the middle and upper vaults. Reduction of the dorsal convexity will create a tendency to deproject the nasal tip to the level of this lowered dorsum or to leave the tip projected beyond the height of the bridge.

This can result in an over-reduced or scooped appearance on the lateral view. If dorsal reduction of the middle vault results in inadequate dorsal septal support, a saddle nose deformity can ensue. On the frontal view, a low dorsum causes less shadowing to the nose and creates an illusion of increased width. At the upper one third of the nose, this may create an appearance of pseudohypertelorism. The amorphous frontal view makes the brow-tip aesthetic lines indistinct and the general appearance of the upper two thirds amorphous. The ideal lateral profile should be straight or slightly concave at the rhinion for women and straight to slightly convex for men. The overall height of the bridge should be determined by the projection of the tip, which should equal just over one half of the nasal length.

Restoring proper bridge height calls for onlay material. In severe saddle deformities, rib cartilage may be necessary (**Fig. 31.5**). The onlay graft should be fashioned into a canoe shape, with the cephalic edge placed into a precise pocket over the upper dorsum. The cephalic edge should terminate roughly at the level of the desired nasal starting point. The caudal edge should terminate in the supratip area; ideally, the domes will project above the graft at its caudal aspect, providing a smooth transition from the dorsum to the tip. All edges of the graft must be tapered to minimize transmission of the graft through the SSTE.

Nasal Starting Point/Radix

A large or improperly placed radix graft or hump reduction short of the patient's wishes can result in excessive dorsal height. A radix graft that is positioned too cephalically will elevate and blunt the nasofrontal angle, creating an illusion of a longer nose. If placed too caudally, the graft may appear as an unnaturally high dorsal hump.

On analysis, the nasal starting point should be at or just below the level of the superior palpebral fissure. The nasofrontal angle should be roughly 120 degrees (although this may vary depending on the plane of the forehead). The degree of radix projection should be harmonious with the rest of the nasal dorsum and tip projection. Byrd and Hobar propose that ideal radix proportion measured from the junction of the nasal bone to the orbit be one third of the overall nasal length.[1] Repositioning or replacing an existing radix graft may restore the correct nasal starting point and nasofrontal angle.

Pollybeak

A pollybeak is an abnormality in which the supratip projects beyond the tip. This causes a rounded appearance to the tip with a lack of definition and an absence of a supratip break or a columellar-lobular break. Although the deformity creates the appearance of supratip fullness, the problem may be caused by one of several processes.

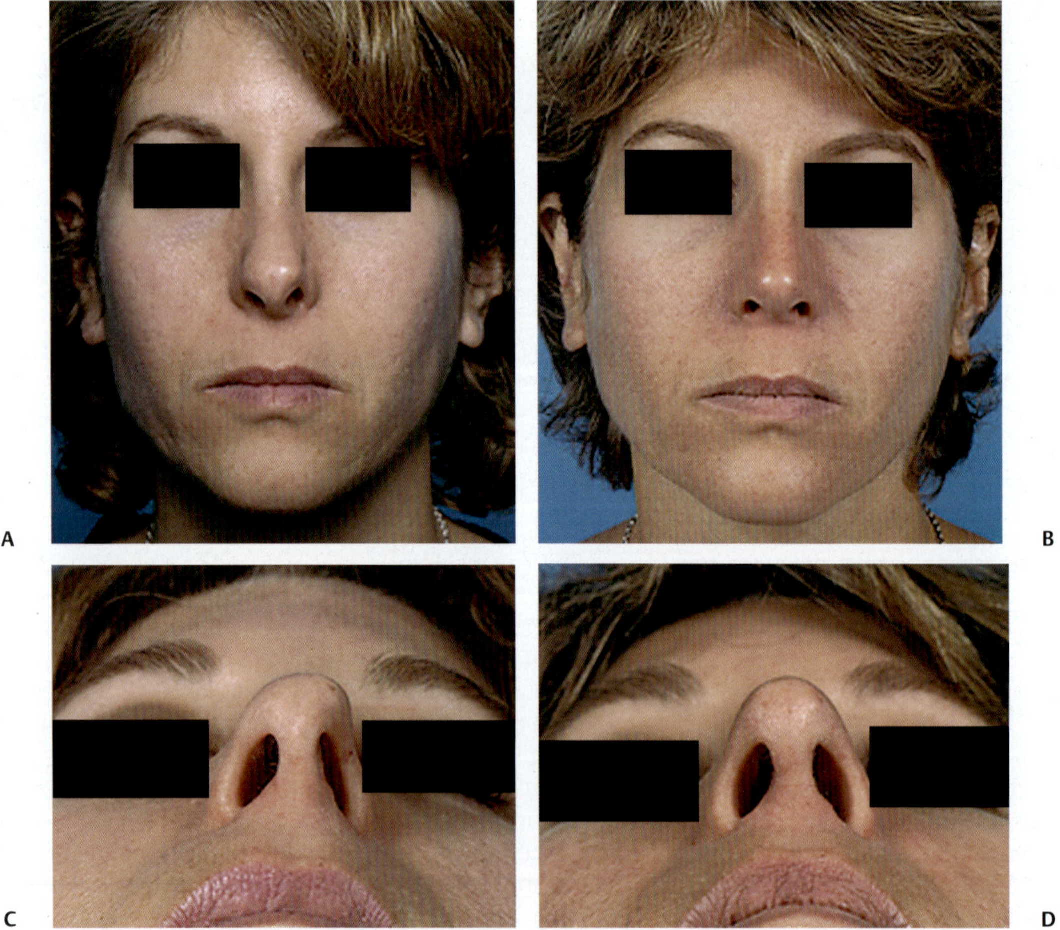

Fig. 31.5 Patient with excessive previous dorsal reduction. The obvious saddle deformity on the lateral view translates into an illusion of increased width on the frontal view. Required costal cartilage graft. Preoperative **(A,C,E)** and postoperative **(B,D,F)** views.

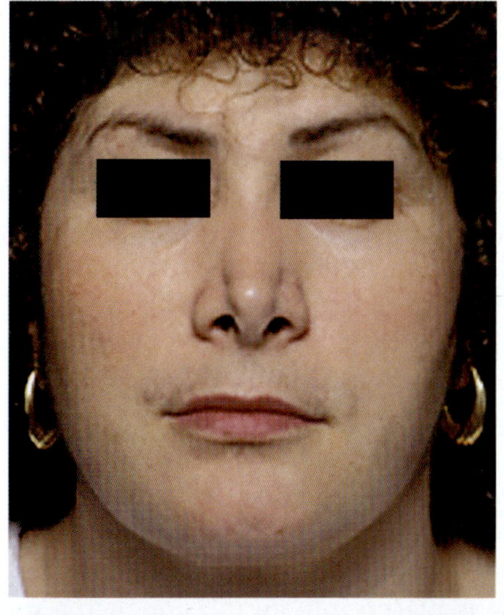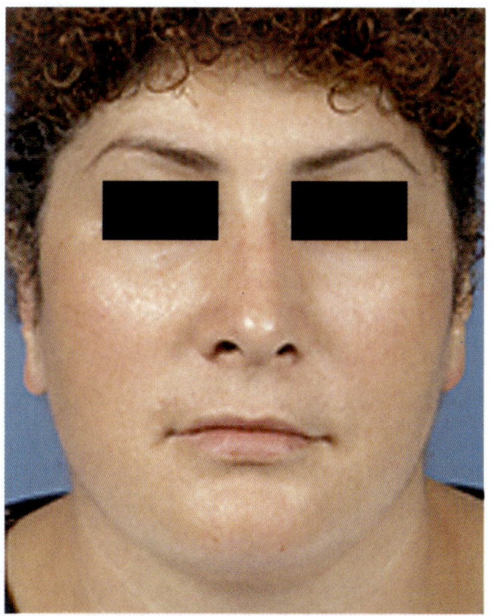

A, B

Fig. **31.6** Soft tissue–type pollybeak caused by the inability of a thick, inelastic skin–soft tissue envelope (SSTE) to drape over the reduced underlying nasal structures. Notice the preoperative poor columellar scar on the base view. Preoperative **(A,C,E)** and postoperative **(B,D,F)** views.

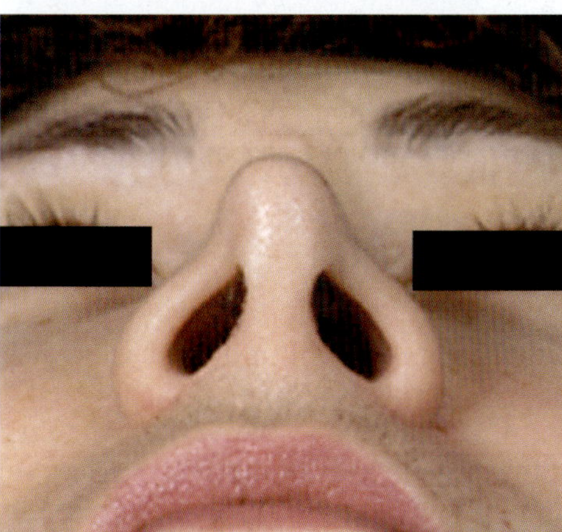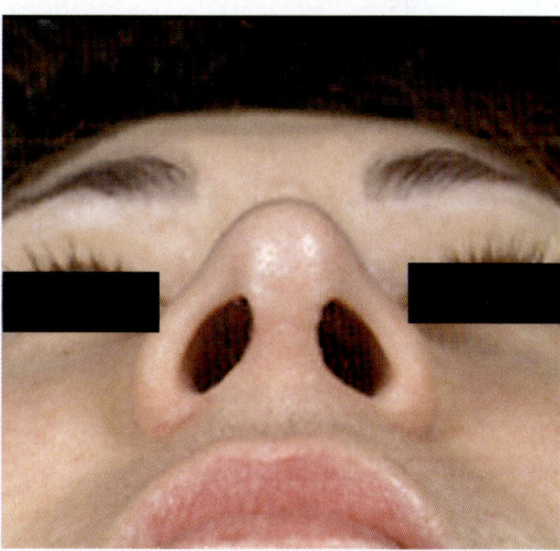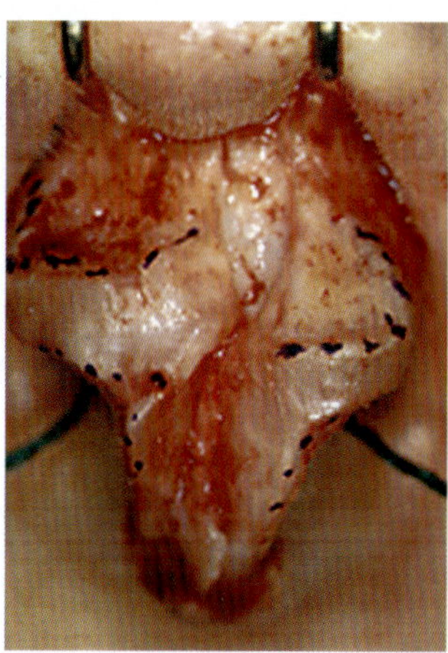

C–E

One possibility is the failure to reduce an overly elevated middle vault and supratip dorsum. In a primary tension nose deformity, the anterior septal angle represents the most projecting point of the nose, with the tip structures "hanging" from this point. Therefore, the dorsum at the level of the anterior septal angle must be reduced or the tip brought out beyond this point to establish a proper tip–supratip relationship. Failure to establish this relationship is an error of omission leading to postoperative pollybeak. Paradoxically, excessive excision of dorsal septal cartilage may result in the same deformity. Particularly in patients with thick, inelastic skin, the SSTE cannot redrape into the area of skeletal reduction. The tissue void fills with scar and fibrosis, resulting in a soft tissue pollybeak. Lastly, if tip support is compromised and not reconstituted, the resultant tip ptosis may lead to deprojection at the tip and an appearance of supratip fullness.[10]

These three different categories of pollybeak deformities require individualized treatments. Correction of the untreated tension nose deformity requires completing the dorsal cartilage reduction and ensuring the presence of a stable nasal base to maintain tip position relative to the dorsum. Correction of the soft tissue pollybeak requires projecting the tip into the thick SSTE beyond the level of the supratip and dorsum (**Fig. 31.6**). The pollybeak caused by tip ptosis requires reestablishing tip support and returning the tip into its appropriate projection. Because these strategies are quite different from each other, it is crucial to understand the etiology of the problem prior to surgery. Palpation is critical to differentiate between soft tissue fullness and cartilaginous excess. An acute nasolabial angle and a weak tip with little recoil will indicate the presence of tip ptosis secondary to loss of tip support.

Middle Vault

The middle vault poses one of the most difficult challenges in rhinoplasty. Separation of the upper lateral cartilages from the septum requires restabilization with spreader grafts to restore the structural relationship. Failure to do this will result in inferomedial collapse of the upper lateral cartilages, pinching of the middle vault, and internal valve airflow obstruction. Particularly in thin-skinned patients with short nasal bones, the collapse and separation of the ULCs from the bony vault may result in a visible and palpable inverted V deformity. Restoring symmetry to a crooked middle vault requires precise placement of asymmetric spreader grafts stabilized between the dorsal septum and ULCs. Small irregularities or asymmetries are apparent on the frontal view, secondary to linear shadowing on the nasal sidewalls. These discrepancies often do not become evident until months or years after surgery.

To identify and diagnose these deformities, the surgeon must perform meticulous examination and analysis of the middle vault. The dimensions of the brow-tip aesthetic line should follow a pattern of relative width at the bony vault, slight narrowness at the middle vault, and width again at the tip. This curve should be subtle. Exaggeration of the curvature may indicate middle vault pinching and/or excessive width at the bony vault or tip.[6,14,15]

In almost all cases, the middle vault width and stability are restored through the placement of spreader grafts. As in primary rhinoplasty, these rectangular grafts are suture stabilized between the dorsal septum and the ULCs. However, in revision cases, a greater degree of collapse or asymmetry may be present. The surgeon must therefore be prepared to insert wider or more numerous spreader grafts than in primary rhinoplasty. In severe cases, the ULCs may be collapsed into the nasal airway. In these situations, the ULCs must be grasped and pulled into the proper dorsal position in alignment with the dorsal margin of the septum prior to placement of spreader grafts.

Alar Base

One of the most difficult rhinoplasty complications to correct is the overly narrowed alar base. Base reduction should be performed conservatively, with the aim of achieving 60 to 70% of an idealized reduction at the time of primary surgery. Unfortunately, excessive or asymmetric reduction is a common mistake during primary surgery. On the frontal or base view, the alar insertion should approximate the intercanthal width with a slight amount of acceptable alar flare, particularly in men. Ethnic variations allow for a greater degree of width and flare, especially in patients of African and Asian descent. Poorly placed incisions or uneven closure may make this problem more conspicuous. Nostril size and shape must be noted on the base view. Meticulous measurements should be made of the width of the columellar pedestal, the width of the nasal sill, and the distance of the outer aspect of the alar insertion to the midline. Repositioning the alar base is a three-dimensional process. The horizontal position of the ala may result in vertical migration of the

alar insertion, which can lead to asymmetry. Comparison of the nose to preoperative photos can help in determining which portion of the alar base was previously removed. A significant reduction in the width of the nostril floor and the interalar distance suggests resection primarily of the sill. Reduction of alar flare suggests resection of the alar sidewall. Reduction of both flare and interalar width suggests excision at the junction of the sill and alar sidewall, possibly through the use of a sliding alar flap. This analysis will help to determine the shape and size of the tissue needed to replace the previous excision.[11]

Composite grafts harvested from the cymba concha work well to correct such deformities. These grafts may be interposed into incisions placed at the areas of maximal narrowing. A common deformity following over-reduction is the overly narrowed or absent nasal sill. In these cases, a composite graft is placed into an incision at the nostril floor, resulting in widening of the sill and interalar distance. Transposition flaps using a superiorly pedicled cheek flap should be avoided as they tend to cause more distortion, vertical alar malposition, and an unsightly scar.

Skin–Soft Tissue Envelope

When the skin has been significantly damaged, the revision rhinoplasty surgeon must be exceedingly cautious in manipulating or undermining the SSTE. If there is any doubt regarding the integrity of the SSTE, surgery should be delayed to allow full recovery. Blue discoloration or cutaneous telangiectasias signify damage and added risk for skin complications. In catastrophic cases where the soft tissue envelope has already been severely compromised, one should consider staged preliminary repair of the SSTE with skin grafts or local or regional flaps prior to any structural nasal surgery.

Conclusion

Secondary rhinoplasty may pose the most difficult challenges of facial plastic surgery. Although many of the tools of analysis and technique are the same as for primary rhinoplasty, these methods may need to be focused toward restoration, reconstruction, and restabilization rather than toward subtle refinement. The ability to correct these problems may be limited by the compromised integrity of the nose, a deficiency of grafting material, and the severity of the individual deformities. Accurate diagnosis, adherence to structural principles, selection of the correct maneuvers based on the category and location of the complication, and meticulous technique will maximize the likelihood of a satisfactory result following revision surgery.

References

1. Byrd HS, Hobar PC. Rhinoplasty: a practical guide for surgical planning. Plast Reconstr Surg 1993;91:642–656.
2. Orten SS, Hilger PA. Facial analysis of the rhinoplasty patient. In: Papel ID, ed. Facial Plastic and Reconstructive Surgery. 2nd ed. New York: Thieme Medical Publishers; 2002:361–368.
3. Tardy ME, Walter MA, Patt BS. The overprojecting nose: anatomic component analysis and repair. Facial Plast Surg 1993;9:306–316.
4. Kim DW, Egan KK. Metrics of nasal tip rotation: a comparative analysis. Laryngoscope 2006;116(6):872–877.
5. Toriumi DM, Becker DG. Rhinoplasty Dissection Manual. Philadelphia: Lippincott; 1999.
6. Toriumi DM. Structure approach in rhinoplasty. Facial Plast Surg Clin North Am 2005;13:93–113.
7. Tardy ME. Rhinoplasty: The Art and Science. Philadelphia: WB Saunders; 1997.
8. Chand MS, Toriumi DM. Treatment of the external nasal valve. Facial Plast Surg Clin North Am 1999;7:347–356.
9. Toriumi DM, Josen J, Weinberger M, Tardy ME Jr. Use of alar batten grafts for correction of nasal valve collapse. Arch Otolaryngol Head Neck Surg 1997;123:802–808.
10. Tardy ME, Kron TK, Younger R, Key M. The cartilaginous pollybeak: etiology, prevention, and treatment. Facial Plast Surg 1989;6:113–120.
11. Becker DG, Weinberger MS, Greene BA, Tardy ME. Clinical study of alar anatomy and surgery of the alar base. Arch Otolaryngol Head Neck Surg 1997;123:789–795.
12. Tardy ME, Toriumi D. Alar retraction: composite graft correction. Facial Plast Surg 1989;6:101–107.
13. Gunter JP, Rohrich RJ, Friedman RM. Classification and correction of alar-columellar discrepancies in rhinoplasty. Plast Reconstr Surg 1996;97:643–648.
14. Park SS. Treatment of the internal nasal valve. Facial Plast Surg Clin North Am 1999;7:333–346.
15. Toriumi DM. Management of the middle nasal vault in rhinoplasty. Plast Reconstr Surg 1995;2:16–30.

Decision tree for complications and treatment of upper lid blepharoplasty

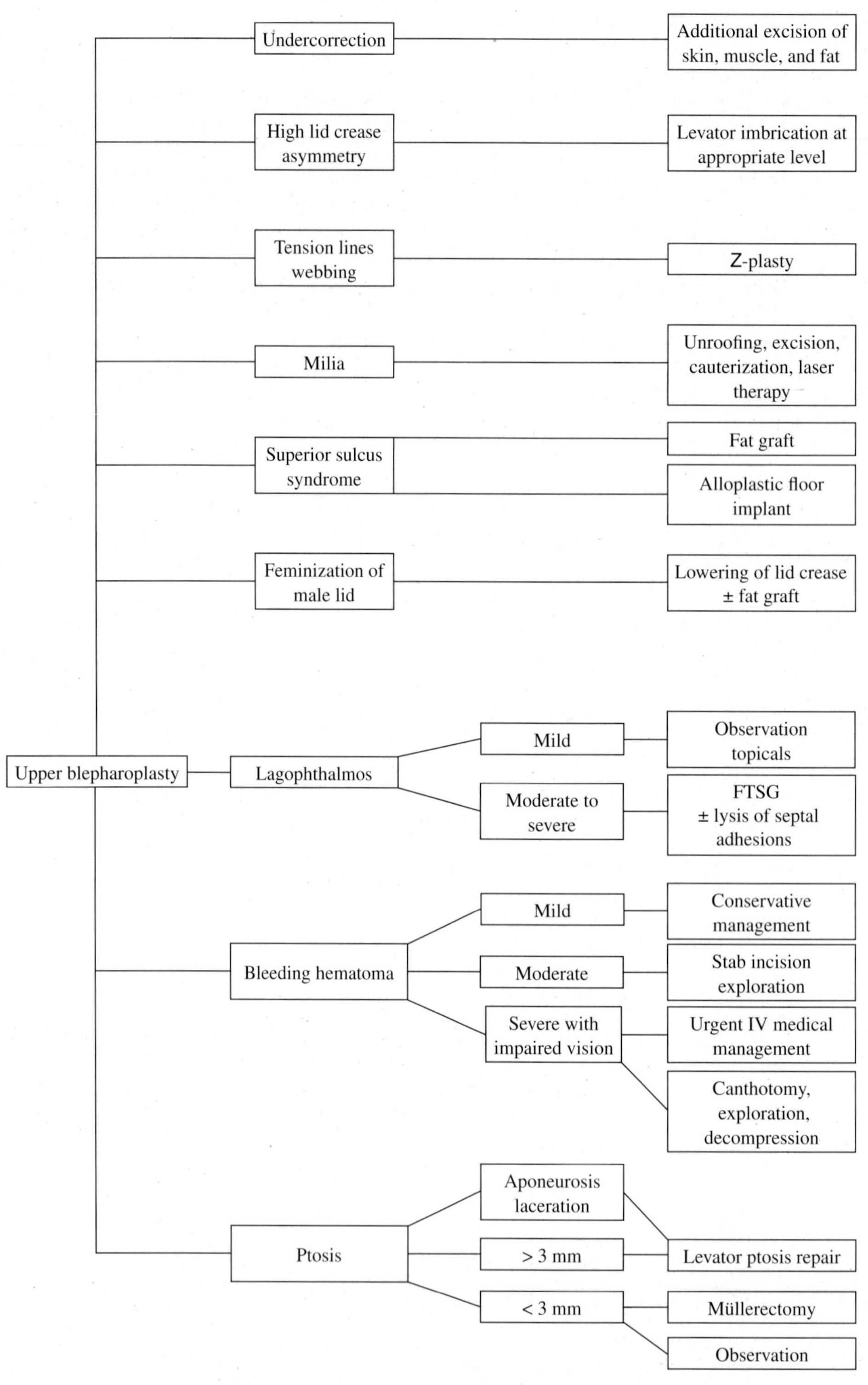

Revision Surgery for Blepharoplasty

Boaz J. Lissauer and Albert Hornblass

This chapter reviews the main anatomical structures involved in eyelid surgery. It discusses complications of upper and lower blepharoplasty and outlines surgical techniques addressing undercorrection, high or asymmetric eyelid creases, nasal tension lines, suture milia, superior sulcus syndrome, feminization of the male eyelid, ptosis secondary to upper eyelid blepharoplasty, lagophthalmos, bleeding, lower eyelid retraction, lateral tarsal strip and horizontal lid shortening, long-standing or severe lower eyelid retraction and lower eyelid ectropion, under- or overexcision of lower eyelid fat, and postoperative skin wrinkling.

Anatomy

Superficial Anatomy

The eyelids are the main protection mechanism for the globe; therefore, it is not difficult to understand why ophthalmic complications can result from any type of eyelid surgery. The eyelids consist of the anterior lamella of skin and orbicularis muscle and a posterior lamella of tarsus and conjunctiva. The precorneal tear film is composed of three layers. The superficial lipid layer is produced predominantly by the meibomian glands and the glands of Zeis and Moll, which aid with lubrication of the cornea by dispersion of the tear film and retardation of tear film evaporation. Any disturbance in the position of the margin or change in palpebral fissure height can precipitate a disturbance in the ocular surface.

The interpalpebral fissure is the exposed zone between the upper and lower eyelids. The normal adult fissure is 27 to 30 mm long and 8 to 11 mm wide. The upper eyelid is more mobile than the lower and can be raised 15 mm by the action of the levator muscle. The frontalis muscle can contribute an additional 2 mm, and the orbicularis oculi muscle is the levator's antagonist. In the adult the upper eyelid rests 1.5 to 2.0 mm below the upper limbus, with the highest point of the lid contour slightly nasal to the pupil. The lower lid is positioned at the lower limbus, with the lowest point of the lid contour slightly temporal. The junction points where the upper and lower eyelids meet are the commissures; the angles the lids form are the canthi.

The upper eyelid crease is most commonly found 8 to 10 mm above the upper lid margin in occidental eyelids. The crease represents insertion of levator fibers in the pretarsal orbicularis and skin. The eyelid crease in Asians is only a few millimeters from the upper lid margin because the superior orbital septum inserts on the levator aponeurosis at the crease, close to the lid margin. The area of skin above the cilia in which the skin and underlying muscle are firmly attached to the tarsal plate is the pretarsal space. The visibility of the pretarsal space is dependent on the amount of skin overhanging the upper lid fold (dermatochalasia). The goal of upper lid blepharoplasty is restoration in the visibility of the pretarsal space, more so in females than in males (**Fig. 32.1**). If the medial canthus is covered by a nasal extension of the upper lid crease, this is termed an epicanthal fold. The lower eyelid crease is less well defined and represents the superficial insertion of the lower lid retractors. The crease is 4 to 5 mm below the lower eyelid margin and has a gradual temporal slope.

Skin and Muscle

The eyelid skin is the thinnest in the body and makes a sharp transition to the thick skin of the brow superiorly and the malar region inferiorly. The subcutaneous tissue in the eyelids is devoid of fat and has loose stroma and attachments to the underlying tissue. This explains the rapid accumulation of fluid in the pretarsal space during hemorrhage or acute allergic response, with an initial sharp demarcation line between the cheek region.

The orbicularis oculi muscle is deep to the dermis and is the protractor of the eyelids (closure muscle). It is divided into three regions: the pretarsal, preseptal, and orbital regions (**Fig. 32.2**).

The pretarsal orbicularis divides into two heads nasally. The superficial head passes anterior to the canaliculi and forms the anterior crus of the medial canthal tendon, inserting into the frontal process of the maxillary bone. The deep head inserts onto the posterior lacrimal crest (Horner muscle). This deep insertion provides a deep anchor and is responsible for the eyelids' convex position on the surface of the globe. The preseptal orbicularis medially inserts into the anterior crus on the medial canthal tendon and temporally forms the lateral horizontal raphe. The orbital orbicularis nasally inserts into the medial canthal tendon, the nasal aspect of the frontal

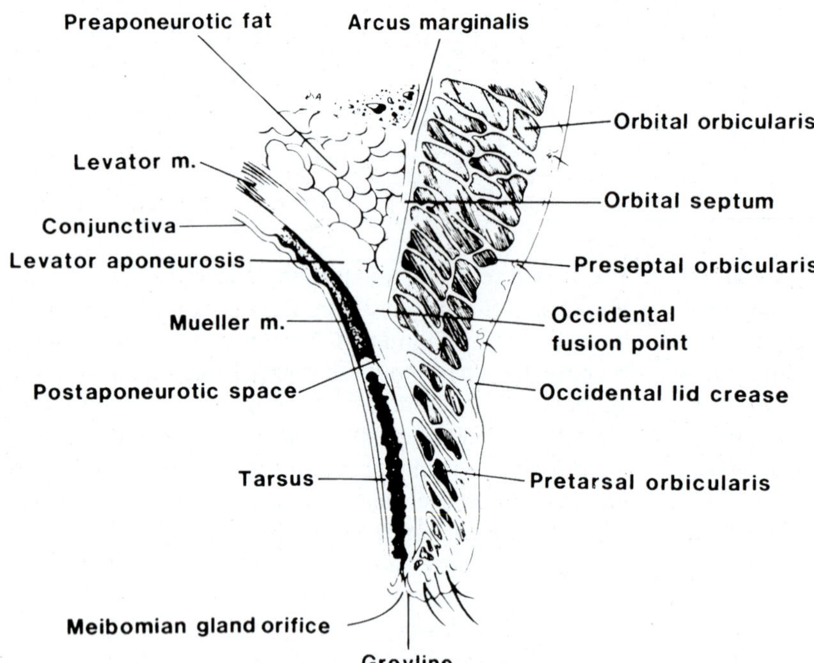

Fig. 32.1 Cross-sectional anatomy of the upper eyelid.

bone, and the inferomedial orbital margin. It then extends laterally around the lateral canthus without insertion into the lateral canthal tendon. The orbicularis muscle provides the lacrimal pump for drainage of tears into the nasolacrimal system. Weakening of the muscle can cause epiphora even in the presence of normal lid position.

Laterally, the pretarsal muscle is attached to the lateral orbital tubercle via the lateral canthal tendon. The preseptal and orbital orbicularis travel along the orbital rim and pass the lateral canthal angle to attach to the zygoma.

Orbital Septum

Deep to the orbicularis muscle is the orbital septum, which is firmly adherent to the arcus marginalis of the

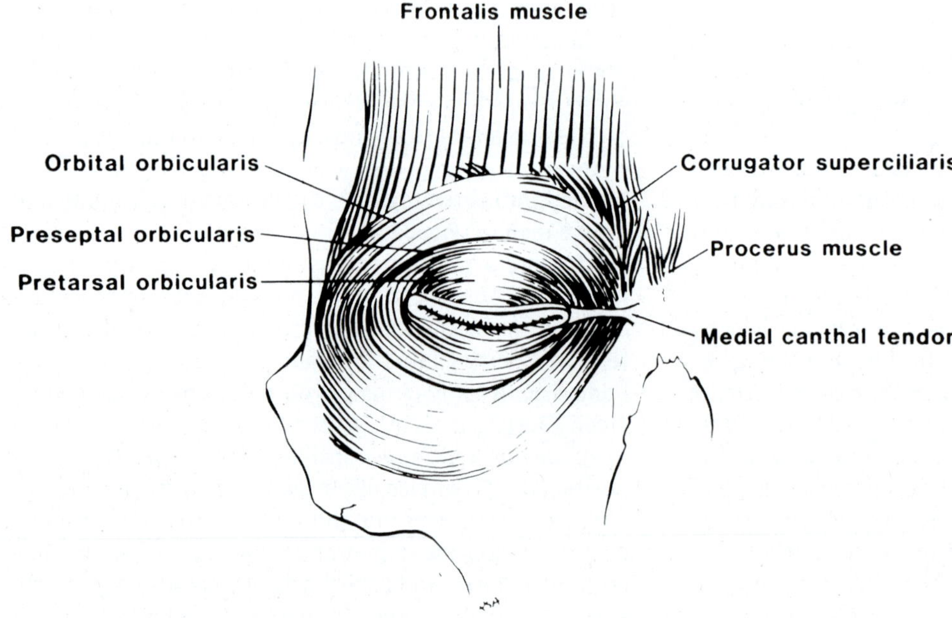

Fig. 32.2 Orbicularis oculi muscle.

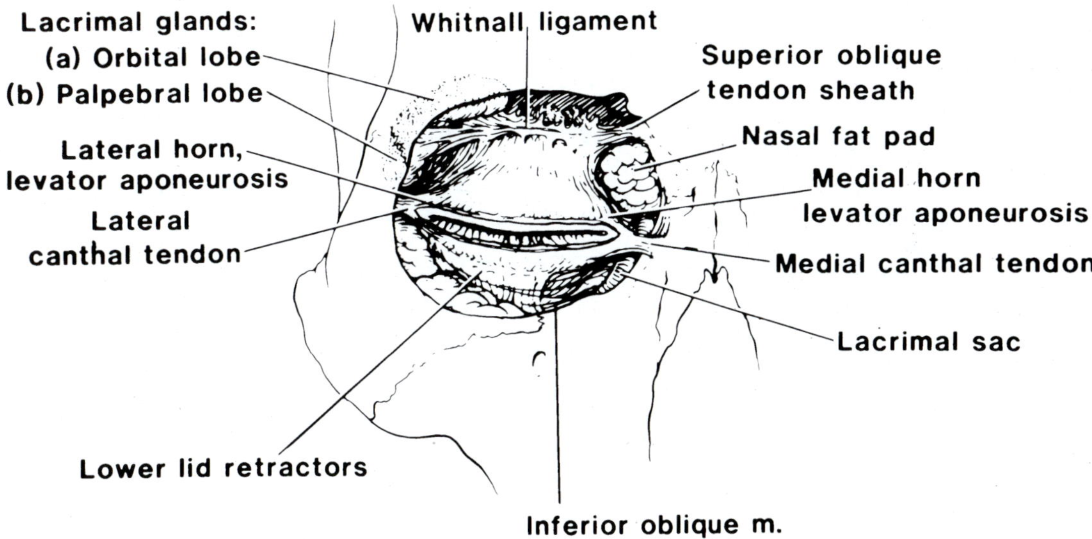

Fig. 32.3 Orbital septum and associated structures.

orbital rim. The septum inserts medially to the posterior lacrimal crest and lacrimal fascia. Laterally, the septum is attached to the lateral canthal tendon and the lateral orbital tubercle. Anteriorly, the orbital septum forms a barrier for the orbital tissues and prevents anterior displacement of the orbital fat.

In the lower eyelid, the septum fuses with the lower eyelid retractors 4 to 5 mm below the tarsal plate, then attaches to the inferior border of the tarsus of the lower lid. In the upper eyelid, the septum fuses with the levator aponeurosis superior to the tarsal plate, ~10 mm above the eyelid margin in occidental eyelids. In Asians, the orbital septum inserts to the levator aponeurosis anterior and inferior to the tarsal plate only a few millimeters from the eyelid margin (**Fig. 32.3**).

Preseptal and Postseptal Eyelid Fat Compartments

The preseptal eyelid fat pad extends in a submuscular plane from the brow region inferiorly beneath the preseptal orbicularis of the upper eyelid. In the upper eyelid posterior to the orbital septum are two fatty compartments. The preaponeurotic fat pad lies anterior to the levator aponeurosis, temporal to the trochlea, and medial to the orbital lobe of the lacrimal gland. Nasal to this fat pad is the nasal fat pad of the upper lid just beneath the trochlea. These fatty deposits can be discerned by their color; the preaponeurotic fat pad is yellow, whereas the nasal fat pad is white.

In the lower eyelid there are three fat pads. The inferior oblique muscle divides the nasal and central fat pads. The central and lateral fat pads are divided by a fibrous

septum anteriorly but connected in the deep tissue posteriorly (**Fig. 32.4**).

Complications of Blepharoplasty

Complications of Upper Blepharoplasty

The most common complication of cosmetic blepharoplasty is dissatisfaction with the surgical results. The easiest way to avoid this complication is by spending time during the preoperative visit explaining to the patient what can be expected. Preoperatively, the patient must be advised of all potential cosmetic outcomes of upper blepharoplasty. including under- and overcorrection, high eyelid creases, asymmetry, nasal tension lines, suture milia, superior sulcus deformity, and feminization of the male upper eyelid. The patient must have realistic expectations even if the procedure progresses as planned. More importantly, the patient must be advised of the functional complications that require surgical revision, including ptosis, hematoma, lid lag or the inability to close the eyelids when sleeping, exposure keratopathy, and vision-threatening retrobulbar hemorrhage.

Complications of Lower Blepharoplasty

Common complications of lower blepharoplasty are fewer and more accentuated than those of upper blepharoplasty. Cosmetic and functional complications include lower lid malposition, retraction with scleral show (**Fig. 32.5**), ectropion, lagophthalmos, bowing deformity, injury to the inferior oblique muscle, worsening of rhytides, improper orbital

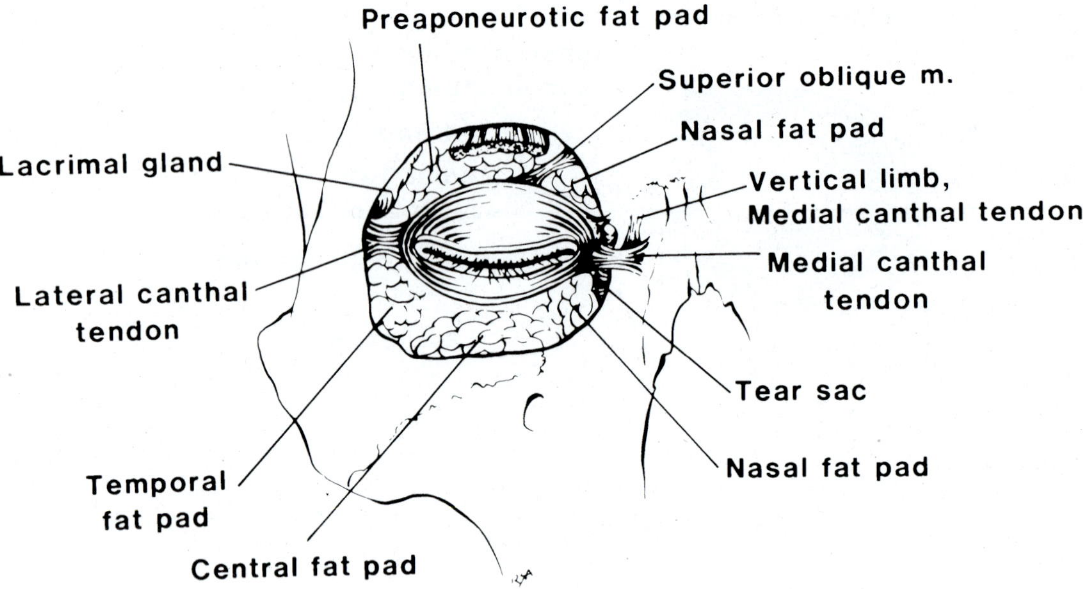

Fig. 32.4 Orbital fat compartments.

fat excision, accentuation of the tear trough deformity, and orbital hemorrhage.

Surgical Revision for Upper Blepharoplasty

Undercorrection

The desired cosmetic result of upper blepharoplasty is a tall, exposed anterior surface of the upper eyelid skin, yielding a youthful appearance. The most common cosmetic complaint of patients is underexcision of skin or dermatochalasia. This complication is very amenable to reoperation, with excision of skin and orbicularis muscle above the previous incision. If the lid crease height is appropriate, the reoperation incision can be made through the original incision along its entire length, maintaining

the lid crease height. Additional orbital fat can be excised to reduce residual bulges, most commonly remaining at the medial fat pad. The skin is then reapproximated, as would any blepharoplasty incision, with interrupted, running, or subcuticular sutures. If the lid crease requires enhancement, the underlying levator aponeurosis is incorporated into each pass of the needle.

High or Asymmetric Eyelid Creases

A common complication of upper eyelid blepharoplasty is inappropriate placement of the upper eyelid crease, most commonly an exaggeratedly high lid crease. This can be a difficult complication to repair, and in cosmetic blepharoplasty it should be avoided, especially in males. A high eyelid crease yields a feminine appearance, and this should be addressed preoperatively in male patients. Maintaining the height of the patient's preoperative eyelid crease height is the best way to avoid this complication unless the patient already has asymmetric eyelid crease height or levator aponeurosis dehiscence with an elevated lid crease. The surgeon should always err on the side of placing the lid crease too low rather than too high, as this is more easily repaired.

The eyelid crease, as previously mentioned, represents the insertion of the levator fibers into the pretarsal orbicularis and skin. To lower the crease surgically, a new blepharoplasty incision should be placed at the desired lid crease height (usually 8–10 mm superior to the eyelid margin). The incision should be carried down through the orbicularis muscle and orbital septum to the levator

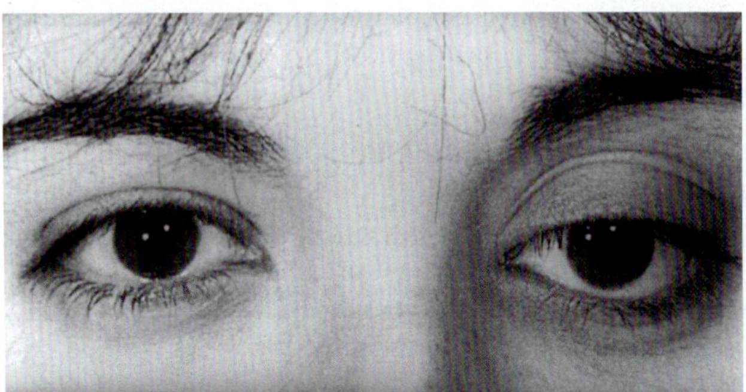

Fig. 32.5 Asymmetric lid creases after blepharoplasty.

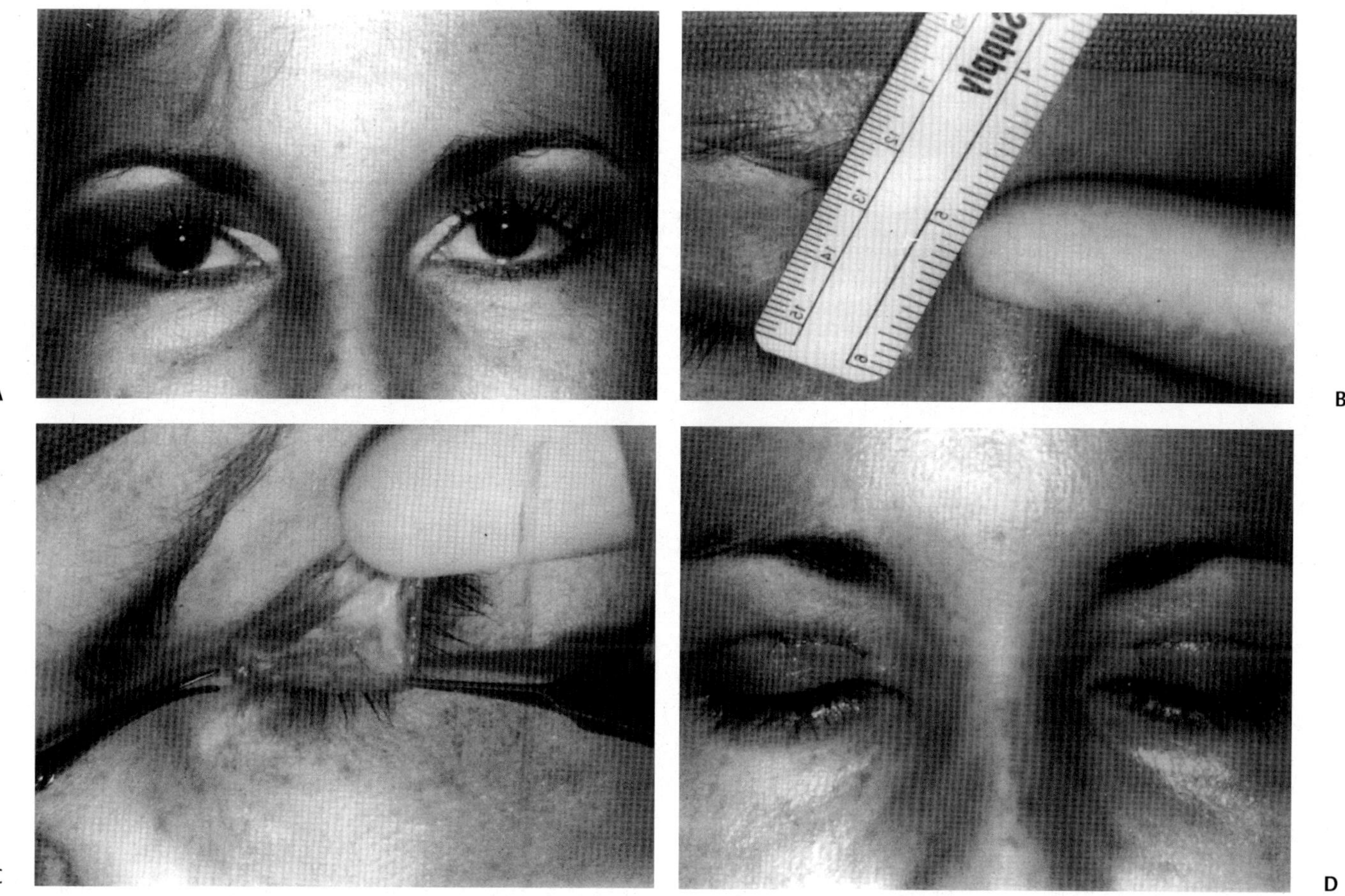

Fig. 32.6 (A) Patient following upper lid blepharoplasty. Note the iatrogenic asymmetric, low eyelid creases. **(B)** The lid creases are almost touching the lashes. On measurement, the lid crease is 4 mm above the lash line. **(C)** To repair the low lid crease, a skin–muscle flap is dissected below the previously formed lid crease. **(D)** Postoperative appearance after reformation of the lid creases. Note the newly elevated, symmetric lid creases.

aponeurosis. If required, a skin–muscle flap and herniated orbital fat may be removed. The incision is then closed with interrupted sutures. The sutures reestablish the new lid crease, as each suture pass incorporates the inferior incisional skin edge and a bite of levator aponeurosis and then the superior skin edge, imbricating the aponeurosis within the skin closure. This allows the upper eyelid skin to slightly hang over the closed incision, re-creating the upper eyelid crease. It should be stressed that taking too much skin laterally in reoperations should be avoided, as it will pull the eyebrows inferiorly.

Asymmetric upper eyelid creases are also encountered after blepharoplasty; this asymmetry is more easily corrected by elevating the eyelid crease that is too low (**Fig. 32.5**). The distance from the lid margin to the lid crease in the eye that is not to be repaired is measured. An ellipse of skin is marked on the eyelid to be repaired above the existing lower eyelid crease, with the inferior incision placed at the same height as the lid crease measured on the opposite eye. The marked ellipse is then excised as a skin–muscle flap along the horizontal length of the eyelid,

and levator aponeurosis adhesions are separated from the previous lower eyelid crease. The incision is closed in a similar manner as mentioned above, with interrupted sutures incorporating the levator aponeurosis into the newly repositioned eyelid crease. The inferior and superior incisional suture passes should be orbicularis and skin together, enhancing the lid crease (**Fig. 32.6**).

Nasal Tension Lines

Nasal tension lines or nasal webbing can be avoided with a W or M incision configuration; however, mechanically created nasal tension lines can also occur during incision closure (**Fig. 32.7**). This can be prevented primarily if tension is noted at the time of suturing. The first pass of the running suture should be placed lateral to the most nasal incision angle (~4 mm), taking a bite of skin and orbicularis inferiorly, then the levator aponeurosis, and then in a parallel vector through skin and orbicularis superiorly (instead of at a meridianal angle). This creates lateral tension on the upper nasal eyelid skin, reducing tension lines. No

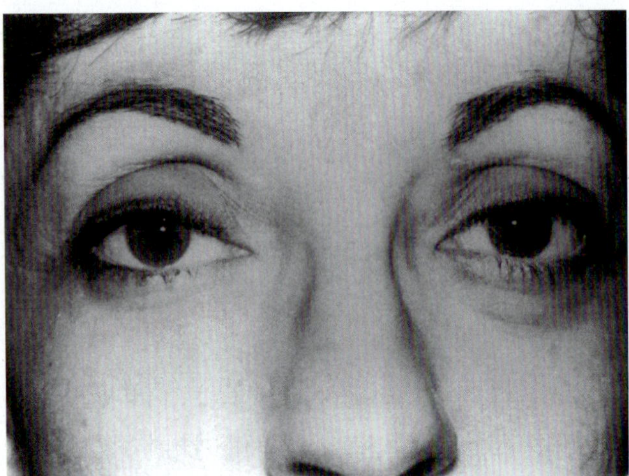

Fig. 32.7 Nasal tension lines after blepharoplasty.

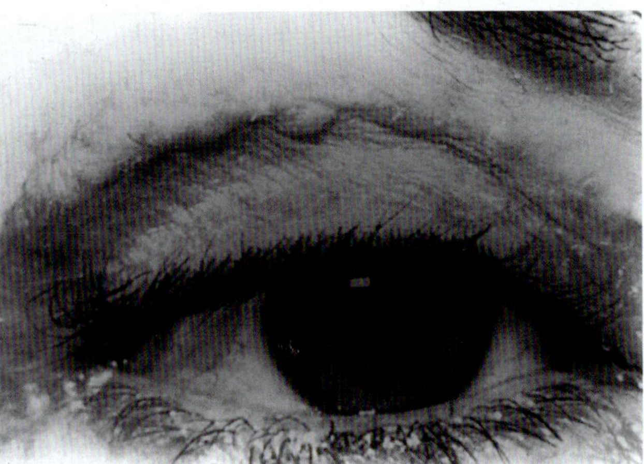

Fig. 32.8 Suture milia after blepharoplasty.

sutures should be placed medial to the first pass of the running suture. If tension lines are still present, remove the first stitch of the running suture and place it even more temporally, again leaving the incision open nasal to the running suture.

Suture Milia

Suture milia are incisional cysts at the area where the suture passes into the skin (**Fig. 32.8**). Associations have been made between the type of suture employed in blepharoplasty closure and the manner in which it is done. Polypropylene sutures appear to have a lower rate of milia occurrence when compared with silk sutures; however, empiric evidence is lacking to corroborate this completely. Also, subcuticular closure appears to decrease milia compared with cutaneous running closure, as the overlying epithelium is not given a fistulous suture track to migrate into. Again, this does not totally eliminate milia. Early suture removal appears to decrease the occurrence as well.

The natural course of milia is they appear typically 1 week postoperatively and usually spontaneously resolve. Their resolution, however, can take weeks to months. Many patients want to hasten their resolution and request intervention. Milia can be unroofed with a needle, excised, or cauterized using hyfrecation (electrotherapy) or laser, usually removing them without recurrence (**Fig. 32.9**).

Superior Sulcus Syndrome

When the area above the pretarsal eyelid appears sunken, this is termed a superior sulcus. Cosmetically, this presents a difficult problem and actually creates a hollow appearance to the superior eyelid, which is seen with physiologic involutional changes of the orbital fat. This is prevented by removing only the preaponeurotic and orbital fat, which freely prolapses into the incision of the orbital septum. Orbital fat should not be pulled out of the orbit, and only gentle retropulsion of the globe should be done to remove herniated orbital fat.

Repair of a pronounced superior sulcus can be done by injection of autogenous fat grafting to the superior orbit. This technique can be unpredictable secondary to fat atrophy and fibrosis of the graft. Obtaining the graft also requires liposuction, with injection into the desired site. Another method of repair is to increase the orbital volume by placement of an alloplastic material subperiosteally on the orbital floor.

Feminization of the Male Eyelid

Careful attention must be paid to male patients undergoing upper eyelid blepharoplasty. The desired cosmetic result in female patients is very different in men. The goal of upper eyelid cosmetic blepharoplasty in women is a high eyelid crease with a smooth, large exposure of the pretarsal upper eyelid. This appearance in men is considered feminizing. Male patients, therefore, are divided into two types: those with prominent eyes and those with enophthalmic, deep-set eyes. In the male patient with prominent eyes, a conservative procedure with excision of skin and orbicularis, not removing orbital fat, and tightening of the superior orbital septum is usually the most appropriate approach. In male patients with enophthalmic eyes and upper eyelid fullness, conservative removal of orbital fat is usually required; however, the vertical excision of skin and orbicularis should be approximately half of what would normally be excised in a female patient. This allows proper draping of the superior eyelid skin

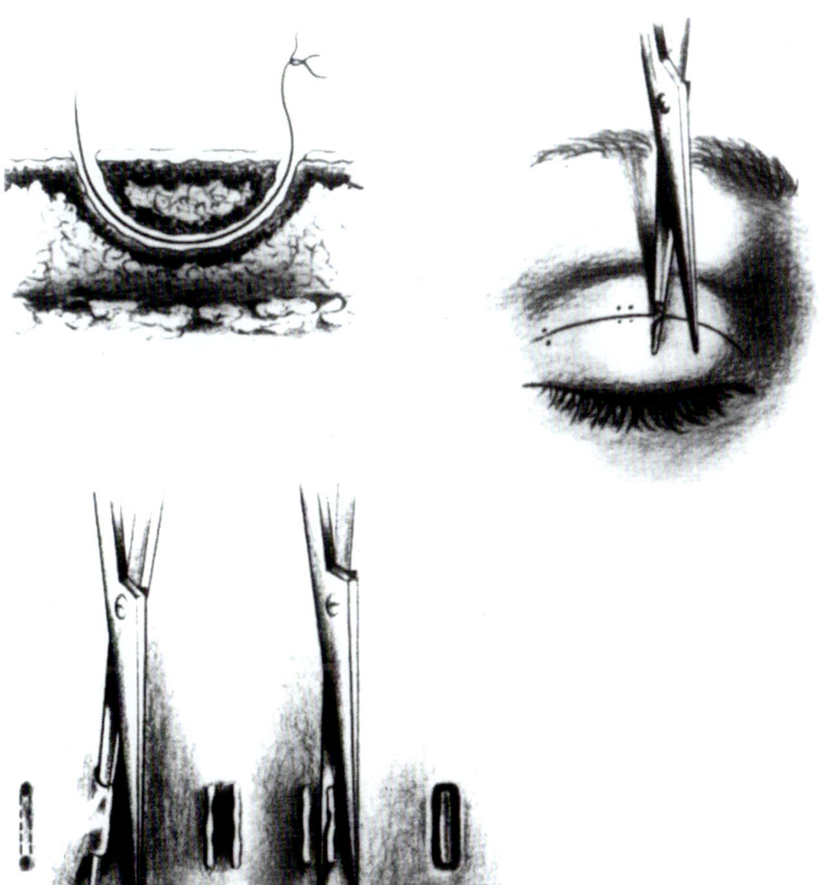

Fig. 32.9 Unroofing of suture milia.

over the eyelid crease while still obtaining a youthful appearance. If necessary, eyelid crease enhancement sutures can be done to emphasize the normally more pronounced eyelid crease seen in men.

Correction of male feminization secondary to upper eyelid blepharoplasty should be aimed at lowering a high eyelid crease, with correction of overexcision of skin, muscle, and orbital fat.

Ptosis Secondary to Upper Eyelid Blepharoplasty

Ptosis after upper eyelid blepharoplasty is seen when there is injury or restriction of the levator aponeurosis. Most commonly this occurs from direct laceration of the aponeurosis during the excision of the skin and orbicularis at the inferior aspect of the incision. Inferior to the preaponeurotic fat pad, the levator aponeurosis fuses with the orbital septum and orbicularis to insert onto the anterior surface of the tarsal plate and anteriorly into the skin to create the lid crease. Any incision into the skin/orbicularis or orbital septum at this point runs the risk of lacerating the aponeurosis. If laceration of the aponeurosis is identified during surgery, repair should be undertaken at that time with elevation of the patient's head during surgery to estimate postoperative lid height. If ptosis is encountered postoperatively, then appropriate ptosis repair should be done with repair of the laceration. The best approach to avoiding laceration of the levator aponeurosis is incising the orbital septum superiorly over the preaponeurotic fat pad, which sits anterior to the aponeurosis and is thus a reliable landmark for identification.

Postoperative ptosis sometimes develops in the absence of a frank aponeurotic laceration but in elongation and dehiscence of the levator aponeurosis insertion. This can result from direct mechanical stretching or from severe postoperative edema or hematoma. This type of ptosis can sometimes improve spontaneously as the edema or hemorrhage subsides, but accompanying fibrovascular ingrowth can cause adhesions and persistent ptosis. One should wait at least 6 months before repairing ptosis, but if this type of ptosis persists, it can be repaired by levator aponeurosis advancement and reattachment, or resection of the fibrotic tissue with reattachment. If the ptosis is small (< 2–3 mm), a tarsoconjunctival müllerectomy may be considered as well, based on the surgeon's preference.

Another possible development of postoperative ptosis is secondary to a leash effect or restriction of the levator aponeurosis by incorporation of the aponeurosis and orbital septum together within the surgical wound during wound closure. To avoid this type of postoperative ptosis, careful attention must be made to not include orbital septum in the suture, placing the suture only through the levator aponeurosis and the skin and muscle edges. Also, placement of the suture bite through the aponeurosis should be made ~1.0 to 1.5 mm above the lower incision edge. If the suture is placed higher, this can leash down the levator to the orbital septum with resulting ptosis.

Treatment of postoperative ptosis < 2.0 to 2.5 mm initially should be observed, as many of these cases can improve spontaneously. The type of ptosis repair is based on the severity of the ptosis, the function of the levator complex, and the amount of fibrovascular tissue present from the initial injury. Selection of the type of procedure is surgeon dependent.

Equally as important as preventing postoperative ptosis in upper eyelid blepharoplasty is recognizing preoperative ptosis. True involutional ptosis should be addressed at the same time as blepharoplasty to avoid unwanted cosmetic and functional results. Again, choice of ptosis repair is surgeon dependent.

Lagophthalmos

Blepharoplasty surgery over the past years has shifted from overzealous excision of skin and orbital fat to conservative skin removal with sculpting of orbital fat and tightening of the orbital septum. When there is overexcision of the upper eyelid skin, the patient may develop postoperative lagophthalmos. The resulting complications of lagophthalmos will be dependent on the patient's ability to protect the eye. Normal tear film mechanisms, Bell phenomenon, absence of ophthalmic external disease, and eyelid function are all important in predicting if a patient will develop exposure symptoms from lagophthalmos. If these mechanisms are compromised, even a small amount of lagophthalmos can produce intractable symptoms and exposure keratopathy. Conversely, with normal mechanisms in place, moderate amounts of lagophthalmos can be tolerated with minimal treatment.

Early mild lagophthalmos can be managed initially with ocular lubrication, such as artificial tears, then progressing to more viscous solutions, gels, and ointments. If symptoms are still persistent, taping the eyelid closed at bedtime can provide additional help in decreasing tear evaporation. With time, many mild cases may improve

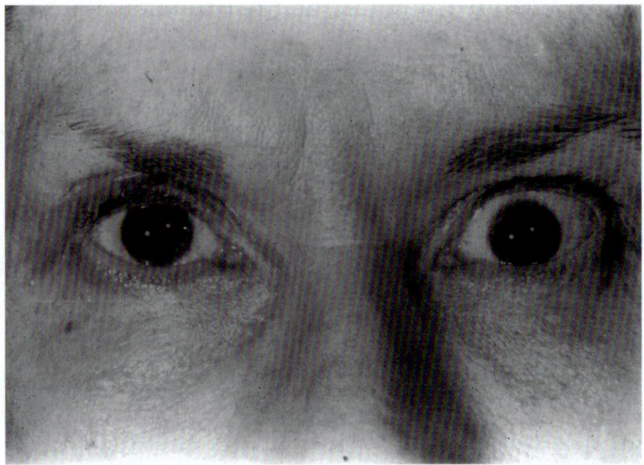

Fig. 32.10 Upper eyelid retraction and lagophthalmos secondary to orbital septal fibrosis and overexcision of the skin after blepharoplasty.

and are tolerated without surgical intervention. In more severe cases, full-thickness skin grafting to the upper eyelid may be necessary, especially if the surface of the eye starts to break down with compromising of vision. The most common donor sites for full-thickness skin grafts to the eyelid are areas with similar thickness, color, and no hair bearing. The contralateral upper eyelid is commonly used in reconstruction; however, if the patient has had a previous blepharoplasty, this site is usually not an option. The retroauricular and supraclavicular areas are both close matches in thickness and color. However, even in the best circumstances, the results are unpredictable, commonly with disappointing cosmetic results and ptosis.

Lagophthalmos can also occur secondary to iatrogenic closure of the orbital septum or septal fibrosis with scarring (**Fig. 32.10**). In these cases, full-thickness skin grafting with lysis of adhesions and removal of scar tissue is important to release any existing cicatrix (**Fig. 32.11**).

Bleeding

Bleeding in most cases does not require surgical revision and postoperatively is usually treated conservatively, especially if the hemorrhage is confined to the preseptal space where there is minimal threat to ophthalmic or visual compromise. If a postoperative hematoma forms, conservative management with cold compresses for the first 48 hours is usually sufficient. If excessive bleeding or hematoma is present, a stab incision and drainage will help to drain the hematoma. Diffuse hemorrhage requires opening of the incision site and exploration with cautery or ligation. The best way to prevent hemorrhage is preoperative discontinuation of medications that can cause excessive bleeding.

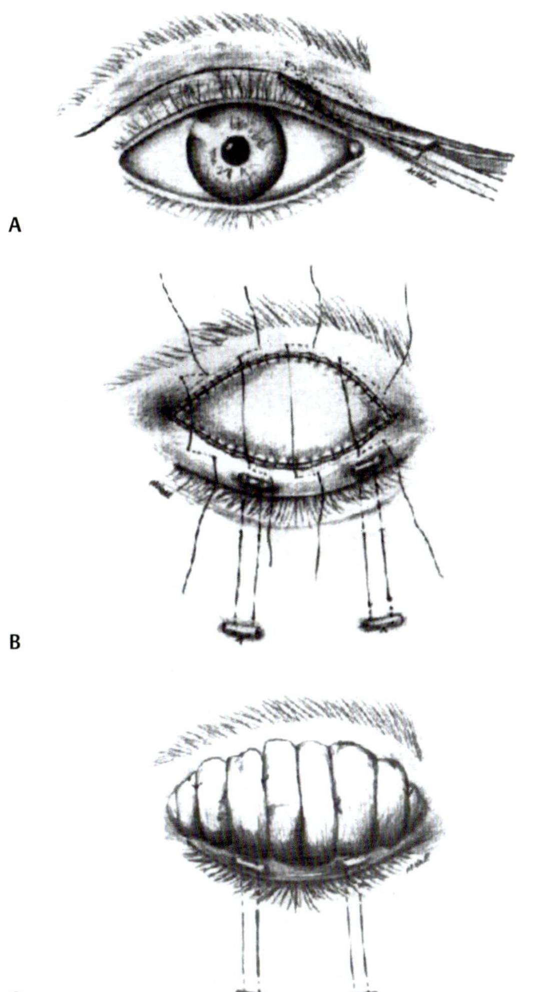

Fig. 32.11 **(A)** A lid crease incision is made through the skin. **(B)** A full-thickness skin graft is placed within the bed and sutured with interrupted and running sutures. **(C)** The dressing is tied over the skin graft.

Hemorrhage in blepharoplasty comes from the orbicularis muscle and the fine vascular plexuses that course throughout the orbital fat. If bleeding persists with extension of preseptal bleeding into the orbit, or direct orbital bleeding, an uncontrolled retrobulbar hemorrhage can result. Development of periorbital ecchymosis, subconjunctival hemorrhage, proptosis, visual loss, and pain with or without an afferent papillary defect are all indicators of uncontrolled hemorrhage. This is a true emergency and should be managed with intravenous (IV) hyperosmotic agents and carbonic anhydrase inhibitors to decrease intraocular pressure and preserve or reestablish optic nerve blood flow. If ocular compromise does not respond to aggressive medication administration, then immediate revision should be undertaken with lateral canthotomy, opening the incision sites, or, if needed, orbital decompression.

Surgical Revision for Lower Blepharoplasty

Lower Eyelid Retraction

One of the most common complications of lower blepharoplasty is eyelid retraction with inferior scleral show (**Fig. 32.10**). This results from fibrovascular tissue or scar formation of the orbital septum with cicatricial changes and contraction of the septum. Clinically, the result is inferior scleral show and blunting or rounding of the lateral canthal angle. This complication is more commonly seen with transcutaneous blepharoplasty than with a transconjunctival approach in which there is no incision made in the septum. Patients with prominent eyes and shallow orbits are also at risk for developing lower eyelid retraction because of greater exposure of the eye. Attention should be paid to the amount of skin excised if a transcutaneous approach is desired in this type of patient. Patients who have had multiple transcutaneous blepharoplasties are also at increased risk, as they already have a shortened anterior lamella and previous incision into the septum with scarring (**Figs. 32.12, 32.13**).

Crucial to optimal treatment of lower eyelid retraction is immediate postoperative recognition. If lower eyelid retraction is seen postoperatively, a Steri-Strip or traction suture can be placed to put the lid on stretch (e.g., Frost suture) for 7 to 10 days. This can resolve lid retraction in some cases. Digital massage can also help break up early septal scar formation. If observation and conservative treatment are not successful, then surgical revision is usually required.

Prior to revision of lower eyelid retraction, a distinction should be made between the component of septal scarring and anterior lamellar shortening. Again, careful attention should be paid to the presence of shallow orbits

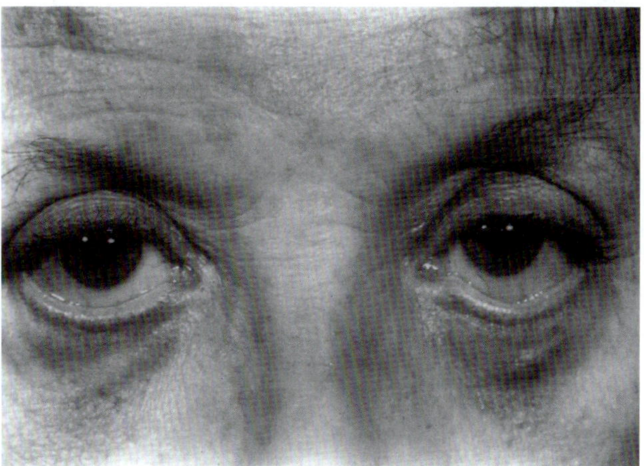

Fig. 32.12 Lower lid retraction after blepharoplasty with scleral show.

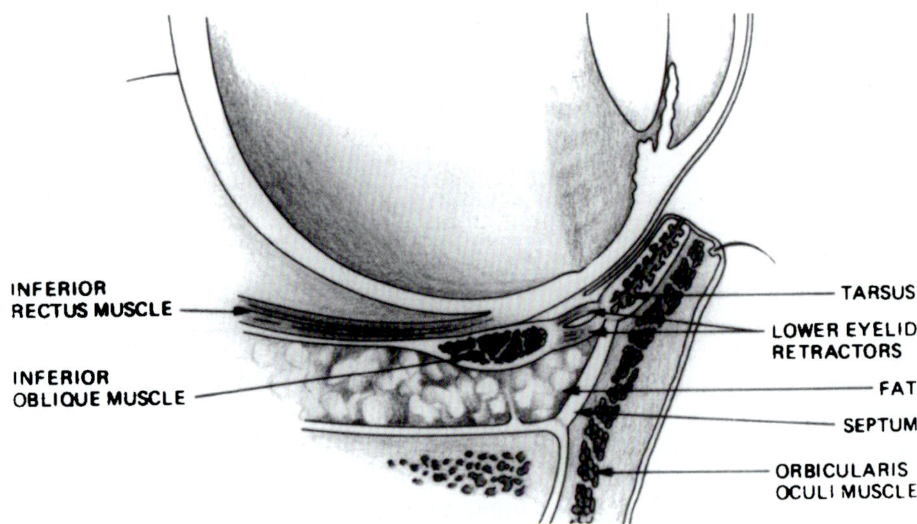

Fig. 32.13 Cross-sectional diagram of lower lid retraction.

and prominent eyes. The surgical revision also varies if the postoperative retraction is recent or old.

If development of postoperative lower eyelid retraction is within 6 months, revision is aimed at lysis of septal and eyelid adhesions with canthotomy, inferior cantholysis, and lateral mobilization of the eyelid from the cicatrizing septum and canthopexy.

The surgeon should measure the amount of vertical traction on the lower eyelid by having the patient look in upgaze and pushing in an upward fashion to palpate the amount of septal adhesions. This helps to localize and quantitate the degree of scarring.

In early lower eyelid retraction revision surgery, a lateral canthotomy and inferior cantholysis are preformed. The lower lid is placed on upward traction, again feeling for the areas of septal adhesions. Scissors are then placed within the free edge of the swinging eyelid, with one blade anterior to the conjunctiva and the other posterior to the skin, in an attempt to divide the orbital septum and vertically limiting adhesions. Lysis of adhesions is assessed while upward traction of the lid is maintained. Upon achieving vertical elevation of the lower eyelid margin with relaxation of the septal cicatrix, attention can be turned toward repositioning the eyelid at the lateral canthus.

With release of adhesions, the lower eyelid is more freely mobile vertically and horizontally. Excess horizontal laxity will create an ectropion, so vertical eyelid tension must be minimized and horizontal eyelid tension maximized. The exception is with the prominent eye with shallow orbits, or thyroid disease. In the prominent eye, if horizontal lid shortening is done, the lower eyelid can retract downward secondary to greater exposure of the globe (e.g., like tightening the belt on a fat man), with horizontal tension not allowing the eyelid to move superiorly

over the inferior aspect of the eye. The lateral edge of the eyelid is placed at its new desired location for canthopexy, usually at the same horizontal level as the pupil, and the lid can be marked as to the amount to be horizontally shortened. The anterior and posterior lamellae of the eyelid are separated using scissors at the gray line of the eyelid margin. Usually in horizontal lid shortening the inferior lid retractors are cut, but this was done previously in lysing the scarred septum and eyelid tissue. A strip of skin of the eyelid margin is removed with scissors from the temporal eyelid to the area marked previously, then a no. 15 Bard-Parker blade is used to scrape the palpebral conjunctival epithelium off the tarsal strip. A straight Stevens scissors is used to create a skin–muscle pocket over the periosteum at the lateral orbital rim. A double-armed permanent suture (our preference is a 4–0 Polydec suture) on a half-curved needle is placed anterior to posterior at the edge of the tarsal strip on the superior and inferior borders. The sutures are then placed just inside the lateral orbital rim, through the periosteum at the level of Whitnall tubercle and tied down. The overlying skin and muscle are closed in either one or two layers.

Lateral Tarsal Strip and Horizontal Lid Shortening

If vertical tension is still noted after releasing the scarred orbital septum, then the temporal orbicularis muscle can also be advanced vertically for added support (**Fig. 32.14**). After the double-armed 4–0 Polydec suture is placed through the periosteum and tied, a skin flap is dissected in the temporal lower eyelid extending to the inferior orbital rim. The orbicularis muscle dissected from the skin flap is advanced superiorly, and two double-armed 6–0 silk

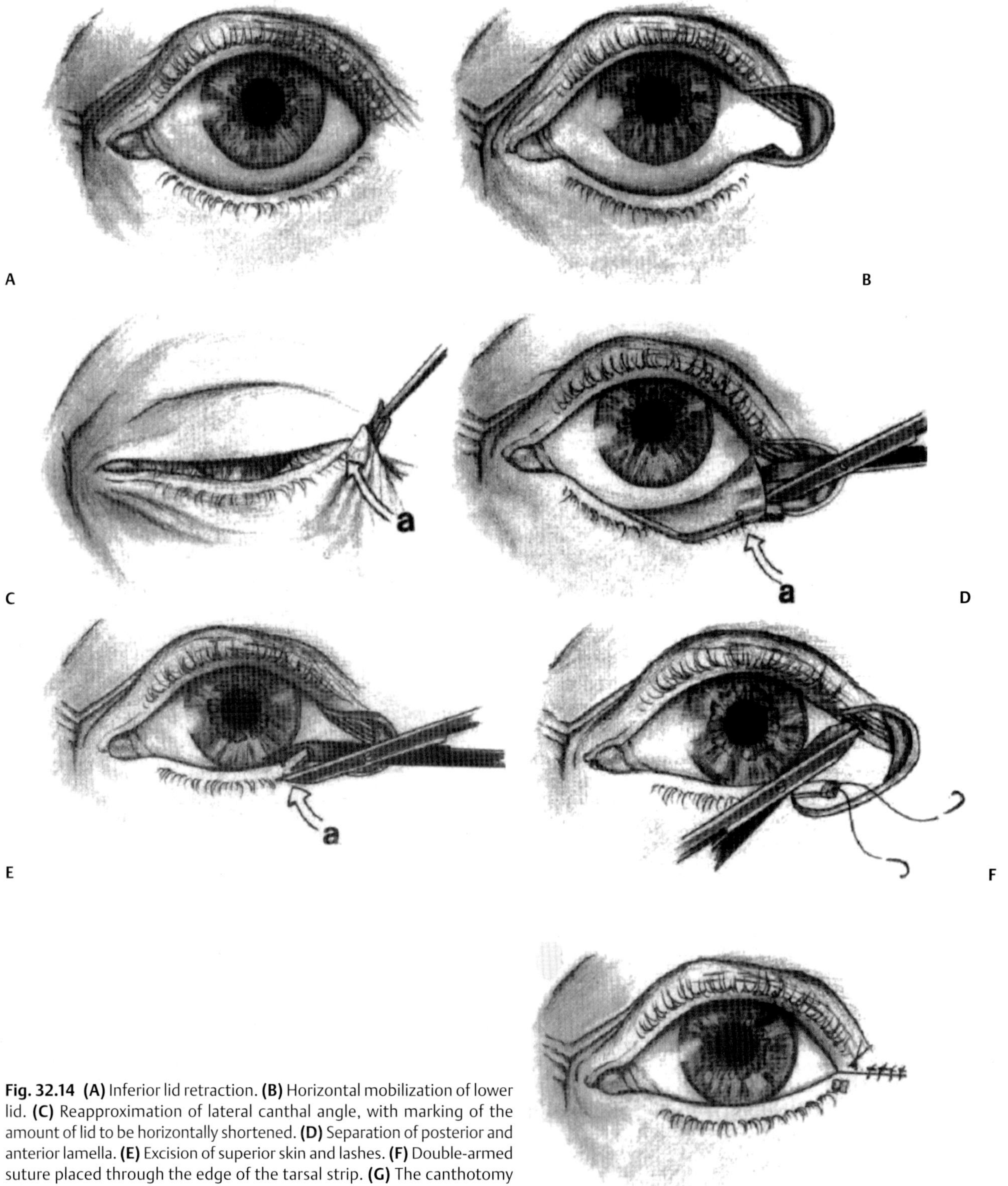

Fig. 32.14 **(A)** Inferior lid retraction. **(B)** Horizontal mobilization of lower lid. **(C)** Reapproximation of lateral canthal angle, with marking of the amount of lid to be horizontally shortened. **(D)** Separation of posterior and anterior lamella. **(E)** Excision of superior skin and lashes. **(F)** Double-armed suture placed through the edge of the tarsal strip. **(G)** The canthotomy incision is closed with interrupted sutures.

sutures are placed through the undersurface of the orbicularis and then through the periosteum of the lateral orbital rim and tied down in a horizontal mattress fashion. At the superior edge of the orbicularis a triangle is resected of the overlapping tissue. The lateral canthal angle is reestablished with an interrupted 6–0 silk suture placed through the gray line of the cut edge of the temporal lower lid and out through the cut edge and gray line of the temporal upper lid. The skin is then closed with interrupted 6–0 silk sutures. A double-armed 4–0 silk traction suture can then be placed through the lateral lower eyelid skin and orbicularis and out through the lid margin and suspended from the lateral eyebrow with skin buttresses.

Long-Standing or Severe Lower Eyelid Retraction

In severe lower eyelid retraction or long-standing cases (blepharoplasty > 6 months ago), severe orbital septum scarring in conjunction with adhesions and shortening of the posterior lamella of the lower eyelid requires a different approach to revision surgery. If prior revision surgery was unsuccessful using the technique previously described, then it is likely that shortening of the posterior lamella is present and needs to be repaired for an acceptable surgical result.

Different options are available for posterior lamellar grafts. Many surgeons prefer autologous grafting to cadaveric or synthetic grafts. Of the autologous grafts, hard palate mucosal grafts provide excellent support and a mucosal surface that similarly matches conjunctiva and adapts well in the eye. Functionally and cosmetically, these grafts heal well with minimal kinking and bumpiness of the overlying tissue. If hard palate grafting is not an option, then ear cartilage can be obtained; however, it provides no posterior mucosal surface and can develop a thickened, bumpy appearance. Other grafting options are AlloDerm acellular tissue (LifeCell Corp., Branchburg, New Jersey), Tutoplast (IOP Inc., Costa Mesa, California), and a Medpor spacer (Porex Corp., Newnan, Georgia) if autologous grafting cannot be done. Each has advantages and disadvantages, and these must be considered when determining the most optimum grafting material.

Once the type of graft has been determined, preparation of the recipient bed is similar regardless of grafting material. A lateral canthotomy and inferior cantholysis may be necessary and are done as previously described to mobilize the eyelid horizontally. The lower eyelid is then mobilized vertically, and the recipient bed is created by a horizontal incision made at the inferior border of the tarsal plate, through the conjunctiva, inferior eyelid retractors, and orbital septum with lysis of septal adhesions. As the scarring is released and vertical tension is placed on the eyelid, the recipient bed will open up, allowing the surgeon to accurately measure the size of the graft that will be required. The graft is then placed into the recipient bed and cut to fit the shape of the bed. The graft is sutured in place superiorly to the inferior border of the tarsal plate and inferiorly to the superior edge of the inferior lid retractors. Interrupted 6–0 chromic gut is used to approximate graft fixation. The lateral canthus is then reestablished and tightened, and the lower eyelid is placed on stretch with tension sutures to prevent graft shrinkage and recurrence of lower eyelid retraction. If eyelid retraction is still present postoperatively, the graft should be allowed to heal in place for 8 to 10 weeks, followed by high resuspension of the lower eyelid to the eyebrow without concern of damaging the graft.

Lower Eyelid Ectropion

Lower eyelid ectropion is a less commonly seen complication than lid retraction. It usually causes more pronounced exposure of the eye with resultant tearing secondary to punctal eversion and defective tear pump function. As compared with lower eyelid retraction, ectropion results from shortening of the anterior lamella of the eyelid, or skin and orbicularis muscle (**Fig. 32.15**). This is seen with transcutaneous lower eyelid blepharoplasty and overexcision of skin. Revision surgery for lower eyelid ectropion repair is aimed at lengthening the vertically shortened anterior lamella, usually through full-thickness skin grafting.

In preparation for a skin graft to the lower eyelid, it must be determined what size skin graft will be required to correct the ectropion. A 4–0 silk suture is placed through the lower eyelid margin to stretch the eyelid, and a subciliary incision is made along the horizontal length of the eyelid. A skin flap is made from the incision to the inferior orbital rim, allowing full relaxation of the inferior

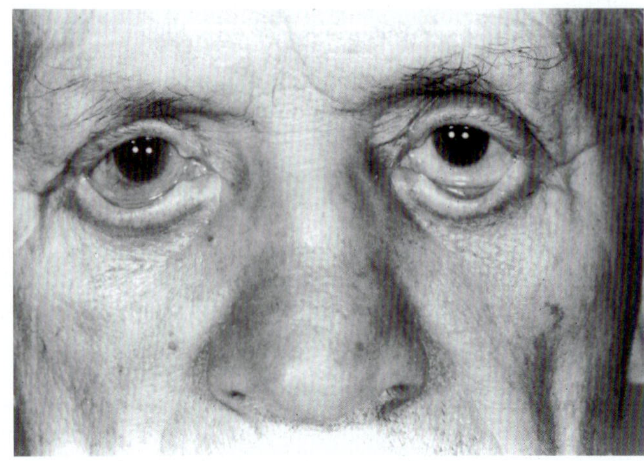

Fig. 32.15 Lower lid ectropion after blepharoplasty.

eyelid skin from underlying vertical tension and expansion of the skin defect. The graft recipient bed can now be accurately measured with tension removed from the skin edges. If horizontal eyelid laxity is also present, contributing to the ectropion, a horizontal lid-shortening procedure or a lateral tarsal strip procedure with or without a base wedge resection should be done at this time, as it will affect the shape and size of the skin graft required.

When ready to obtain the skin graft, with the eyelid on stretch, a metal ruler or calipers can be used to measure the horizontal and vertical size of the defect. A piece of sterile filter paper can be used to draw a template over the recipient bed. There are many sites that can be used for full-thickness skin grafting for the eyelid, keeping in mind that the eyelid skin is not hair bearing and is the thinnest in the body. The contralateral upper eyelid, posterior auricular, preauricular, supraclavicular, and medial upper arm are all reasonable sites for full-thickness skin grafts. The graft is outlined 10% larger than the recipient bed to allow for graft shrinkage. Depending on the site, the underlying subcutaneous fat should be removed to create as thin a graft as possible. The graft is placed in the bed, and multiple 6–0 silk sutures are used to fixate the graft, with one end left long to tie over a bolster. Multiple stab incisions can be made within the graft to prevent hematoma formation beneath the graft, causing graft failure. The lower eyelid should remain on stretch postoperatively to prevent skin graft shrinkage and recurrence of ectropion (**Fig. 32.16**).

It should be noted that, although lower eyelid retraction and ectropion are described as separate entities above, in many cases there are components of both that need to be repaired during surgical revision. Preoperative assessment and recognition of these components are essential in planning surgical revision.

Under- or Overexcision of Lower Eyelid Fat

As approaches to orbital fat removal continue to evolve in blepharoplasty surgery, the desired cosmetic result is a smooth, short lower eyelid contour with single convexity of the lower eyelid and cheek. Fat removal is now shifting to fat repositioning in cosmetic blepharoplasty. As a rule of thumb, it is better to underexcise nasal orbital fat and to overexcise temporal orbital fat. Overexcision of nasal orbital fat accentuates the palpebrojugal fold (tear trough deformity), which creates a hollow, deskeletonized appearance similar to the superior sulcus defect seen in the upper eyelid. Revision surgery for overexcision of nasal fat can be approached by free fat injection or tear trough implant.

Free fat injections into the tear trough deformity are not always predictable because of fat absorption and atrophy. As a result, tear trough implants are a predictable approach to repairing tear trough deformity.

Prior to blepharoplasty, orbital fat repositioning can be considered in a patient who has prominent lower eyelid fat pads with a prominent tear trough deformity. Removing orbital fat alone in these patients accentuates the tear trough deformity. Instead, sculpting of the prominent lateral fat pad with central and nasal subperiosteal fat pad repositioning into the tear trough deformity can provide long-lasting improvement in the deformity. Typically, this procedure cannot be done after blepharoplasty, as the pronounced orbital fat has already been removed. It also provides a less dramatic effect compared with alloplastic implants.

Tear trough implants such as the Flowers implant (Implant Tech, Van Nuys, California) or Medpor medial cheek implant (Porex) are specifically designed to fit the medial concavity seen in suborbital deficiency. In many patients the tear trough deformity is secondary to maxillary hypoplasia with poor support for the lower eyelid and cheek soft tissues. If these same patients have lower lid blepharoplasty with nasal fat excision, this further accentuates the lack of bony support. The tear trough implant addresses this lack of bony support and is inserted subperiosteally posterior to the tear trough deformity. Different approaches can be used to place the implant. Preoperatively, the patient is given IV antibiotics, and the implant is soaked in an antibiotic solution (e.g., gentamicin). A central notch is carved out of the implant not to distract the infraorbital neurovascular bundle. A transconjunctival lower lid approach is performed inferiorly to the orbital rim. The periosteum is incised and dissected beneath the tear trough deformity. The implant is placed in the subperiosteal pocket, with the implant flush with the inferior orbital rim. If the implant extends superiorly over the rim, it should be trimmed. The implant is then sutured to the cut edge of the arcus marginalis. The suborbicularis oculi fat can be lifted over the implant if desired for a more accentuated result. The conjunctival incision is then closed with interrupted 6–0 chromic gut sutures, and the lateral is canthus resuspended if needed.

Underexcision of the temporal lower eyelid fat is common. The orbital fat shifts superiorly and posteriorly when the patient is supine, usually causing underexcision. The lateral orbital fat pad of the lower eyelid is more easily approached from the transcutaneous approach; however, the risk of lower eyelid retraction is much higher in this approach than in a transconjunctival approach even if minimal skin is excised. If underexcision of fat occurs, then revision surgery via a transconjunctival approach can be done with more aggressive fat excision.

Postoperative Skin Wrinkling

In transconjunctival blepharoplasty, the main cosmetic result is reduction in herniated orbital fat. This procedure does not appreciably change the appearance of the skin.

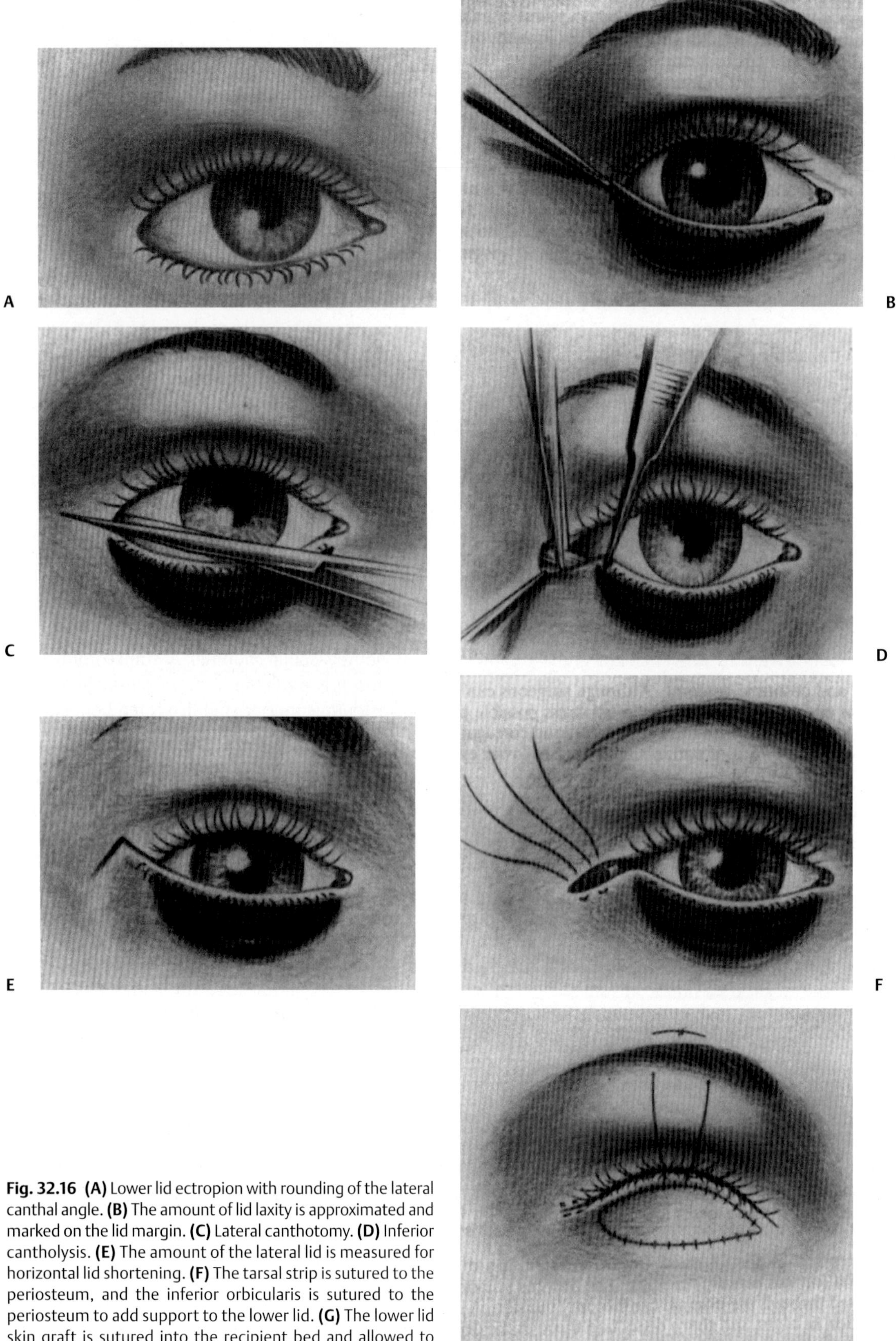

Fig. 32.16 **(A)** Lower lid ectropion with rounding of the lateral canthal angle. **(B)** The amount of lid laxity is approximated and marked on the lid margin. **(C)** Lateral canthotomy. **(D)** Inferior cantholysis. **(E)** The amount of the lateral lid is measured for horizontal lid shortening. **(F)** The tarsal strip is sutured to the periosteum, and the inferior orbicularis is sutured to the periosteum to add support to the lower lid. **(G)** The lower lid skin graft is sutured into the recipient bed and allowed to remain on stretch with a traction suture.

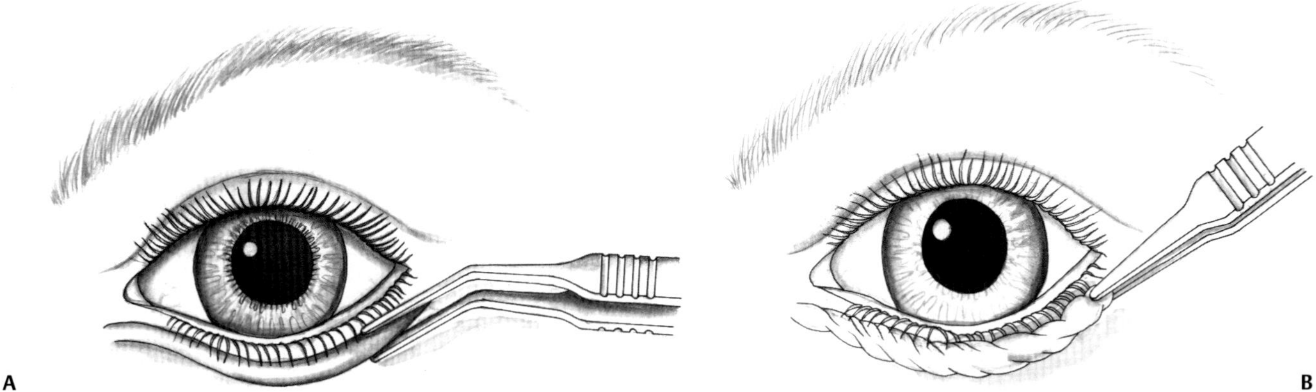

Fig. 32.17 (A,B) Skin pinch technique for excess lower lid skin.

Skin wrinkling is still present postoperatively and in some instances can be made more prominent. One of the most common solutions today is to address the skin wrinkling at the same time as the lower eyelid blepharoplasty with CO_2 or erbium laser resurfacing or dermabrasion. This can also be done postoperatively as a revision surgical procedure.

Another approach to skin wrinkling is the skin pinch technique; this can be done only if a distinct skin fold is identified on the lower eyelid. After injecting the skin with local anesthetic, the excess skin is pinched between the teeth of a forceps, delineating the skin to be excised. The skin is then excised along the crush marks. The incision is closed with running 6–0 nylon sutures (**Fig. 32.17**).

Suggested Reading

Baylis HI, Long JA, Groth MJ. Transconjunctival lower eyelid blepharoplasty: technique and complications. Ophthalmology 1989;96:1027–1032.

Baylis HI, Nelson ER, Goldberg RA. Lower eyelid retraction following blepharoplasty. Ophthal Plast Reconstr Surg 1992;8:170–175.

Goldberg RA. Transconjunctival orbital fat repositioning: transposition of orbital fat pedicles into a subperiosteal pocket. Plast Reconstr Surg 2000;105:743–748.

Hornblass A. Oculoplastic, Orbital and Reconstructive Surgery. Vol 1. Baltimore: Williams & Wilkins; 1988.

McCord CD. Eyelid Surgery Principles and Techniques. Philadelphia: Lippincott-Raven; 1995.

Putterman AM. Cosmetic Oculoplastic Surgery: Eyelid, Forehead, and Facial Techniques. 3rd ed. Philadelphia: WB Saunders; 1999.

Zarem HA, Resnick JI. Expanded applications for transconjunctival lower lid blepharoplasty. Plast Reconstr Surg 1991; 88:215–220.

Decision tree for revision ptosis repair

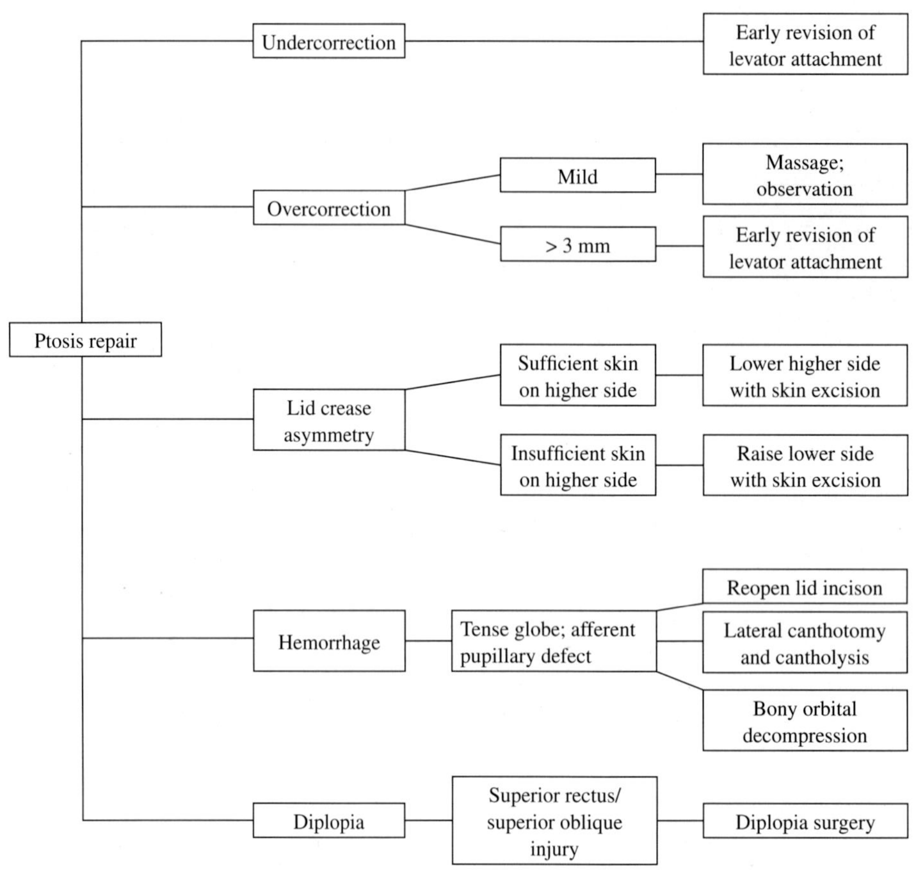

33 Revision Ptosis Surgery

*Michael T. Yen and Richard L. Anderson**

The surgical correction of blepharoptosis is one of the most challenging procedures in facial plastic surgery. Not only must the desired functional and aesthetic outcome of upper eyelid elevation be achieved, but adequate eyelid closure and corneal protection, vital to avoiding exposure keratoconjunctivitis and corneal ulceration, must also be maintained. Other complications of ptosis surgery include undercorrection, overcorrection, asymmetry, eyelid margin contour deformity, lash ptosis, entropion, ectropion, lagophthalmos, poor upper eyelid crease, superior rectus or superior oblique paresis, suture granuloma, infection, hemorrhage, and loss of vision. Historically, unpredictable results in ptosis surgery were common, and it is no surprise that revision surgery was often necessary. However, by taking a systematic approach with careful respect of eyelid anatomy, most complications after ptosis surgery can be improved or corrected. In this chapter, we describe our logical approach to revision ptosis surgery.

Preoperative Assessment

Prior to any surgical intervention, thorough evaluation of and consultation with the patient are mandatory, especially when the patient has already had complications requiring revision surgery. Eyelid height, eyelid fold, margin contour, eyelid crease position, abnormalities (e.g., eyelid notching), and symmetry should be carefully noted during the preoperative evaluation (**Fig. 33.1**). The original cause for the ptosis should be determined (aponeurotic, traumatic, neurogenic, mechanical, or congenital). Slit-lamp examination of the cornea with assessment of tear production and eyelid closure should also be performed prior to surgery to determine if the patient is prone to developing a dry eye. Visual acuity documentation and preoperative photographs are very important for the record and for medicolegal documentation. If the ptosis is functional and to be covered by insurance, visual field examinations are also essential.

Equally important is evaluating the prior surgical procedures performed on the eyelids. Was the prior ptosis surgery performed through an external or internal approach? Was the procedure combined with upper blepharoplasty

and fat excision? Intraoperative complications should be noted. The eyelid should be everted to evaluate the condition of the tarsus and whether a prior shortening has been performed. If the eyelid initially achieved a good height after surgery and recurred with time, neurologic or neuromyopathic conditions should be considered. Careful and thorough discussion with the patient should occur prior to surgery so that he or she understands the goals and limitations of revision ptosis surgery.

Anatomical Review

Successful and predictable results in ptosis surgery require precise knowledge of eyelid anatomy. Eyelid elevation is normally a function of the levator palpebrae muscle and the sympathetically innervated Müller muscle.[1] In most cases of acquired ptosis, defects in the levator aponeurosis can be observed. These defects include disinsertion, dehiscence, and rarefaction of the levator aponeurosis (**Fig. 33.2**).[2,3] They may result from age-related changes or be associated with orbital swelling or excessive eyelid squeezing. Successful surgical correction of ptosis should be directed toward strengthening the existing eyelid elevators.[4] In revision ptosis surgery, where the normal eyelid anatomy may be distorted from prior surgery or scarring, identification of the levator aponeurosis is crucial for successful revision surgery. The preaponeurotic fat pad is key to identifying the

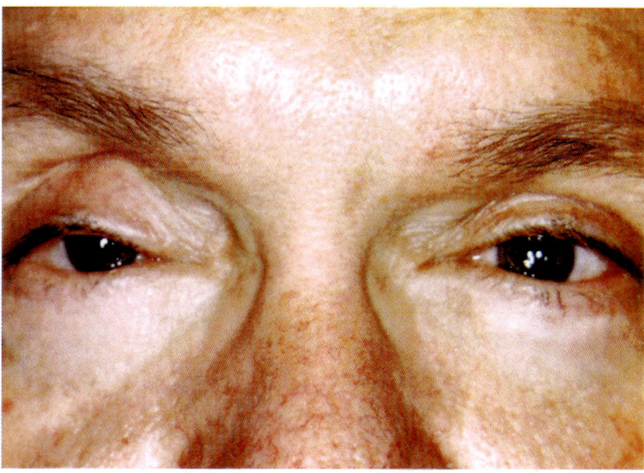

Fig. 33.1 A 52-year-old man after two attempted ptosis repairs of the right upper eyelid. Note the persistent ptosis and high, asymmetric eyelid crease on the right.

*The authors have no financial interest in the techniques described herein.

309

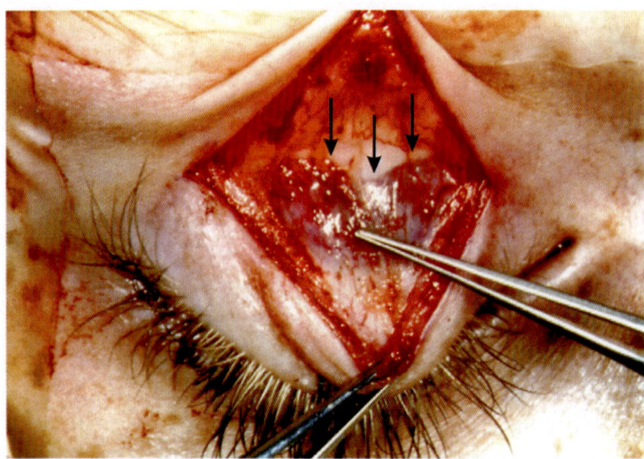

Fig. 33.2 Disinsertion of the levator aponeurosis as the cause of ptosis. Arrows outline the edge of the disinserted aponeurosis. Müller muscle is below the disinserted edge of the aponeurosis. The forces point to the peripheral arcade in Müller muscle, which helps identify this structure.

levator aponeurosis, as the aponeurosis is immediately behind the fat pad, and scar tissue may obscure other natural landmarks.

The levator muscle originates above the anulus of Zinn in the apex of the orbit. It runs anteriorly in the orbit just inferior to the orbital roof.[5] The levator becomes aponeurotic below the Whitnall ligament (superior transverse ligament),

then descends posterior to the preaponeurotic fat pads and inserts onto the anterior surface of the tarsus.[3] Anterior fibers of the aponeurosis attach to the skin through the pretarsal orbicularis muscle to form the eyelid crease. The Müller muscle originates from the levator ~12 mm above the tarsus and inserts onto the superior border of the tarsus.

The orbital septum is a multilaminated fibrillar membrane that can be mistaken for the levator aponeurosis in ptosis surgery.[6] The septum and its relationship with the levator aponeurosis is also the key anatomical distinction between the Caucasian eyelid and the Asian eyelid.[7] In the Caucasian eyelid, the orbital septum fuses with the levator aponeurosis above the superior tarsal border (**Fig. 33.3**). At the inferior border of the fused septum/aponeurosis, anterior fibers pass through the orbicularis muscle and attach to the skin to form the eyelid crease. In the Asian eyelid, the orbital septum fuses with the levator aponeurosis below the superior tarsal border (**Fig. 33.4**). This allows preaponeurotic fat to extend inferiorly and produce a thickened, full-appearing eyelid. The inferior extension of the orbital septum also prohibits the superficial attachments of the levator aponeurosis from attaching to the skin. The eyelid crease is subsequently poorly developed or, if present, is much lower than in the Caucasian eyelid. Appreciation of the anatomical distinctions between the Caucasian and Asian eyelid is important for all surgeons performing ptosis surgery.

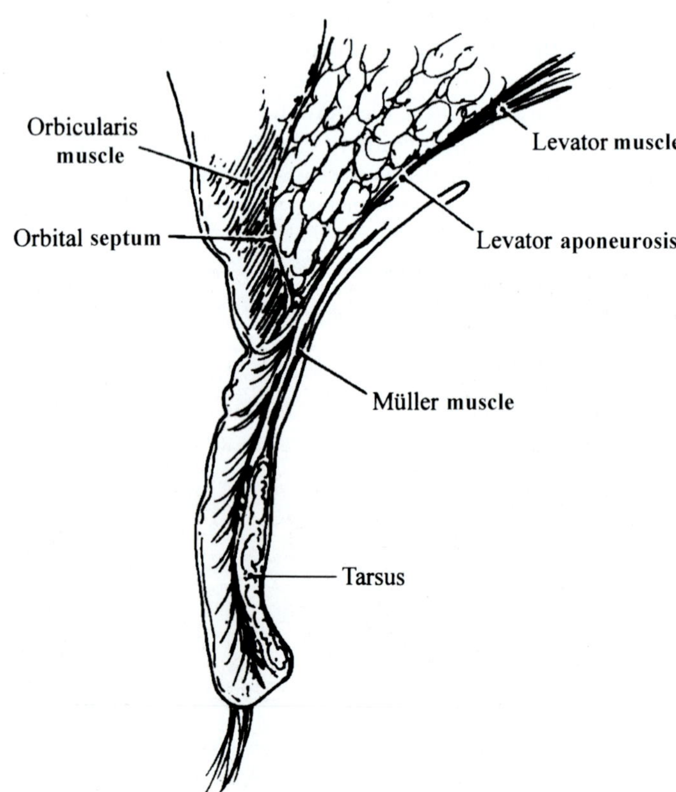

Fig. 33.3 In the Caucasian eyelid, the orbital septum fuses with the levator aponeurosis above the superior tarsal border.

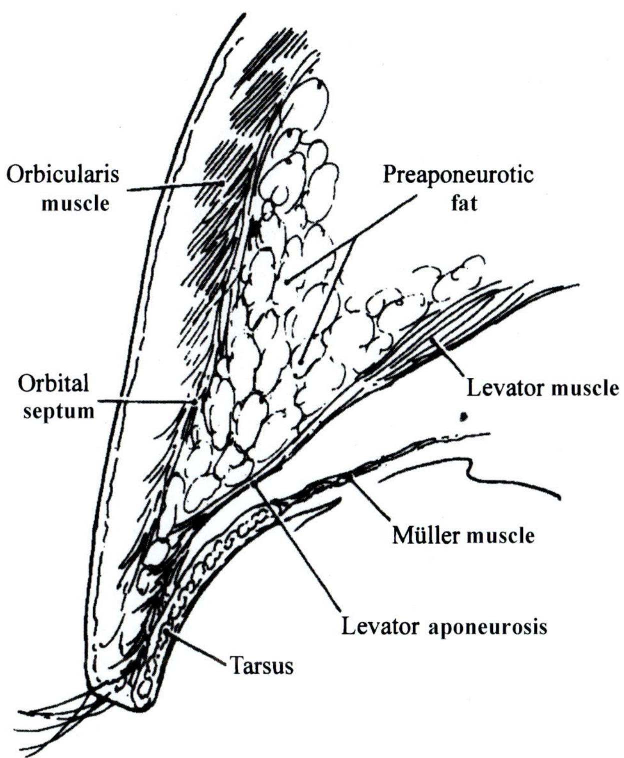

Fig. 33.4 In the Asian eyelid, the orbital septum fuses with the levator aponeurosis below the superior tarsal border.

Surgical Approach

In most cases of blepharoptosis, surgery directed toward tightening of the levator aponeurosis is required for successful correction.[4] The exception would be for patients with poor levator function (<4 mm of levator excursion from downgaze to upgaze), such as in some cases of congenital ptosis.[8] These patients usually require a superior tarsectomy or frontalis suspension for adequate correction of their blepharoptosis.[9] Patients with moderate or good levator function achieve the best postoperative results with levator aponeurosis tightening.[10]

Many techniques have been described for the surgical correction of blepharoptosis. Bowman first described levator shortening through a transconjunctival approach in 1857.[11] Eversbusch described the anterior approach to levator shortening in 1883.[12] Some surgeons have advocated surgical correction of ptosis with resection and advancement of the Müller muscle and conjunctiva alone or with a superior tarsectomy.[13,14] Unfortunately, the amount of eyelid elevation achieved is often limited and unreliable. We prefer an external approach to the levator aponeurosis in revision ptosis surgery as described by Anderson and Dixon in 1979.[4] They presented a reliable and practical approach to aponeurosis surgery that could be easily modified for patients with congenital as well as acquired ptosis, except

for those with poor levator function. The advantages of the external approach during revision ptosis surgery include (1) reestablishing and maintaining normal anatomical planes during dissection; (2) preserving all elevating structures, including the Müller muscle; (3) easy intraoperative adjustment of overcorrections and undercorrections; and (4) preserving tear-producing structures within the conjunctiva of the superior fornix.

Surgical Technique

Prior to injection of local anesthetic, the patient should be evaluated in a seated, upright position to determine the exact amount of ptosis and dermatochalasis. The level of the desired eyelid crease is then marked. The eyelid crease is usually made ~10 mm above the eyelid margin in women, 2 mm lower in men. The amount of excess skin and orbicularis muscle is then demarcated in a similar fashion as when performing upper eyelid blepharoplasty. Caution should be taken when determining the amount of skin to be excised, as patients undergoing revision ptosis surgery may already have had large amounts of skin excised from the upper eyelids. If excess skin is not present, then only the eyelid crease incision should be made.

Local anesthesia is strongly recommended for revision ptosis surgery, as this allows for intraoperative assessment of eyelid height and contour. If intravenous sedation is also administered, the anesthesiologist should be informed when to allow the patient to awake for assessing eyelid height and contour. We infiltrate 2% lidocaine with 1:100,000 epinephrine subcutaneously into the eyelid only where incisions are to be made. Excessive infiltration of local anesthetic can partially paralyze the levator muscle and result in significant overcorrections. When operating without an assistant, a 4–0 silk traction suture may be placed through the eyelid margin and secured to the drapes with a hemostat.

After creating skin incisions, the lateral corner of the skin and orbicularis to be excised is elevated, and a full-thickness cut is made with Stevens scissors. Entry into the avascular postorbicular fascial plane allows the skin and muscle to be excised en bloc. The key to finding the levator aponeurosis is to identify the preaponeurotic fat, as this may be the only reliable landmark in previously operated eyelids (**Fig. 33.5**).[15] Gentle pressure on the globe may aid identification by pushing the preaponeurotic fat pad anteriorly. The orbital septum is then opened, allowing the preaponeurotic fat to prolapse forward (**Fig. 33.6**). Scarring between the orbital septum, the levator aponeurosis, and the preaponeurotic fat pad may be encountered, and sharp dissection may be required to enter the fat pad. The levator aponeurosis is usually seen as a white structure under the preaponeurotic fat. All adhesions should be

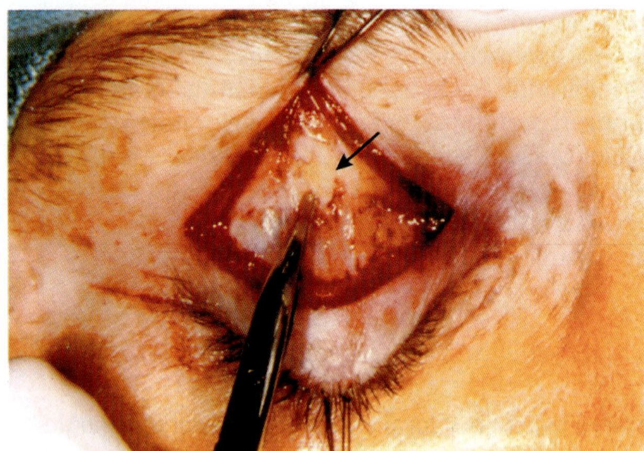

Fig. 33.5 The preaponeurotic fat pad can be seen behind the orbital septum (*arrow*). The levator aponeurosis lies just below the preaponeurotic fat pad.

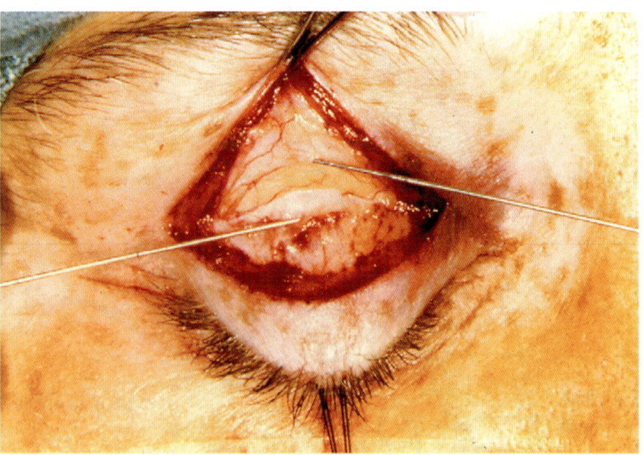

Fig. 33.6 After opening the orbital septum, the preaponeurotic fat pad prolapses forward between the edge of the disinserted aponeurosis (*lower pointer*) and the cut edge of the orbital septum (*upper pointer*).

released to allow the levator aponeurosis to move freely without restriction.

In difficult revision cases where the levator aponeurosis may not be distinct from the surrounding fibrotic tissues, asking the patient to open and close the eyes while grasping the suspected tissues may be helpful. Tension should be felt if the levator is grasped while the patient attempts to open his or her eyes. Occasionally, the septum or scarring may be mistaken for the levator aponeurosis. In these situations, firm attachments to the superior orbital rim can be felt, and no increased tension is appreciated when the patient attempts to open the eyes. Again, the key to locating the levator aponeurosis in difficult revision cases is to first identify the preaponeurotic fat pad.

Once the levator aponeurosis has been identified and separated from all adhesions, appropriate adjustments to its position can be made. In correcting undercorrections, we prefer to create a fresh edge to the aponeurosis by resecting a small amount just above the tarsal border. This will result in permanent scarring for good fusion between the aponeurosis and the tarsal plate.[4] The levator aponeurosis is then advanced and secured to the tarsus with several 5–0 polyglactin 910 sutures on a spatula needle (**Fig. 33.7**). We prefer not to use permanent sutures here to avoid the risk of suture granulomas and posterior erosions, which can lead to corneal irritation and ulceration. The first suture is usually placed just medial to the pupil corresponding to the natural high point of the upper eyelid.[16] Additional sutures are placed medially and laterally as needed to provide the desired eyelid contour. In correcting overcorrections, the levator aponeurosis is recessed and secured to the underlying Müller muscle and conjunctiva to prevent postoperative advancement of the aponeurosis.[17] Use of a spatula needle will reduce the risk of full-thickness eyelid perforation and penetrating globe injuries.

The amount of eyelid elevation, eyelid contour, and symmetry between the two eyelids should be assessed

intraoperatively with the patient seated upright. Adjustments to the sutures can be made until the desired height and contour are achieved. Although many surgeons have attempted to calculate the amount of resection or advancement to be performed based on the degree of ptosis and levator function, we feel that these calculations are often imprecise. The best results require intraoperative assessment and adjustment to the amount of resection and advancement performed.

Once meticulous hemostasis has been confirmed, the eyelid crease incision is then closed with interrupted 6–0 plain catgut sutures. For most patients with optimum levator function, a good lid crease will form without aponeurotic fixation of the skin sutures, especially if any skin and orbicularis muscle were excised in conjunction with the ptosis surgery. This usually also provides better symmetry between the two upper eyelids. However, if lash ptosis is present, or if a poor lid crease existed preoperatively, or if the levator function is poor, then skin–aponeurosis–skin

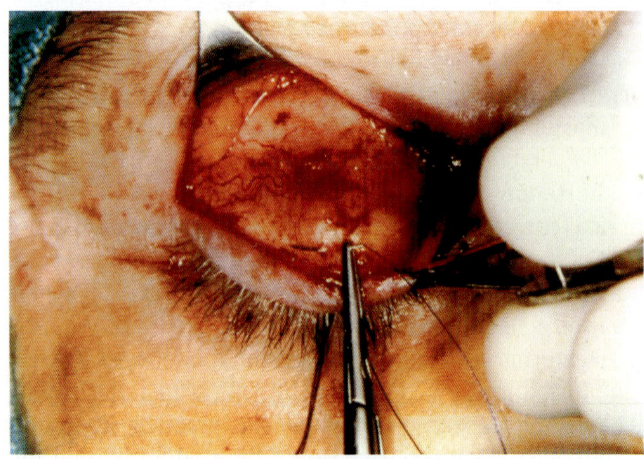

Fig. 33.7 Polyglactin sutures are placed in a lamellar fashion through the tarsus to secure the advanced levator aponeurosis.

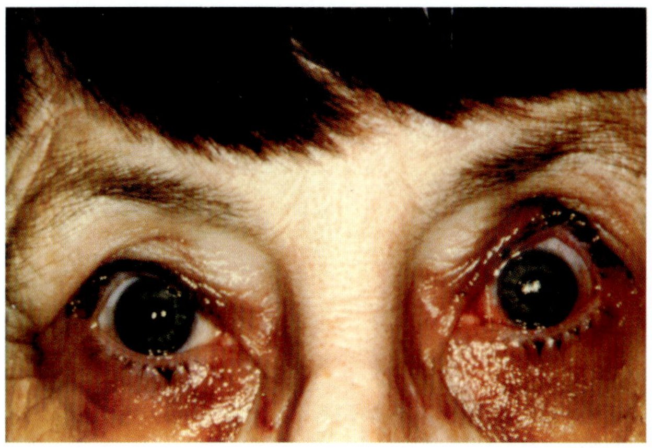

Fig. 33.8 Marked overcorrection of ptosis noted postoperatively. Note the irregular light reflex in the left eye. This is indicative of corneal drying and epitheliopathy. Recession of the levator aponeurosis should be performed urgently to prevent corneal ulceration.

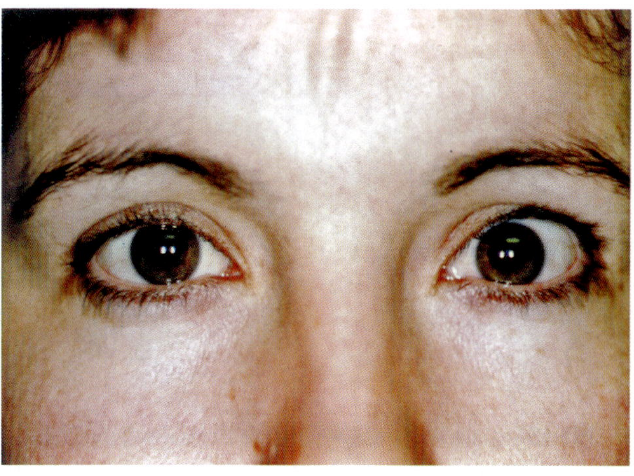

Fig. 33.9 Temporal overcorrection of ptosis in the left upper eyelid at 3 weeks postoperatively.

sutures should be placed to enhance the upper eyelid crease and fixate the anterior lamella to the tarsus. With this technique, each pass of the needle takes a bit of skin along the lower wound edge, then a bit of the levator aponeurosis, then a bit of skin along the upper wound edge.[4] Care should be taken not to incorporate the orbital septum in the wound closure, as this may lead to tethering and restriction of the levator function.

Management of Complications

Undercorrections and Overcorrections

Fat resection should be avoided in unilateral cases to prevent the creation of asymmetry; the best symmetry and cosmesis are usually provided with bilateral surgery. Many cases of apparent overcorrection are actually related to a contralateral ptosis made more apparent by unilateral surgery. Mild overcorrections can usually be managed with eyelid massage to stretch the levator and loosen the sutures securing the aponeurosis to the tarsus. Overcorrections >3 or 4 mm, however, usually require surgical revision (**Fig. 33.8**). When performed within 3 weeks of the previous surgery, the wound can be separated, and the sutures are easily identified and released (**Figs. 33.9, 33.10**). The levator aponeurosis is then reattached more superiorly on the tarsus or to the underlying Müller muscle or conjunctiva.[18]

Postoperative edema can give the appearance of undercorrection. However, after the swelling has subsided, if an undercorrected ptosis remains, revision surgery should be performed promptly to avoid difficult surgery associated with fibrosis (**Fig. 33.11**). In the first few weeks, the wound can be easily pulled apart, and the levator aponeurosis can be identified, advanced, and secured to the tarsus as previously described.

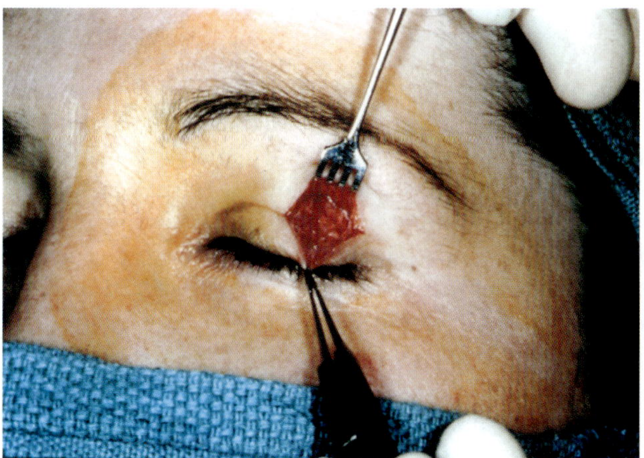

Fig. 33.10 Same patient in **Fig. 33.9**. At this time, the wound can still be separated with relative ease to expose the sutures securing the levator aponeurosis to the tarsus.

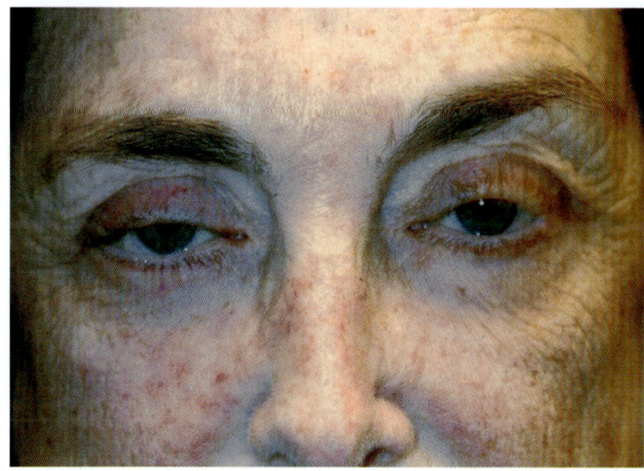

Fig. 33.11 Undercorrection of a right upper eyelid ptosis. This patient will require revision ptosis surgery.

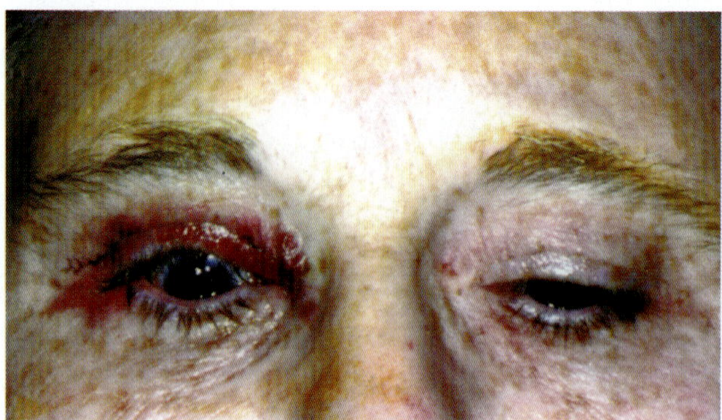

Fig. 33.12 Mild eyelid lagophthalmos of the right upper eyelid, especially prominent in downgaze, is noted on postoperative day 1.

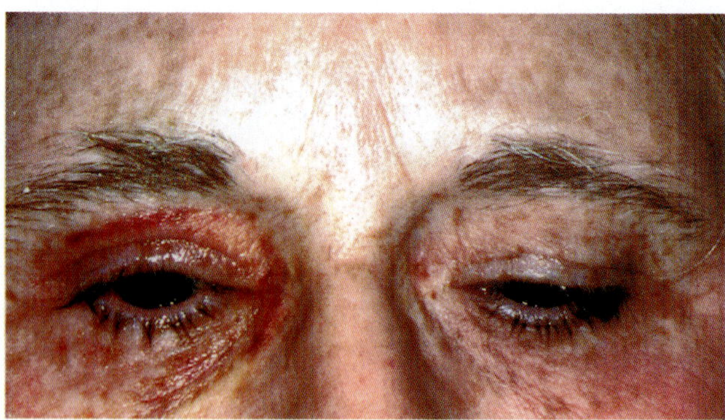

Fig. 33.13 Same patient in **Fig. 33.12.** By postoperative day 7, the eyelid lagophthalmos has resolved.

When an excessive amount of eyelid skin has been excised, or if a large levator resection has been performed, a postoperative lagophthalmos may be present (**Fig. 33.12**). With mild lagophthalmos and good tear production, the patient may be asymptomatic or only mildly symptomatic. Lubrication with ointment and artificial tears, along with eyelid massage, can lead to improvement with time (**Fig. 33.13**). However, larger lagophthalmos or poor natural ocular lubrication can lead to severe complications, including exposure keratoconjunctivitis and corneal ulceration (**Fig. 33.14**).[19] The levator aponeurosis may need to be recessed to lower the upper eyelid, or a full-thickness skin graft may be necessary to prevent these complications. The contralateral upper eyelid skin provides the best match for thickness and color. If the contralateral upper eyelid skin is insufficient, then pre- or postauricular skin can be used as a donor site.

Asymmetric Eyelid Creases

Asymmetric eyelid creases are relatively common after surgery, especially if aponeurotic fixation of the skin sutures was done asymmetrically. In correcting asymmetric eyelid creases, the easiest approach is to lower the high lid crease if enough upper skin is present. An ellipse of skin is marked below the high crease, with the lower line of the ellipse representing the new eyelid crease symmetric with the other eyelid. The ellipse of skin and orbicularis is then excised, and any attachments to the aponeurosis below the new crease are dissected free. The incision is closed with aponeurotic fixation to match the contour of the contralateral eyelid crease. If insufficient skin is available on the eyelid with the higher crease, then the lower eyelid crease can be raised.[20] An ellipse of skin is marked above the low crease, with the lower line of the ellipse representing the new eyelid crease symmetric with the other eyelid. The incision is then closed with aponeurotic fixation. The disadvantage of raising a low eyelid crease is that a double crease may frequently result.

Hemorrhage

Although rare, the most devastating complication of ptosis surgery is permanent vision loss caused by postoperative bleeding.[21] Retrobulbar orbital hematomas may cause optic nerve compression and central retinal artery and vein occlusion. Patients usually complain of significant pain, and examination reveals significant periorbital ecchymosis and subconjunctival hemorrhage. The orbit is tense, and an afferent pupillary defect may be present. Under these circumstances, the eyelid incisions should be opened immediately (**Fig. 33.15**). If this is insufficient, a lateral canthotomy with cantholysis or even bony orbital decompression should be performed to relieve the orbital tension.[22] Although vision loss is an extremely rare complication, accurate preoperative assessment of visual acuity

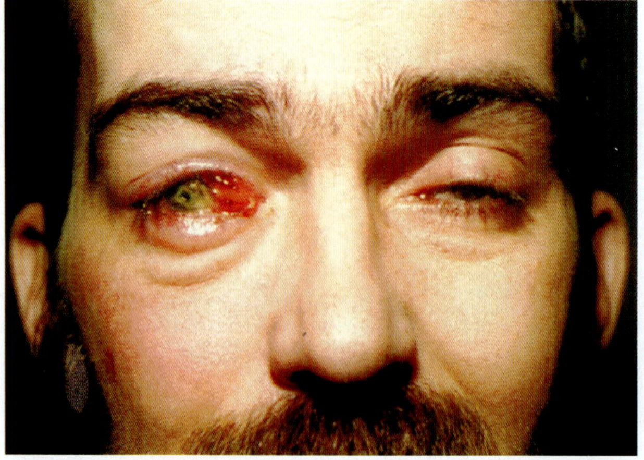

Fig. 33.14 After unilateral ptosis repair of the right upper eyelid, this patient was lost to follow-up and developed corneal exposure with subsequent corneal ulceration.

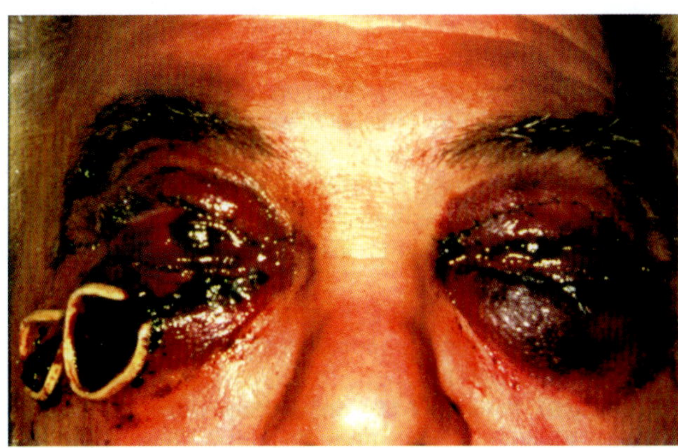

Fig. 33.15 Massive orbital hemorrhage after bilateral upper eyelid ptosis repair and lower eyelid blepharoplasty. This patient required opening of incision and placement of drains in the right orbit because of compressive visual loss.

and optic nerve function should be obtained for medicolegal documentation.

The most common cause of intraoperative and postoperative bleeding is the use of aspirin or other anticoagulating products. We ask that all patients discontinue aspirin for 2 weeks prior to their surgery, and all nonsteroidal anti-inflammatory agents for 1 week prior to surgery. This allows adequate time for platelet aggregation to return to normal. During surgery, most of the bleeding comes from the orbicularis muscle, and meticulous cautery should be applied prior to closing the incisions. If excision of the medial fat pocket is to be performed, particular attention should be paid to the medial palpebral vessels to avoid inadvertent transection. If bleeding from these vessels does occur, gentle pressure on the globe will cause the orbital fat to prolapse forward, and the bleeding vessels can be cauterized under direct visualization.[23] Postoperatively,

blood pressure should be monitored in the recovery area, and hypertension should be appropriately treated. All patients are instructed to apply cold compresses for 2 days and avoid heavy exertion for 1 week.

Diplopia

Injury to the superior rectus muscle and superior oblique muscle can occur during surgery of the upper eyelid. When dissection of the levator aponeurosis extends superior to Whitnall suspensory ligament, care must be taken not to damage the superior rectus muscle, which lies just inferior to the muscular levator. The common sheath is the structure between the levator and superior rectus muscle and provides support to the superior fornix. Injury to the common sheath should also be avoided. Injury to the trochlea of the superior oblique muscle has been reported after eyelid surgery.[24] This usually occurs when bleeding is encountered during dissection of the superior medial fat pad, and blind cauterization is applied, damaging the trochlea. Careful dissection to expose the medial palpebral vessels should be done to prevent significant hemorrhage in this area.

Conclusion

The best postoperative results in ptosis surgery are usually obtained when complications are avoided during the primary repair. When revision ptosis surgery is required, a thorough understanding of eyelid and orbital anatomy is a prerequisite for surgical exploration. With advances in our understanding of eyelid anatomy, more anatomical approaches have been developed for revision ptosis surgery. These approaches allow for improvement or correction of most complications of ptosis surgery.

References

1. Jones LT. The anatomy of the upper eyelid and its relation to ptosis surgery. Am J Ophthalmol 1964;57:943–959.
2. Dortzbach RK, Sutula FC. Involutional blepharoptosis: a histopathological study. Arch Ophthalmol 1980;98:2045–2049.
3. Anderson RL, Beard C. The levator aponeurosis: attachments and their clinical significance. Arch Ophthalmol 1977;95:1437–1441.
4. Anderson RL, Dixon RS. Aponeurotic ptosis surgery. Arch Ophthalmol 1979;97:1123–1128.
5. Lemke BN, Stasior OG, Rosenberg PN. The surgical relations of the levator palpebrae superioris muscle. Ophthal Plast Reconstr Surg 1988;4:25–30.
6. Meyer DR, Linberg JV, Wobig JL, McCormick SA. Anatomy of the orbital septum and associated eyelid connective tissues. Ophthal Plast Reconstr Surg 1991;7:104–113.
7. Doxanas MT, Anderson RL. Oriental eyelids: an anatomic study. Arch Ophthalmol 1984;102:1232–1235.
8. Anderson RL, Jordan DR, Dutton JJ. Whitnall's sling for poor function ptosis. Arch Ophthalmol 1990;108:1628–1632.
9. Holds JB, McLeish WM, Anderson RL. Whitnall's sling with superior tarsectomy for correction of severe unilateral blepharoptosis. Arch Ophthalmol 1993;111:1285–1291.
10. Jordan DR, Anderson RL. The aponeurotic approach to congenital ptosis. Ophthalmic Surg 1990;21:237–244.
11. Bowman WP. Report of the chief operations performed at the Royal London Ophthalmic Hospital for the quarter ending September 1857. R Lond Ophthalmol Hosp Rep 1859;1:34.
12. Eversbusch O. Zur operation der congenitalen blepharoptosis. Klin Monatsbl Augenheilkd 1885;21:100–107.
13. Putterman AM, Urist MJ. Müller muscle–conjunctiva resection: technique for treatment of blepharoptosis. Arch Ophthalmol 1975;93:619–623.

14. Fasanella RM, Servat J. Levator resection for minimal ptosis: another simplified operation. Arch Ophthalmol 1961;65: 493–496.
15. Barker DE. Dye injection studies of intraorbital fat compartments. Plast Reconstr Surg 1977;59:82–85.
16. Dutton JJ. The eyelids and anterior orbit. In: Atlas of Clinical and Surgical Orbital Anatomy. Philadelphia: WB Saunders; 1994:113–138.
17. Harvey JT, Anderson RL. The aponeurotic approach to eyelid retraction. Ophthalmology 1981;88:513–524.
18. Jordan DR, Anderson RL. A simple procedure for adjusting eyelid position after aponeurotic ptosis surgery. Arch Ophthalmol 1987;105:1288–1291.
19. Daut PM, Steinemann TL, Westfall CT. Chronic exposure keratopathy complicating surgical correction of ptosis in patients with chronic progressive external ophthalmoplegia. Am J Ophthalmol 2000;130:519–521.
20. Baylis HI, Goldberg RA, Wilson MC. Complications of upper blepharoplasty. In: Putterman AM, ed. Cosmetic Oculoplastic Surgery: Eyelid, Forehead, and Facial Techniques. Philadelphia: WB Saunders; 1999:411–428.
21. Anderson RL, Edwards JJ, Wood JR. Bilateral visual loss after blepharoplasty. Ann Plast Surg 1980;5:288–292.
22. Liu D. A simplified technique for orbital decompression for severe retrobulbar hemorrhage. Am J Ophthalmol 1993; 116:34–37.
23. Sutcliffe T, Baylis H, Fett D. Bleeding in cosmetic blepharoplasty: an anatomical approach. Ophthal Plast Reconstr Surg 1985;1:107–113.
24. Wesley RE, Pollard ZF, McCord CD. Superior oblique palsy after blepharoplasty. Plast Reconstr Surg 1980;66: 283–287.

Secondary Rhytidectomy

Stephen W. Perkins and Shervin Naderi

Rhytidectomy, or facelift, has been part of plastic surgery for over a century. And for probably just as long, patients have been unhappy with the results; hence the need for secondary procedures. We begin this chapter with an overview of the history of surgical techniques, focusing on the conflict in perceptions between surgeons and patients. We look at patient expectations and facelift limitations as well as patient selection as a predictor of revision facelift. Next, we review the types of revision surgery, particularly submentoplasty and cheek-only tuck-up facelift, and end with a discussion of new techniques that can reduce the incidence of revision or tuck-up procedures.

Improving or Maintaining the Primary Facelift Results: Conflicting Perceptions

Trying to enhance one's appearance by "turning back the clock" surgically has been a pursuit of individuals for at least the past century. Cosmetic surgeons began to develop rejuvenation surgery procedures, particularly facelift surgery, in the early 1900s. Some of the early efforts were pioneered by German and French surgeons. In 1906, Lexer was thought to have performed surgery to treat wrinkles, but it was Hollander in 1912 who was the first to report a surgical case. Other European physicians, including Joseph (1921) and Passot (1919), developed their own techniques to treat the sagging, aging face.[1] Early facelifting techniques consisted of very limited subcutaneous dissections, with skin elevation and tightening relying solely on the skin layer itself (**Fig. 34.1**). Unfortunately, this often resulted in a very temporary improvement, and occasionally an overzealous tightening of the skin resulted in an obvious operated look. Samuel Fomon, who was a pioneer in facial cosmetic surgery, recognized the limits of this type of facelifting procedure and of facelifts in general. According to Fomon, "The average duration of the beneficial effects, even with the best technical skill, cannot be expected to exceed 3 or 4 years."[2]

Many of the early surgical techniques were not well publicized or talked about by plastic surgeons, as there was a prevailing attitude against vanity surgery. However, beginning in the late 1950s, and certainly by the early 1970s, there was a significant effort made to develop a surgical procedure that would offer long-lasting results yet leave the patient with a cosmetically pleasing, natural look. From a surgeon's perspective, the ultimate facelift would be one that was predictable, had a low instance of complications, was technically feasible, and could be performed in a relatively short, efficient period of time. From a patient's perspective, the surgical technique would be minimally invasive yet effective and last as long as possible, leaving the individual with a natural appearance. This difference between a more invasive procedure that created a fundamentally altered appearance but offered long-lasting results and a shorter, less invasive operation that improved the patient's appearance with minimum recovery time but with short-term results emphasized the conflict in perceptions between the surgeon and patient as well as misconceptions about what can be expected from a facelift.

It is interesting to note that the original facelifts performed were skin lifts only. Some of the most recent literature describing such "S-lifts" seem to advocate a return to these same early procedures that were found to be of limited benefit over a long period of time.[3] Often "new" techniques such as S-lifts, or mini-facelifts, attract patients because they are minimally invasive, require only a short period of recuperation, and are reasonably low cost. However, they rarely satisfy the expectations of the patient or the surgeon.

From a surgeon's perspective, the pursuit of the ideal facelift procedure has created a great deal of different opinions and philosophies as to how to achieve natural, long-lasting results and a satisfied patient population. Much of this problem is due to the inherent limitations of the facelift procedure, no matter which technique is employed. It is an expensive operation, is technically involved, requires significant recovery time for the patient, and is inherently flawed. Both the patient and the surgeon are less than completely satisfied no matter how good the results may be for the given individual.

Early discussions in the literature compared short skin flap elevations with long complete flap elevations. Cosmetic surgeons such as Richard Webster realized and demonstrated that lifting the underlying fascia and muscular layer often gave a nice improvement in the jaw- and neckline with fewer skin complications and a more natural appearance.[4] This fascial layer was anatomically described by Mitz and Peyronnie in 1976 as the superficial muscular aponeurotic system (SMAS) (**Fig. 34.2**).[5] Webster performed a comparison of plication (folding over

Decision tree for secondary rhytidectomy

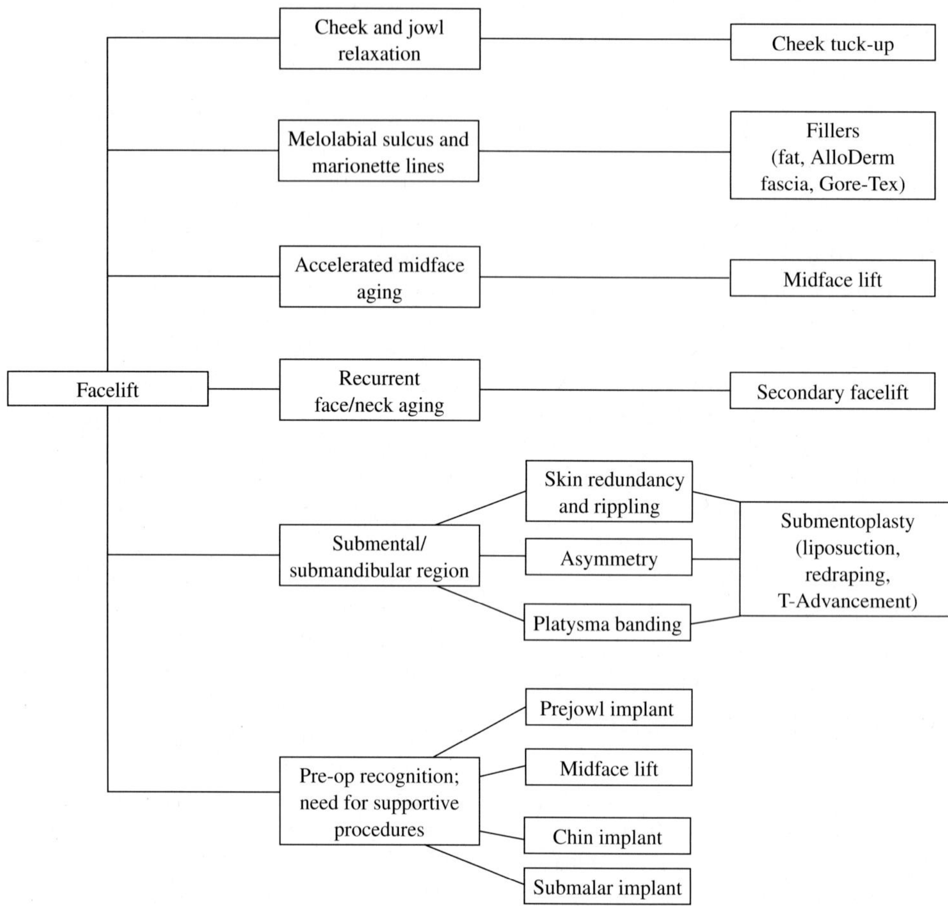

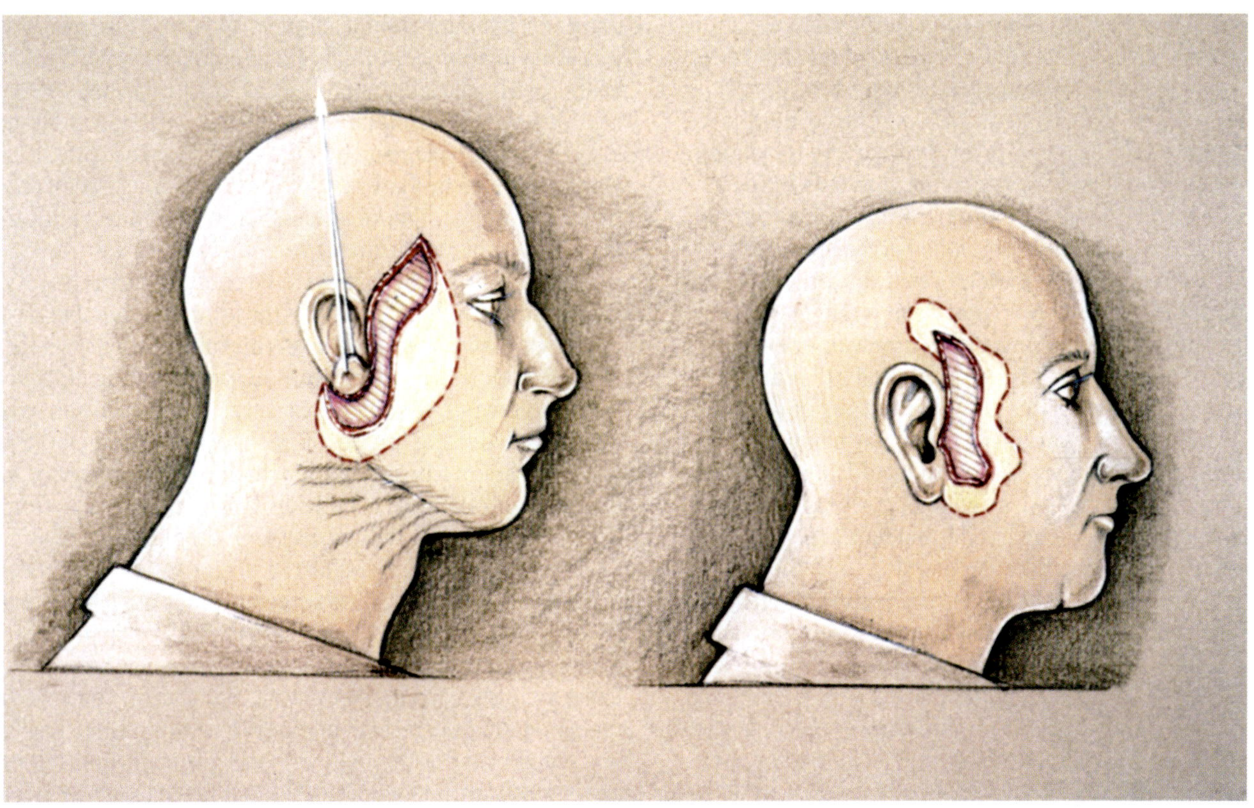

Fig. 34.1 Passot's 1910 "skin only" lift with limited or no undermining.

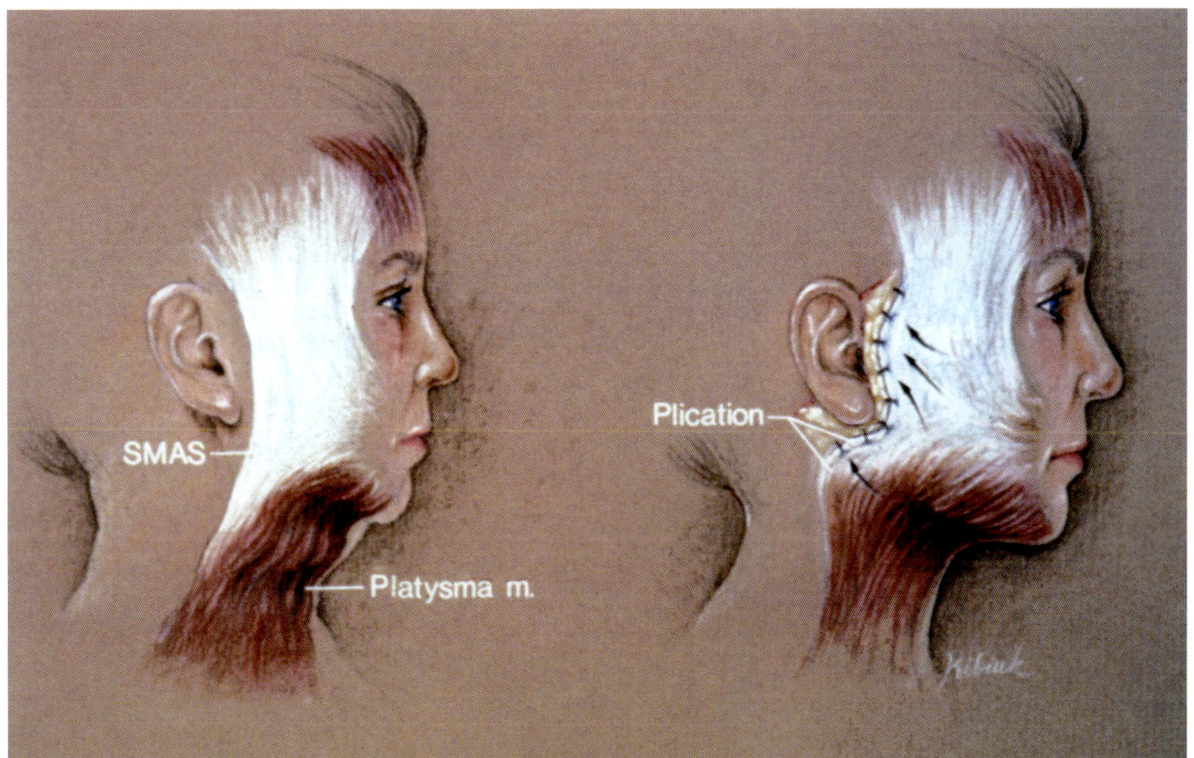

Fig. 34.2 Plication of superficial muscular aponeurotic system (SMAS).

and suture suspension) of this layer with relatively short skin flap elevation to large skin elevation with skin lifting only. Surgeons such as Skoog realized the benefits of the subfascial plane dissection as well and performed large elevations below the SMAS layer, treating the movement of the SMAS and the overall skin subcutaneous tissue as a sliding tectonic plate.[6] This imbrication (advancement, shortening, and suturing) technique became the mainstay of facelift surgery and has been recently repopularized through the extended SMAS and deep plane techniques.

With the advent of liposuction, direct lipectomy and sculpting of fatty tissues in the submandibular and submental areas became safer with less chance of potential complications to the marginal mandibular nerve. This improved the overall neck result with facelifting. However, this can lead to asymmetries due to uneven fat removal or recurrent lipoptosis, as well as dermal banding and skeletonization of the submandibular gland.

Over time, surgeons were observing in their patients not only recurrent sagging of the skin and SMAS tissues but also significant recurrent banding of the platysma muscle in the neck (**Fig. 34.3**). Techniques not only to correct the platysmal banding but also to prevent it from recurring were developed, including anterior plication techniques, various anterior border muscular myectomy techniques, and direct transection of each playtsma muscle from side to side.[7] Each of these techniques, however, fails to prevent recurrent

platysmal banding in some patients and can create ridges of platysma or submental "cobralike" appearances. In recent years, with the development of the extended SMAS rhytidectomy,[1] the biplane and triplane rhytidectomy of Baker,[8] the deep plane techniques of Kamer,[9] the composite rhytidectomies by Hamra,[10] and the subperiosteal dissections by Ramirez,[11] more aggressive surgical interventions were driven by the desire of surgeons to achieve a fundamental improvement that could be counted on to last for a significant length of time. As these techniques became more aggressive, increased levels of complications by relatively less experienced surgeons began occurring. In addition, the greater the degree of surgical intervention, the longer the healing phase or recuperation time for the patient. Patients became disenchanted with 6 weeks to 6 months of healing to achieve a "natural appearance" from their facelift. Increased competition among surgeons for facelift patients has brought the entire range of surgical techniques full circle. Some surgeons today are advocating "neck only" facelifts, midfacelifts, "laser" facelifts, and even endoscopic facelifting with essentially no skin redraping. There are increasing marketing claims of facelifts that allow the patient to fully recover and return to work over a weekend. Each of these procedures has significant limitations and significant incidences of recurrence of sagging with return of the aging face appearance, creating a dissatisfied patient population.

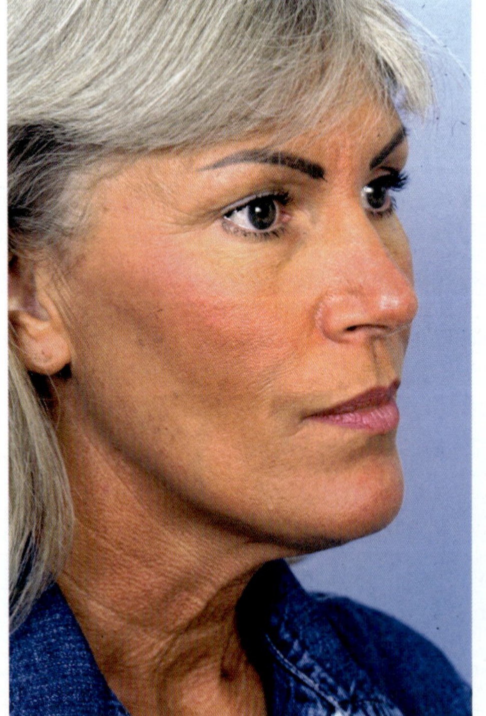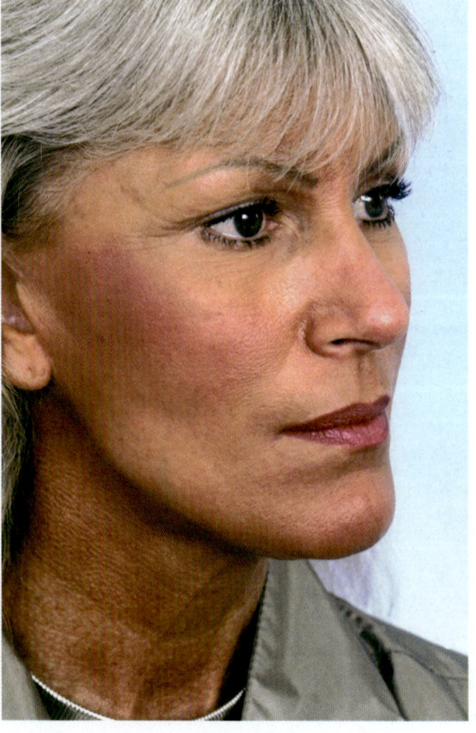

Fig. 34.3 **(A)** Preoperative platysmal banding and **(B)** postoperative recurrent platysmal banding.

There is no "perfect" facelift operation, and no matter the technique, there is significant healing time required. Fortunately, there are secondary procedures that can retighten the skin, the SMAS, and even the platysma, as well as repeat some liposculpting techniques to improve the overall initial result and maintain a longer lasting natural appearance for the patient.

Each patient asks his or her potential surgeon this fundamental question: How long is my facelift result going to last? It is generally expected that a given facelift procedure should last for at least 8 to 10 years. However, there are significant variations from patient to patient and preexisting condition to preexisting condition that can affect this average. There are certainly cases that one would expect to have significant recurrence of laxity and platysmal banding based on the preexisting condition, and these recurrences may be visible to the patient within the first 1 to 2 years. This creates relative dissatisfaction in an otherwise happy patient. There are also certain patients on whom a facelift result may last 12 to 15 years or longer in terms of a rejuvenated jawline and neckline compared with the preoperative condition. This mostly has to do with the preexisting elasticity, or lack thereof, and the patient's individual hereditary tendency. Photoaging and smoking, for example, will at least accelerate, or even partially cause, a premature loss of elasticity, increased wrinkling, and early relapse of the prefacelift conditions with a significant diminution of the aesthetic result. Still, patients can be told that, following a facelift, they will continue to look younger, by 5 to 10 years, even though they will continue to age in a normal fashion because of their hereditary tendency, preexisting conditions, and lifestyle choices.

Fundamentally, each patient, and, for that matter, each surgeon, desires a long-lasting improved jawline with minimum jowling, a well-contoured neckline with minimum to no platysma banding, and a naturalness to the overall look with relatively smooth skin. Therefore, secondary or tuck-up facelift procedures are required and are necessary to improve and maintain the primary facelift results.

Patient Expectations and Facelift Limitations

One of the more common areas of patient misunderstanding as to what facelifts will and will not do is the cheek–lip groove and fold, or the melolabial groove and fold. A standard cheek–neck facelift has very little effect on the upper third to upper half of this fold. There are techniques involved in midfacelifting, with particular attention to repositioning the middle cheek fat pad, that have some effect on this groove. Unless these are added to the operative procedure, patients need to understand that this is an area where very little improvement will be noted at the 6-month to 1-year postfacelift mark (**Fig. 34.4**). Another area of concern is the downward turn to the corner of the

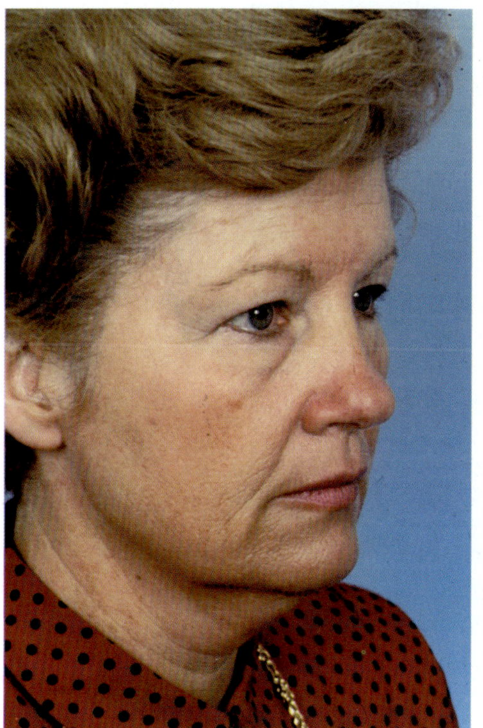
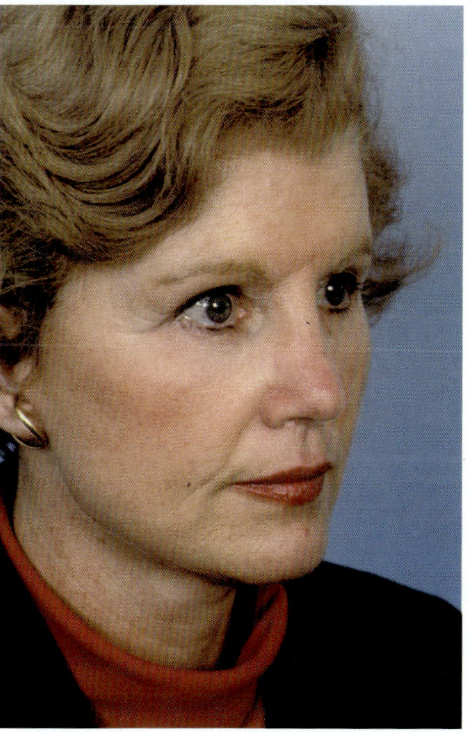

Fig. 34.4 **(A)** Preoperative cheek–lip groove and fold and **(B)** postoperative persistent cheek–lip groove and fold.

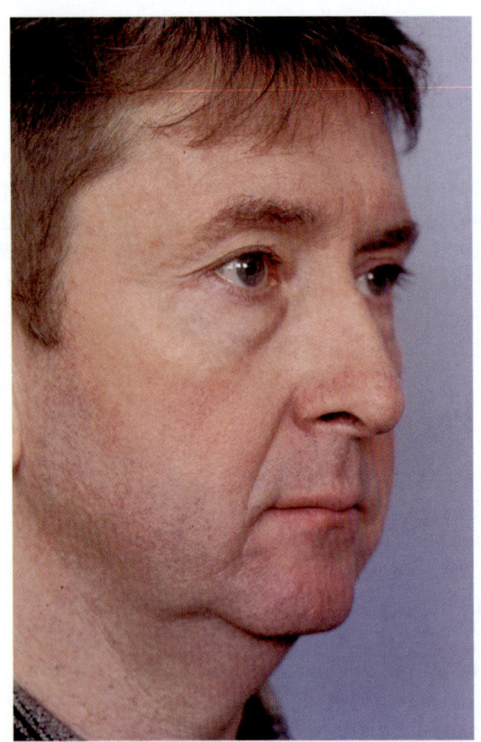
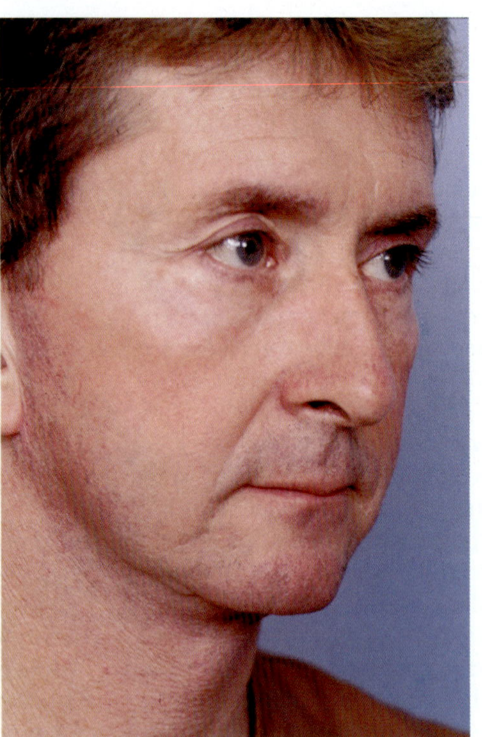

Fig. 34.5 **(A)** Preoperative chin–cheek groove, or "marionette line," and **(B)** postopeartive partial correction of chin–cheek groove.

mouth. This oral commissure groove, which can extend to a significant "marionette line," is only partially corrected with standard facelifting techniques (**Fig. 34.5**). By lifting the jowl and soft tissues of the lower third of the cheek, the marionette line is significantly effaced. However, the oral commissure itself is not affected by standard facelifting techniques (**Fig. 34.6**). Recurrence or persistence of this can be an area of dissatisfaction for the patient. Wrinkles

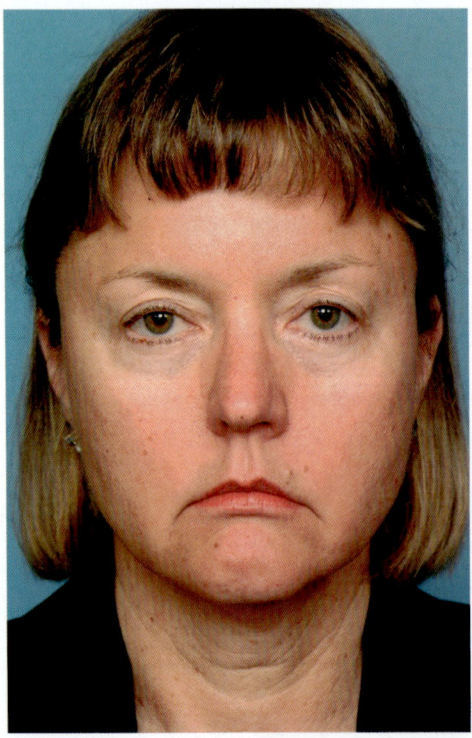
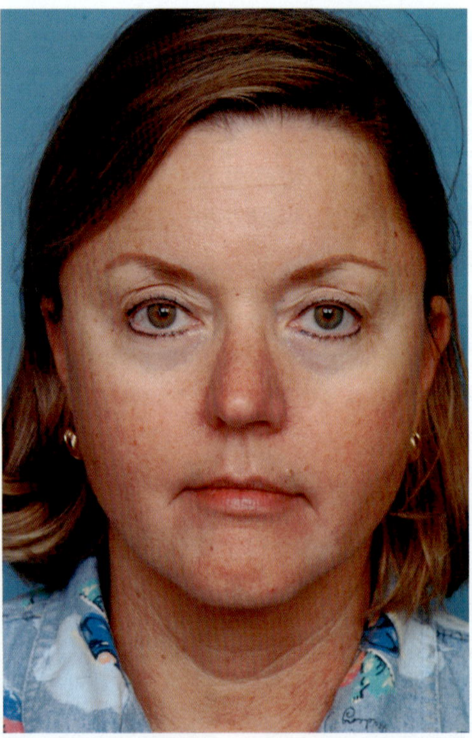

Fig. 34.6 **(A)** Preoperative downward turn of the corner of the mouth and **(B)** postoperative persistent partially corrected downward turn to the corner of the mouth.

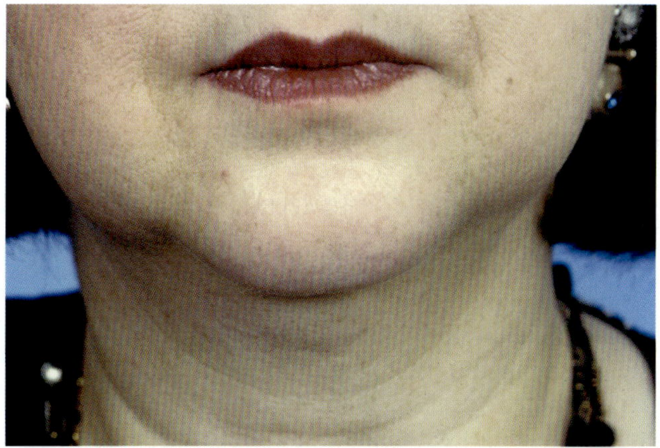

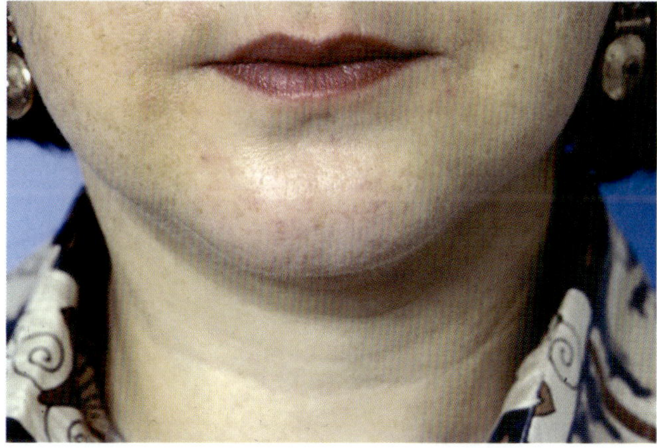

Fig. 34.7 **(A)** Preoperative square jawline with prejowl grooves and **(B)** postoperative facelift with prejowl implants.

or rhytides that exist within the surface of the skin may look better, if not significantly better, with facelifting. However, when the edema resolves and the tissue rebound relaxation occurs, most of these rhytides will still be present, and the patient needs to be educated about this fact in the preoperative consultation. None of these issues relate to a need for secondary or revision facelift surgery. They are just related to the limits of the procedure itself, and the patient's expectations must be in concert with this prior to surgery.

The issues that may result in the need for revision or secondary procedures have to do with the inherent elasticity or hereditary elastosis of the patient's skin, acquired loss of elasticity due to smoking or ultraviolet light exposure, and inherent "give back" or rebound relaxation of both the skin and the deeper subcutaneous tissues.

Areas that often result in the need for a secondary tightening or tuck-up procedure include persistence or recurrence of the jowl, recurrence or persistence of lipoptosis in the submental and submandibular area, and recurrence or persistence of platysmal banding and skin laxity of the cervical mental angle. It is worthwhile to note that the anatomical existence of a prejowl sulcus or geniomandibular groove may need additional augmentation to get a satisfactory result from facelifting and repositioning of the jowl.[12] A person with a heavy jowl and a square jawline with a forward chin, as well as a significant prejowl groove, needs to be aware that this will not be corrected, and may even be accentuated, with facelifting (**Figs. 34.7, 34.8**).

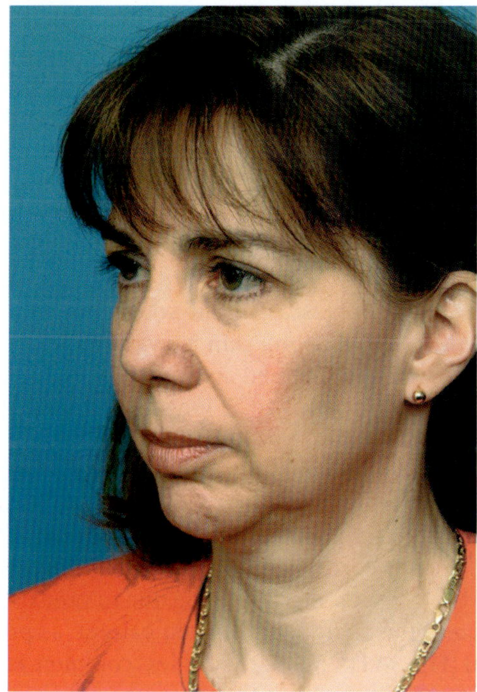

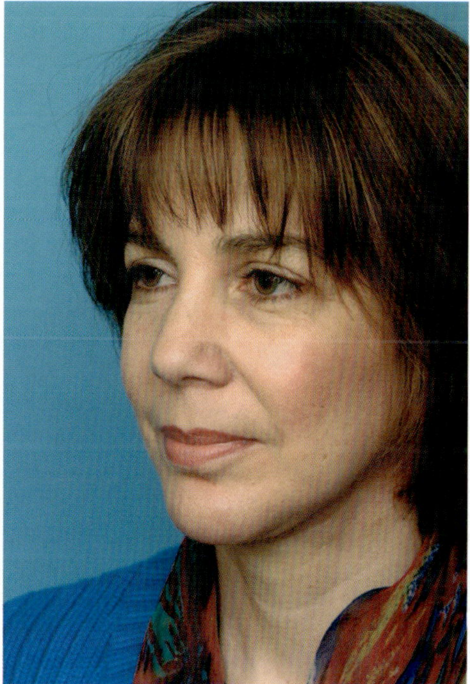

Fig. 34.8 **(A)** Preoperative oblique view showing prejowl grooves and **(B)** postoperative oblique view after prejowl implants and facelift.

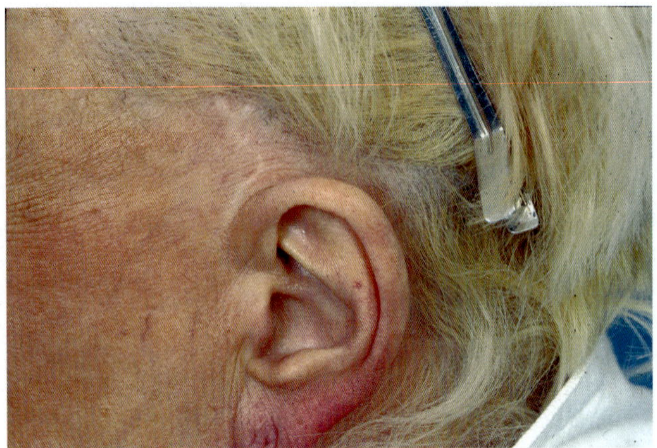

Fig. 34.9 Loss of sideburn hair tuft.

Other sequelae from facelift surgery that may require revision, but not specifically secondary facelifting or tuck-up procedures, are skin rippling, dimpling, and subcutaneous scar band formation in the submental and cervical neck. Additionally, overskeletonization with relaxation of the submandibular glands creates a fullness that may not be obvious preoperatively. This is a condition that is very difficult to correct satisfactorily. Alterations in the hairline are potentially avoidable but can necessitate revision surgery with hair grafting and/or small hair flap repositions (**Fig. 34.9**). Small areas of alopecia, if persistent, can be directly removed. Scarring that is visible in the pre- and postauricular areas is often avoidable by scar placement planning techniques, but adverse healing, whether small skin sloughs or infection, may create scarring that is visible, requiring revision surgery (**Fig. 34.10**).

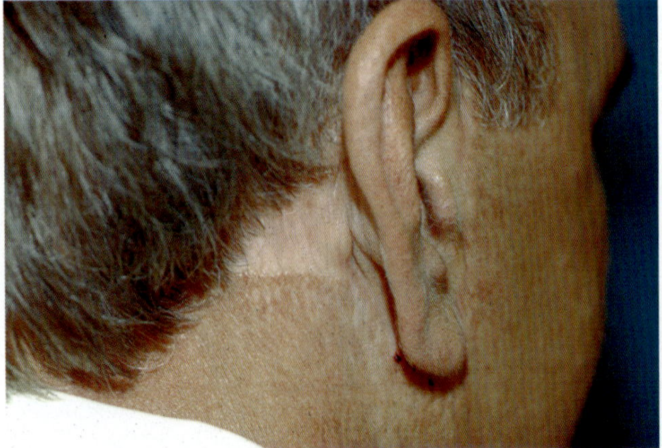

Fig. 34.10 Wide, visible postauricular scar.

Patient Selection as a Predictor of Revision or Tuck-up Facelift

A patient's preexisting conditions may preclude a good result or at least may predict a very short-term result with the need for further surgery, sooner rather than later. Any of these preexisting conditions are easily graded based on the patient's own anatomy. Dedo offered a classification system of the chin and neck that is clinically applicable here.[12] For example, patients with weaker, hypoplastic mentums, low or anterior hyoids, obesity, and significant lipoptosis, as well as patients with significant elastosis of the skin, can be expected to have poor initial results. Patients who have been smokers and have abused their skin in the sun will shorten their overall long-term results as well.

The skin itself has an inherent "creep" phenomenon, which includes rebound relaxation of both the skin and the subcutaneous tissues. As Perkins and Dayan noted, "It is inevitable that [patients] will experience a certain degree of rebound relaxation in superficial tissues of the face and neck."[1]

Types of Surgery in Revision and Secondary Facelifting

Revision surgery, by definition, involves revising something that otherwise did not heal as expected. This may involve revising a scar, removing an area of alopecia, correcting a skin slough problem, or tightening one side of the jawline or neckline that is asymmetrical to the other side. A "tuck-up" is defined as a lesser procedure that is generally performed anywhere from 6 to 18 months after the original facelift. This may involve tightening the submental area or relifting both cheek and jowls (a cheek-only tuck-up). The secondary facelift involves essentially the same standard facelift incisions and most likely involves a similar set of procedures, including SMAS dissection, skin elevation, and skin redraping. It can be performed anywhere from $1\frac{1}{2}$ to 2 years after the first facelift to as long as 15 to 20 years later.

There are planned versus unplanned revisional and tuck-up procedures.[13] In the first 6 to 18 months postfacelift, it is not uncommon to require retightening of the submental area or correction of the recurrent platysma band. This is often a predictable issue due to preexisting conditions and the anatomy of a given patient, as previously noted (**Fig. 34.11**). Similarly, but less common, is the repeat lifting of the cheek and jowl tissues, as these tissues will have settled and rebound relaxation will have

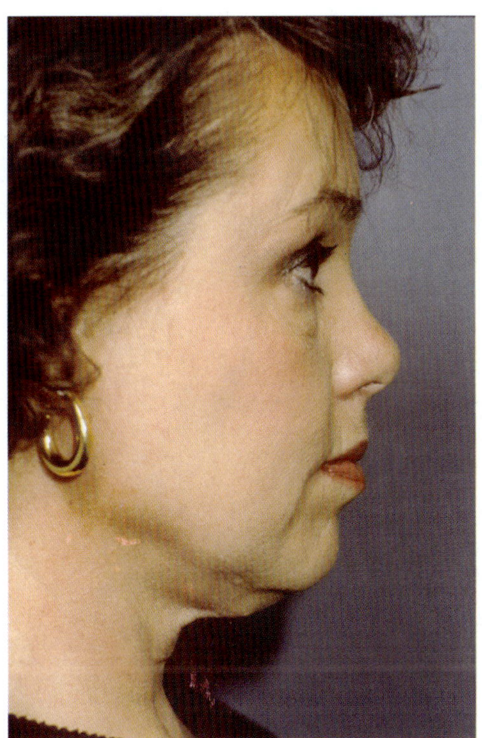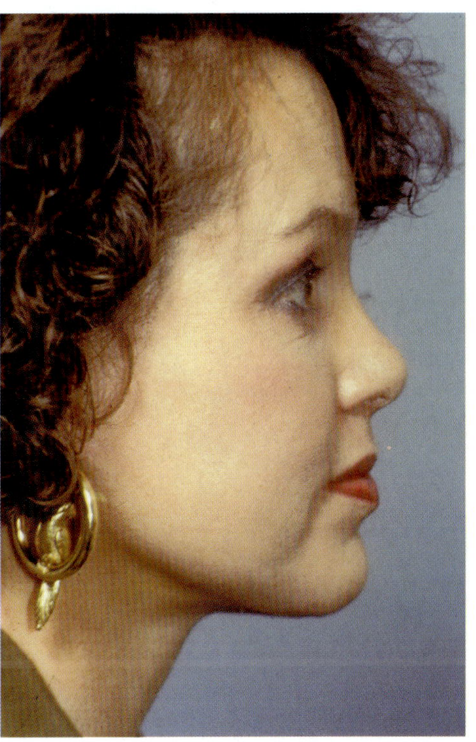

A   B

Fig. 34.11 (A) Preoperative facelift and **(B)** 1-year postoperative facelift with recurrent submental fat and laxity.

occurred, and the effect of gravity and loss of elasticity continues even in the early postoperative period. This, again, can be predicted based on the "cherub cheek" patient or full, heavily jowled patient, especially with a weak chin and ill-defined mandibular margin (**Fig. 34.12**). Either one of these procedures can be unplanned or unexpected and require intervention to maintain or achieve a satisfactory facelift in the relatively early postoperative period.

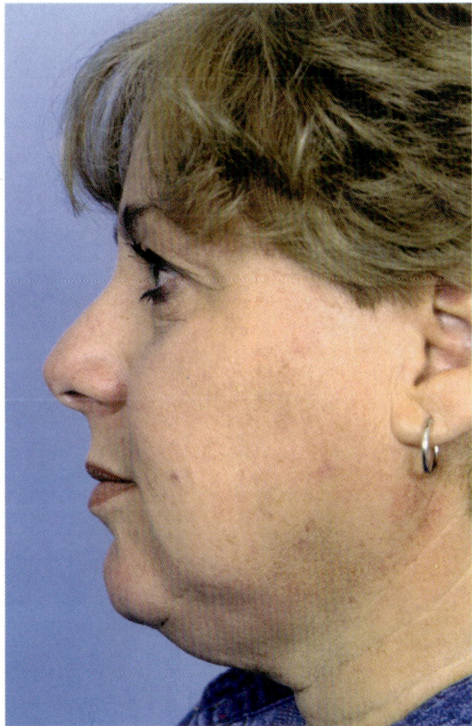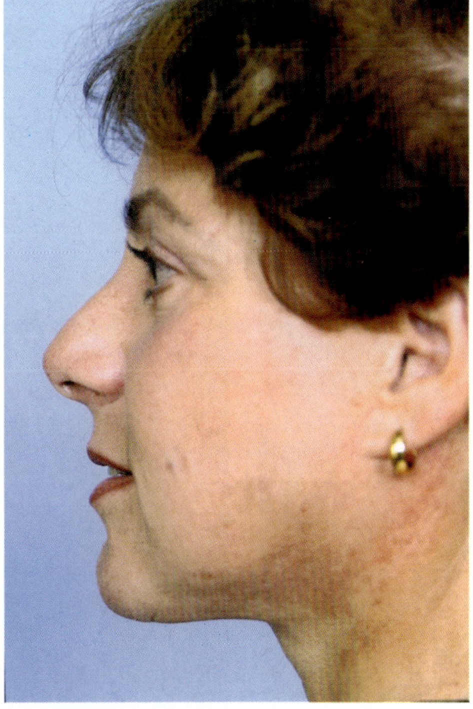

A   B

Fig. 34.12 (A) Preoperative "cherub cheek" facelift and **(B)** 1-year postoperative facelift.

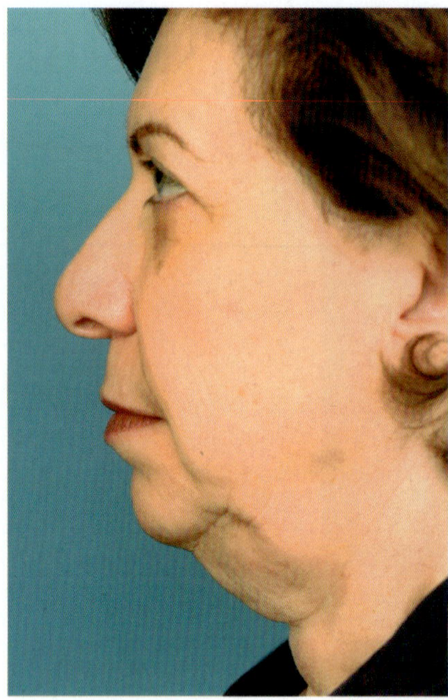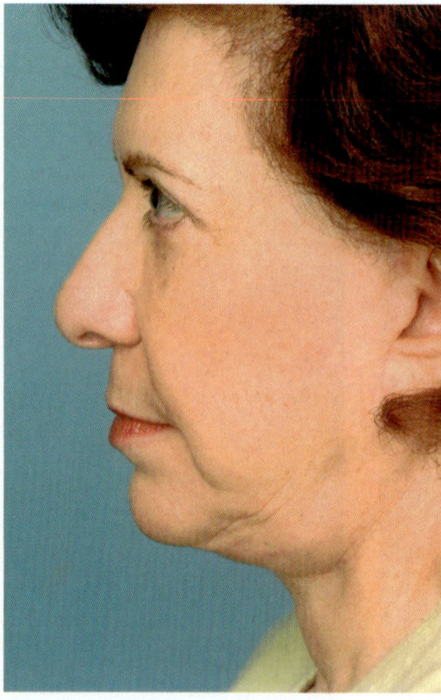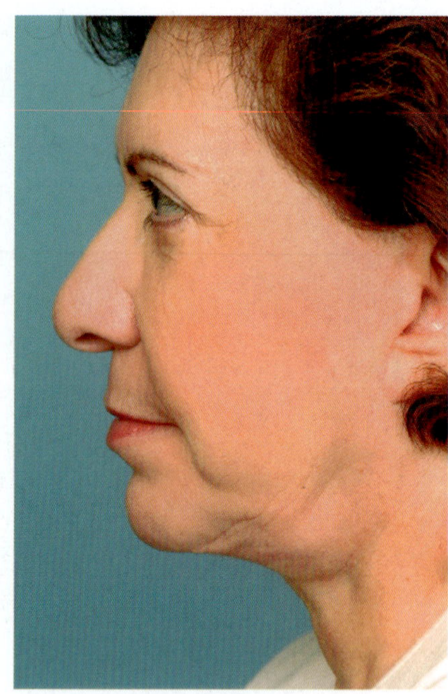

A–C

Fig. 34.13 **(A)** Preoperative "heavy neck" facelift; **(B)** 1-year postoperative facelift; **(C)** postoperative submentoplasty tuck-up operation.

Submentoplasty

A submental tuck-up or modified submentoplasty can involve one of three tissues:

1. Repeat liposuction only for reaccumulation or resettling of an asymmetrical area of fatty tissue (lipoptosis) in the submandibular or submental area (**Fig. 34.13**)
2. Skin redraping due to rebound relaxation of the skin itself, premature loss of elasticity, or rippling in the skin texture itself. This is often caused by or aggravated if the patient has had a seroma in the early postoperative period (**Figs. 34.14, 34.15**).

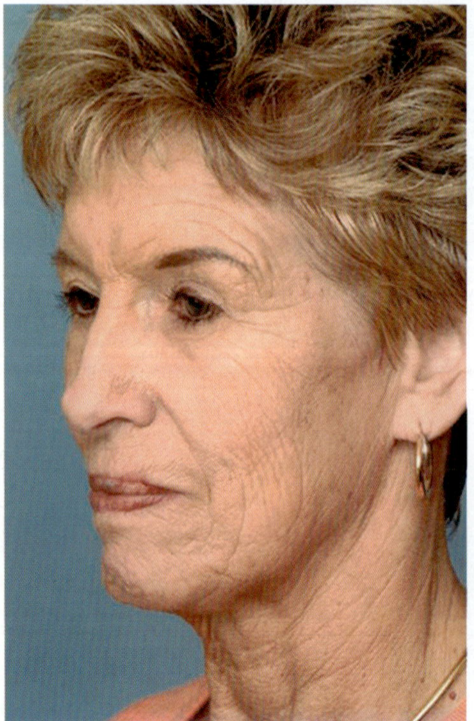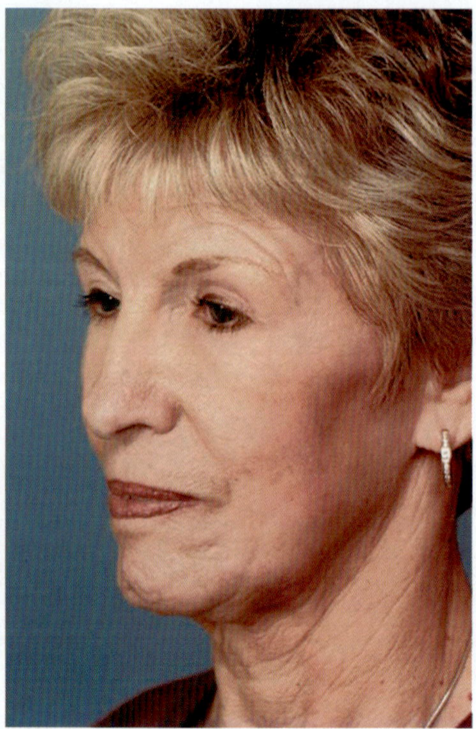

A

B

Fig. 34.14 **(A)** Preoperative severe neck skin rippling and photodamage and **(B)** 1-year postoperative facelift with "recurrent" rippling.

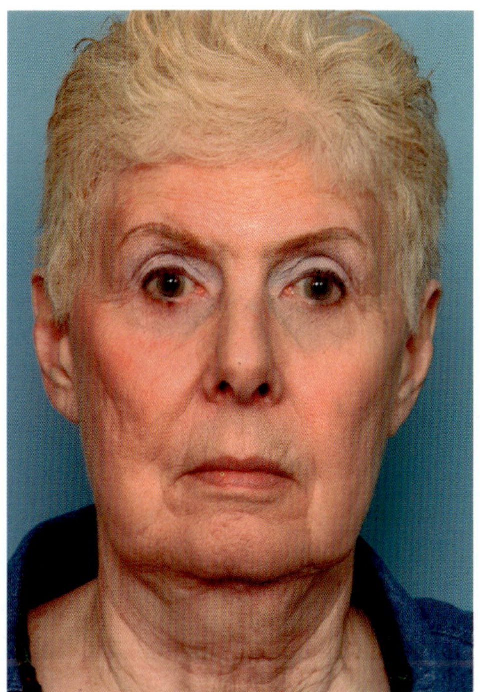
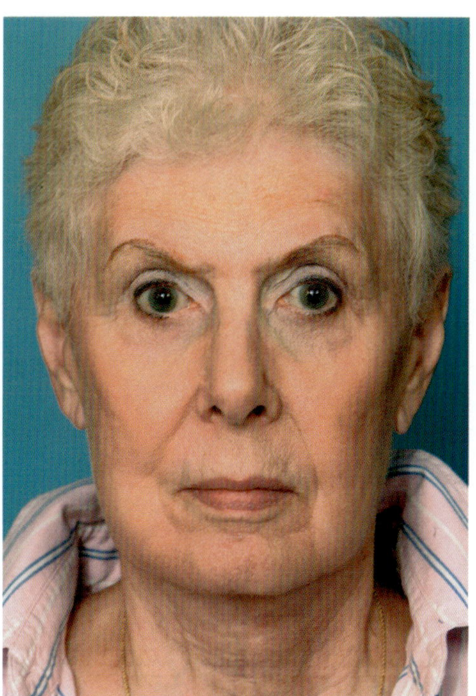

Fig. 34.15 (A) Unhappy patient 1-year postoperative facelift and postoperative seroma done elsewhere; **(B)** postoperative facelift repeat with full neck skin undermining and redraping.

3. Platysma band correction that may involve replication and undermining with redraping of the skin (**Fig. 34.16**)

In an article written by Perkins and Gibson in 1993 comparing patients from the senior author's practice, of the original facelifts, 96% of patients had liposuction of the submental area, 10% had direct excision, 31% had anterior platysmal resection, and 13% had a midline plication of platysma; 89% had SMAS plication, and 11% had SMAS imbrication.[14] Of this total patient group, postoperatively,

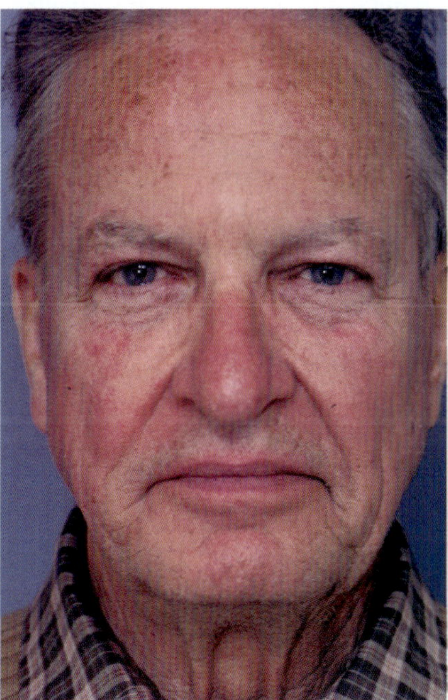
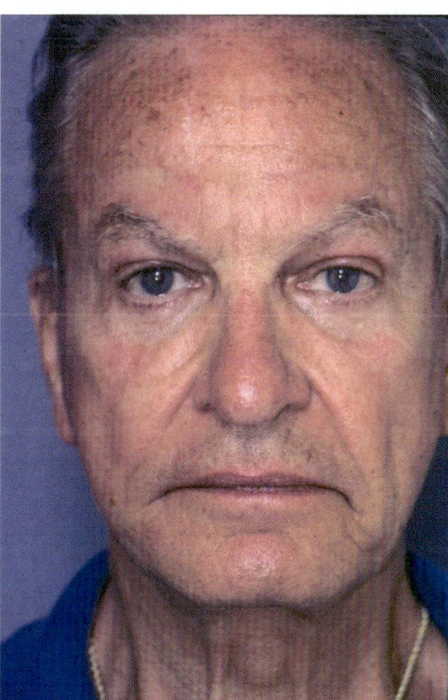
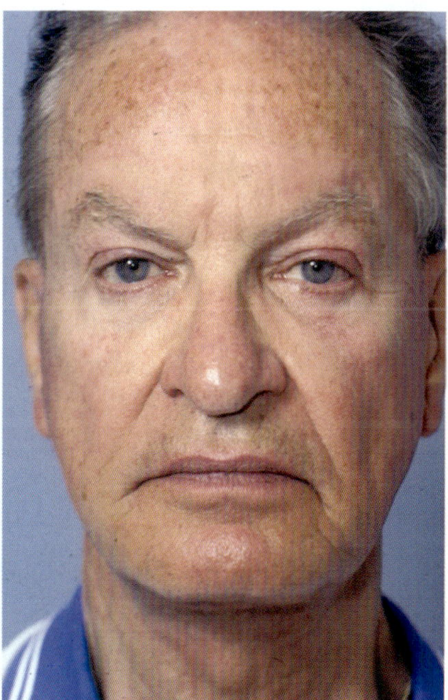

Fig. 34.16 (A–C) Patient with severe platysmal banding that recurred 1 year after facelift improved by submentoplasty tuck-up.

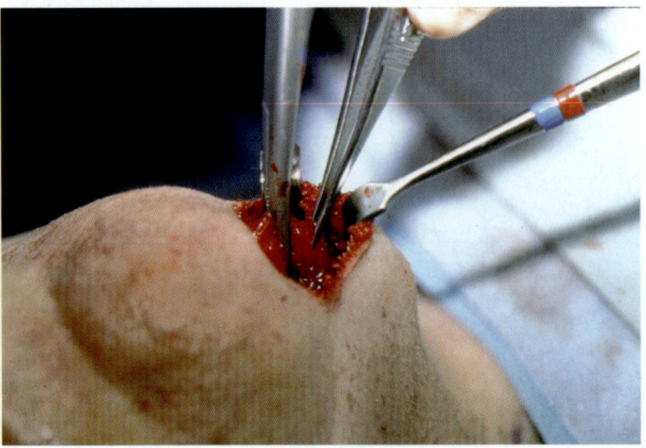

A

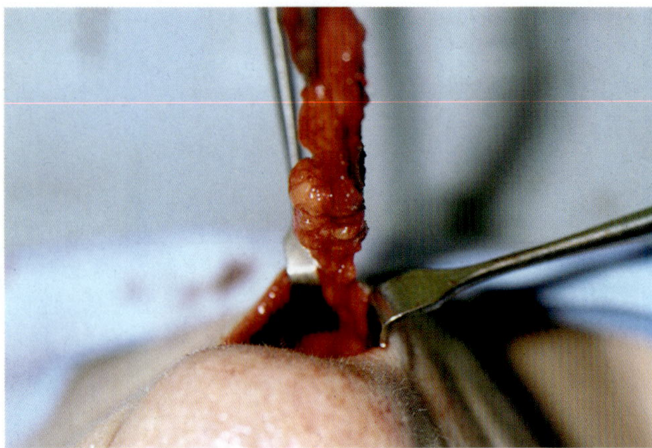

B

Fig. 34.17 (A,B) Kelly clamp technique for platysmaplasty.

60% had platysmal banding; 5% had recurrent or residual fat in the follow-up 6 to 18 months, and 15% of the overall group required a submental tuck-up procedure. Perkins and Dayan reviewed the same authors' facelift patients and noted that the revision submentoplasty had been reduced to 2 to 3%.[1] These senior authors' primary facelift procedures have been modified and enhanced. Currently, 98% of the patients have liposuction, and the "Kelly clamp technique" is used for direct excision of both fat and platysma banding in about 60% of patients (**Fig. 34.17**). Midline plication was done in 100% of these patients. Additionally, 100% of the patients had SMAS elevation, imbrication, and deep plane techniques in the midcheek region. Eight-five percent of patients had long flap elevations in the neck and medium flap elevations in the face (**Fig. 34.18**). This compares to Perkins and Gibson's findings that only 61% of patients had medium flaps and 39% had long flaps.[14]

The submentoplasty tuck-up procedure is usually performed at least 6 months but before 18 months after the initial facelift. It is a procedure that revises the submental area through the previous submental crease incision. This horizontal crease incision is often converted to a short T-shaped incision, as shown in **Fig. 34.19.** This allows for undermining of the skin, repeat liposuction, and repeat platysma plication. Most importantly, it allows for redraping of the skin in a lateral to medial direction, as well as from posterior to anterior. The surgeon must be careful not to develop redundancy of tissue underneath the mandibular margin at either end of the incision bilaterally. By advancing the tissues posterior to anterior, the vertical length of the T incision is shortened by approximately 50%. At no time would the vertical limb extend to or even past the anterior cervical mental angle. Normally, the vertical limb of this incision is no more than 3.0 cm long, ending up 1.0 to 1.5 cm in length at the time of closure. Generally, patients are quite accepting of this extended incision because they realize a small operation will actually further correct and improve the results they expected from their previous facelift. As is the

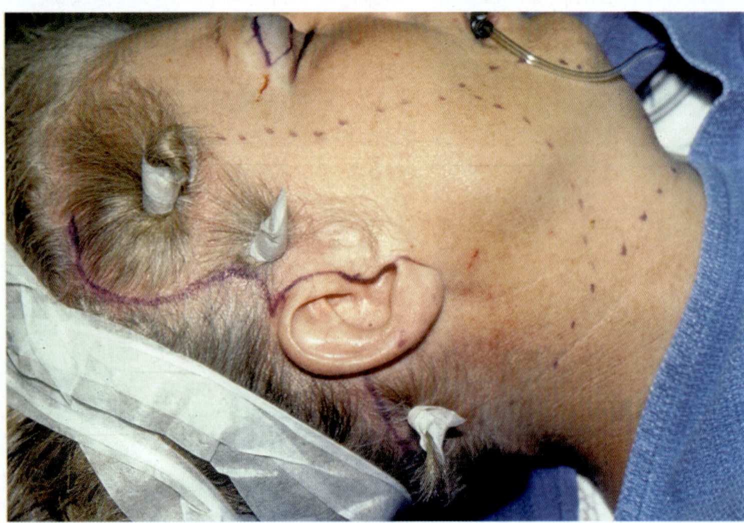

Fig. 34.18 Preoperative marking of patient for medium-length flap elevation of cheek and long flap elevation of neck.

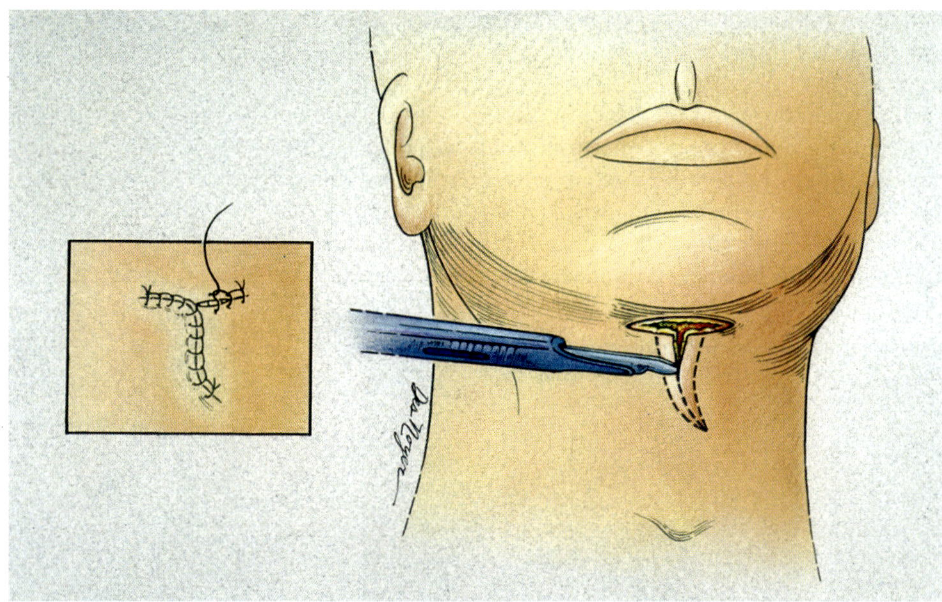

Fig. 34.19 T-shaped incision used in tuck-up operation for isolated submentoplasty after primary facelift.

case with any scar, for those patients who depigment the actual scar itself, it can become a visible issue for them, particularly if their surrounding skin is of a more sallow color. A lot of these scars will blend in with natural skin tones, however. This procedure takes approximately a half hour to 45 minutes of operating time and can be done under intravenous (IV) sedation in the office or ambulatory operating suite. Currently, I perform this procedure in approximately

1 to 2% of all facelift patients in the first 6 to 18 months following the primary procedure (**Fig. 34.20**).

Cheek-Only Tuck-up Facelift

A cheek-only tuck-up facelift is indicated for a patient on whom I have performed the initial facelift procedure but who has had some exaggerated rebound relaxation of the

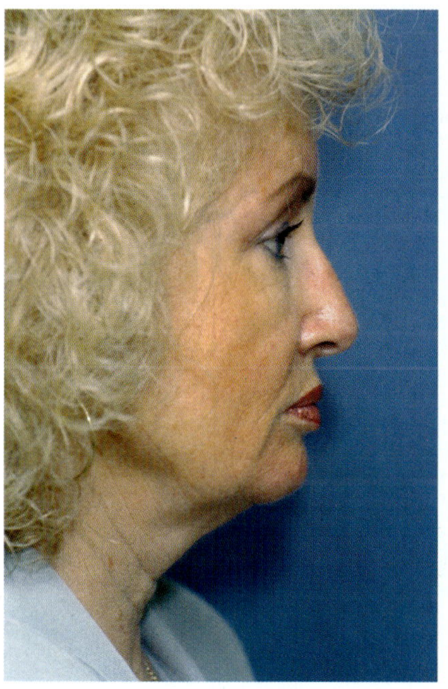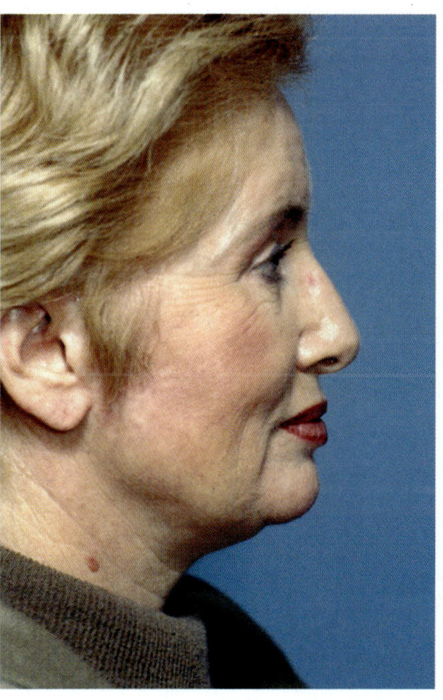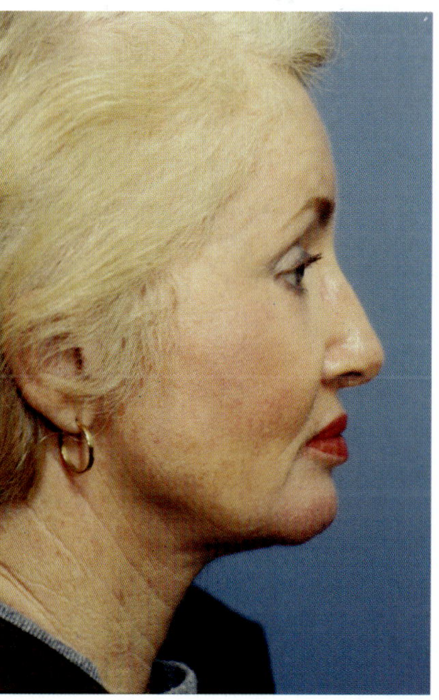

A–C

Fig. 34.20 (A) Pre- and **(B)** postoperative views of patient who underwent primary facelift and **(C)** secondary submentoplasty tuck-up at 14 months post-op.

midcheek or jowl tissues. This creates a disappointment in the patient who is otherwise pleased with their jawline and neckline. These tissues are the most affected by gravity and are the least improved by liposuction techniques. It is a challenge surgically to permanently suture fixate the cheek and jowl soft tissues in the posterosuperior direction where they were repositioned during the facelift. Re-elevating the skin for a medium flap length, retightening the SMAS layer, either by a short imbrication technique or by a plication-foldover technique, significantly improves the overall long-term effect of the original facelift. Currently, for the cheek tuck-up, I use a permanent suture such as 3–0 Tevdek to support the SMAS layer, as opposed to a completely absorbable 3–0 Vicryl or 3–0 PDS (polydioxanone) suture used in the primary facelift. Skin redraping is also an issue, and the incision has to be extended along the postauricular sulcus back to the posterior hairline, but not extending posteriorly into the postauricular hair, as in

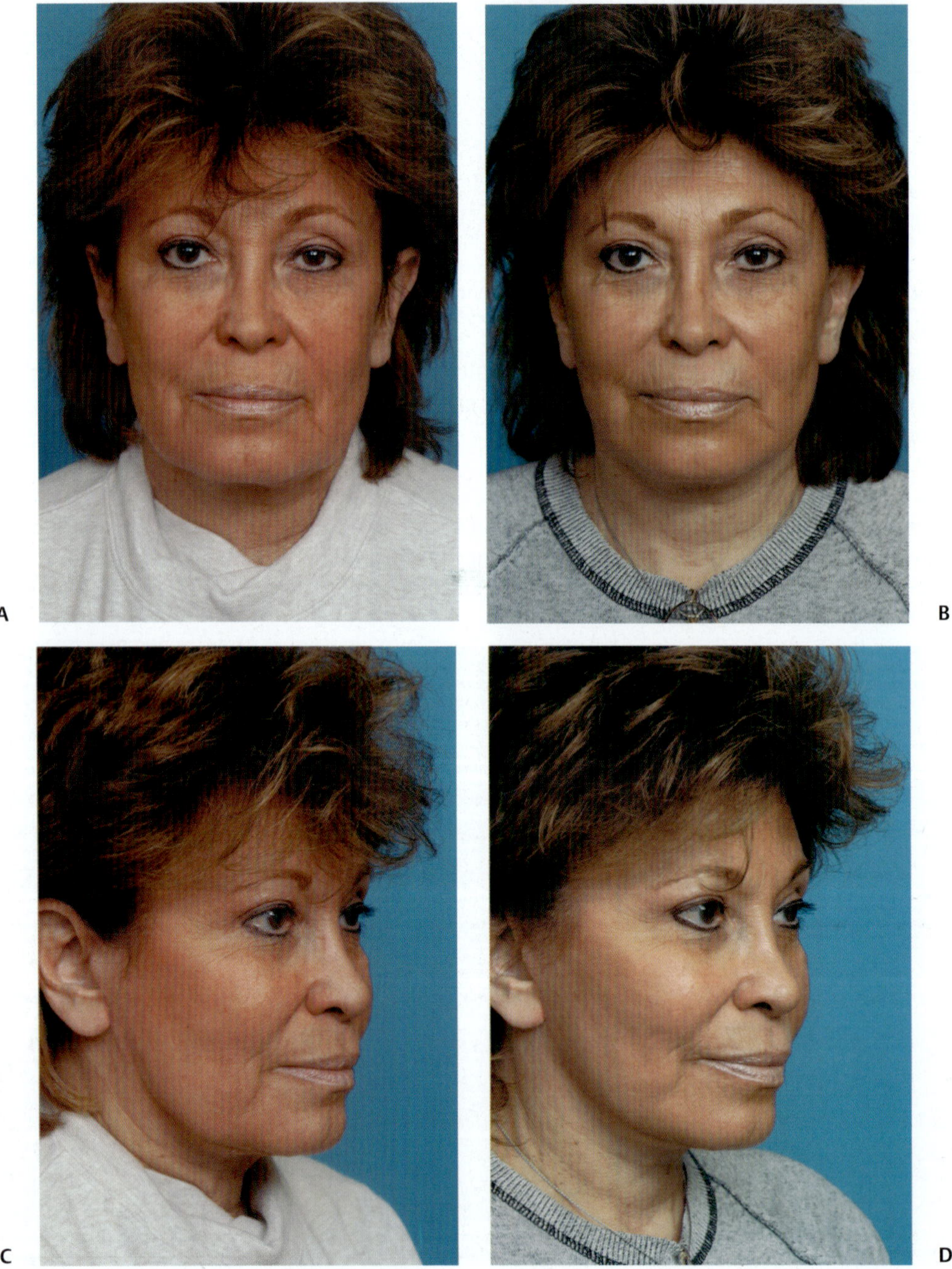

Fig. 34.21 **(A)** Pre- and **(B)** postoperative views of patient who underwent primary facelift and **(C,D)** secondary cheek-only tuck-up at 18 months post-op.

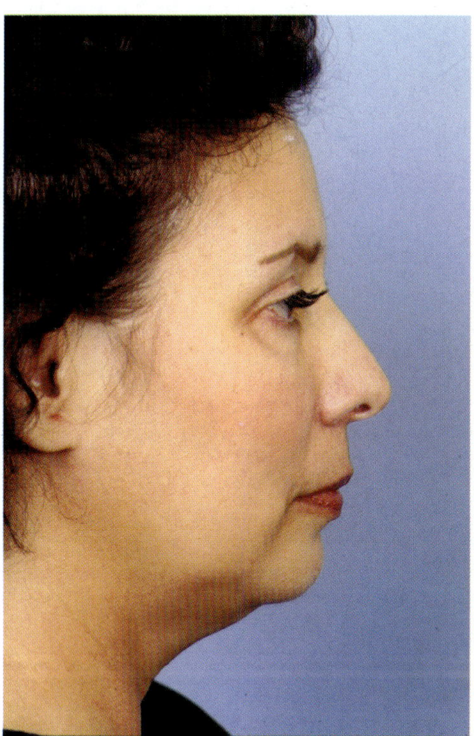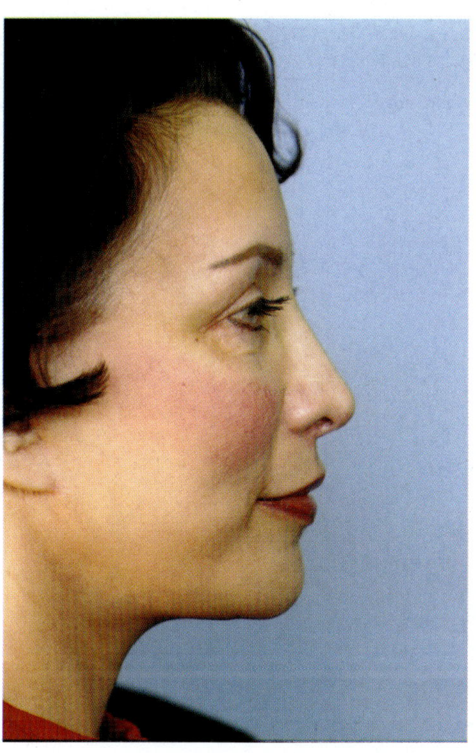

A   B

Fig. 34.22 (A) Pre- and **(B)** postoperative views of patient who underwent a facelift and chin augmentation.

the original facelift. A short degree of undermining in the infra-auricular area is required, but not full neck undermining. Two to 3 cm of SMAS is elevated and imbricated in the preauricular area and just below the level of the angle of the mandible. A re-elevation in the midface deep plane below the SMAS is generally not required. Because of the limited undermining, a smaller 2 mm drain may be all that is required, or no drain at all. Primary facelifts are drained with a 4 or 7 mm flat, perforated drain. The procedure takes approximately $1^1/_2$ hours of operating time and can be done under IV sedation in the operating suite. This procedure is done in approximately 1 to 2% of all facelift patients in the first 18 months (**Fig. 34.21**).

Additional Procedures

Adding new procedures to the primary facelift can further reduce the incidence of revision or tuck-up procedures in the first 6 to 18 months. These procedures include chin augmentation, prejowl implants for the geniomandibular sulcus, and midfacelifting of the cheek–lip fold and midfacial malar tissues (**Fig. 34.22**).

There are instances when new techniques added to the rejuvenating process are actually separate and distinct procedures. These procedures, which technically are considered secondary facelifts or revision surgery, become necessary once the cheek and jawline are adequately rejuvenated and the patient still thinks he or she has a sagging face. This is often related to the persistence of cheek–lip folds and grooves, sagging midcheek tissues with midfacial hollows, a tired lower eyelid look, and a sagging of the lateral brow and midglabellar tissues. One of the procedures that is commonly performed today in concert with facelifting to improve the cheek–lip fold and groove involves augmenting this groove at the time of facelift (**Fig. 34.23**). Occasionally, this is done in lieu of facelifting when the patient is not quite ready. It can be done as a secondary procedure to improve the otherwise persistent groove that was not going to be corrected by the initial facelift procedure.[15] Augmentation of this groove as well as the downward turn of the oral commissure or marionette region can be done with a person's autologous fat. Autologous fat transfer will improve both of these areas at the time of the original facelift, and the fat can easily be obtained from the submental and submandibular liposuction. This auto-reinjection of fat has variable persistence, but generally it is not considered to be a permanent improvement. It may last from 6 to 18 months, depending on the patient. Further augmentation materials include AlloDerm (acellular dermal graft that is micronized human cadaveric collagen; LifeCell Corp., Branchburg, New Jersey)[16] and SMAS fascia or temporalis fascia. None of these tissues has longevity that is persistent past 1 year. The one material that has shown persistence and a great tolerance in the soft tissues is Gore-Tex (expanded polytetrafluoroethylene).[17] This will provide some degree of augmentation, but it does not correct the cheek–lip fold or sagging midfacial tissues. If one recognizes

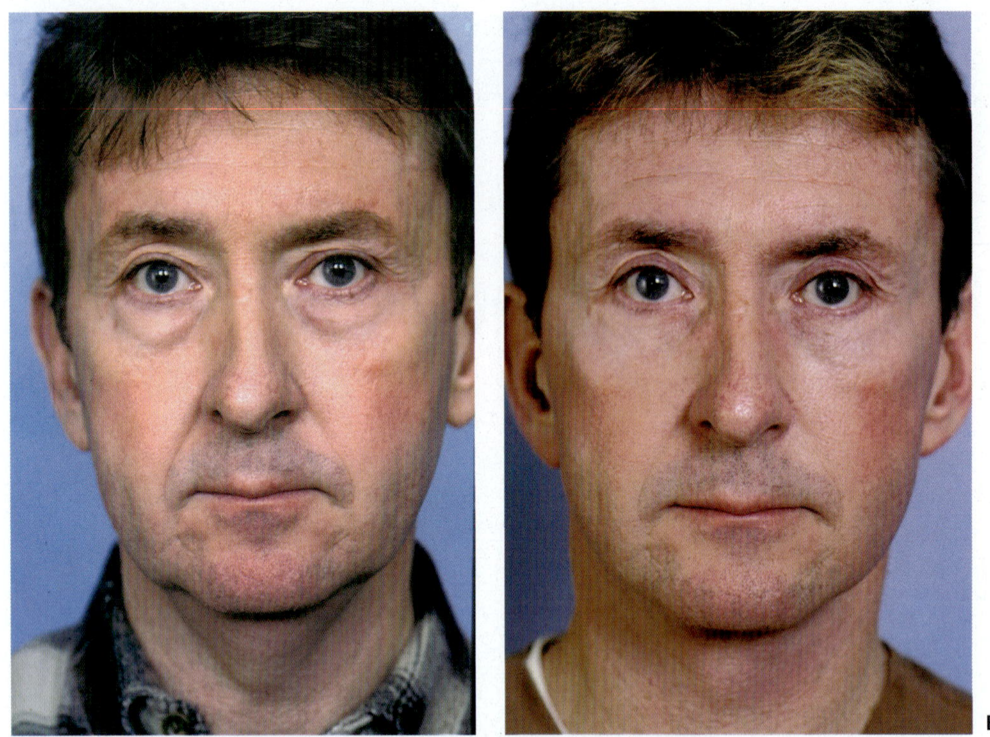

Fig. 34.23 **(A)** Pre- and **(B)** postoperative views of facelift combined with augmentation to cheek–lip grooves.

the hypoplasia or loss of subcutaneous fat tissue and atrophy in the midface, one can suggest augmentation materials at the time of the initial facelift. The augmentation of the midface with a submalar implant often will improve the overall facelift result and ensure a happier patient with the initial procedure[18] (**Figs. 34.24, 34.25**).

Patients often wonder how many facelifts are possible or how many facelifts constitute too many. They also ask

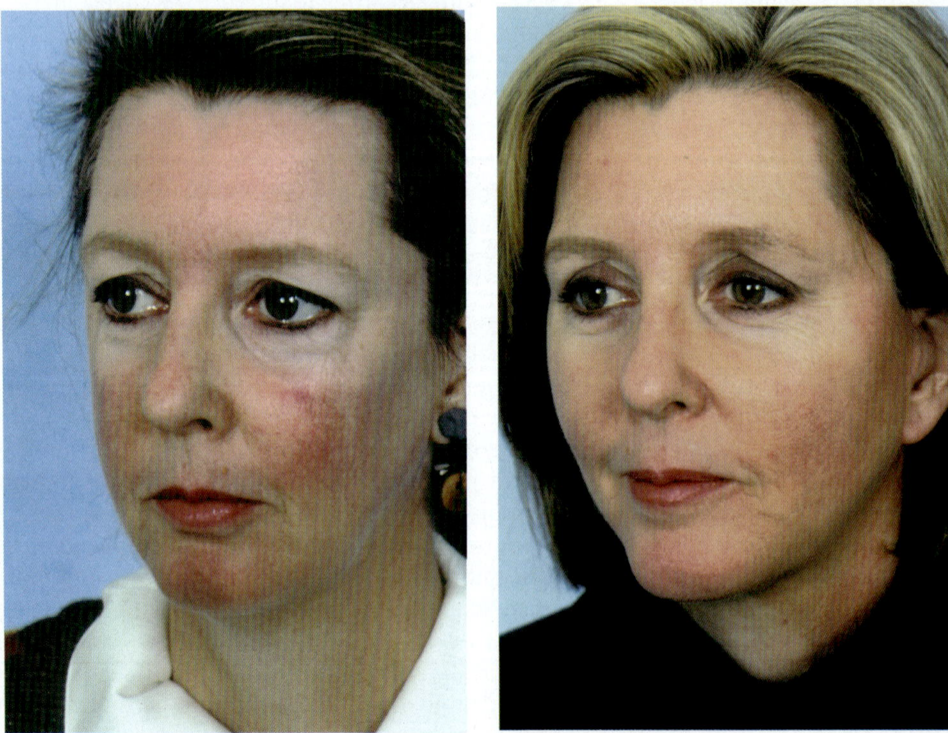

Fig. 34.24 **(A,B)** Patient who underwent facelift combined with cheek or malar implants and chin implant.

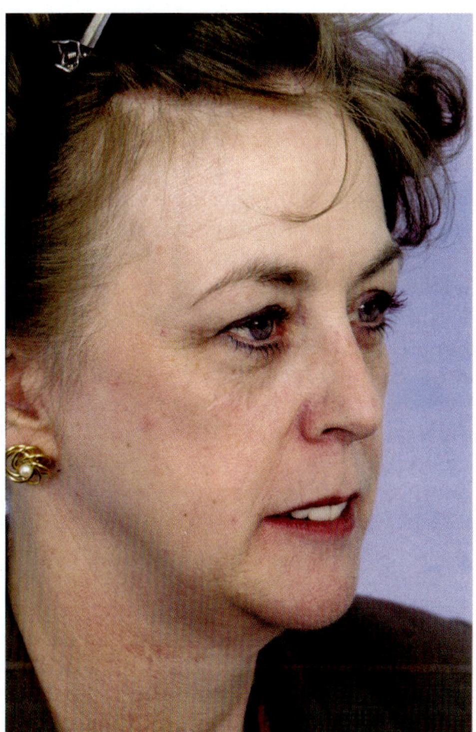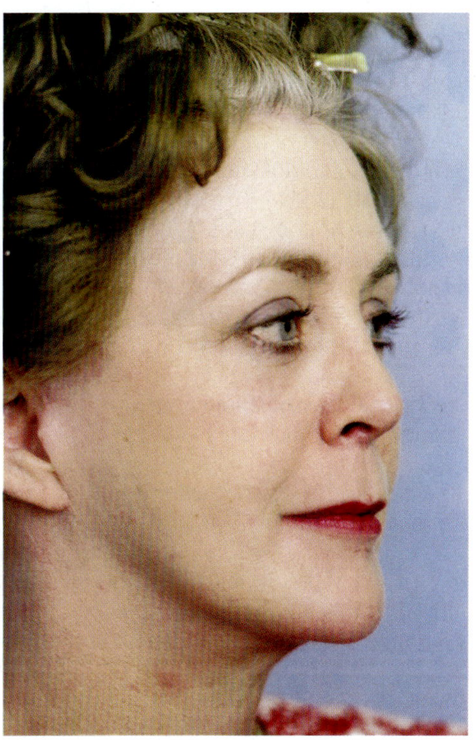

Fig. 34.25 (A,B) Patient who underwent facelift combined with submalar implants.

the question, once you have had a facelift, do you have to have another one? There certainly is a limit to the stretch ability and skin elasticity with rebound relaxation. Some of the rebound relaxation of the skin tissues themselves can add to the natural look of the overall facelift result. However, once the skin itself is tightened, there is a limit to the elasticity, and the skin becomes taut and will not rebound. These patients often can be identified as having had a facelift as they have an unnatural look in the mid-cheek tissues pulled posterosuperiorly, and the rhytides that accompany the skin are redirected laterally. This is an unnatural appearance, and most patients want to avoid it at all costs. Using deep plane techniques, which rely on repositioning the foundation tissues of the face rather than on skin tightness itself, is a good way to avoid this problem. Retightening the SMAS tissues themselves does have limits and, despite a scar tissue plane that forms between the SMAS and subcutaneous tissues of the skin, there is a limit to which the SMAS can be tightened, as it will finally thread thin and shred at the time of secondary facelifting. Certainly, patients need to be told that once they have had a facelift, they do not have to have another and that they will continue to age gracefully. The one exception to this is the patient who is aging faster in the midface than in the lower face; this sets up an unnatural appearance, creating laxity in the lateral cheek/jowl region that needs to be lifted with a different approach rather than a standard cheek–neck facelift.[19]

Cost to the patient is generally an issue when dealing with your own patient population on whom you have done the primary facelift. They at least have some expectation that further revision may be needed. It is very important to identify patients in preoperative consultation who most likely will need a tuck-up procedure in the first year to 18 months. You can then prepare the patients for additional costs that may be required. Generally, there is no surgeon's fee to do these modifications if they are done within the first year to 18 months after the primary facelift. If the patient elects to put this off for 2 years or longer, the costs begin to escalate based on the degree of work that needs to be done and the length of time he or she has "enjoyed" the benefits of the primary facelift. A cheek-only tuck-up involves more time and effort and may even generate a physician's practice fee of approximately one fourth the previous facelifting fee. Generally, submentoplasty is done at no additional cost. However, the patient must be aware that both these procedures require at least a level of anesthesia with IV sedation in an accredited operating facility. This will generate a cost that is the patient's responsibility. It is generally the goal of any surgeon to ultimately have a satisfied patient who is willing not only to refer other patients for facelifting but also to return for other procedures in the future. By entering into a mutually acceptable financial relationship for this secondary procedure, one can maintain a satisfied patient population while doing facelifts on all types of individuals.

References

1. Perkins SW, Dayan SH. Surgical rhytidectomy: facelift and the endoscopic forehead lift. In: Kaminer MS, Dover JS, Arndt KA, eds. Atlas of Cutaneous Cosmetic Surgery. St. Louis: Mosby; 2002.
2. Fomon S. The Surgery of Injury and Plastic Repair. Baltimore: Williams & Wilkins; 1939:1344.
3. Fulton JE, Saylan Z, Helton P, Rahimi AD, Golshani M. The S-lift facelift featuring the U-suture and O-suture combined with skin resurfacing. Dermatol Surg 2001; 27(1):18–22.
4. Webster RC, Smith RC, Papsidero MJ, et al. Comparison of SMAS plication with SMAS imbrication in face lifting. Laryngoscope 1982;92:901–912.
5. Mitz V, Peyronnie M. The superficial musculoaponeurotic system (SMAS) in the parotid and cheek area. Plast Reconstr Surg 1976;58:80–88.
6. Skoog T. Plastic surgery: the aging face. In: Plastic Surgery: New Methods and Refinements. Philadelphia: WB Saunders; 1974:300–330.
7. Guerrero-Santos J. The role of the platysma muscle in rhytidoplasty. Clin Plast Surg 1978;5:29–49.
8. Baker SR. Tri-plane rhytidectomy. Arch Otolaryngol Head Neck Surg 1997;123:1167–1172.
9. Kamer FM. One hundred consecutive deep plane facelifts. Arch Otolaryngol Head Neck Surg 1996;122:17–22.
10. Hamra ST. Composite rhytidectomy. Plast Reconstr Surg 1992;90(1):1–13.
11. Ramirez OM. The subperiosteal rhytidectomy: the third generation face lift. Ann Plast Surg 1992;28:218–232.
12. Dedo DD. Preoperative classification of the neck for cervicofacial rhytidectomy. Laryngoscope 1980;40:1894–1896.
13. Kamer FM. Sequential rhytidectomy and the two-stage concept. Otolaryngol Clin North Am 1980;13:305–320.
14. Perkins SW, Gibson FB. Use of submentoplasty to enhance cervical recontouring in facelift surgery. Arch Otolaryngol Head Neck Surg 1993;119:179–183.
15. Mittelman H. Geniomandibular groove implant—an adjunct to facelift surgery. Paper presented at: American Association of Facial Plastic and Reconstructive Surgeons Fall Meeting; September 22–24, 1988; Washington DC.
16. Kridel RWH. Acellular human dermis for facial soft tissue augmentation. Facial Plast Surg Clin North Am 2001;9:413–437.
17. Dyer WK II, Robertson KM. Expanded polytetrafluoroethylene (Gore-Tex) augmentation of deep nasolabial creases. Arch Otolaryngol Head Neck Surg 1999;125:456–461.
18. Binder WJ. A comprehensive approach for aesthetic contouring of the midface in rhytidectomy. Facial Plast Surg Clin North Am 1993;1:231–255.
19. Sclafani AP. The multivectorial subperiosteal midface lift. Facial Plast Surg 2001;17:29–36.

35 Hair Replacement and Revision Surgery

Jeffrey S. Epstein

In a practice devoted to hair restoration, a considerable percentage of individuals presenting for treatment are those who have had prior procedures and are seeking to improve appearances. For this 30% of the practice's patients, the goals are sometimes as high as expressed by those with virgin scalps (a completely undetectable restoration), but for the majority of revision surgery patients, the goals are somewhat tempered (a less detectable restoration). And for the overwhelming majority of revision surgery patients, in fact it is possible to overcome the limitations incurred by less than optimal work and significantly improve appearances.

A Relevant History of Hair Transplantation

An understanding of the evolution of hair transplantation provides a framework on which to evaluate the results from prior procedures and to decide upon a course of treatment. Since the early days of hair transplantation, beginning in the late 1950s in the United States with the use of large plug grafts, the evolution of techniques has been toward the goal of achieving undetectability. Although the current technique follicular unit grafting is indicated in most hair restorations performed today, in some revision cases the final result may best be achieved using more conventional techniques, but incorporating some of the technical aspects of follicular unit grafting.

Hair transplantation involves the surgical moving of "permanent" hairs from one part of the scalp to areas of baldness or hair thinning, and remains the only "permanent" treatment for male and female pattern hair loss, not curing the process but improving upon its manifestations. Several other conditions are also treatable with hair transplantation, the most common being alopecic scarring from prior surgical or other trauma.

In the original technique of plug grafting, the graft consisted of a 3 to 4 mm circle of scalp containing as many as 20 hairs. When punched out from the back of the scalp and placed into a similarly sized hole in the front or other part of the scalp, some or most of the hairs from the graft grow. Because hair does not naturally grow in groups of 15 or more hairs, plug grafting results in an unnatural appearance best described as doll's hair. Other problems with plug grafting include scarring in the donor area and the often poor growth of the transplanted hairs. Another significant problem is scarring of the skin surrounding the grafts. Most commonly presenting as hypopigmentation and/or hypertrophic scarring, it is a result of the large amount of skin transplanted along with the hairs. Improved aesthetic outcomes from plug grafting relied upon staged procedures, usually three to four, performed at 4-month intervals, to fill in all surrounding areas, essentially creating a solid wall of hair. The total amount of bald scalp that could be covered using this solid coverage technique was limited, leaving the scalp behind the solid hairline to be bald or transplanted with spread-out plug grafts. At its best, plug grafting provided coverage that relied on careful hair grooming. At its worst, the patient looked as if he had doll's hair.

More natural-appearing results became possible with the use of smaller grafts. Dividing a 4 mm plug graft in half or quarters, or using 3 and 2 mm punches for graft harvesting, created minigrafts containing four to eight hairs. Appearances certainly improved with these smaller grafts, which relied less on the creation of a solid wall and more on a spread-out distribution. Micrografts, small grafts typically containing one or two hairs, when placed in front of the minigrafts along the hairline significantly improved results. Their use, which was popularized in the early 1990s, permitted the creation of a softer, more natural-appearing hairline.[1]

Improvements in appearance came not only through the use of smaller grafts. Techniques of donor site harvest improved with several innovations, including suturing of the punch graft sites (facilitated by the excision of the skin between the individual punch graft holes), which evolved into the harvesting of the donor tissue as a single strip rather than individual punches. This single strip, no more than 10 to 12 mm wide and easily reapproximated with a simple running suture, remains the technique of choice. Enhanced appreciation of the aesthetics of hair transplantation evolved as well. Recognition of the proper direction and position of hair growth significantly improved appearances. Developments in hairline design, the scope of which is beyond the content of this chapter, but which is nicely reviewed in the literature,[2] and more anteriorly angled direction of grafts are two of the more important areas of improvement.

But perhaps no advancement in hair transplantation was more important than the recognition of the lifetime

Decision tree for revision hair restoration

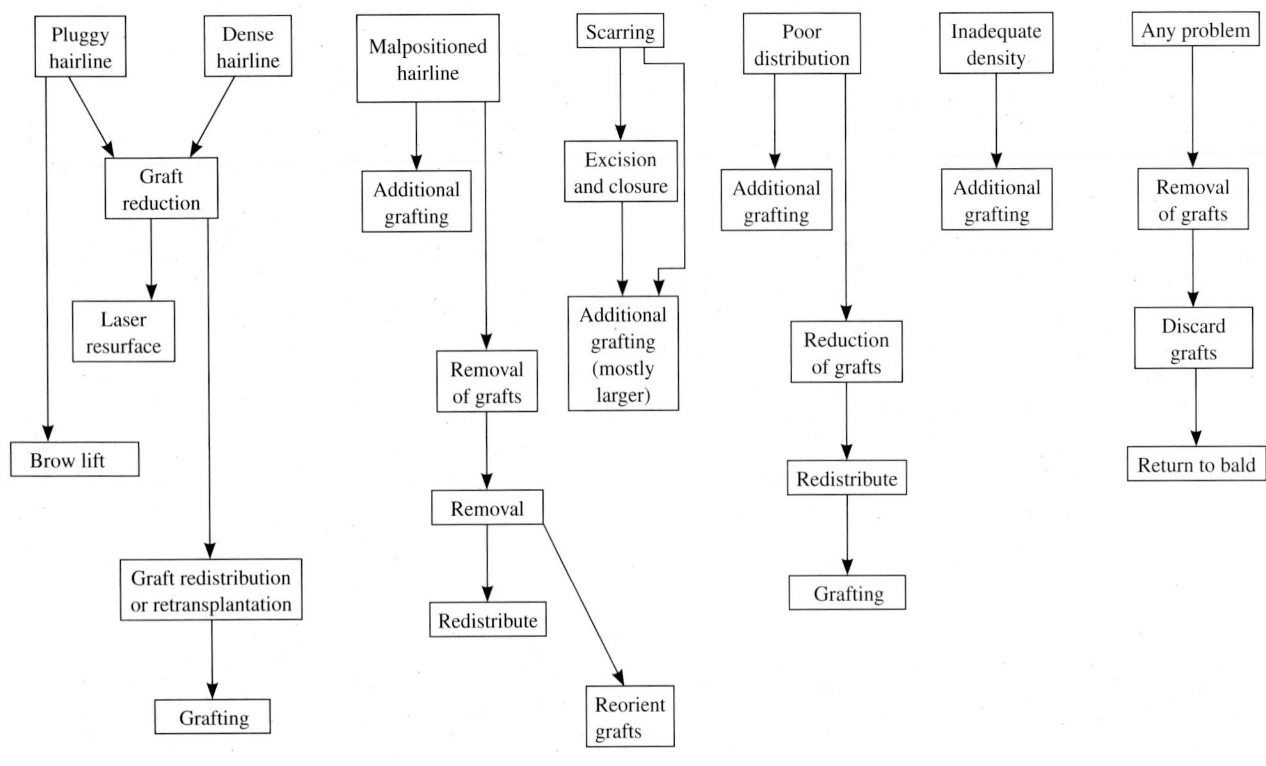

progressive nature of male pattern hair loss. With this knowledge, the responsible hair transplant physician could better plan the restoration and counsel for the possible need for more transplantation in the future.

Today, the culmination of advancements in hair transplantation has produced what nearly all leading hair transplant surgeons agree is the state-of-the-art technique, follicular unit grafting.[3] This technique relies on microscopic dissection to create grafts, each containing a single follicular unit. The follicular unit, as described originally by Headington, is the naturally occurring grouping of one to four hairs, most commonly two or three hairs, and the supporting glandular elements, surrounded by a fine adventitial sheath.[4] The use of the microscope is required to more accurately identify the individual follicular units, and to remove all the non-hair-bearing tissue (which can constitute as much as 50% of the total donor tissue). Although it is a technically demanding procedure, requiring a team of trained assistants to dissect and assist in the planting of as many as 3500 grafts, the natural results justify the effort.

The advantages of follicular unit grafting are many, most due to the smaller size of the grafts. Because the recipient sites are smaller, they can be placed closer together to maximize density, while minimizing trauma to already existing hairs in the areas being transplanted. In addition, healing is quicker, and there is minimal to no scalp scarring in the areas of the transplanted hair. Other advantages include less trauma to the hair follicles during graft dissection, resulting in as much as a 20% greater growth of hair, and more accuracy in dividing grafts by the number of hairs they contain, therefore assuring the placement of only one hair graft along the anteriormost hairline. But the most important advantage of the technique is that, because the grafts contain hairs as they grow naturally in the scalp, the results are the most natural. This explains why follicular unit grafting is the procedure of choice for most of the leading hair transplant surgeons in North America.

Indications for Revision Surgery

Individuals seeking reparative procedures present with a variety of concerns and problems with the results from prior transplants. Often the patient simply complains of "unnatural appearances," while other times identifying the reason for dissatisfaction with the transplant. It is the job of the revision hair transplant surgeon to both identify the problem(s) and counsel the patient as to what can realistically be achieved. Given the disappointment these patients feel with the results of prior procedures, it is critical to reestablish trust in the doctor–patient relationship.

The following is a review of the most common indications for performing revision surgery.

- Pluggy hairline: the classic "doll's hair" appearance, with the hairline composed of large grafts with intervening non-hair-bearing scalp
- Dense hairline: similar to the pluggy hairline, except that multiple procedures were performed of usually large grafts to create a solid wall of hairs. Commonly, the density decreases significantly just a few centimeters behind this hairline.
- Malposition of the hairline: including several situations, often occurring simultaneously:
  - Inadequate frontotemporal recessions: a flat or broad hairline, which in its extreme can create a simian appearance due to the caudal position of the lateral hairline
  - Asymmetric hairline: whereby one side of the hairline is lower than the other, giving an off-balance appearance
  - Too low a hairline: commonly seen when the hair transplant had been performed on a young man, at which time a lower hairline seemed appropriate, but with advancement in age that hairline is inappropriately low. These too low hairlines often create challenges of filling in the remainder of the scalp (see Poor Distribution of Transplants).
- Misdirection of hair growth: one of the more common errors, usually the result of recipient incisions made at a more perpendicular angle, rather than the cosmetically appropriate more anterior acute angle. This is a problem almost inherent in plug grafts because of the difficulty in making larger punches at a sharp angle, but it often occurs with slit grafting. Besides looking less natural, the more perpendicular direction of hair growth results in a coarser appearance that is the result of the human eye looking at the base of the transplanted hair shafts, a phenomenon avoidable when the hairs grow in the viewer's direction.
- Scarring of the recipient scalp: fibrosis, cobblestoning, ridging, and altered pigmentation of the recipient site are forms of scarring that largely result from the skin of the graft that gets transplanted along with hairs. Healing of large grafts is often associated with scar formation, sometimes resulting in hyperfibrosis and ridging.[5] Larger grafts, especially plug grafts, but even conventional micro- and minigrafts where a large cuff of skin is often present, are at high risk of causing these forms of scarring.
- Poor distribution of transplants: because of poor planning for the progression of hair loss, older transplant procedures often used many of the donor hairs, not leaving enough donor hairs to cover areas of further hair loss. One result is a fully transplanted crown region

that with further hair loss leads to the development of a cuff or halo of bald scalp around the crown transplants with not enough donor hairs available to further transplant and extend the area covered. Another problem can be the result of transplanting into the frontotemporal recessions, creating in the future with further hair loss a bald central forelock surrounded by filled-in frontotemporal recessions. Typically, it is those areas that lose hair later in the balding process that are the most critical to transplant to achieve a natural-appearing restoration.

- Inadequate density: probably the most common complaint of patients transplanted with modern techniques. This is usually the result of insufficient or deceptive pre-op counseling. Unrealistic expectations of density leave the patient dissatisfied. Poor growth of transplanted hairs can also result in a less than anticipated density. Rough handling and desiccation of grafts are two of the most common reasons believed to result in this poor hair growth.
- Scarring of the donor site: with plug grafting, the donor site defects that healed by secondary intention result in multiple circular scars. For donor site defects closed primarily, wide incision scars can result from incisions placed too low or closed under excessive tension. This scarring is more visible when donor site incisions or punches were made too cephalic, close to regions that eventually undergo pattern hair loss.
- Pitting: characterized by small, depressed areas of scalp out of which grow the transplanted hairs. This commonly results from placing grafts too deep, in that the skin around the graft was placed below the surface of the surrounding recipient site skin. With healing, the surrounding scalp skin contracts, creating a pit at the base of the transplanted hair shafts.
- Two, three, and more hair grafts growing along the hairline: unlike plug grafting, where the goal is the creation of a "wall" of hair, with micro-/minigrafting, the goal is the creation of a feathered hairline, created by the placement of one and occasionally two hair grafts most anterior. This attempt at a natural-appearing hairline is disrupted when grafts containing two, three, or more hairs are placed most anterior.
- Scalp reduction sequelae: the best known of these sequelae is incision scarring that is worsened by the often-occurring stretchback. Another sequela is slot formation, whereby the hairs from the opposite sides of the head are brought together, creating a deformity.
- Scalp flap surgery sequelae: rarely performed today, scalp flap surgery is unsurpassed in its ability to create a dense hairline, but it is associated with several deformities. Most common of these is scarring along the donor defect as well as along the leading edge of the flap. Another significant problem is the lack of density

posterior to the flap or flaps, requiring further transplantation to fill the midscalp and crown regions.

Approaching the Patient

Reestablishing trust in the doctor–patient relationship and establishing realistic expectations in the patient are the first steps in the reparative process. Education is essential to restoring confidence in the patient, who can be skeptical or mistrusting of the hair restoration process. Recognition of the limitations in undertaking reparative work is critical for formulating a plan for repair. In spite of these limitations, however, significant improvement in appearance is possible for most patients using a variety of techniques.

The most important limitation in repairing prior work is the limited supply of donor hair. Especially in those patients who had large numbers of grafts in the past, the number of available donor hairs is reduced. Scarring of the donor region reduces the compliance of the tissue, further limiting the ability to harvest additional hairs.

Another limitation to reparative hair work is that circulation to the scalp is compromised. This impairment is due to scarring and fibrosis in the recipient areas, and possible transection of the occipital and/or postauricular arteries that supply blood to the scalp due to prior donor harvesting.

Before establishing a treatment plan, the patient's concerns and priorities must be understood. Some patients desire a more natural-appearing hairline, others seek more density or coverage, while others are concerned about donor site scarring. The occasional patient may seek to return to a bald scalp, hoping to have prior placed grafts removed.

Options in Repair

The surgeon has available three basic corrective techniques: further grafting; the removal, reduction in size, or redistribution of prior placed grafts; and scar repair. These techniques have all been described in the scientific literature.[6–10]

With further grafting, the goal is to fill in those areas requiring more hair, including the creation of a new hairline. The hair used for grafting in this case comes from the donor area of the scalp. Graft removal, reduction, and redistribution all involve manipulation of prior placed grafts. Graft removal is applied to grafts placed in a wrong position, or in those patients who desire a return to a balding scalp. It can be applied to all sized grafts. Graft reduction is usually performed on large plug grafts where only a portion of the graft is removed to reduce its size and associated pluggy appearance. Graft redistribution, because it involves the retransplanting of hairs previously transplanted, is performed on the material obtained by graft reduction or removal. Finally, direct scar repair usually involves the excision and closure of donor site scars and is often performed with further grafting. A combination of techniques is often used for the most aesthetic results.

Further Hair Grafting

In the majority of reparative cases, further transplanting is the approach of choice. The hairs are transplanted to those areas where additional coverage is most beneficial. Typically, this involves the placing of follicular unit grafts containing one and two hairs along the hairline and grafts containing two to four hairs in other parts of the scalp that require more hair.

Hairline grafting is performed to correct several problems, including a pluggy appearance, an abruptly dense hairline, an asymmetric hairline, and unaesthetic direction of transplanted hairs. When transplanting along the hairline, the goal is to minimize its lowering while softening it in its appearance. Restoring a more aesthetic anterior direction of hair growth, filling in and lowering that part of the hairline that is asymmetrically higher than its opposite side, and grafting into and/or in front of scarred scalp are all achievable with further grafting.

Hair grafting may also be used to repair the alopecic scarring from prior bald scalp reductions and scalp flap surgery procedures. With scalp reductions, the visible scar along the incision(s), accentuated by the stretchback and slot formation that often occur, can be improved with further hair grafting. Similarly, alopecic scarring that can occur along the donor site and edges of a scalp flap can be effectively treated with further hair grafting. As a general rule, growth of hair when transplanted into scar tissue is less than the 90% of hair growth when transplanted into normal scalp. The anticipated reduction in hair growth can be compensated for by placing slightly larger grafts into areas of scarring to ensure adequate coverage.

Because the donor supply is usually limited, it is critical to transplant hairs where they will provide the greatest aesthetic benefit. Usually this is in the anterior to midscalp region, especially along the central forelock, where the greatest density is desirable. A maximally dense central forelock serves not only to frame the face and give the appearance of coverage, but also to create a denser backdrop to soften any pluggy appearance of the region anterior to it.

Technique

With revision surgery, the choice of the donor site may be limited. Many times, the donor strip will incorporate areas of prior scarring, allowing for the removal of unsightly scars, but reducing the numbers of hairs that can be harvested. Graft dissection is best performed under the microscope, where the enhanced visualization allows for maximal preservation of hairs. In cases where an old donor site scar is excessively caudal (usually defined as below the nuchal ridge), because of the high risk of widened scar formation, it is best, if possible, to harvest from a more cephalad portion of the scalp. It is important to maintain an adequately wide strip of hair-bearing skin between the old and the new donor sites, leaving sufficient numbers of hairs to cover the caudal prior donor site scar. If necessary, donor material can be harvested from the sides of the head. In fact, a surprising number of excellent grafts can be harvested from the temporal region, a place that is avoided as a donor site by many surgeons.

Anesthetizing the scalp is usually more difficult in revision cases because scarring interferes with the distribution of the anesthetic solution. Like most of the hair transplant cases I perform, the patient is given oral diazepam and Ambien for relaxation and some amnesia. The hair in the donor region is cut to 2 mm, then the surrounding hair taped out of the way. Under sterile technique with the patient sitting upright, the donor strip is harvested with a single no. 15 scalpel blade, cutting parallel to the hair follicles to minimize transection (a common theme throughout the graft preparation process). Removal of the strip by dissecting in the subcutaneous fat plane is often more difficult due to scarring. Any bleeding is secured with electrocautery. The donor site is then closed with a single running 3–0 polypropylene suture placed superficial to the hair follicles, supplemented if necessary with interrupted subcutaneous 3–0 Vicryl sutures.

The donor strip is then dissected out under the binocular microscope. This step is usually performed by the hair technicians, of whom there may be as many as 10 to 12 working on a single patient. The dissection process first involves the vertical subsectioning of the donor strip into individual slivers, one or two follicular units wide. From these slivers are dissected out follicular unit grafts that contain a minimum amount of surrounding non-hair-bearing skin that, in these secondary cases, usually includes scar tissue.

In classical follicular unit grafting, the size of the grafts is determined by the natural grouping of hairs, most commonly two hairs, then one hair, then three and four hairs. It is sometimes advantageous to use grafts containing more than one follicular unit in the region of prior plug grafting. Rather than transplanting one, two, or three hair grafts that will get "lost" when placed adjacent to grafts containing eight or more hairs, a more natural appearance is best achieved with the transplanting of grafts containing three to four hairs. These grafts can be created by combining follicular units, resulting in follicular unit "family" grafts (**Fig. 35.1**).

The recipient sites are made simultaneously with the microscopic dissection. The recipient sites along the

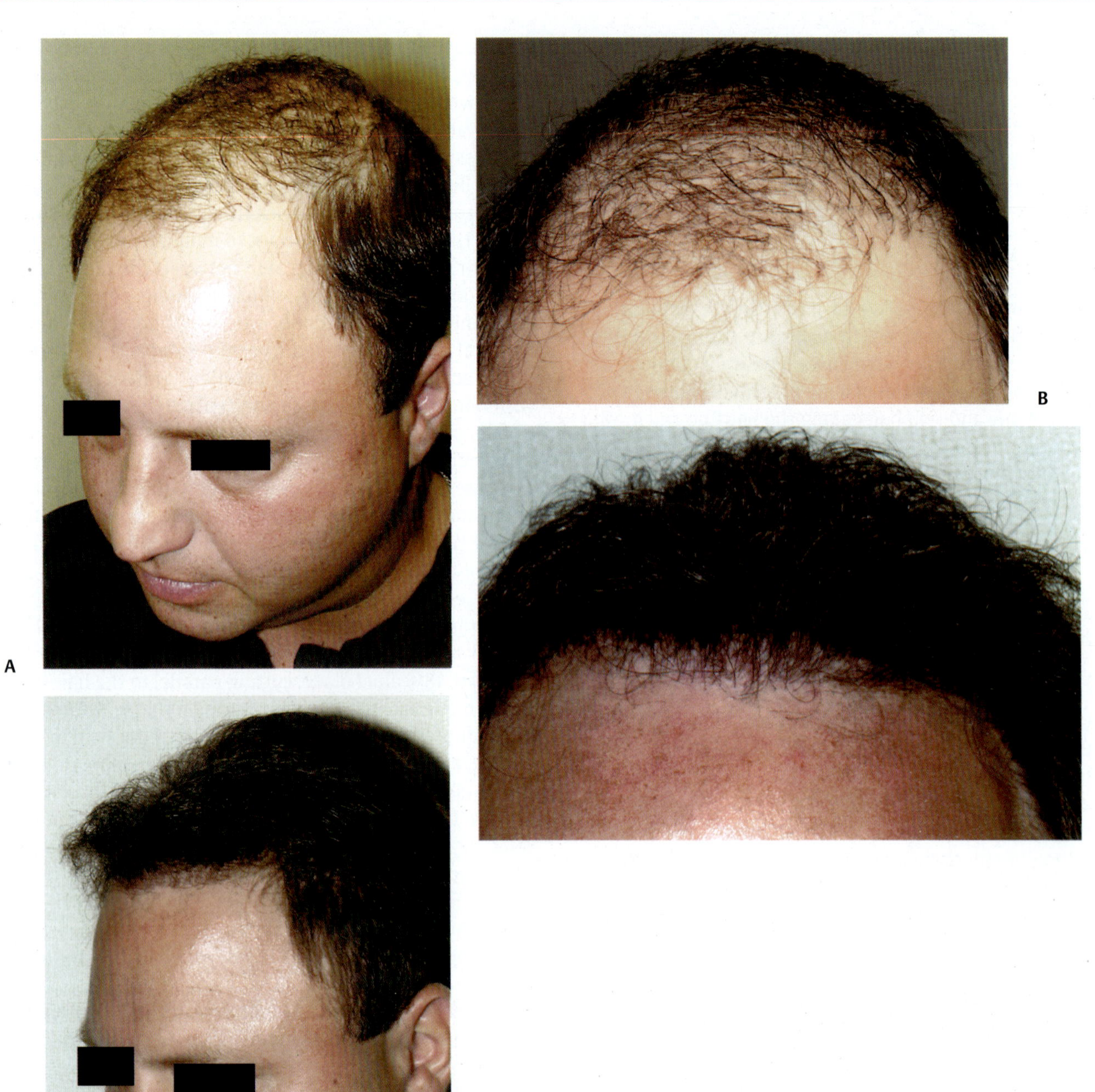

Fig. 35.1 A 35-year-old patient, following two procedures 4 and 7 years prior for a total of 1000 grafts, shown **(A,B)** before and **(C,D)** after a single reparative procedure of further hair grafting. In total, 1560 grafts were placed to improve the hairline and fill in between large grafts.

hairline, where the smallest grafts will go, are made with specially designed microblades 0.6 to 0.9 mm and smaller. Anterior direction of hair growth is achieved by angling the recipient sites, but the degree of angulation must not be considerably out of line with the direction of any prior placed hairline grafts, otherwise a parting will occur between the hairs placed previously and those placed with the reparative procedure. In revision cases where there is poor circulation and/or considerable scarring, it is often beneficial to make the recipient sites slightly larger than would be made normally, both to induce at least minimal bleeding to ensure graft nourishment and to minimize graft damage during placement into fibrotic tissue. However, this benefit of larger recipient sites must be balanced with the problem of compromising circulation to the more central scalp by these larger and/or deeper recipient sites.

The making of recipient sites proceeds from anterior to posterior as indicated, using larger blades or needles as necessary. Similar to grafts along the hairline, it is possible to make more anteriorly directed recipient sites than the direction of prior transplanted hairs in the midscalp region, but the angle must not be significantly different from already existing hair grafts so as to avoid awkward, difficult-to-style hair growth. The proximity of recipient sites must maximize density while minimizing the compromise of scalp circulation.

Once the recipient sites are made, the grafts are planted. Alternatively, some surgeons use a stick-and-plant technique, whereby the recipient sites are made one at a time and then filled with a graft before the next recipient site is made. With this technique, the hair technicians usually make a considerable percentage of recipient sites. This is as opposed to the technique of separating the two steps, whereby the surgeon makes all the recipient sites, then the surgeon and hair technicians plant the grafts. It is always possible to use a stick-and-plant technique to place any extra grafts after all recipient sites are filled.

Alteration of Prior Grafts

Certain alterations can be undertaken on prior grafts, including reduction in size, complete removal, and relocation. There are several indications for altering grafts. When a hairline was made too low or has hairs that grow completely in the wrong direction, it is best to remove the graft(s) completely. These hairs can then be discarded or, if further hair coverage is desired, retransplanted. Large plug grafts in the crown region are sometimes best reduced in size, at other times completely removed. Some patients will want to have a "normal" bald scalp again; in this case, the grafts are removed and discarded (**Fig. 35.2**). If the grafts are not to be transplanted to provide further coverage in the regions of pattern hair loss, it may be beneficial to transplant the removed graft material into donor site scars that may be present, essentially returning the hairs to their original site.

Occasionally, rather than removing grafts individually, it may be preferable to excise an entire strip of prior transplanted scalp and suture close the defect. This technique is usually reserved for elevating an overly low hairline

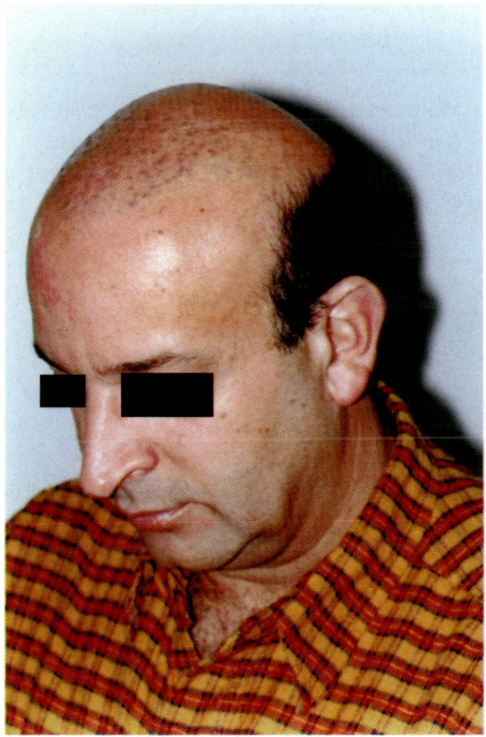
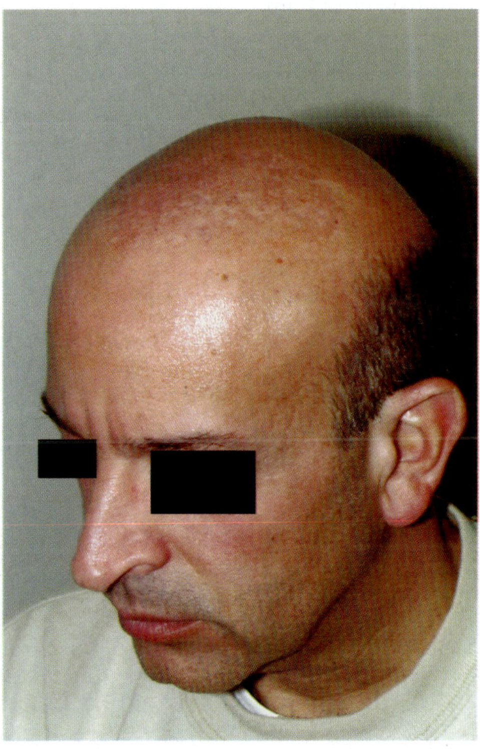

Fig. 35.2 A 43-year-old patient, following plug grafts 20 years prior for a total of 144 grafts, shown (**A**) before and (**B**) after removal of all the grafts using the punch technique. Four procedures in all were required.

of plug grafts or minigrafts. With this technique, a brow lift is usually performed simultaneously.

Reducing the size of prior grafts is an effective technique for reducing a pluggy appearance, especially along the hairline or crown region when additional grafting will not be sufficient for improving appearances. Typically performed on grafts of six or more hairs, the goal is to remove a portion of the graft, follicles included. The portion removed can be retransplanted into another recipient site on the scalp.

Technique

Graft removal is usually best performed by the same technique that was used to place the graft the first time: by punching out the entire cylinder of skin and removing it in its entirety. The size of the graft determines the size of the punch, typically a standard dermatologic biopsy punch. Effort must be taken to remove the entire graft, otherwise retained follicles can potentially continue to grow hair.

As a general rule, to minimize scar formation any hole on the scalp > 1.5 mm in diameter must be sutured closed, whereas those 1.5 mm or smaller can be allowed to close secondarily. One or two simple interrupted 4–0 or 5–0 nylon sutures are used to reapproximate the punch defects. Because of the limit in scalp compliance, when large numbers of punch removals are to be performed on grafts close to each other, to minimize scarring it is best to stage the removals at 3- to 4-month intervals, typically removing no more than 40 or so grafts in a single procedure.

Occasionally, it may be beneficial to laser resurface the scalp after punch plug removal. This technique has been necessary only when excessive tension on the sutured-closed punch defects has resulted in scarring, a situation usually avoidable by staging the removals as necessary.

The technique of strip removal with brow lift is similar to that of traditional trichophytic brow lift. At or just posterior to the hairline, a beveled incision is made so that the leading edge of the forehead portion of the flap has an overhang of skin, allowing for hair growth through the scar. Undermining in the subfrontalis plane is taken down to the eyebrows, where the glabellar musculature and subbrow portion of the orbicularis oculi can be divided, providing additional mobility if necessary of the forehead portion of the flap and permitting maximum width of graft-bearing skin to be excised. After determining the desired position of the brows, the corresponding excess amount of frontal scalp containing the undesirable hairline grafts is excised, and the defect is reapproximated in a layered fashion.

Punch reduction of large grafts is best performed with standard dermatologic punches 1.5 to 2.0 mm in diameter. The ideal size is determined by the amount of hair-bearing plug tissue that is to be excised. Similar to the technique of complete plug removal, effort must be taken to remove the entire portion of the hairs. It is not necessary to suture close the residual defect, unless a 2 mm or greater punch is used.

Once removed, the follicles from the removed grafts can be retransplanted. The excised cylinder of tissue is dissected out under the microscope to create the desired graft size. Many times, because of partial hair follicle damage, a 1.5 mm punch will yield only a one- or two-hair graft, whereas a 2.5 mm punch will provide two or three of these similarly sized grafts. Retransplantation of the graft is performed according to standard techniques.

Scar Repair

Several techniques are available for treating scalp scars from prior hair restoration procedures. These scars may be due to fibrotic tissue growth where prior plug grafts were placed. Also, scarring may occur with bald scalp reductions

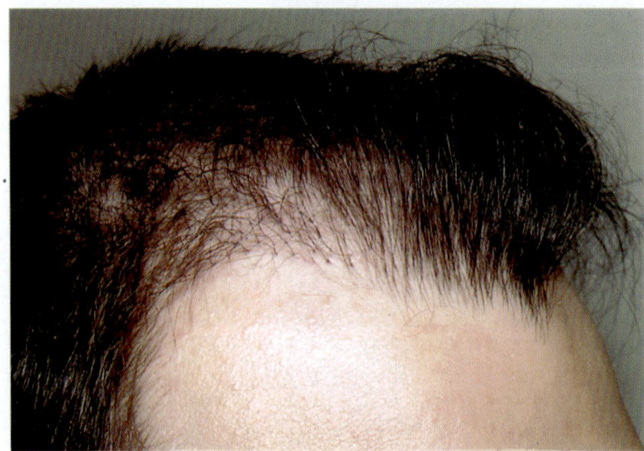
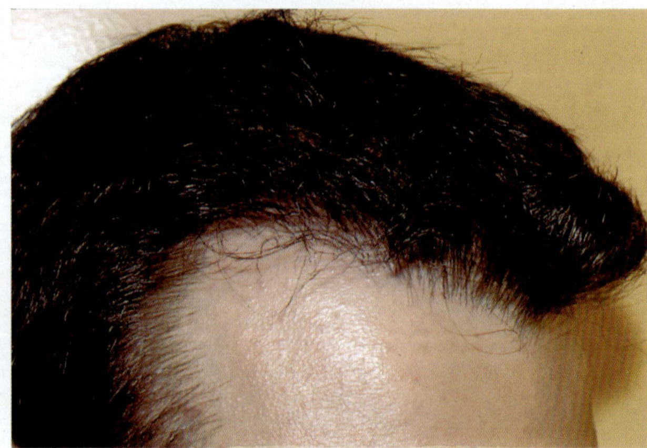

Fig. 35.3 A 36-year-old patient, following hair grafts 2 years prior with poor hairline design characterized by rounded frontotemporal recessions and two to four hair grafts placed anteriorly with pitting, shown **(A)** before and **(B)** after a single reparative procedure of further grafting and removal of malpositioned grafts on each side. In total, 1460 grafts were placed to improve the hairline and fill in the anterior and midscalp region.

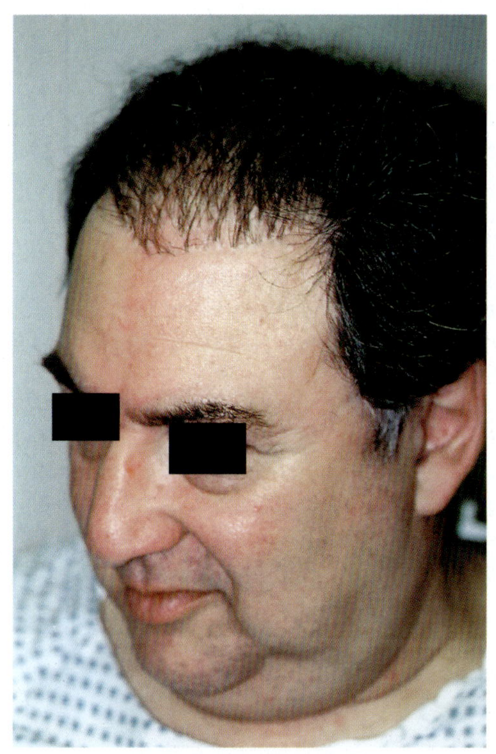
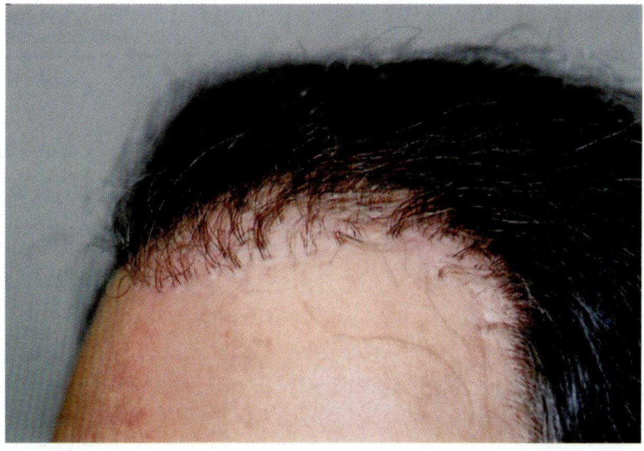
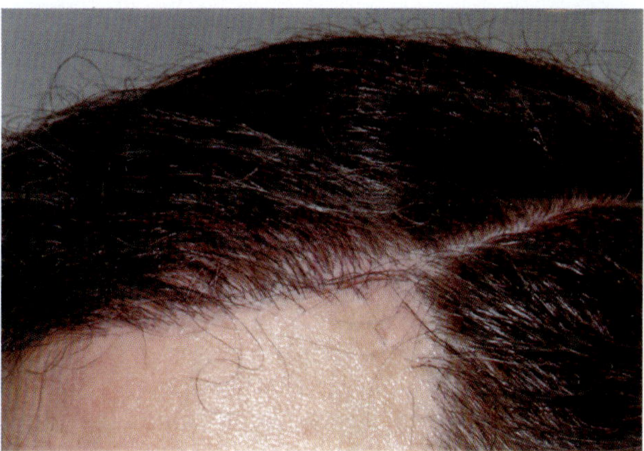
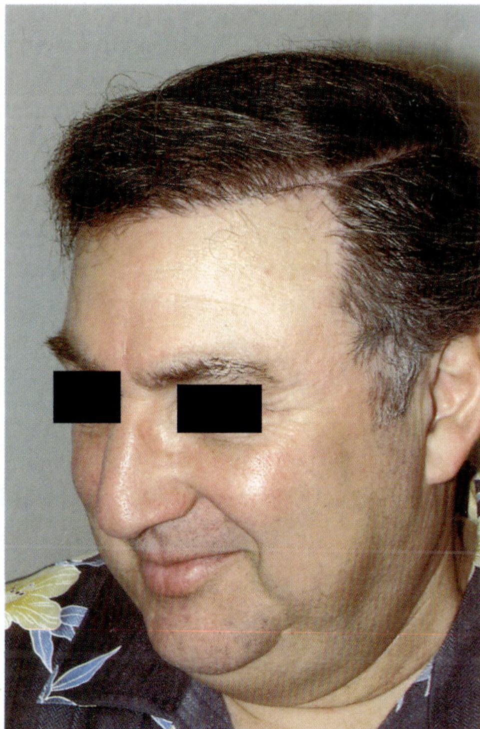

Fig. 35.4 A 62-year-old patient, following plug grafts 30 years prior, and a minigraft procedure of 250 grafts 8 years prior, shown **(A,B)** before and **(C,D)** after a single reparative procedure of further grafting and removal of visible plug grafts along the left hairline. In total, 1800 grafts were placed in the anterior portion to improve the hairline and fill in between large grafts.

along the incisions where stretchback occurs, or with scalp flaps along the donor site incisions, the hairline edge of the flap where healing resulted in hypopigmentation, or the distal end of the flap when poor circulation resulted in partial loss of the flap.

Scarring also occurs in the donor site region of prior hair grafts. Prior plug graft donor sites allowed to heal by secondary intention result in multiple circular alopecic scars 2 to 3 mm in diameter (**Fig. 35.3**). Wide donor site scars may also be present in cases where a donor site strip was closed primarily under excessive tension or made too caudal so that it widened due to the action of the occipitalis muscles in the area.

Technique

The two options for treating scars are to remove them or to transplant into them. Excision and closure of scars along the scalp can be challenging because the original conditions that contributed to their formation, such as poor location or excessive tension, are usually still present. Wide undermining in the subgaleal plane is of little to no benefit, due to the noncompliant nature of the fibrotic galea. Galeotomy, the making of incisions through the galea in a horizontal direction, may be of some benefit, but it carries the risk of impaired circulation and scalp necrosis. For scars in the lower occipital region, wide undermining into the nape of the neck may provide some limited benefit, but caution must be taken to avoid compromising the occipital circulation. Layered closure is best performed using 3–0 or 2–0 long-lasting absorbable or even nonabsorbable sutures for the galeal and subcutaneous layers. Galeal to periosteal sutures can be effective in minimizing stretchback when repairing prior scalp reduction scars.

Further hair grafting into scalp scars is usually the most effective technique. In most cases, the goal is not complete coverage with equivalent density to that of the surrounding scalp, but rather sufficient hair growth to conceal the presence of the scars. Although most commonly performed along the top and upper sides of the scalp, hair grafting may be performed into donor site scars in the occiput. This technique reduces the number of hairs that could be used to treat areas of pattern baldness; however, a relatively small number of grafts can significantly improve the area that is often of greatest preoccupation.

As discussed earlier, hair growth is often compromised when transplanting into scars. To compensate for the anticipated poorer hair growth, it is best to use grafts containing 30 to 50% more hair (e.g., using a three-hair graft when it is hoped that two hairs will grow) (**Fig. 35.4**).

Conclusion

As a discipline, reparative hair transplantation has many challenges. Because of the limited donor supply of hairs and potentially compromised scalp circulation, it is important to use state-of-the-art techniques such as microscopic dissection and follicular unit grafting to preserve every potential donor hair. Equally as important as surgical technique is thorough preoperative counseling to restore confidence and trust in the patient.

Finally, the importance of preventing untoward or undesirable results of hair transplantation cannot be understated. It is much easier to prevent complications or undesirable results than it is to repair them after they have occurred.

References

1. Marritt E. Single-hair transplantation for hairline refinement: a practical solution. J Dermatol Surg Oncol 1984;10: 962–966.
2. Stough DB. Hairline placement. In: Stough DB, Haber RS, eds. Hair Replacement: Surgical and Medical. St. Louis: Mosby Year Book; 1996:170–172.
3. Limmer BL. Elliptical donor stereoscopically assisted micrografting as an approach to further refinement in hair transplantation. J Dermatol Surg Oncol 1994;20:789–793.
4. Headington JT. Transverse microscopic anatomy of the human scalp: a basis for a morphometric approach to disorders of the hair follicle. Arch Dermatol 1984;120:449–456.
5. Unger M. Hyperfibrotic transplants. Hair Transplant Forum Int 1993;3(4):8,9.
6. Epstein JS. Revision surgical hair restoration: the repair of undesirable results. Plast Reconstr Surg 1999;104(1): 222–232.
7. Bernstein RM, Rassman WR, Rashid N, et al. The art of repair in surgical hair restoration: 1. Basic repair strategies. Dermatol Surg 2002;28:783–794.
8. Vogel JE. Advances in hair restoration surgery. Plast Reconstr Surg 1997;100:1875–1885.
9. Unger WP. Correction of poor transplanting. In: Unger WP, ed. Hair Transplantation. 3rd ed. New York: Marcel Dekker; 1995:375–388.
10. Leavitt ML. Corrective hair restoration. In: Stough DB, Haber RS, eds. Hair Replacement: Surgical and Medical. St. Louis: Mosby Year Book; 1996:306–314.

36 Auricular Reconstruction, Revision, and Salvage

E. Fred Aguilar

Since the advent of autologous cartilage for use in the repair of congenital microtias, numerous authors have published their results and recommendations for managing this deformity. Brent's publication detailing 1200 cases serves as the gold standard for all surgeons.[1–3] The need for this repair continues, as the incidence of this condition is not lessening and remains at 1 in 6000 births. Aguilar published the Integrated Auricular Reconstruction Protocol (IARP), which encourages plastic surgeons to consider the repair of the aural atresia (that usually accompanies this condition) as an integral part of the staged reconstruction.[3] In this protocol, the individual stages correspond to fixed procedures, and our descriptions of these stages remain constant. Stage III is the correction of the aural atresia; this stage may not be done in all patients. In this protocol, stage IV is tragal reconstruction, and stage V represents auricular elevation.

This chapter will focus on eight cases that represent individuals presenting with congenital mocrotiz/atresia in a variety of age groups with standard and unusual considerations. The discussion that follows specifies issues concerning surgical timing, materials, drains and dressings, hairline, atresia repair, and problem areas associated with this type of reconstruction, as well as complications associated with revision surgery.

Case Studies

Case 1

This 29-year-old Hispanic male patient finally sought treatment after many years of ridicule and embarrassment (**Fig. 36.1**). Stage I reconstruction with rib cartilage graft was accomplished on October 7, 1998. The cartilaginous framework was larger and thicker than standard, measuring 6.5 cm long, 3.5 cm wide, and 20.0 mm high. The procedure was tolerated well without tissue necrosis, and a second procedure to transfer the lobule was accomplished on February 9, 1999. A computed tomography (CT) scan of the temporal bones determined that he was not a candidate for atresia repair due to a congenital absence of the

ossicular chain. Therefore, a stage IV reconstruction, or creation of the tragus, was performed on May 5, 1999. Following this procedure, the patient developed an infection, causing resorption of the cartilage graft. This was subsequently revised on December 4, 2000. The elevation, stage V, was completed on October 10, 2000.

Case 2

This patient had been followed since birth for a bilateral complete aural atresia with a grade III microtia of the left ear and a grade II microtia of the right (**Fig. 36.2**). He was fitted with a bone-conducted hearing aid, and reconstruction was begun at age 5. Preoperative CT scans showed the patient to be a good candidate for atresia repair on the right, more completely formed ear and a marginal candidate on the left. Stage I reconstruction was done on the left ear on December 16, 1994, with framework measuring 5.0 cm long, 2.8 cm wide, and 15.0 mm high. Stage II was accomplished on the left in conjunction with atresia repair on the right ear by the otologist. A later hearing test confirmed a 20 dB speech reception threshold with a 96% speech discrimination score. The remaining two stages were completed by December 27, 1996. Photographs taken during subsequent follow-up visits showed no resorption of cartilage graft and hearing in the normal/near-normal range without benefit of a hearing aid.

Case 3

This patient is a 6-year-old white female with an almost complete anotia of the right ear with a severe hemifacial microsomia (**Fig. 36.3**). Preoperative CT scans determined that she was not a candidate for atresia repair due to malposition of the facial nerve and malformation of the ossicular chain. External reconstruction was begun on July 8, 1992, and the appropriate stages were completed on July 12, 1993. Note the addition of pierced earrings following the final procedure. This patient also had mandibular distraction.

Decision tree for microtia

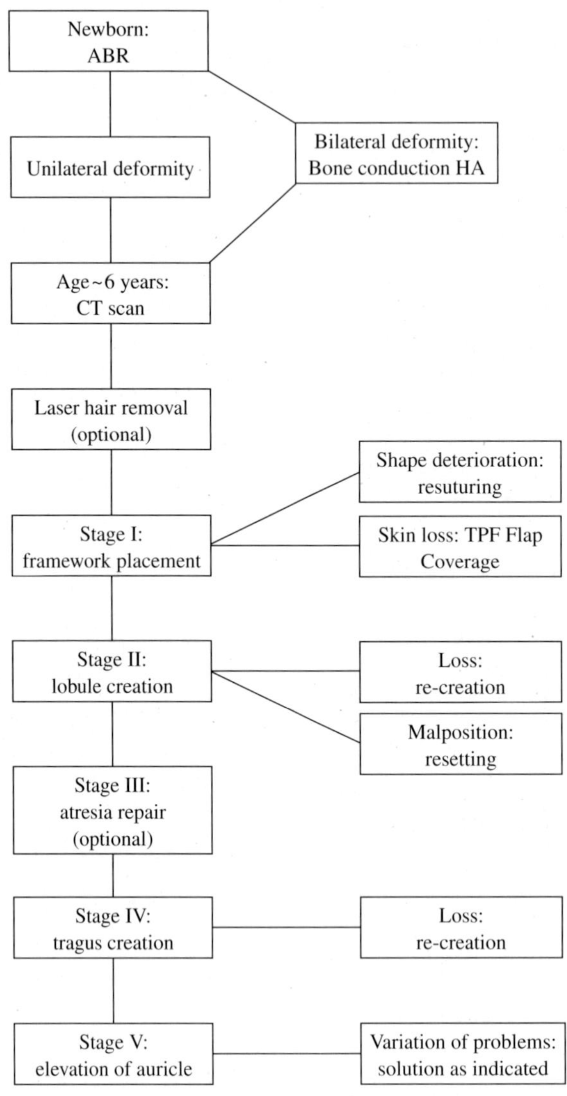

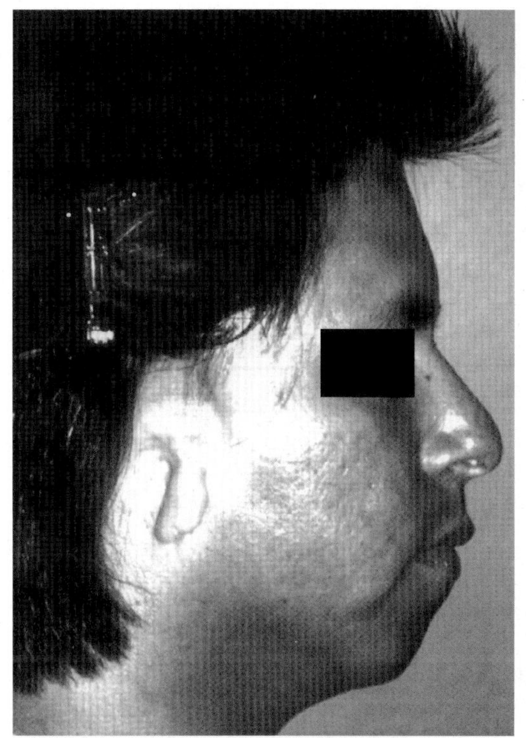

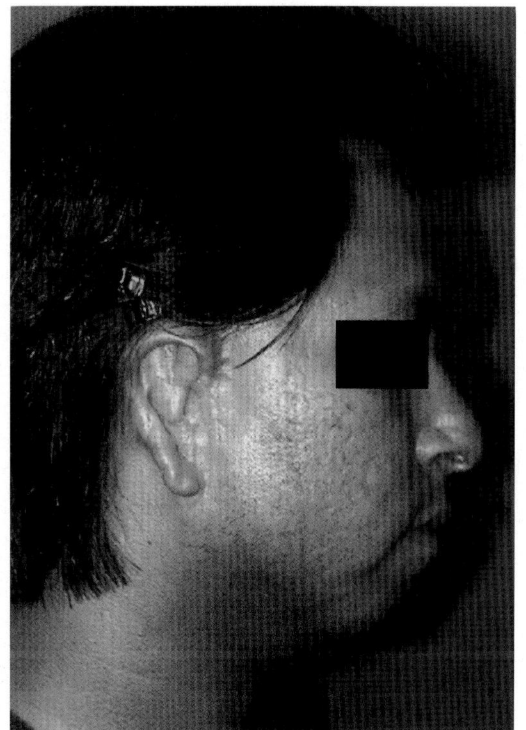

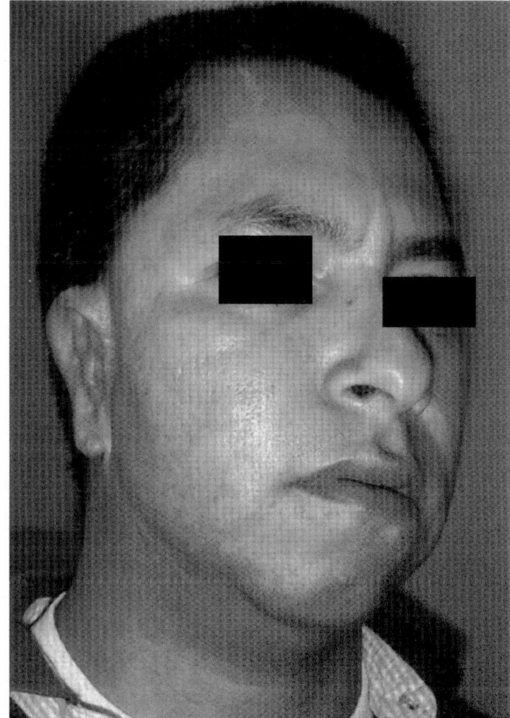

Fig. 36.1 Case 1. A 29-year-old male. **(A)** Preoperative photograph. **(B)** The postoperative photograph shows an early result following stage V. **(C)** Note the change in hairstyle following full reconstruction.

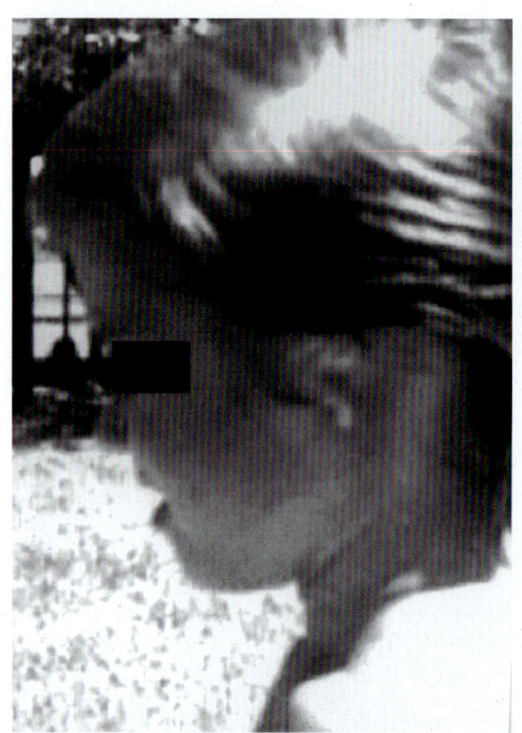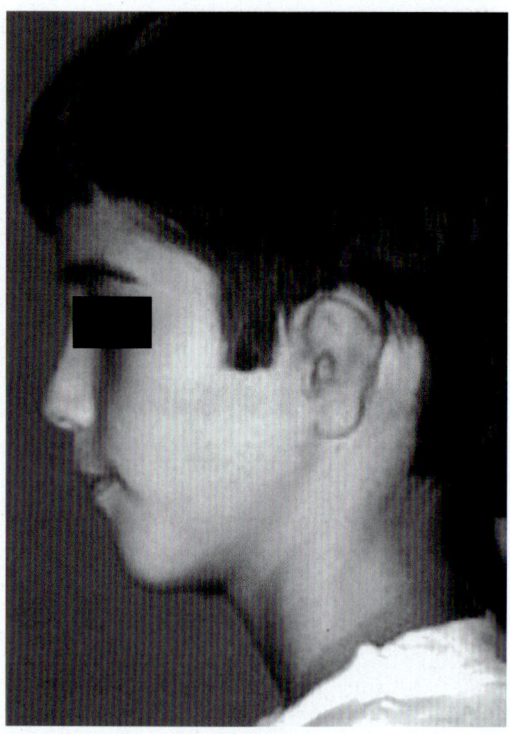

A

B

Fig. 36.2 Case 2. **(A)** Preoperative photograph of left grade III microtia/atresia. **(B)** Postoperative photograph taken 4 years after reconstruction. The patient was not a candidate for atresia repair on the left.

Case 4

This 6-year-old Asian male had a unilateral microtia with atresia of the right ear (**Fig. 36.4**). Reconstruction was begun on September 8, 1993, with the standard rib cartilage graft. Preoperative CT scans showed the patient to have a fused malleus/incus head and an incus that was two thirds of the normal size. Atresia repair was performed on February 9, 1994, and hearing was improved to normal range. All procedures were accomplished on June 16, 1994.

Case 5

This Hispanic male patient presented at age 13, when the family was advised that surgical reconstruction was possible (**Fig. 36.5**). A stage I procedure was performed on August 8, 1988, with a framework measuring 5.1 cm long, 3.2 cm wide, and 13.0 mm high. Transfer of the lobule was performed December 13, 1988. Preoperative CT scans showed satisfactory structures for the atresia repair, done on July 19, 1989. Postoperative speech reception threshold was improved to 15 dB with a speech discrimination score of 92%. All procedures were completed by December 13, 1991. Photographs taken 10 years following reconstruction showed no resorption of cartilage framework. This

patient continues to have normal hearing, is married, and has a 6-year-old son with normal ears.

Case 6

This is a 6-year-old white female with a left microtia/ atresia (**Fig. 36.6**). Staged reconstruction was begun on June 16, 1998, with a cartilaginous framework. All procedures were completed by June 2, 1999.

Case 7

This 32-year-old Hispanic female presented due to peer pressure and a desire to wear her hair in current fashion (**Fig. 36.7**). She also stated that she always had extreme difficulty with sound location and hearing when in crowds or on the telephone, which her job required. Stage I was performed on May 22, 1998, with framework measuring 5.2 cm long, 3.5 cm wide, and 14.0 mm high. The lobule was transferred on July 24, 1998, and later revised on September 17, 1998, due to migration of the pedicle flap off the lower end of the thicker framework necessary in adult rib. The preoperative CT scans showed the patient to be a good candidate for atresia repair. All procedures were accomplished when the patient requested ear piercing on March 22, 2001.

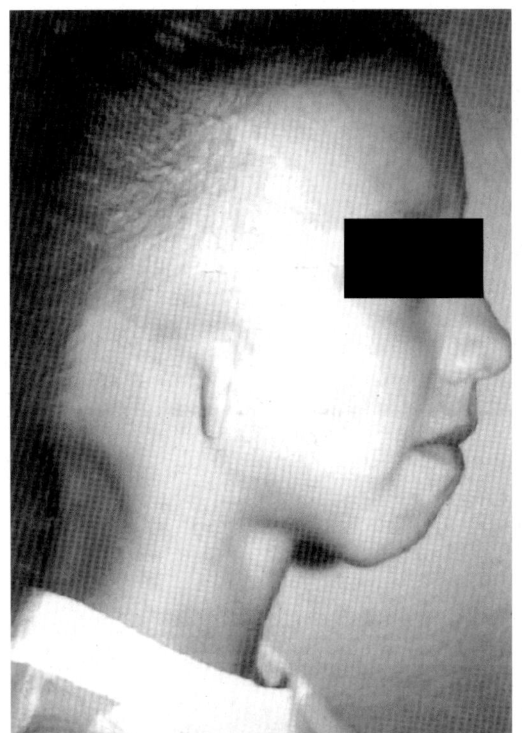

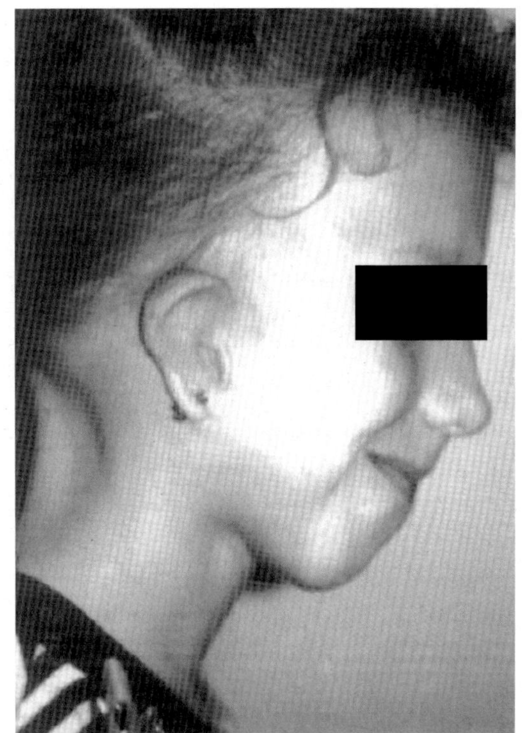

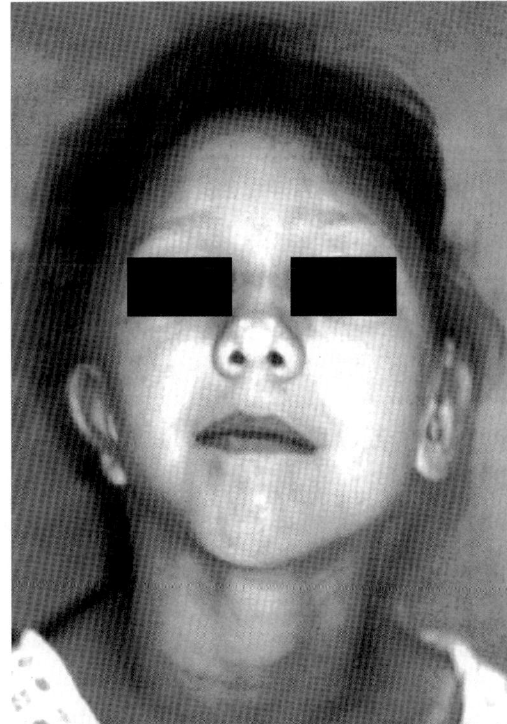

Fig. 36.3 Case 3. **(A)** Preoperative photograph of almost complete anotia of the right ear. **(B)** Postoperative view of the patient with pierced earrings. **(C)** Preoperative photograph prior to distraction surgery 3 years later.

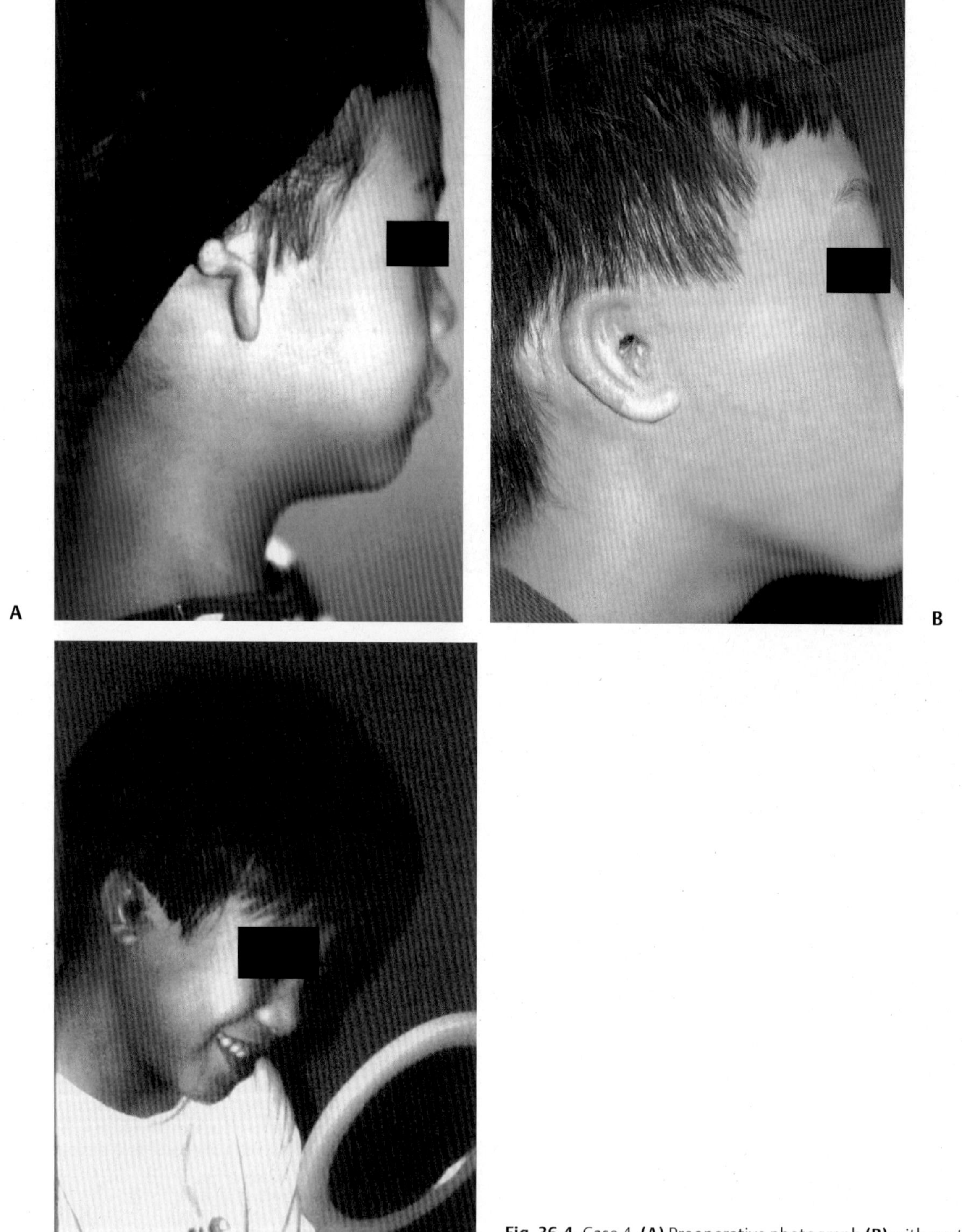

Fig. 36.4 Case 4. **(A)** Preoperative photograph **(B)** with postoperative result. **(C)** Note the delighted smile.

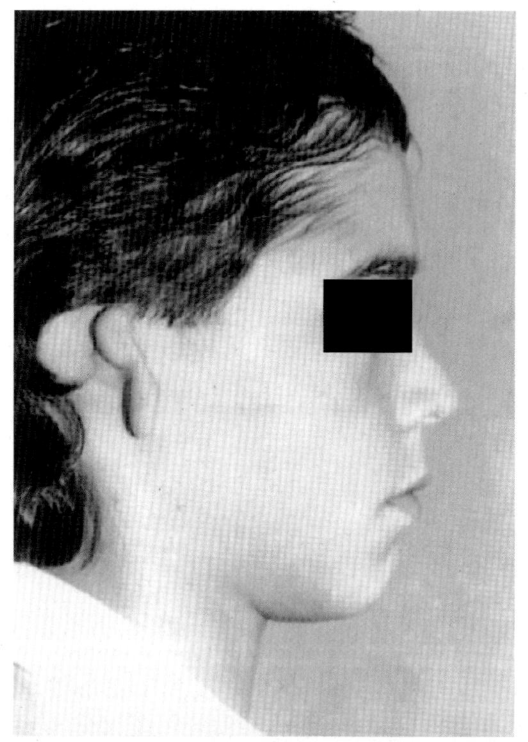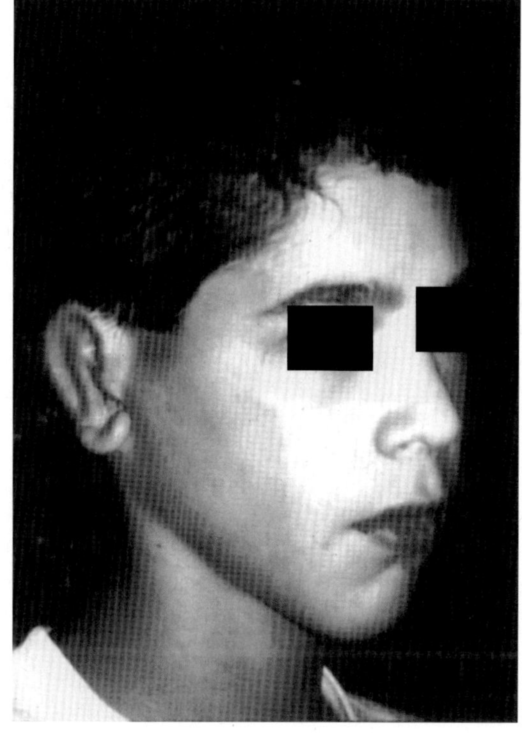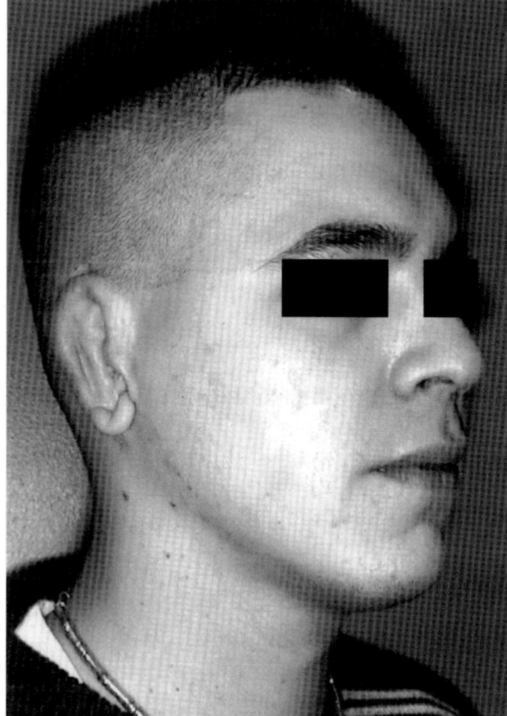

Fig. 36.5 Case 5. **(A)** Preoperative photograph **(B)** with early postoperative result. **(C)** Long-term follow-up photograph taken 10 years later.

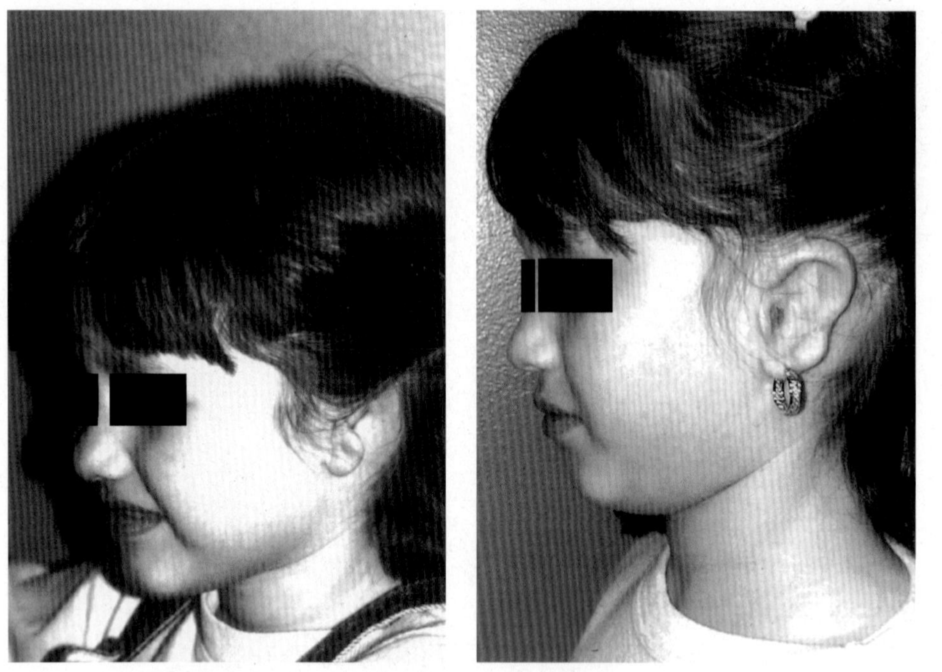

Fig. 36.6 Case 6. **(A)** Preoperative photograph **(B)** with postoperative photograph taken following ear piercing. Note deepening of the conchal bowl, although patient was not a candidate for atresia repair.

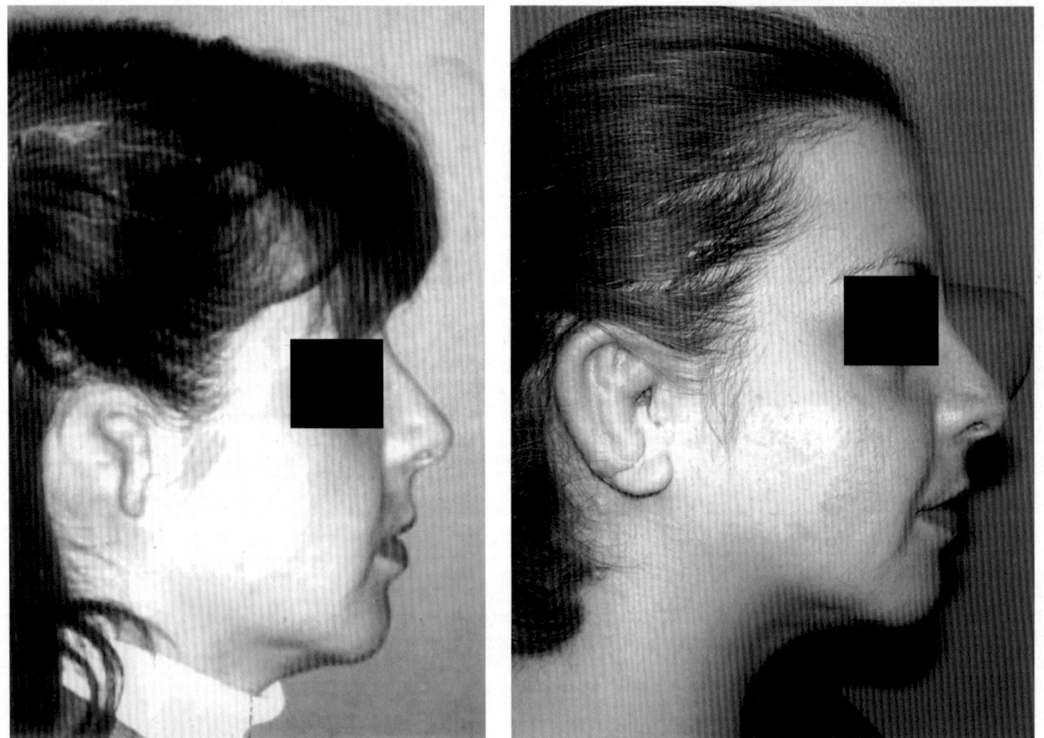

Fig. 36.7 Case 7. **(A)** Preoperative photograph of 32-year-old patient with **(B)** postoperative photograph after all stages were completed. Note the relationship of the ear canal to the framework.

Case 8

This patient, who resides in Peru, was presented when his mother came pleading for help to correct a severely deformed right ear that was previously reconstructed (**Fig. 36.8**). Multiple surgeries (12) had been performed at age 5, beginning with the implantation of a Silastic framework, resulting in infection, wound dehiscence, unsightly skin graft, and lobule malposition. The 21-year-old was brought to the operating room for removal of the Silastic implant and rib graft reconstruction. Implantation was performed on August 22, 1997, and initially went well. However, the previous insult to the skin flaps caused tissue necrosis of the helical rim skin, and the patient was returned to the operating room on September 9, 1997, for a temporoparietal graft. Healing was accomplished without loss of cartilage framework, and an elevation was performed with full-thickness skin graft on March 17, 1998. Follow-up photographs show early results.

Discussion

As these cases reveal, the process of auricular reconstruction is intricate and often involves a convoluted path to full repair. There is no simple case, and the details that a family must know are many. Patients seek reconstructive procedures of the external ear for a variety of reasons. These range from social to psychological and affect the entire family unit. These patients are seen from infancy to late adulthood. Often their childhood is filled with multiple reconstructive attempts. Sadly, this compromises their faith in surgeons as well as their hope for a decent result, not to mention the trauma to the entire auricular area. This type of surgery is not cosmetic, but instead is inherently linked to the patient's self-esteem and body image. This is a reconstructive procedure that corrects congenital deformities. Often families must battle third-party payers to cover this important reconstructive surgery. Furthermore, carriers will send patients to in-network providers who do not have the necessary skills, placing the patient at risk. The author maintains that these patients are entitled to the best arsenal available to the experienced surgeon; hence this surgery is not for the novice.

Timing

It has long been thought that institution of reconstructive efforts should begin when the patient is approximately age 6. By that time the patient will have achieved enough stature to support the cartilage graft necessary to match the size of the contralateral ear, as

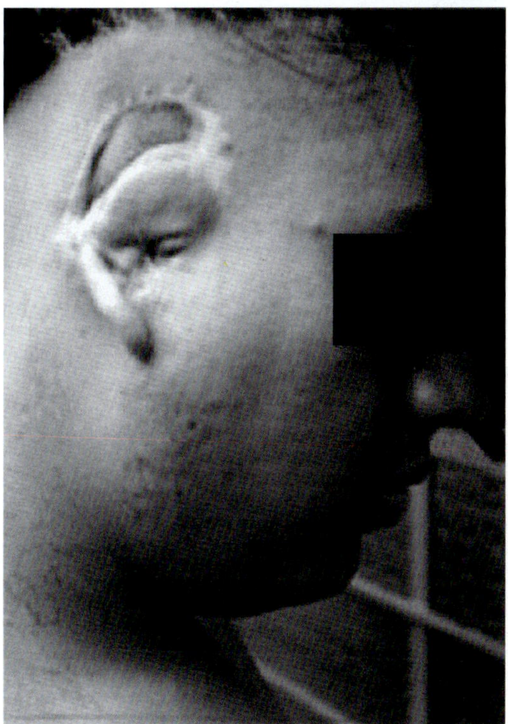
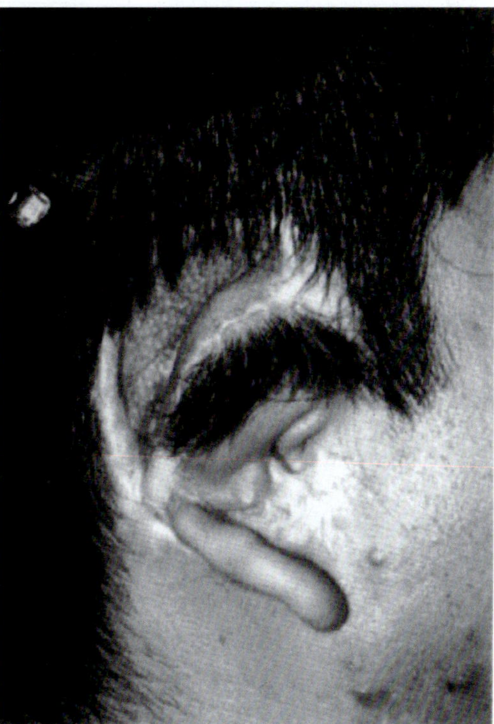

Fig. 36.8 Case 8. **(A, B)** Preoperative photographs of patient with Silastic framework.

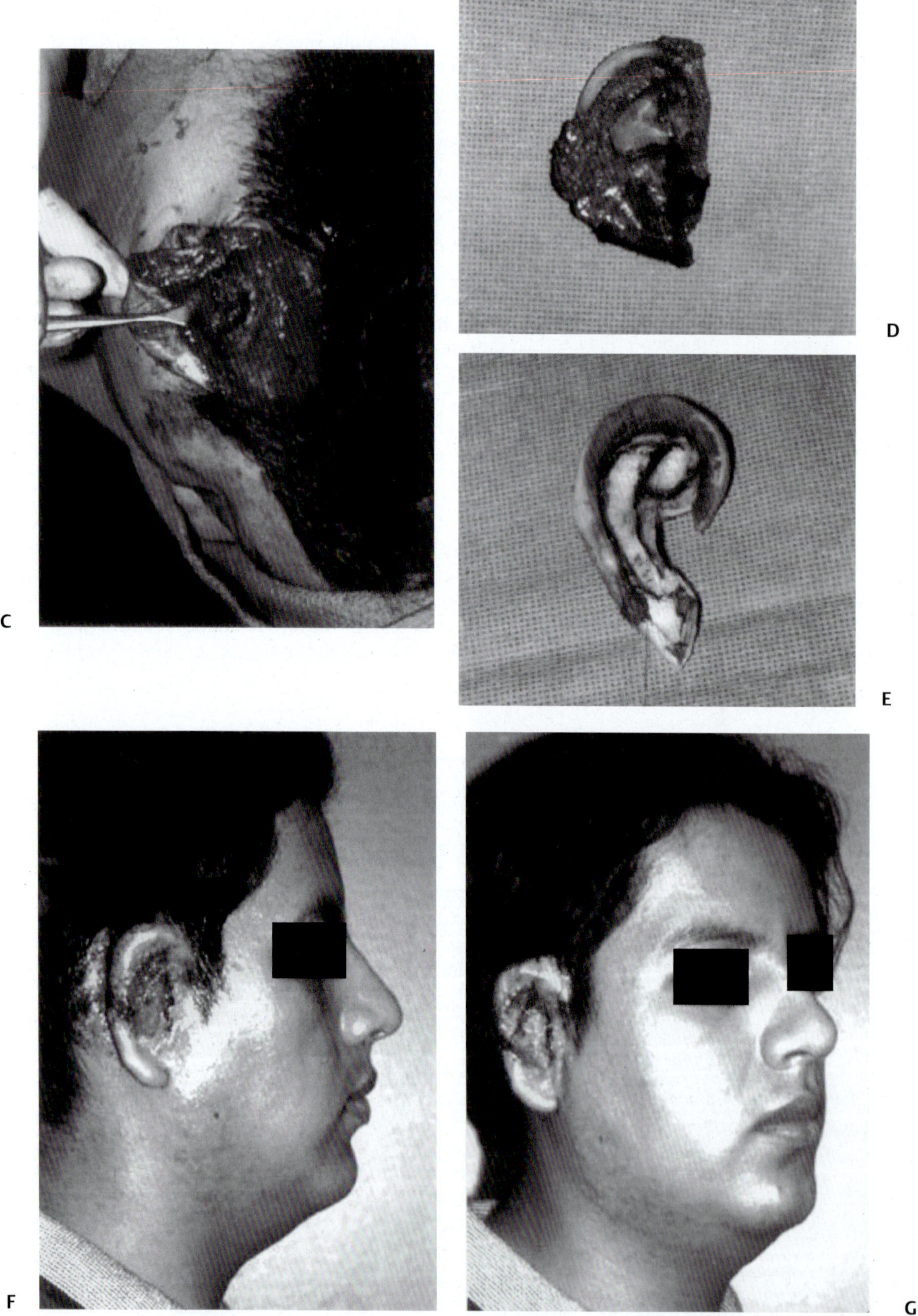

Fig. 36.8 *(Continued)* Case 8 **(C,D)** Intraoperative photographs showing exposure of Silastic implant and explantation. **(E)** Rib cartilage framework. **(F,G)** Early postoperative photographs.

well as the maturity to cooperate during the postoperative phase. This also allows the patient to benefit from total reconstruction prior to age 8, when peer pressure is more greatly internalized. However, greater experience with more predictable results has allowed for a much later attempt at successful reconstruction. The cases discussed here show that an artificial prosthesis may not be the only option in the adult or previously reconstructed patient. In bilateral cases of microtia/atresia, it remains imperative that the child be supplied with a bone-conducting hearing aid after auditory brainstem response (ABR) testing is obtained within days of birth. In unilateral cases, an ABR should be obtained within the same span of days. This can put the family and doctors at ease regarding the potential hearing of the child. The role of high-resolution CT scans of the temporal bone has no place in these neonates if the ABRs reveal normal neural pathways. These CTs are best performed at the time of planned surgical intervention by the plastic surgeon (age 5 or 6). The anatomy is, quite simply, easier to interpret. The first stage of the surgical repair should begin at age 5 in bilateral cases and at age 6 to 8 for primary unilateral cases. The framework carving best suited for this is the technique already outlined by Tanzer, Brent, and Aguilar. The use of Silastic is not advised. DellaCroce et al reported studies on the issue of cartilage growth.[4] Framework carving spares perichondrium, which allows it to receive nourishment. Cartilage growth after placement was documented. Length and width grew, paralleling the opposite ear. The placement of cartilage frameworks slightly larger than the other side or at a later age to compensate for growth was therefore not necessary.

Materials

The author believes that autogenous cartilage is still the very best material available for congenital microtia. Synthetic materials from the Silastic implant to the newer Medpor implant (Porex Surgical Products Group, Newnan, Georgia) result in an increased frequency of extrusion. Creating an external os during atresia repair becomes very problematic with these synthetic implants in place. Exposure of these implants to the bacterial milieu of an external ear canal certainly increases the risk of infection and subsequent extrusion. Studies regarding the use of Medpor do not have the benefit of long-term follow-up.[5] The author has seen two cases of extrusion of the Medpor implant that have ruined a perfectly beautiful anatomical area by leaving scar and

compromised tissue behind. The skin in the periauricular area is extremely delicate and will provide excellent contour for ear reconstructions without the need for a temporoparietal fascia (TPF) flap or Medpor implant. Park's contribution outlining use of tissue expanders is must reading by every student of auricular reconstruction.[6] He uses the capsule of the tissue expander to cover the back of the framework, and the skin covers the front of the framework. A skin graft is then done, with elevation of the ear at the same time. Park's early results appear promising. In the United States, the use of tissue expanders led to too thick of a covering for the framework, with less than optimal results. The use of a TPF flap as a first-line tool eliminates it for consideration should there be necrosis of the skin and fascia, necessitating salvage of the cartilage framework. The TPF flap should be held in reserve. The author still supports the staging of procedures at an interval of at least every 3 months. The added risk of skin loss, lobule loss, and cartilage loss makes one- or two-stage reconstructions less desirable.

Drains and Dressings

Initially, in the author's practice, one drain was placed, and a dressing was used for 5 days. When two drains were used, the amount of suction was improved, but skin ischemia seemed to be higher, and the long-term result showed no significant difference between the two methods. In this practice, we have begun to take the dressings off on post-op day 1 so that the nursing staff and family can monitor the skin. Leaving the dressing entirely off on two patients resulted in the drains being accidentally pulled out in the immediate (within hours) postoperative period. Therefore, the ear dressing is important for the 1st day. By the 2nd day, the patient is usually awake enough to avoid this embarrassing complication. Many of our patients are discharged by the 3rd or 4th postoperative day. All drains are kept in for a total of 5 days and removed in the office.

Hairline

The problem with low hairlines is well documented. We have attempted laser hair removal prior to and after stage I reconstruction. Laser removal prior to stage I has seemed to leave the skin unscarred and its blood supply unaffected. Furthermore, the compliance of the patient was better if the laser removal was performed well in advance. This may be because after the stage I is performed; children are instinctively hypersensitive to any further manipulation of the area either manually or by laser. The aesthetics are enhanced if a stage I surgery can be performed on hairless skin.

Atresia Repair

The author strongly supports the inclusion of an experienced otologist in the correction of the child with microtia/atresia. The independent surgical intervention by either the plastic surgeon or the otologist without regard for the final functional result of the patient is to be avoided. It is also this author's experience that completion of the external ear through stage V prior to atresia repair can detrimentally affect success of the tragal graft and/or the elevation procedure. Therefore, recommendation of the atresia repair as the stage III reconstruction is highly recommended.

Problem Areas

Adequate elevation remains elusive. Using the traditional four-stage approach invariably leads to an ear closely adherent to the side of the head. Authors have attempted blocks of cartilage, fascia rolls, and stents to keep the ears out. The one- or two-stage procedures seem to allow for a better separation of the ear from the side of the head, but long-term follow-up is lacking.[7] Family involvement is key from the onset of the operations. We begin answering questions and reassuring families with the initial consult. Their involvement in postoperative care can become an integral part of a good result aesthetically and can be an emotional support system for the children. We encourage hands-on involvement, sharing potential problems and allowing them to speak to other families as well. Carving a good framework is not the only important part of the reconstructive process. Other areas are just as crucial to the success of the procedures. The thickness of the auricular skin flap, for example, is crucial. When too thick, the framework may look ill defined; if too thin, it may result in necrosis and loss of a portion of the framework. The subdermal plexus is vitally important, and scissor dissection is the gentlest way to elevate the flap. Skin injury can occur by too forceful an elevation. The appearance of the flap after the placement of the framework is important. If the surgeon notices severe blanching, wider undermining may be useful. The use of nitropaste in the postoperative time has proved invaluable.

Complications

The major complications in this type of reconstruction are usually not limited to the carving of the rib framework. The complications from carving fall into two categories: insufficient strength of the sutures, leading to collapse of the structure or aberration in its shape (cracking, warping), and insufficient detail. The former is difficult to correct and may require redoing of the sutures; this will necessitate removal of the implant from the pocket. I have done this on two patients who had been operated on elsewhere and on one of my own. It is best to do this type of revision before the second stage. Insufficient detail is very hard to correct, and the only improvement can require direct excision of fibrous tissue in the sulci of the framework.

Complications of the second stage are lobule loss and malposition of the lobule. Malposition can be corrected by reoperating and resetting the lobule. Sometimes this is better achieved at the elevation, when the entire ear can be visualized easily. Lobule loss is devastating, and the only way to restore this would be to use other accepted methods of earlobe creation, such as the Gavello flap. These other methods, however, are far from satisfactory.

The fourth stage often is compromised by improper location of the tragus and loss of cartilage secondary to infection. If the cartilage dies, the only correction is to redo the procedure. Other sources of cartilage are septum and the framework itself.

The fifth stage has many potential problems. The skin graft behind the ear can die and leave exposed fascia. The ear can reattach to the postauricular area. The framework can collapse and mar a good result. The framework can be exposed, become infected, or resorb. There has been one case where the patient, age 8, kept scratching at the skin graft even after the second time it was placed. The ear was put back down, and the elevation was deferred for 3 years.

Conclusion

Auricular reconstruction remains an area of frustration, even among experienced surgeons. Searching for the perfect result, combining form with function, makes any choice difficult. Yet it is a rewarding area. Correcting mistakes requires dedication to thought and purpose. The skills of the surgeon will be taxed in this difficult reconstructive field.

References

1. Tanzer RC. Microtia: a long term follow-up of 44 reconstructed auricles. Plast Reconstr Surg 1978;61: 161–166.
2. Brent B. Technical advances in ear reconstruction with autogenous cartilage grafts: personal experiences with 1200 cases. Plast Reconstr Surg 1999;104:319–334.
3. Aguilar EF III. Auricular reconstruction of congenital microtia (grade III). Laryngoscope 1996;106(12, Pt 2, Suppl 82):1–26.
4. DellaCroce FJ, Green S, Aguilar EA III. Framework growth following microtia reconstruction: is it real and what are the implications? Plast Reconstr Surg 2001;108(6): 1479–1486.
5. Romo T III, Fozo MS, Sclafani AP. Microtia reconstruction using a porous polyethylene framework. Facial Plast Surg 2000;16(1):15–22.
6. Park C. Subfascial expansion and expanded two flap method for microtia. Plast Reconstr Surg 2000;106:1473–1487.
7. Nagata S. Modification of the stages in total reconstruction of the auricle, I: Grafting the three-dimensional costal cartilage framework for lobule-type microtia. Plast Reconstr Surg 1994;93:221–230.

Decision tree for contour scar revision surgery

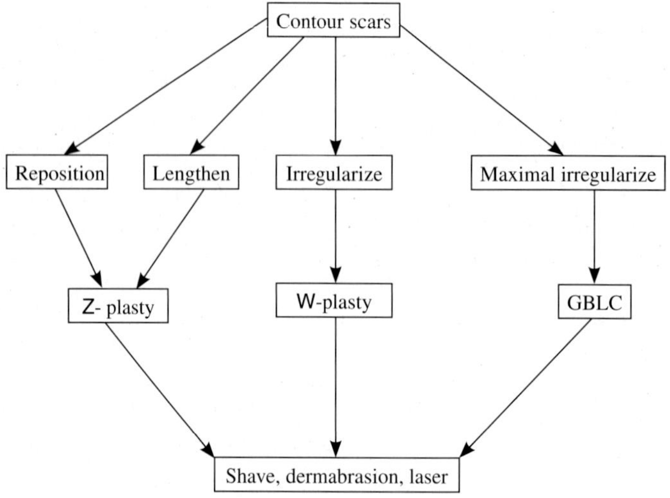

Decision tree for small scar revision surgery

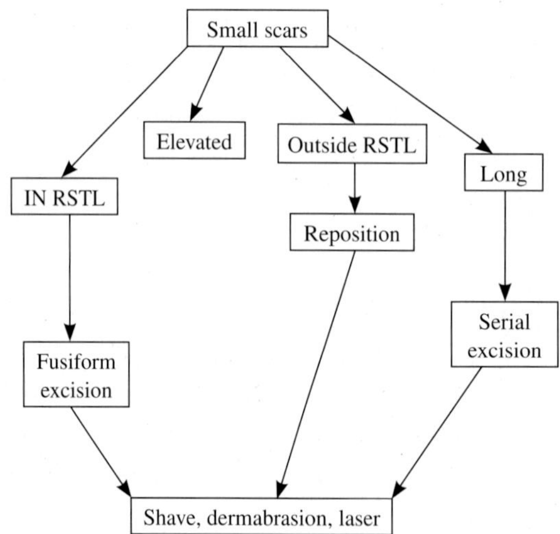

Scar Revision Surgery

J. Regan Thomas and Stephen Prendiville

A wound that is allowed to heal under favorable conditions is most likely to produce an acceptable scar. The first documentation concerning scar formation is found in the Smith papyrus (1700 bc).[1] The physicians of ancient Egypt, Greece, and India empirically appreciated the need to maintain clean wounds, minimizing wound irritation. Harsher methods such as hot cautery and boiling oil were later employed without scientific basis in Europe during the Middle Ages. The concepts of foreign body removal and sterility were largely ignored in favor of wound irritation and "laudable pus." Obviously, such techniques resulted in slower healing and a disfiguring scar. Knowledge of wound healing has since been refined to minimize characteristics that might draw attention to a scar.

The predictability of facial scarring depends partly on the etiology of injury. Causes of facial wounds include trauma, burns, elective procedures, and emergency surgery. Scars resulting from collisions or from tribal ceremonies will often contain varying amounts of debris and fibrosis. A well-planned sterile surgical incision is more likely to heal favorably than an avulsion injury sustained in a motor vehicle accident. Ideally, planned procedures should require lower rates of scar revision than traumatic injuries. However, improper tissue handling techniques, poorly designed incisions, and uneven wound edges can lead to unacceptable scars. Adverse wound-healing factors such as infection, excessive tension, presence of a foreign body, and prolonged presence of suture material may also contribute to the formation of obvious and unsightly scars.

In certain situations, unappealing scars can develop despite a surgeon's best efforts and optimal wound-healing conditions. Some individuals, particularly those of African, Hispanic, or Asian descent, are predisposed to keloid formation or hypertrophic scars. Information regarding a patient's personal healing characteristics should be sought preoperatively.

Wound healing is a dynamic process that undergoes numerous transformations before achieving a steady state. Prior to reaching its final appearance at approximately 1 year after tissue injury, a wound progresses through the phases of coagulation, inflammation, fibroplasia, and remodeling. The remodeling phase represents the stage of maturation during which intense fibroplasia, inflammation, and angiogenesis have subsided. Subsequently, a cycle of collagen deposition and lysis develops that continues in perpetuity. A scar will ultimately reach 80% of the tensile strength of normal skin.[2]

Scar Analysis

Scarring is a normal biologic reaction to tissue injury; no incision or cutaneous injury will heal without forming a scar. Therefore, the question regarding the nature of scarring after surgery does not pertain to if, but instead to what, extent. Failure on the part of the surgeon to adequately convey this fact may encourage the patient to foster unrealistic expectations. In scar revision surgery, the original scar should be carefully assessed for the amount of improvement that can be realistically obtained.

The ideal scar should be flat, narrow, level with the surrounding skin, of good color match, within or parallel to relaxed skin tension lines, and sinuous.[3] These properties make a scar less distinguishable from the expected skin contour, effectively camouflaging it. Obviously, there are limits to which a scar can be made less noticeable. With this in mind, attempts to further camouflage a scar that has met most of the above criteria are not advisable.

There are many situations in which the patient and surgeon mutually agree that the appearance of a scar can be improved. Traditionally, an arbitrary waiting period of 6 to 12 months has been proposed prior to revision, allowing for scar maturation. However, appropriate early intervention is sometimes justified. Six to 9 weeks after tissue injury, a high degree of intrinsic fibroblastic activity exists. This serves as the basis for early dermabrasion of a wound.[4]

Certain scars show signs of functional compromise and/or unacceptable appearance at an early stage and will almost definitely require later revision. Precocious intervention is warranted in such situations. Examples include scars that are perpendicular to relaxed skin tension lines or facial anatomical landmarks such as the melolabial crease.

Techniques in Scar Revision

The decision to revise a scar, the timing of this revision, and appropriate nonsurgical options should be discussed with the patient. If surgical intervention is decided upon, the manner in which it is accomplished depends on several factors: the position and orientation of the scar, its

359

relationship to important anatomical sites, the thickness and quality of surrounding skin, and the size of the scar. A description of each technique and a critical analysis of its indications, benefits, and disadvantages are included below.

Excisional Techniques

The most important concept to be considered in excisional techniques is that of scar position. An ideally placed scar does not draw undue attention from surrounding facial features. Incisions should be placed within or parallel to relaxed skin tension lines (RSTLs), within lines separating facial anatomical subunits, or within the hairline to allow for appropriate camouflage. A basic principle of surgical therapy applies: the least complex form of therapy with acceptable results is frequently the best.

Fusiform Excision

A scar that lies within an RSTL or in a similar favorable position can be managed by fusiform excision (**Fig. 37.1**). Incisions that are perpendicular to RSTLs and those requiring opposing angles of > 60 degrees are not suitable for this technique. The superficial portion of the scar is excised in a fusiform shape, with opposing angles of 30 degrees or less. It is frequently helpful to leave the deeper component of the scar intact. This firm, mature scar tissue may augment the depth of the wound and help prevent a depressed surface to the scar. Excessively long incisions, those abutting important functional structures, or requiring angles between 30 and 60 degrees can be managed with an M-plasty. The M-plasty technique can prevent unnecessary removal of tissue or scar lengthening.

Adequate undermining is often necessary to approximate wound edges in an even and tension-free manner. Subcutaneous and dermal closure is achieved using absorbable suture (usually 5–0 polygalactic acid suture), followed by cuticular closure with a monofilament suture (usually 6–0 polypropylene). The external monofilament sutures should be removed within 1 week.

Shave Excision

The cosmetic deformity caused by a scar can be simple or complex. A superficial irregularity can be tangentially shaved using a flexible razor blade or scalpel. Narrow scars with raised or uneven wound edges and small standing cutaneous deformities are suitable for this form of treatment. Shave excision can be done in conjunction with other scar revision techniques for portions of a scar. The excision should be superficial enough to level the scar with the surrounding skin, yet avoid entry into the deep

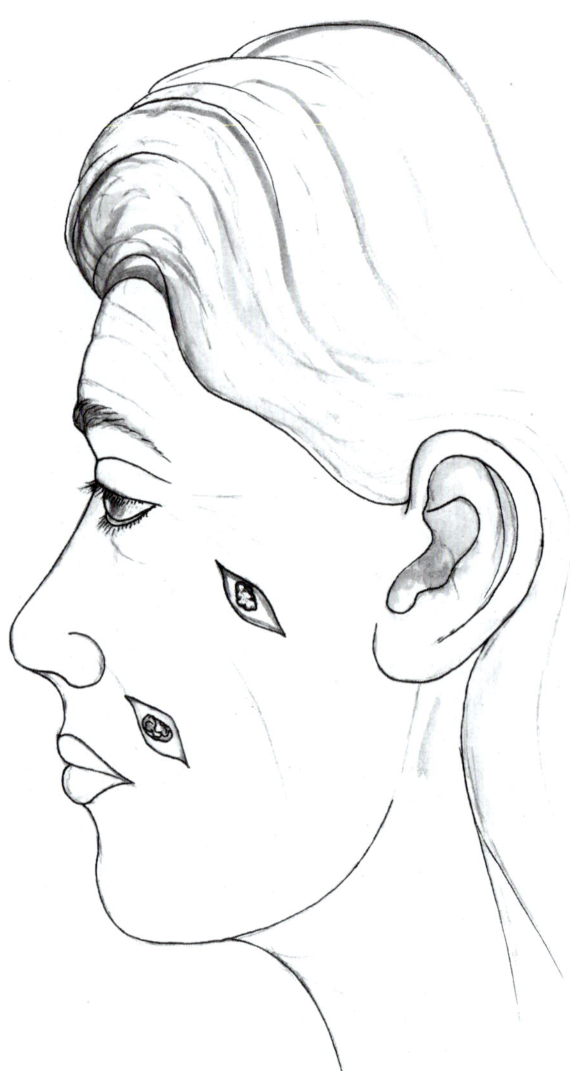

Fig. 37.1 The dynamic action of the facial musculature is responsible for the formation of relaxed skin tension lines (RSTLs). RSTLs are perpendicular to the underlying facial muscles. Placement of incisions should be within or parallel to RSTLs for optimal cosmesis in wound healing. The simplest form of scar revision involves excision of a scar in the form of an ellipse followed by primary wound closure.

dermis. After excision, the wound is allowed to heal by secondary intention.

Scar Repositioning

The appearance of a scar may be more noticeable or even objectionable due to its location. Some small scars lie close to RSTLs, important lines separating anatomical subunits, or the hairline and can be appropriately repositioned with excision of a small amount of intervening normal tissue. For example, selected scars can be repositioned into a nasolabial fold, preauricular crease, glabellar crease, or horizontal forehead rhytid.

Serial Partial Excision

Size and anatomical considerations of a scar can prevent single-stage excision and reconstruction. However, a scar can be sequentially excised using adjacent skin to be advanced into the area of deficit. The number of procedures required depends on the size of the scar, its location, and the relative elasticity of the surrounding skin. Techniques using acute and chronic tissue expansion may provide an alternative approach to serial partial excision and may at this time be preferable.

Scar Irregularization

Scars that distract attention from the normal facial contour are undesirable. Scars likely to do this include those that are long and straight, cross into an adjacent anatomical subunit, distort anatomical relationships, or have a webbed appearance. For such situations, techniques are required to break up or irregularize the line of the scar to provide greater camouflage.

Z-plasty

Z-plasty scar can be used to lengthen a contracted scar, efface a web or cleft, reposition distorted facial landmarks, or break up a long, straight scar. If irregularization alone is the goal, however, other techniques may be more useful.

Based on transposition of triangular skin flaps, Z-plasty helps to diffuse the forces acting on a scar and to diminish contractile distortion in the healing process. A primary feature of Z-plasty is scar lengthening, which varies with the angles used in designing the triangular skin flaps and with the elasticity of the surrounding skin. The classic Z-plasty technique uses three limbs equal in length (**Fig. 37.2**). The central limb represents the original line of incision or scar. The first and third limbs are parallel to each other and extend from the ends of the central limb at 60 degrees. A line drawn between the ends of the first and third limbs represents the final position of the central limb after transposition of the skin flaps. Z-plasty using angles of 60, 45, and 30 degrees will lengthen the incision by 75, 50, and 25%, respectively. Angles of < 30 degrees may lead to flap necrosis and create only minimal lengthening or effacement of the scar. Angles of > 60 degrees cause large standing cone deformities and are difficult to transpose.

In addition to lengthening or repositioning a scar, other applications of Z-plasty exist.[5] Because Z-plasty changes the direction of a scar, it can be used for functional benefits. For example, facial landmarks such as a distorted oral commissure or webbed medial canthus can be repositioned with this technique. In addition, multiple Z-plasties can improve the pincushioned appearance of a circular scar or "trapdoor" deformity.

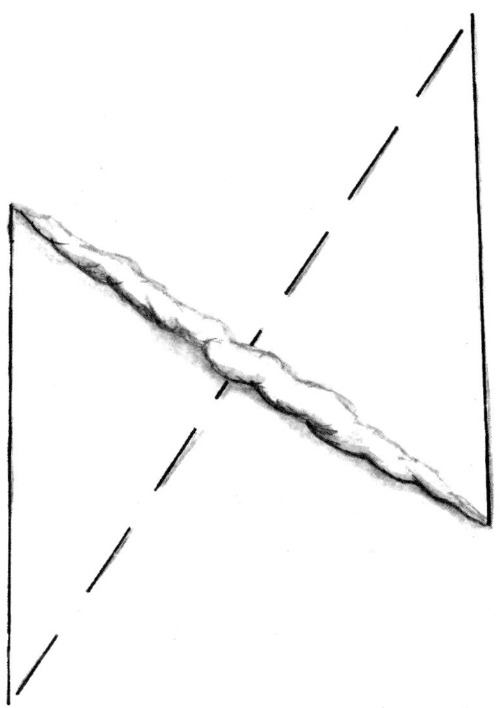

Fig. 37.2 Z-plasty uses two additional limbs designed parallel to relaxed skin tension lines and equal in length to the scar. The angle made between the scar and the limbs determines the amount of scar lengthening that will result (30-degree angle: 25% increase in wound length; 45-degree angle: 50% increase in wound length; 60-degree angle: 75% increase in wound length). A line drawn between the ends of the Z-plasty limbs represents the new position of the reoriented scar.

It is unwise to use Z-plasty in the reconstruction of keloids, due to the substantial recurrence rate and potential for further disfigurement. Measures that do not involve scar lengthening should be chosen preferentially.

W-plasty

The running W-plasty technique described by Borges uses a series of small interdigitating triangular skin flaps to irregularize a scar.[6] Several small Ws are positioned along either side of the wound such that the two lines will interpose precisely following scar excision and local undermining (**Fig. 37.3**). Because the components of a running W-plasty are interposition flaps rather than transposition flaps (as in Z-plasty), there is no lengthening of the scar.

W-plasty is ideal for long, straight scars that are perpendicular to RSTLs and traverse areas of convex curvature such as the mandibular border, cheek, and forehead. The "regularly irregular" incision pattern of W-plasty helps hide a scar, but it does not provide optimal camouflage in some scars due to its predictability. Because of the necessary excision of small amounts of normal skin, wound closure may be problematic in areas without a great deal of skin laxity. Ideally, the components of W-plasty should parallel RSTLs as much as possible. A preplanned second-stage

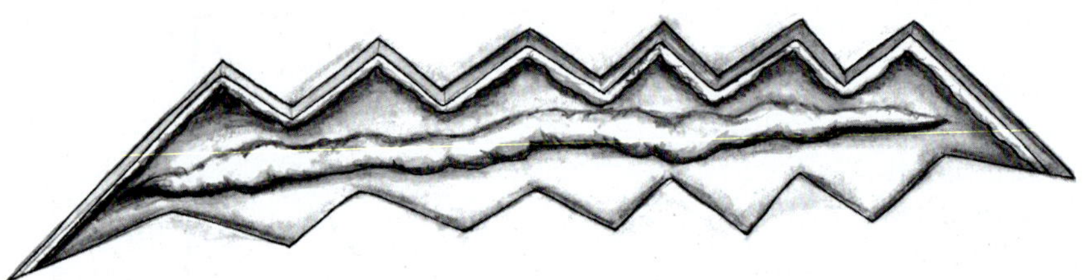

Fig. 37.3 A running W-plasty irregularizes a straight-line scar with a regular pattern of interdigitating Ws. Several small Ws are positioned along either side of the wound such that the two lines will interpose precisely following scar excision and local undermining.

dermabrasion should be part of the treatment plan and may ideally be scheduled at 6 to 8 weeks postoperatively.

Geometric Broken Line Closure

Geometric broken line closure (GBLC) is the most sophisticated of the scar irregularization techniques. Unlike Z-plasty, it camouflages a scar without scar lengthening. The "irregularly irregular" pattern is less predictable and therefore less obvious to the untrained eye than W-plasty. GBLC utilizes a series of varying geometric shapes on one aspect of the wound designed to precisely interlock with a mirror image on the other side (**Fig. 37.4**). It is ideal for long or straight scars that traverse RSTLs. As with W-plasty, a preplanned second-stage dermabrasion is performed 6 to 8 weeks postoperatively.

The geometric shapes used in GBLC should be < 5 to > 7 mm in size. If the individual shapes are < 5 mm, the components are difficult to work with, and the final scar may not have an irregularized appearance. If the figures are > 7 mm, they will be too obvious to provide adequate camouflage.

When performing GBLC, a general rule of scar revision applies: the deeper portion of the old scar should not be excised to allow for wound effacement with closure.

Both W-plasty and GBLC are closed in two layers. A 5–0 or 6–0 polygalactic acid suture is used in the dermal layer, and a running, locking 6–0 fast-absorbing gut suture (or 6–0 mild chromic) is used for the cutaneous closure. The suture line is covered with Steri-Strips, which are removed in 1 week. Residual gut suture remnants are removed, and Steri-Strips reinforce the wound for 1 to 2 more weeks.

Ablative Techniques

Certain scars can be treated with nonexcisional camouflaging techniques.

Dermabrasion

Dermabrasion is a method of controlled skin ablation useful for smoothing skin surface contour irregularities. The appearance of certain scars is made unacceptable by an irregular or uneven surface. Dermabrasion is a form of "sanding" of the skin to create a smoother, more even surface. This technique was first used in the early part of the 20th century prior to World War I.[3] Dermabrasion can be used primarily for treatment of a raised scar, or it can be used 6 to 8 weeks after scar excision as a secondary procedure.

Dermabrasion uses a motor-driven hand piece (20,000 to 30,000 rpm) with an attached diamond fraise to produce a controlled injury over a broad area. The fraises vary in quality from fine to coarse. The acceptable depth of penetration is generally the mid- or deep-papillary dermis. Preservation of the reticular dermis and adnexal structures therein is essential for reepithelialization without scarring.

The procedure can often be performed with appropriate local regional anesthesia. Intravenous sedation or general anesthesia may be used as indicated. Certain authors have advocated the use of tumescent local anesthesia to increase skin turgor and rigidity.[7,8] Refrigerant agents have been used to produce a firm anesthetized surface without distorting skin topography. The dermabrader should be held at 90 degrees to the direction of wheel rotation and should be advanced in the direction of wheel rotation. A sterile metal spoon may be used as an eye shield. Loose gauze should be kept away from the path of the wheel to prevent entanglement with the dermabrader. The periphery of the dermabraded area should be feathered to allow for a smooth transition between treated and untreated areas.

Patient selection is critical when performing elective procedures. All skin ablative procedures carry the risk of hyper- or hypopigmenation. The former is more likely to occur in olive-skinned individuals or those with a darker complexion. Systemic Accutane (13-*cis*-retinoic acid) treatment

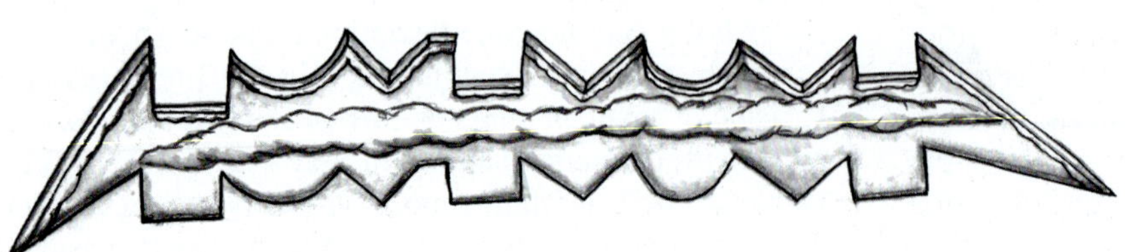

Fig. 37.4 Geometric broken line closure (GBLC) uses a regularly irregular pattern of half circles, rectangles, and triangles to irregularize a scar. The geometric shapes used in GBLC should be < 5 to > 7 mm in size.

within the preceding year is a contraindication to dermabrasion due to the potential for scarring.

If a history of past herpetic infection is elicited, antiviral therapy should be considered. A procedure on a patient with active herpetic lesions should be postponed to a later date.

Patients can be expected to reepithelialize within 5 to 7 days postoperatively. A period of erythema lasting up to 2 to 3 months is normal. The occurrence of milia in the treated areas is not uncommon. These areas can be removed with mild abrasives or with unroofing.

Dermabrasion is a very technique-dependent procedure, and results vary with experience. However, in most circumstances the likelihood of scar improvement with dermabrasion is greater than doing nothing at all.

Laser

The use of lasers in scar revision is well documented. Although not typically utilized as first-line therapy, this modality often plays an adjunctive role in scar camouflage. CO_2 laser ablation has much the same effect as dermabrasion, with response related to depth of ablation. However, in our experience, results obtained with dermabrasion are frequently superior.

The 585 nm pulsed dye laser is a newer application of laser technology in scar revision. Several clinical reports have documented success in flattening hypertrophic scars and keloids.[9,10] However, changes in pliability, erythema, and pruritis are generally more remarkable with pulsed dye laser therapy than changes in scar width.[9,10] The end point of therapy at the treatment site is the appearance of purpura. Prophylactic treatment of traumatic incisions with pulsed dye laser therapy has also been suggested to decrease the incidence of unfavorable scars.[11] Bench research on a rat model appears to support the inhibitory effect of the pulsed dye laser on the growth of implanted hypertrophic scar tissue.[12] The mechanism of action of the pulsed dye laser appears to result from selective damage to the microvasculature of scar tissue and subsequent inhibition of fibroblastic activity.[13]

When discussing pulsed dye laser therapy as a treatment option with patients, emphasis should be placed on the fact that some elements of a scar will be made less conspicuous. However, the proportions of a scar are not likely to change appreciably.

Adjunctive Techniques

Steroids

Intralesional steroid injections are frequently used to soften keloids and hypertrophic scars and to prevent recurrence. Steroids can also be used to enhance the cosmetic result of a local flap with persistent edema.

The most commonly used form of injectable steroid is triamcinolone (10 mg/mL), injected intradermally or at the dermal–subcutaneous junction. Unsightly deformity due to fat atrophy can occur if steroid is injected into the subcutaneous fat or if excessive amounts are used.

Topical steroids are best used in the subacute setting after dermabrasion or CO_2 laser of a scar. Application of steroid (hydrocortisone 2.5%) can diminish postablative erythema when applied 2 to 3 weeks after surgery.

Dressings, Topical Ointments, and Cosmetics

In the immediate postoperative period, topical antibiotic ointments help moisten surgical incisions and create a hydrophobic ointment that is less favorable to bacterial growth. Such conditions promote reepithelialization of the incision.

In general, dressings should not be relied upon to provide wound strength. They may serve as a reminder to keep the incisional area immobilized for 24 to 48 hours postoperatively. Reinforced tape strips can provide additional support at the time of primary closure or after suture removal. A newer form of surgical adhesive, Dermabond (octyl-2-cyanoacrylate), can also provide additional support to suture lines at the time of primary closure or after suture removal.[14] The efficacy of both of these modalities is diminished by petroleum-based antibiotic ointments.

Silicone sheeting has been used to help diminish pruritis, erythema, and contour irregularities in keloids and hypertrophic scars.[15] Likewise, pressure stockings have been used with moderate success to immobilize and apply pressure to scars. However, the time required to achieve results encourages noncompliance.

Application of vitamin preparations, emollients, and other topical preparations should be discouraged for the 1st week after surgery. After this point, the decision to use such preparations is left up to the patient, with the caveat that there is no proof of efficacy.

Scar massage is encouraged once epithelial healing is complete. This helps collagen fibers to realign and possibly to prevent adhesions to deeper structures.

In the early stages of healing, the patient may find cosmetics and alterations in hairstyling of benefit in camouflaging scars. This is best accomplished with the assistance of an aesthetician in the community or within the office.

Conclusion

Scar revision is indicated in certain situations for cosmetic and functional reasons. Improvement is not feasible with all scars; expectations must be tempered and realistic goals set. There is no "one size fits all" approach for the timing or technique in scar revision. Certain scars will benefit from revision at 6 to 12 months after the inciting traumatic event, others from much earlier intervention. Most scars will show degrees of improvement for up to 1 year. However, many may benefit from earlier treatment, including dermabrasion. The decision to revise a scar must be reached by both patient and surgeon, with realistic expectations and the end point clearly established. The simplest and most direct approach should then be taken to reach this goal.

References

1. Madden JW, Arem AJ. Wound healing. In: Sabiston DC, ed. Textbook of Surgery. 14th ed. Philadelphia: WB Saunders; 1991:164–175.
2. Terris DJ. Dynamics of wound healing. In: Bailey BJ, ed. Head and Neck Surgery–Otolaryngology. 2nd ed. Philadelphia: Lipincott-Raven; 1998:219–234.
3. Thomas JR, Holt GR, eds. Facial Scars: Incision, Revision, and Camouflage. St. Louis: CV Mosby; 1989.
4. Thomas JR, Hochman M. Scar camouflage. In: Bailey BJ, ed. Head and Neck Surgery–Otolaryngology. 2nd ed. Philadelphia: Lipincott-Raven; 1998:2026–2033.
5. Thomas JR, Ehlert TK. Scar revision. In: Papel ID, Nachlas NE, eds. Facial Plastic and Reconstructive Surgery. St. Louis: Mosby; 1992:45–55.
6. Borges AF. Improvement of anti-tension line scars by the "W-plastic" operation. Br J Plast Surg 1959;12:29–43.
7. Goodman G. Dermabrasion using tumescent anesthesia. J Dermatol Surg Oncol 1994;20:802–807.
8. Connell AF, Boyd JB. Dermabrasion. In: Blitzer AB, Binder WJ, Boyd JB, Carruthers A, eds. Management of Facial Lines and Wrinkles. Philadelphia: Lippincott Williams & Wilkins; 2000:55–72.
9. Alster TS. Improvement of erythematous and hypertrophic scars by the 585-nm pulsed dye laser. Ann Plast Surg 1994; 32:186–190.
10. Alster TS. Laser treatment of hypertrophic scars, keloids, and striae. Dermatol Clin 1997;15(3):419–429.
11. McCraw JB, McCraw JA, McMellin A, Bettencourt N. Prevention of unfavorable scars using early pulse dye laser treatment: a preliminary report. Ann Plast Surg 1999; 42(1):7–14.
12. Reiken SR, Wolfort SF, Berthiaume F, Compton C, Tompkins RG. Control of hypertrophic scars using selective photothermolysis. Lasers Surg Med 1997;21(1):7–12.
13. Anderson RR, Parrish JA. Microvasculature can be selectively damaged using dye lasers: a theory and experimental evidence in human skin. Lasers Surg Med 1981;1(3): 263–276.
14. Greene D, Koch RJ, Goode RL. Efficacy of octyl-2-cyanoacrylate tissue glue in blepharoplasty prospective controlled study of wound healing characteristics. Arch Facial Plast Surg 1999;1(4):292–296.
15. Katz BE. Silicone gel sheeting in scar therapy. Cutis 1995; 56:65–67.

Skin Resurfacing: Laser Revision Surgery

Dee Anna Glaser and Paul J. Carniol

Complications following ablative laser and other resurfacing procedures are relatively infrequent, but when they do occur, they need to be treated quickly and efficiently to minimize patient anxiety and long-term morbidity. Obviously, patient selection, surgical management, and postoperative care are necessary to help prevent complications, but even in the best of cases, complications do occur. In this chapter, we will try to address some of the more commonly seen complications and discuss options for their treatment. An updated approach to revision is necessary, and the surgeon must be diligent in keeping up with the latest technologies.

Pigmentary Abnormalities

Hypopigmentation

Lightening of the skin is desirable for most patients undergoing facial rejuvenation. Mottled hyperpigmentation, lentigines, and the sallow yellow tones that photodamaged skin develops are lessened or removed with the various resurfacing techniques, including carbon dioxide (CO_2) laser, erbium:yttrium aluminum garnet (Erb:YAG) laser, and other resurfacing, as well as medium and deep chemical peels and dermabrasion. Some patients will present just for treatment of lentigines and other pigmentary problems.

Patients who undergo resurfacing of cosmetic units, such as the perioral area or periocular area, may exhibit a lighter noticeable difference between the "new" treated skin and the untreated skin that exhibits the various dyschromias associated with photoaging. In these cases, treating the remaining skin will lighten the hyperpigmentation and help to blend in the differences. Although topical agents such as retinoids and hydroquinones can be used, visible results take months and are not practical for most patients.

Although nonablative technology can also yield improvements, revision resurfacing is the most efficient way to improve a patient's appearance in these cases and to blend in pigmentary alteration left by the resurfacing. Depending on the severity, a chemical peel such as a Jessner's/35% trichloroacetic acid (TCA) peel may be sufficient, or laser resurfacing can be performed. When superficial resurfacing is all that is required for blending, the Er:YAG laser is an effective device. This superficial erbium resurfacing typically has a brief associated recovery period. Postresurfacing, pinkness resolves and reepithelialization occurs in a few days to a week. The goal of this procedure is to remove the epidermis; depending on the laser, one or two passes may be all that are required. This usually heals rapidly and with minimum risks.

Other options that may be useful include the newer vascular and pigmented lasers, as well as intense pulsed light sources and fractionated lasers of varying wavelengths. These are discussed in more detail in the following sections. The goal is to improve the appearance of the skin and blend it with adjacent untreated skin.

In the very sun-damaged patient, it may be difficult to find a good stopping point, due to diffuse actinic changes. In these instances, treating the full face may only accentuate the neck's discoloration. If rejuvenation of the neck is performed, it may accentuate the chest's skin changes. With some of the more recent technology and techniques, skin can be treated in the neck and chest area, extending onto the breast, but there is a risk that this may accentuate the actinic changes of the arms and forearms. In these patients, a combination of modalities can be used: topical agents as described above for the entire area, laser resurfacing of the face, lighter resurfacing of the neck and chest (we generally use chemical agents such as 20 to 30% TCA or 70% glycolic acid, but Er:YAG laser resurfacing has been used successfully by some physicians), and chemical resurfacing of the arms, forearms, and hands with 20 to 30% TCA or 70% glycolic acid (**Fig. 38.1**). More recently a shorter wavelength fractionated laser has become available (Microspot VariLite, Iridex, Mountain View, California) that can be judiciously used to treat chest lentigines and vascular lesions. As there is a paucity of sebaceous glands and adnexal structures in the chest and neck compared with the face, any procedure, including resurfacing, should be performed cautiously to help prevent scarring.[1,2]

Another option is the use of nonablative intense pulsed light devices for a "photofacial" technique. To minimize complications, it is important to adjust the setting for each patient's skin. One system, available through Lumenis (Santa Clara, California), uses a broad spectrum intense pulsed light source with changeable crystals attached to the handpiece to filter out undesirable wavelengths. Similar devices are available from other manufacturers. This modality has been applied to the face, neck, chest, and upper

Decision tree for laser surgery complication

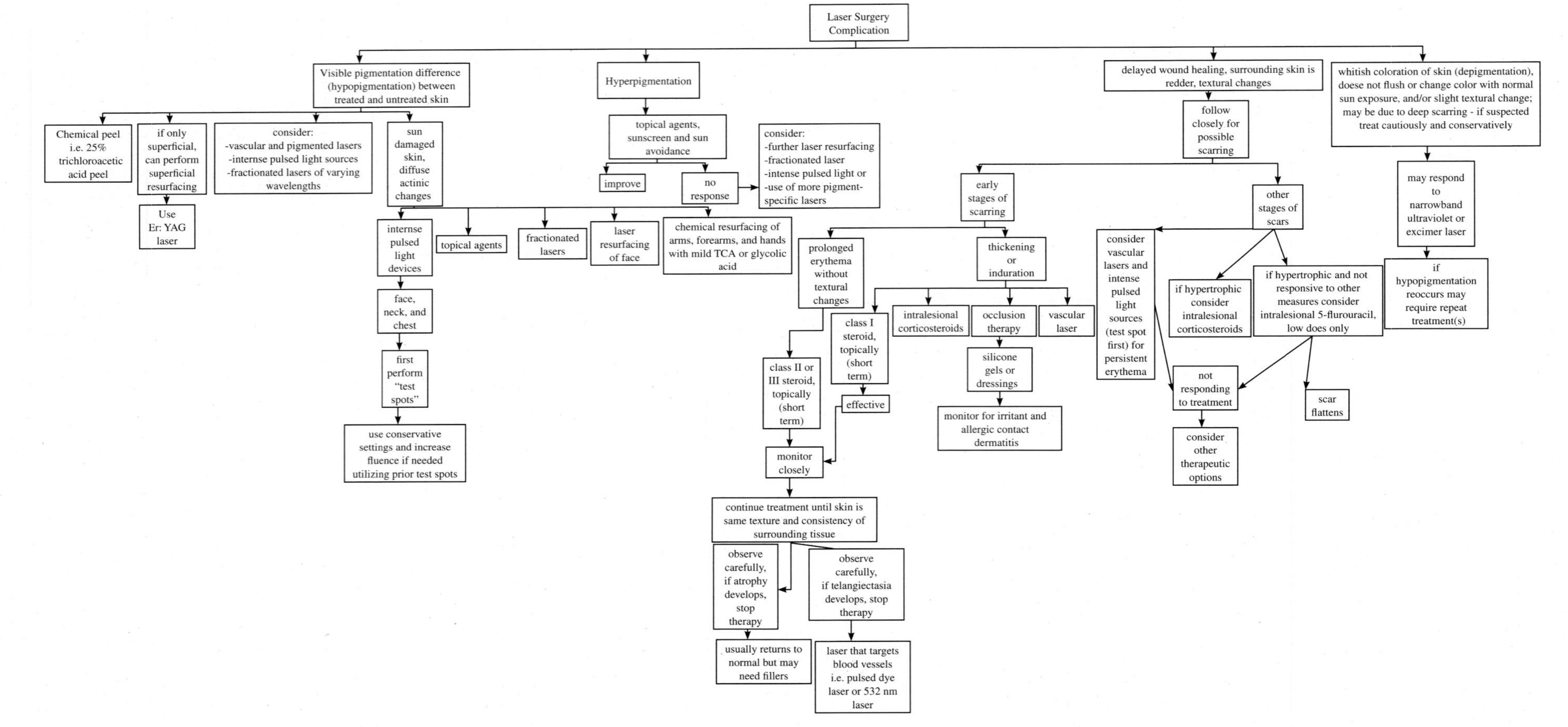

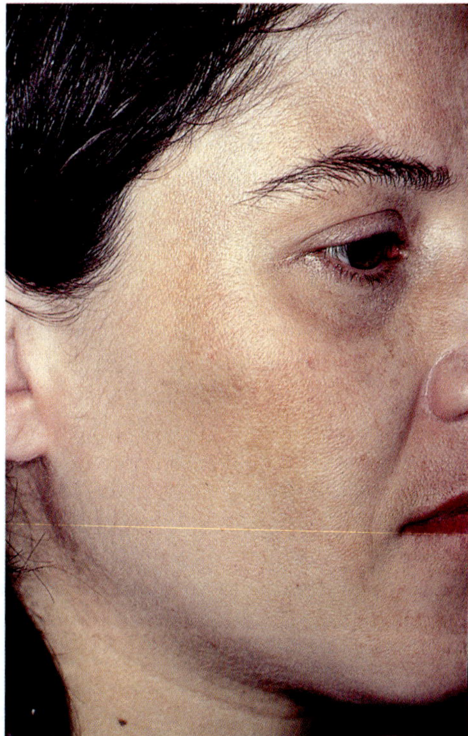
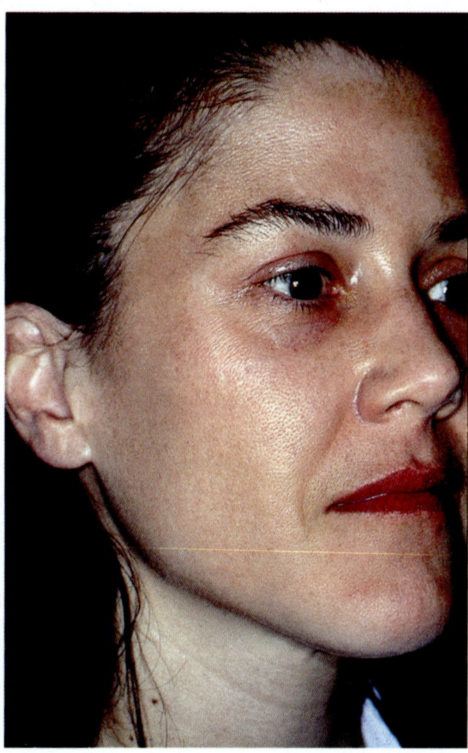

Figure 38.1 (A) A 33-year-old woman approximately 1 year after an erbium: yttrium aluminum garnet (Er:YAG) laser resurfacing of the periocular area resulting in local hypopigmentation and accentuation of her melasma and surrounding facial hyperpigmentation. She had been treated with tretinoin solution and an unknown "bleaching" agent at the time of consultation. **(B)** Nine months after the use of tretinoin cream, hydroquinone, sunblock, and monthly glycolic acid peels 50 to 70%.

extremities. Numerous treatment sessions are required but are generally well tolerated, with little to no "healing time" for the patients. The parameters used must be adjusted for each patient's skin. As described, the neck has fewer pilosebaceous units and would generally be treated more conservatively, using lower fluences. Furthermore, the lower neck has a greater tendency to scar, and if treated, an even more conservative setting should be used.

A chilled gel is applied to the area prior to treatment. This helps to protect and cool the epidermis during the treatment. It is important that the operator carefully place the filters to avoid overlapping but also to prevent skipped areas or "footprinting." These types of systems have a fairly high learning curve for the surgeon. This is particularly the case as there are different parameters that can be changed depending on the skin type, what is being treated, and individual patient variability. These devices have computer settings to assist in selecting the optimal parameters. Performing "test spots" can be useful before treating an entire area. Depending on the patient's response during successive treatment sessions, deeper wavelengths may be chosen, and fluences can be increased.

The 532 nm wavelength of the VariLite laser (Iridex, Mountain View) with a scanner can also be used to achieve a "photofacial" effect. This also requires a few treatments and the use of cooling gel. Typically for a "photofacial," a scanner coverage of 45% is used with a thin layer of protective cooling gel. Before each treatment test spots should be performed to determine the optimum settings. After treatment some patients will have mild pinkness for up to a few hours. One of us (PJC) has been pleased with the results of this technique.

Depigmentation

True depigmentation of the skin following laser resurfacing is more difficult to treat than the relative pseudohypopigmentation described above. The skin acquires a whitish coloration and does not flush or change color with normal sun exposure. A slight textural change can even be noted at times such that the patient will complain that makeup does not "stick" to the skin well or does not last as long as the makeup applied to other areas. It can occur after any form of resurfacing, but it has been our experience that it is more commonly encountered with CO_2 laser resurfacing and is less commonly seen following Er:YAG laser resurfacing. Considering the lower risk of complications and short recovery, the first author uses this laser more frequently than the resurfacing CO_2 laser.

Like pseudohypopigmentation, depigmentation seems to be more evident when cosmetic units are treated individually or when a cosmetic unit such as the upper lip is treated more aggressively than the surrounding skin.

When hypopigmented areas are evaluated histologically, there has been a varying quantity of epidermal melanin present. Typically, residual epidermal melanocytes are present, indicating that repigmentation should be possible. Mild perivascular inflammation has been noted in 50% of biopsies, and superficial dermal fibrosis was present in all biopsies.[3] This suggests that the pathogenesis of the laser-induced hypopigmentation may be related to a suppression of melanogenesis and not destruction of the melanocytes.

Grimes and colleagues have reported the successful treatment of hypopigmentation following CO_2 laser resurfacing using topical photochemotherapy twice weekly.[3] Seven patients were treated with topical 8-methoxpsoralen (0.001%) in conjunction with ultraviolet A (UVA) therapy. Moderate to excellent repigmentation was demonstrated in 71% of the patients. This pilot study suggests that phototherapy may be a viable therapy of laser-induced hypopigmentation.

Using the same reasoning, narrowband ultraviolet B (UVB) and the excimer laser may both be effective. Narrowband UVB, which emits 311 to 312 nm, has been reported to be efficacious for vitiligo and may have fewer adverse effects than topical phototherapy.[4,5] At the time of this writing, there are no published reports on narrowband ultraviolet therapy treating laser-induced hypopigmentation. The excimer laser emits 308 nm wavelength and can be targeted to a given site. Friedman and Geronemus have reported two patients who were treated for laser-induced leukoderma using the excimer laser.[6] The first patient had > 75% improvement in pigmentation and the second patient had ~50% improvement after 10 treatment sessions to her upper lip. The average cumulative UVB dose was 1750 mJ/cm², and there were no complications. The researchers speculate that repigmentation is related to the stimulation of melanocyte proliferation and migration along with the release of cytokines and inflammatory mediators in the skin. A later study by Geronemus looking at hypopigmented scars and stria found that the excimer laser was beneficial in the 31 subjects studied. Treatments were initiated at the minimal erythema dose (MED) minus 50 J/cm². Treatments were performed biweekly and eventually every 2 weeks. Hypopigmentation can recur; post-treatment and maintenance therapy may be required.

Potential disadvantages of any of these therapies include the time necessary to see repigmentation, which ranged from 13 to 38 treatments (mean 25) for the topical psoralen plus UVA (PUVA), and a mean of 19 treatments was needed by Scherschun et al to successfully repigment vitiligo.[4] Other potential problems with the use of phototherapy include costs, travel to a center for the treatments, erythema and pruritus during therapy, and hyperpigmentation of skin immediately surrounding the treated skin, which can take months to return to normal. This technology is not available in all communities. Results are mixed at this time, with only one patient achieving 100% repigmentation in Grimes et al's report, and 29% of the patients achieved only 25 to 50% repigmentation.[3] Also, loss of the pigmentation can be seen at the end of PUVA therapy as reported in two patients (29%) in Grimes et al's series who lost 25 to 50% within 6 to 8 weeks after discontinuing photochemotherapy.[3] The two patients who received the excimer laser had no loss of pigmentation at their 4-week follow-up.[6]

Repigmentation of depigmented skin following laser has been an unrealistic goal, and until more data are available on investigative tools such as phototherapy, an honest discussion must take place with the patient. Additional resurfacing of the unaffected skin may be helpful to reduce any hyperpigmentation or dyschromia if present, but it will only help to reduce the differences of adjacent areas (**Fig. 38.2**). Once again, care should be taken not to re-treat too aggressively.

Hyperpigmentation

Hyperpigmentation following the various resurfacing techniques is most common in darker skin types and frequently related to sun exposure during the postoperative period. Sun avoidance, sunscreens, and the use of bleaching agents are often employed before and after resurfacing to prevent this complication. The role of lasers to treat hyperpigmentation following laser resurfacing is quite minimal. Diligent use of topical agents such as those already mentioned and sun avoidance generally are sufficient. This may be combined with topical retinoids and mild exfoliants to provide gradual improvement. Several pigmented lasers are available, but when used in this situation, they can induce a greater inflammatory reaction and more subsequent postinflammatory hyperpigmentation. This can be especially true of persons with melasma. Further laser resurfacing or the use of more pigment-specific lasers should only be used as a last resort, in the opinion of the authors. New laser technology such as fractionated lasers may be of value, but to date, it has not been studied in this population.

Scarring

The development of scarring following laser surgery is perhaps the most feared and distressing complication encountered. Deeper wounds are more likely to result in scarring and are usually not encountered unless the wound extends

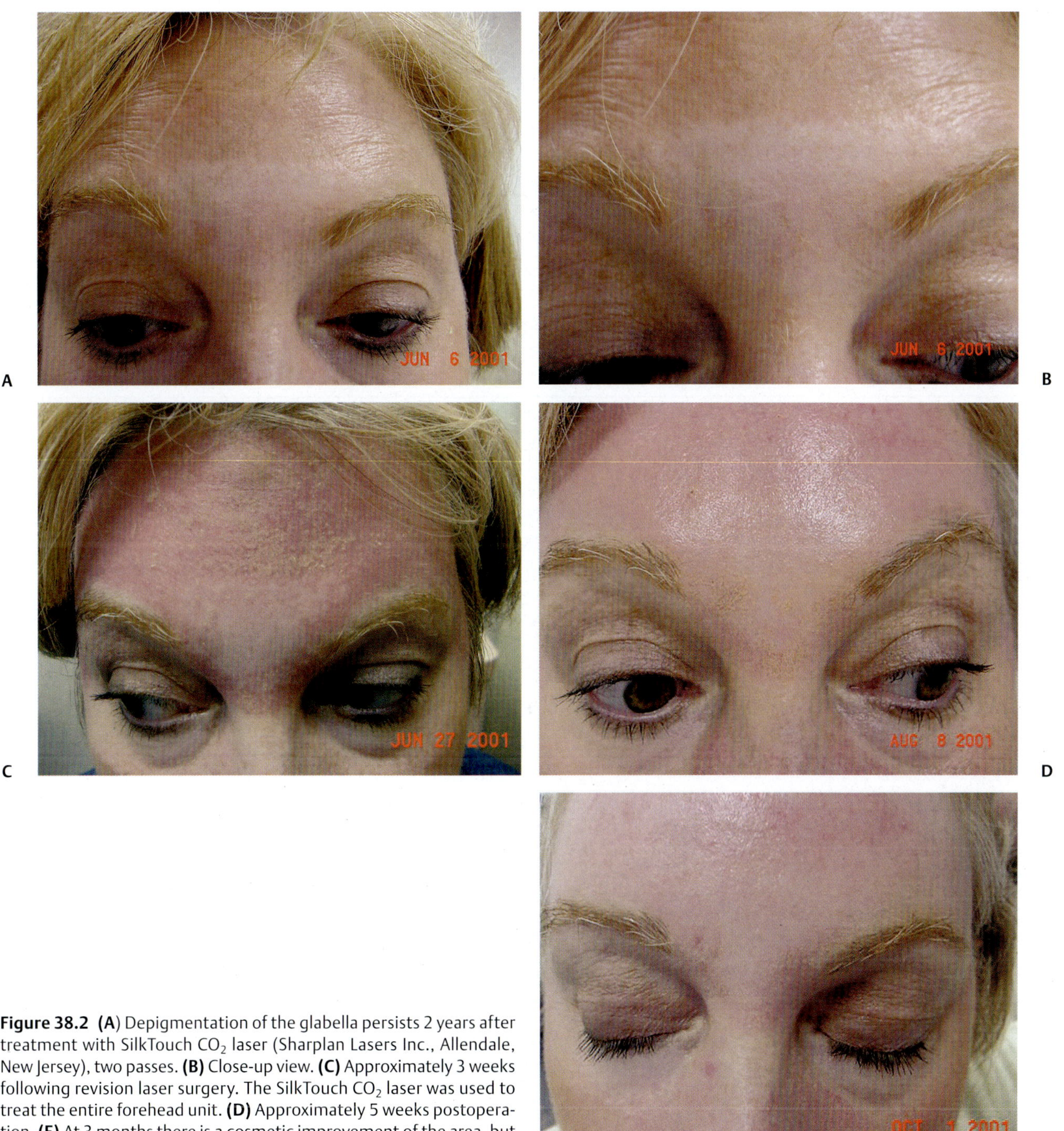

Figure 38.2 (**A**) Depigmentation of the glabella persists 2 years after treatment with SilkTouch CO_2 laser (Sharplan Lasers Inc., Allendale, New Jersey), two passes. (**B**) Close-up view. (**C**) Approximately 3 weeks following revision laser surgery. The SilkTouch CO_2 laser was used to treat the entire forehead unit. (**D**) Approximately 5 weeks postoperation. (**E**) At 3 months there is a cosmetic improvement of the area, but the patient sill notes some texture changes.

into the reticular dermis. However, because this is the level that is generally targeted with the CO_2 laser, dermabrasion, and the deeper chemical peels to eradicate wrinkles, acne scars, and varicella scars, cosmetic surgeons will be faced with scarring if they perform enough procedures. Hypertrophic scars can develop anywhere, but they are most likely to occur around the mouth, chin, and mandibular margin and less often over other bony prominences, such as the malar and forehead regions. Nonfacial skin is also more likely to develop scarring due to the relative paucity of pilosebaceous units and adnexal structures.[7,8] It has been the experience of one of us (DAG) that patients with a history of acne scarring, regardless of prior isotretinoin use, are more likely to develop delayed wound healing and hypertrophic scarring when compared with the average "photoaged" laser patient.

The surgeon should be alerted to possible scarring when there is delayed wound healing for any reason. Infections need to be treated early and aggressively. Candida, bacterial, and herpetic infections can delay healing, prolong the inflammatory stage, and increase the chance that the wound will heal with scar development. Likewise, contact dermatitis that is not controlled early and poor wound care are potential precursors for postoperative scarring. Wound care has been discussed in detail in other texts.[9]

Early on in scar formation, the skin may appear redder than the surrounding skin. As the process continues, textural changes can be discerned with palpation of the area.

As time progresses, a mature scar will develop. In the early stages, topical steroids may have a role. A medium to potent steroid should be used only in the area of concern twice daily (**Table 38.1**). If prolonged erythema alone is noted without any discernible textural changes, a class II or III steroid may suffice, but if thickening or induration is present, a class I steroid may be used. The patient's progress should be monitored closely to prevent the development of steroid-induced atrophy, stria, or telangiectasia.

Intralesional glucocorticosteroids are probably more effective than topical steroids if texture changes and induration have developed. We typically use triamcinolone

Table 38.1 Classification of Topical Steroids

Generic Name	Brand Name
Class I	
Clobetasol propionate 0.05%	Cormax cream, ointment, and tape
Augmented betamethasone dipropionate 0.05%	Diprolene lotion and ointment
Diflorasone diacetate ointment 0.05%	Psorcon cream and ointment
Clobetasol propionate 0.05%	Temovate cream and ointment
Halobetasol propionate 0.05%	Ultravate cream and ointment
Class II	
Amcinonide 0.1%	Cyclocort ointment
Augmented betamethasone dipropionate 0.05%	Diprolene AF cream
Betamethasone dipropionate 0.05%	Diprosone ointment
Diflorasone diacetate 0.05%	Florone ointment
Halcinonide 0.1%	Halog cream and ointment
Fluocinonide 0.05%	Lidex cream, ointment, and gel
Diflorasone diacetate 0.05%	Maxiflor ointment
Desoximetasone	Topicort 0.25% cream and ointment, 0.05% gel
Class III	
Triamcinolone acetonide 0.5%	Aristocort cream and ointment
Fluticasone propionate ointment 0.005%	Cutivate ointment
Amcinonide 0.1%	Cyclocort cream and lotion
Betamethasone dipropionate 0.05%	Diprosone cream
Mometasone furoate 0.1%	Elocon ointment
Diflorasone diacetate 0.05%	Florone cream
Diflorasone diacetate 0.05%	Maxiflor cream
Desoximetasone 0.05%	Topicort emollient cream
Class IV	
Mometasone furoate 0.1%	Elocone cream
Triamcinolone acetonide 0.1%	Kenalog ointment
Fluocinolone acetonide 0.025%	Synalar ointment
Flurandrenolide 0.05%	Cordran ointment
Hydrocortisone valerate 0.2%	Westcort ointment

(Continued on page 371)

Table 38.1 *(Continued)* **Classification of Topical Steroids**

Generic Name	Brand Name
Class V	
Flurandrenolide 0.05%	Cordran cream and lotion
Fluticasone propionate 0.05%	Cutivate cream
Betamethasone dipropionate 0.05%	Diprosone lotion
Triamcinolone acetonide 0.1%	Kenalog cream and lotion
Hydrocortisone butyrate 0.1%	Locoid cream
Fluocinolone acetonide 0.025%	Synalar cream
Hydrocortisone valerate 0.2%	Westcort cream
Class VI	
Aclometasone dipropionate 0.05%	Aclovate cream and ointment
Desonide 0.05%	DesOwen cream, lotion, and ointment
	Tridesilon cream
Fluocinolone acetonide 0.01%	Synalar solution

acetonide diluted to a concentration of 2.5 to 5.0 mg/mL for facial scars. A 30-gauge needle is used to minimize further trauma to the area, and the injection is given into the superficial dermis of the scarred area. The end point is a small wheal and blanching of the scar. Injections can be repeated every 4 to 6 weeks, depending on the response or progression of the scar. The concentration of the steroid can be increased to 7.5 to 10.0 mg/mL for very thick or indurated scars. Treatment should be continued until the skin returns to the same texture and consistency of the surrounding tissue. Overtreatment can result in atrophy. Hypopigmentation and/or telangiectasia can develop with glucocorticoid steroid treatment. Atrophy, if it develops, will usually return to normal without further treatment, although a dermal filler can be used in a patient who needs immediate correction of the atrophy. Should telangiectasia develop in a treated area, a laser that targets blood vessels, such as a pulsed dye laser, or a 532 nm laser can be employed. One to three treatments spaced approximately 4 weeks apart will be helpful for most.

Some surgeons will use occlusion therapy in the early stages of scarring. The number of silicone gels and dressings available has exploded over the past few years. Some are self-adhering, whereas others, such as ReJuveness (RichMark International Corp., Ballston Spa, New York), require the use of tape. They should be applied to the scar daily and worn for 12 to 24 hours per day as tolerated. We prefer the silicone gels to dressings. A mild dishwashing detergent can be used by the patient to clean the area. An onion skin extract, Mederma (Merz Pharmaceuticals, Greensboro, North Carolina), is also marketed to improve and prevent scarring. It is available as a cream and contains Cepalin. The manufacturer suggests applying the

product 3 or 4 times daily for 2 to 3 months for new scars. Patients using any of these products need to be monitored for irritant and allergic contact dermatitis.

Another option for scars following laser surgery is 5-flurouracil (5-FU).[10] This antimetabolite is a pyrimidine analogue and works by inhibiting fibroblast proliferation. A concentration of 50 mg/mL is injected into the scar, and a total dose of 2 to 100 mg is used at each injection session. Although effective, the injections are quite painful. The addition of triamcinolone should be considered and is mixed such that 0.1 mL of triamcinolone 10 mg/mL is added to 0.9 mL of the 5-FU (45 mg 5-FU). Greater efficacy and less pain are associated with the latter solution. Approximately 0.05 mL is injected per site at 1 cm intervals within the scar tissue. Injections should be performed 2 or 3 times weekly initially, and only the indurated portions of the scar should be injected. Side effects include pain with injection, purpura, and, rarely, superficial tissue slough.

Flashlamp pumped dye laser (FLPDL) therapy is effective and was first described by Alster in 1993.[11,12] The settings typically used with the 585 nm FLPDL are 5.0 to 7.5 J/cm^2 with a 7 mm spot size or 4 to 5 J/cm^2 with a 10 mm spot size. Newer vascular lasers and intense pulsed light sources are also being used to treat surgical scars. As the area is already scarred, we recommend that low but adequate fluences be used. The VariLite (Iridex, Mountain View) has a long-pulse 532 nm wavelength laser that has also been used for treatment of hypertrophic scars (PJC). The Vbeam (Candela Corp., Wayland, Massachusetts) with a wavelength of 595 nm and a cryogen spray to help cool the epidermis has also been used to treat hypertrophic scars.

Broad spectrum, intense pulsed light such as the VascuLight (Lumenis), has also been effective. As with lasers, low fluences should be initiated and can be increased with subsequent treatments as tolerated, if necessary. In general, with any of these devices, the laser/light spots should be applied in an adjacent, nonoverlapping pattern. Treatments are administered at 4- to 6-week intervals and generally will require at least two to four treatment sessions for maximum benefit. These devices are most effective with new pink scars and less effective for older, flesh-colored scars.

Patients may develop anxiety about having "more laser surgery" if they have already developed a scar from previous laser surgery, but these techniques are generally well tolerated and have minimal risks. Because of the low fluences used, purpura usually does not develop. There may be some pain with the treatment, but topical anesthesia is usually sufficient. Although well accepted as an effective treatment, not all studies have demonstrated good results using the pulsed dye laser for scars.[11] In a study by Wittenberg, the FLPDL and silicone gel sheeting showed improvement in scar blood flow, volume, and pruritus, but the results were no different than the controls.[12] Silicone gels can also be used.

Combining modalities will ensure the best results in scar volume, erythema, and texture. Laser therapy can be added to the regimen after the scar has begun to show flattening with 5-FU or steroids.[13] Thus fibroblast activity is suppressed by 5-FU, inflammation is suppressed by corticosteroids, and pulsed dye laser suppresses angiogenesis and endothelial cell growth factors.

Concomitant use of the CO_2 laser and the pulsed dye laser has been described for nonerythematous scars.[14] The CO_2 laser is used to deepithelialize the scar; total vaporization of the scar is not suggested. The 585 nm PDL is used with fluences of 6.0 to 6.5 J/cm^2 with a 7 mm spot.

Finally, resurfacing can be tried for scars that have not responded to the treatment modalities already described. This, however, can result in further scarring and should be used judiciously and more as a "last ditch effort." The patient needs to be counseled extensively on the potential risks. The scarred area and a small amount of normal-appearing skin surrounding the scar should be anesthetized with local anesthesia. Either a CO_2 or Er:YAG laser can be used, but we prefer the Er:YAG system because it provides ablation with little thermal injury. The scarred area should be ablated superficially with an additional pass to blend with the surrounding skin. Wound care is performed in the standard fashion.

Less commonly, hypertrophic scars are hyperpigmented. One author advocates the use of a pigment-specific pulsed dye 510 nm laser and a 532 nm frequency-doubled neodymium-doped (Nd):YAG laser to lighten this type of scar. According to this author, the immediate end point is the production of an ash-white color.[14]

Conclusion

Revision laser surgery should be approached with an open mind and serious consideration of the patient's needs and goals. Although lasers and light devices are excellent tools, several different modalities may need to be used for optimal improvements.

References

1. Fulton JE, Rahimi DA, Helton P, Dahlberg K. Neck rejuvenation by combining Jessner/TCA peel, dermasanding, and CO_2 laser resurfacing. Dermatol Surg 1999;25:745–750.
2. Goldman MP, Marchell M. Laser resurfacing of the neck with the combined CO_2/Er:YAG Laser. Dermatol Surg 1999;25:923–925.
3. Grimes PE, Bhawan J, Kim J, Chiu M, Lask G. Laser resurfacing-induced hypopigmentation: histologic alterations and repigmentation with topical photochemotherapy. Dermatol Surg 2001;27:515–520.
4. Scherschun L, Kim JJ, Lim HW. Narrow-band ultraviolet B is a useful and well-tolerated treatment for vitiligo. J Am Acad Dermatol 2001;44:999–1003.
5. Westerhof W, Nieuweboer-Krobotova L. Treatment of vitiligo with UV-B radiation vs topical psoralen plus UV-A. Arch Dermatol 1997;133:1525–1528.
6. Friedman PM, Geronemus RG. Use of the 308-nm excimer laser for postresurfacing leukoderma. Arch Dermatol 2001;137:824–825.
7. Fitzpatrick RE, Goldman MP. Resurfacing of photodamage of the neck using the Ultrapulse CO_2 lasers. Lasers Surg Med 1997;21:33.
8. Goldman MP, Fitzpatrick RE, Manuskiatti W. Laser resurfacing of the neck with erbium:YAG laser. Dermatol Surg 1999;25:164–167
9. Bridenstine JA. Laser resurfacing techniques and postresurfacing management. In: Carniol PJ, ed. Facial Rejuvenation. New York: Wiley-Liss; 2001;313–325.
10. Fitzpatrick RE. Treatment of inflamed hypertrophic scars using intralesional 5-FU. Dermatol Surg 1999;25:224–232.
11. Alster TS, Kurban AK, Grove G. Alteration of argon laser-induced scars by the pulsed dye laser. Lasers Surg Med 1993;13:368–373.
12. Alster TS. Improvement of erythematous and hypertrophic scars by the 585-nm flashlamp-pumped pulsed dye laser. Ann Plast Surg 1994;32:186–190.
13. Connell PG, Harland CC. Treatment of keloid scars with pulsed dye laser and intralesional steroid. J Cutan Laser Ther 2000;2:147–150.
14. Alster T. Laser treatment of hypertrophic scars and striae. In: Manual of Cutaneous Laser Techniques. Philadelphia: Lippincott Williams & Wilkins; 2000:89–107.

V
Nasal and Sinus Surgery

Decision tree for revision septal surgery

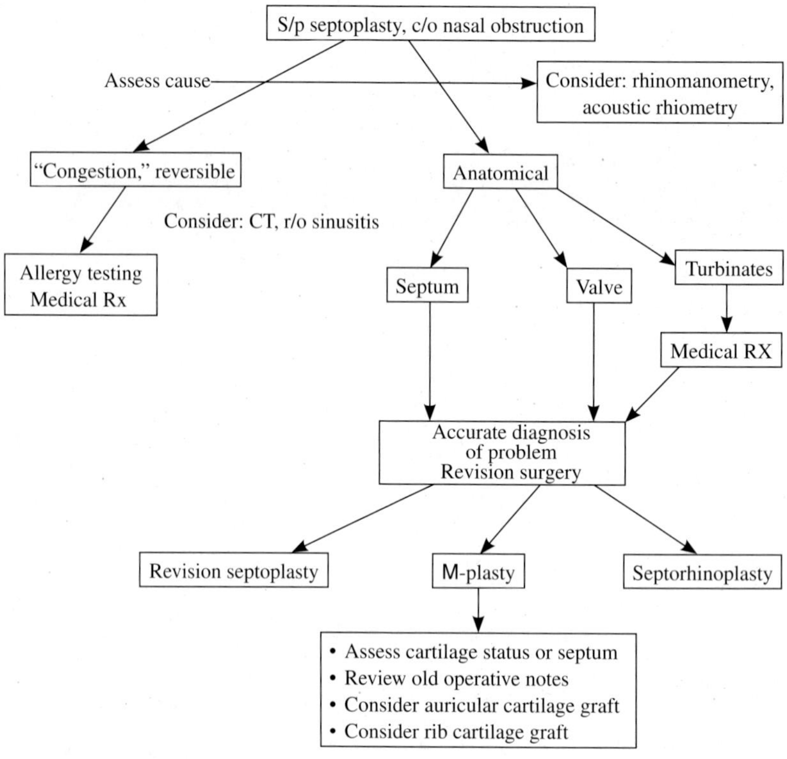

Revision Surgery of the Nasal Septum

Nissim Khabie and Eugene B. Kern

Nasal obstruction and difficulty breathing in a patient who has had a previous nasal operation present a major challenge to rhinologists. This chapter offers some suggestions regarding the diagnosis and surgical treatment of this problem. The key to successful revision surgery is to accurately diagnose the cause for surgical failure. The three categories of surgical failure are

1. Failure to properly diagnose and treat preexisting pathology of the septum (failures to correct a caudal end deformity [area 1] or valve pathology [area 2] are common findings)
2. Partial treatment of correctly diagnosed pathology
3. Sequelae, such as septal perforations, over-resection, scarring, adhesions, and atrophy, as a result of the previous operation

The goal of the surgery is to "reconstitute normality." The challenge is to decide what is normal. There are three options available to the surgeon to address this challenge, namely, by adding, removing, or repositioning septal structures as indicated by the preoperative and intraoperative evaluation and findings.

Evaluation

Ideally, an evaluation of a patient with a history of previous surgery begins with the collection of surgical records, clinical notes, and preoperative photographs. These data contain clues as to the etiology of the surgical failure. Although surgical reports are frequently incomplete and lack surgical details, information such as materials used for repair, planes of dissection used, and difficulties encountered by the previous surgeon may be gleaned from these reports. Technical difficulties may have been encountered, such as excessive bleeding, torn mucosal flaps, or intraseptal scarring, and these notes may give an indication as to the cause for the residual nasal airway obstruction.

Physical Examination

The physical examination should emphasize three critical sites: the mucosa and soft tissue, the septum, and the valve region. **Figure 39.1** demonstrates abnormalities of these three areas.

Soft Tissue and Mucosal Changes

Patient history and physical examination are the bedrock of clinical medicine and require attention to detail. Mucosal disorders such as allergic rhinitis, nasal atrophy, chronic rhinosinusitis, nasal polyposis, Wegener granulomatosis, and even hypothyroidism are commonly encountered and therefore must be properly diagnosed and treated. Most mucosal disorders are treated medically, although submucosal cauterization and radiofrequency ablation of enlarged turbinates are becoming common practices.

Nasal Septum

The septum is inspected for obstructing bends, impactions, perforations, and structural integrity. The septum must be palpated with the gloved finger and a cotton-tipped applicator to discern where tissue is missing and/or displaced. No examination is complete without topical decongestion. The prior surgeon may have overlooked spurs or impactions, especially when a cosmetic procedure was performed without sufficient intranasal examination. The caudal end of the septum, anterior nasal spine, and premaxilla may not have been corrected. Palpation of the caudal end and the external nose is important in determining tip support. The amount of cartilage and bone remaining in the intraseptal space should be determined, because this tissue is often necessary for reconstructive purposes. Nasal deformities may occur as a result of an overzealous nasal septoplasty, most notably a saddle-type deformity resulting from the failure to leave an adequate dorsal strip. Nasal tip ptosis or weakness can result from manipulations

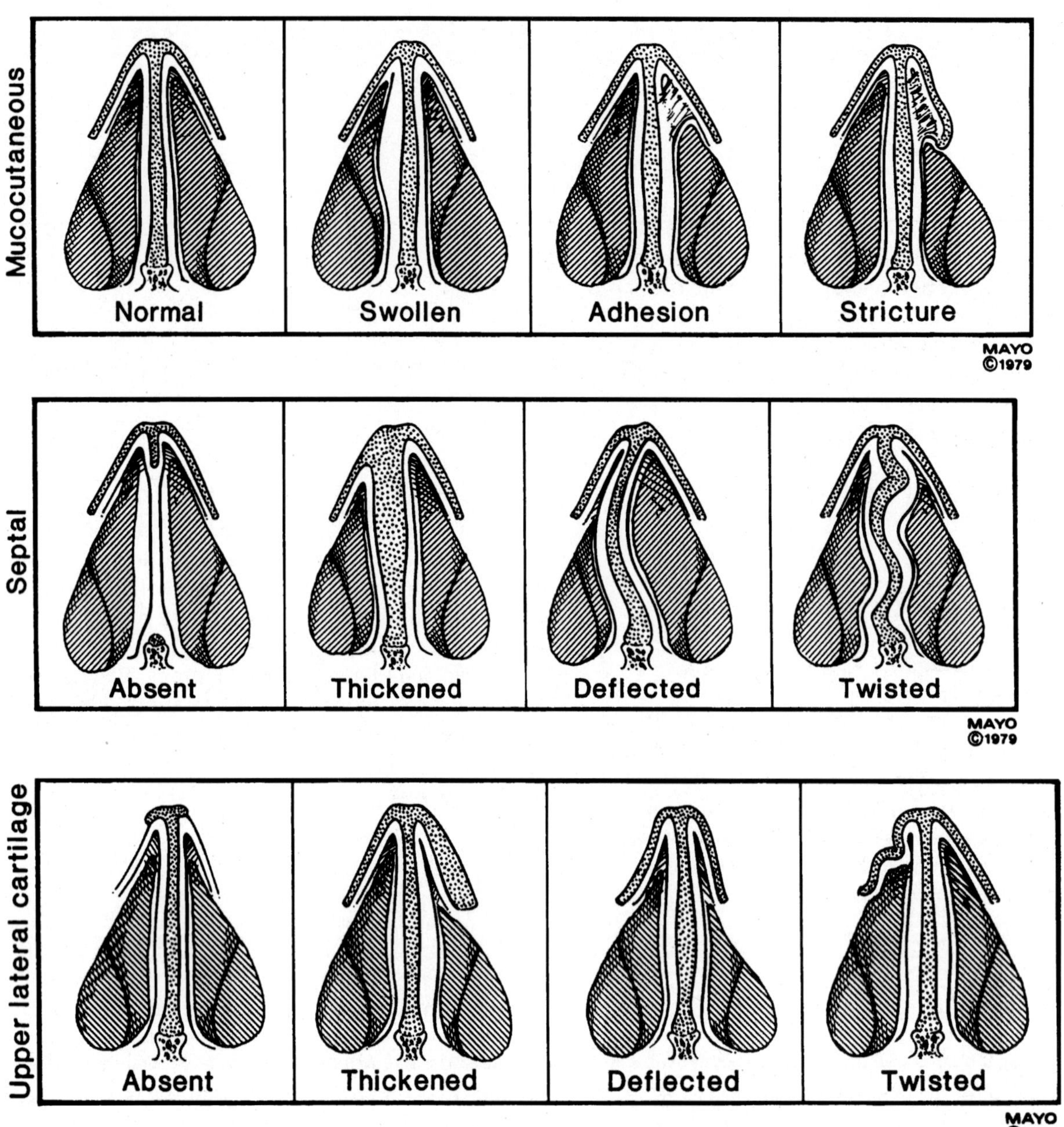

Fig. 39.1 Common abnormalities of the intranasal soft tissues (*top*), septum (*middle*), and upper lateral cartilage (*lower*) that can contribute to nasal obstruction.

of the caudal end and can result in functional and cosmetic deficits.

The Nasal Valve

Particular attention is given to the valve angle and the valve area (**Fig. 39.2**). This entire region is inspected for pathology. The examination begins without using a nasal speculum, as the tines of this instrument can obstruct important pathology in the nasal valve region. A nasal lobular elevator designed by Fausto Infante-Lopez (**Fig. 39.3**) is useful for inspection. Areas to be inspected include the septum, upper lateral cartilage, premaxillary wing, floor of the pyriform aperture, and head of the inferior turbinate. Dynamic evaluation is necessary, as collapse with inspiration may indicate a weakening of the upper lateral cartilage. A Cottle maneuver (**Fig. 39.4**) is used to determine the contribution of upper lateral collapse to nasal airway obstruction due to narrowing of the valve angle. Attention needs to be paid to both the internal and

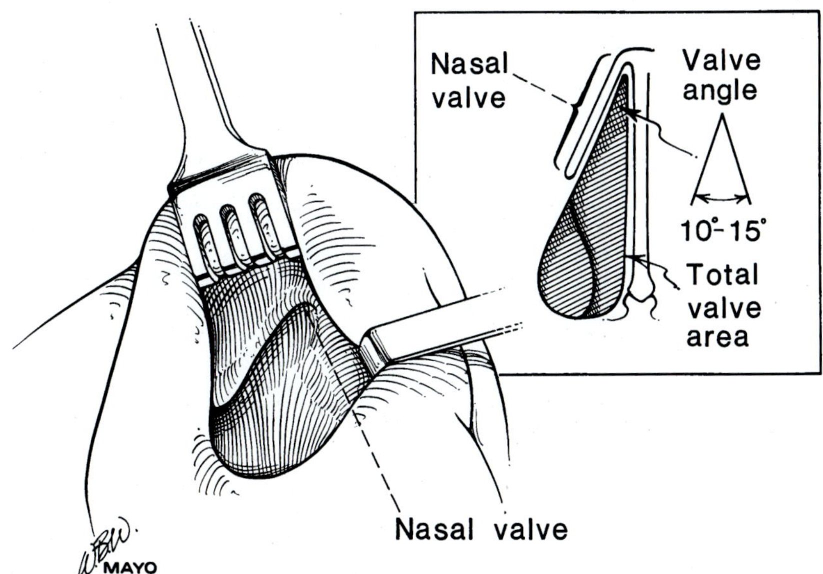

Fig. 39.2 Anatomy of the nasal valve. The junction between the caudal end of the upper lateral cartilage and the septum creates the valve angle. This angle is normally 10 to 15 degrees. The valve is best inspected by retracting the lobule without a nasal speculum. Pathology in the valve angle, septum, or head of the inferior turbinate can all contribute to valvular nasal obstruction.

external valves formed by the nasal lobule and lower lateral cartilage.

Ancillary Testing

Preoperative tests include olfaction testing, rhinomanometry, and photographs. Allergy testing, acoustic rhinometry, and computed tomography (CT) scans can also be of aid to the surgeon. Rhinomanometry provides quantitative evidence of obstruction to nasal airflow. These pressure measurements allow the surgeon to calculate nasal airway resistance before and after decongestion, which helps determine the relative contributions of mucosal versus structural abnormalities toward nasal obstruction. These data are consistent enough to provide for postoperative comparison.

CT scans are most helpful in determining concomitant sinus pathology and may also demonstrate residual skeletal, structural, and soft tissue abnormalities. Acoustic rhinometry may aid the surgeon in localizing an abnormality. We believe that photographs are necessary even for noncosmetic procedures. These serve to properly

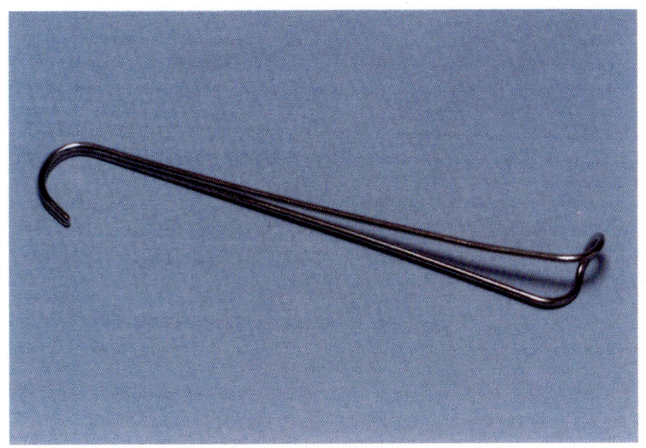

Fig. 39.3 The Fausto nasal lobule elevator.

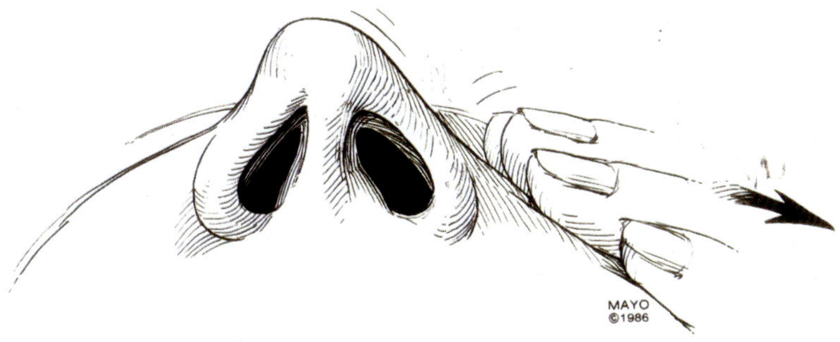

Fig. 39.4 Demonstration of the Cottle maneuver. The cheek is pulled away from the midline, which pulls the upper lateral cartilage laterally, thus opening the valve angle. The patient is asked if this reduces the nasal obstruction; an affirmative answer indicates a positive test.

document the preoperative appearance of the nose to avoid any misunderstandings or legal consequences if a previously unnoticed cosmetic defect is noted by the patient postoperatively.

Preoperative Discussion

Preoperatively, the surgeon must have a detailed discussion with the patient and his or her family regarding the goals and risks of the procedure as well as the possibility of additional surgery. The preoperative discussion is an opportunity for the surgeon to review photographs and tests, to explain the procedure, and to demonstrate the pathology by video endoscopy and CT scans. This is also an opportunity for the patient and family to ask questions. The surgeon must address the expected benefits of surgery, the chance for complete versus partial relief of symptoms, and cosmetic concerns. All of the standard risks should be discussed, including bleeding, infection, pain, and discomfort. The surgeon should explain the postoperative recovery and appointment schedule, including the timing of dressing and stent removal. Patients undergoing revision surgery should understand that a further revision is possible. The risks of septal perforation, nasal deformity, and persistent obstruction should also be discussed.

Surgical Treatment

Once a diagnosis is made, a proper preoperative evaluation has been performed, and consent is obtained from the patient, the surgery may proceed. Either general or local anesthesia may be used, based on both the surgeon's and the patient's preferences. In either case, local anesthetic agents with vasoconstrictive additives are used to provide immaculate hemostasis during the procedure. Exposure is crucial to revision surgery; therefore, bleeding must be minimized.

Elevating Flaps

In revision surgery, especially following a "submucous resection," identification of the intraseptal space can be difficult. The maxilla-premaxilla approach is an excellent means of exposure in this situation. Essentially, this approach is used to go superiorly or inferiorly on the native, undisturbed septum to find the proper plane for dissection. This approach involves a hemitransfixion incision to expose the caudal end of the septum. The proper plane of dissection is found by following the cartilage along the dorsal strut that usually remains. Often, bilateral inferior

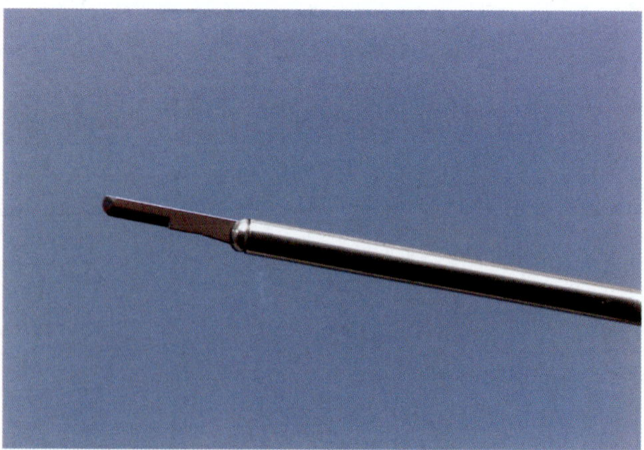

Fig. 39.5 A no. 64 Beaver blade.

tunnels, exposing the premaxilla, are helpful in continuing the dissection posteriorly. Once the proper plane is reached, dissection becomes much easier. As the dissection is performed into the previously operated site, where cartilage or bone may be missing, scarring is inevitable and ubiquitous. To avoid tearing the mucoperichondrial flap, sharp dissection is necessary. Improved visualization is obtained when the surgeon uses 2 × magnifying surgical loupes. The no. 64 Beaver blade (**Fig. 39.5**) is very useful for this dissection. This technique allows the surgeon to maintain the proper plane without excessive shearing and tearing forces on the flaps, minimizing the chance for mucosal tears.

As the proper exposure is obtained, the surgeon reassesses the nature of the pathology and the steps needed for correction. **Table 39.1** outlines the "seven sine qua nons" of septal surgery according to Cottle. As in primary septal surgery, bony and cartilaginous abnormalities are addressed, resected, repositioned, reconstructed, replaced, and fixated as required by the pathology and extent of the surgery. Several areas require special attention.

Table 39.1 Seven Sine Qua Nons of Nasal Septal Surgery According to Cottle

There are seven sine qua nons when extensive or revision nasal surgery is performed for cosmetic or breathing problems.
1. Ability to perform the maxilla-premaxilla approach
2. Continuing diagnosis
3. Ability to operate through scar, because of scar and in spite of scar
4. Ability to sew septal mucosal tears
5. Ability to move the pyramid if needed to improve the airway
6. Ability to operate on children if necessary
7. Ability to perform total nasal septal reconstruction

The Caudal End of the Septum

The caudal end of the septum may often be deflected yet completely ignored in the "classic" submucous resection (SMR) approach. A hemitransfixion incision and bilateral anterior mucosal tunnels allow for full assessment of the caudal end of the septum. Often, a conservative resection can be performed with transplantation of posterior cartilage or bone to the caudal end as necessary to treat airway obstruction and provide postoperative nasal tip support. Furthermore, it is necessary to ensure that the inferior angle of the septum remains secured to the nasal spine when it has become dislocated during surgery or "wandered off" due to scarring from the previous surgery. A 3–0 polydioxanone suture (PDS) secured in a figure-of-eight fashion between the cartilage and the prespinous fascia is helpful in maintaining the proper relationships (**Fig. 39.6**).

Septal Perforations

Septal perforations are common sequelae of the old SMR technique, with incidence ranging from 2 to 8%. The Cottle

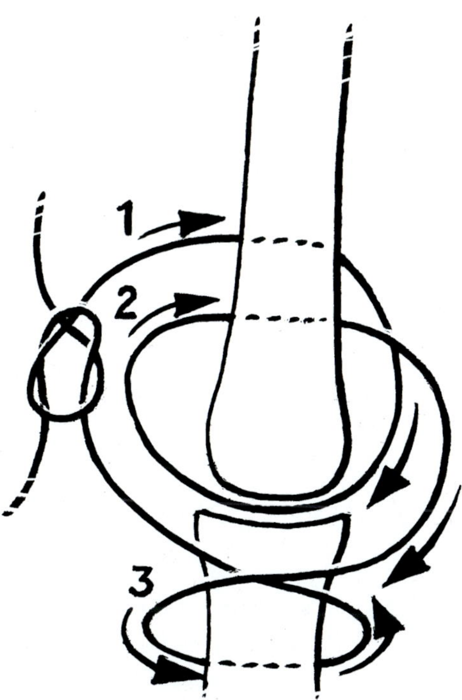

Fig. 39.6 Fixating the caudal end to the prespinous fascia using a figure-of-eight suture. A 3–0 polydioxanone (PDS) suture is passed through the inferior aspect of the caudal end of the septal cartilage from right to left, then brought under the cartilage and again passed from right to left to lock the suture. After the prespinous fascia is identified, the suture is passed from right to left through the fascia and tied on the right side, locking the septum on the maxillary crest.

technique of septal reconstruction greatly reduces this complication because mucosal tears are repaired and bone and cartilage is replaced into the intraseptal space. Patients with a perforation may experience nasal obstructive symptoms as well as crusting, bleeding, headaches, and whistling. Small (<10 mm) perforations may be closed when symptomatic by local mucosal advancement flaps and primary closure. Our preference for larger perforations is the placement of a Silastic septal button. This button can be custom made for the patient to the exact dimensions of the perforation based on CT scans. The button is placed under general or local anesthesia in the operating room or the office, depending on the size and accessibility of the perforation and whether additional septal surgery needs to be performed. One flange is sutured together to allow it to fit through the perforation. Once in place, the suture is cut, and the button should fit snugly against the septum (**Fig. 39.7**). Any excess Silastic can be trimmed.

Valve Scarring

Scarring or narrowing of the nasal valve may be a consequence of previous surgical or nonsurgical trauma and may have existed previously but was never adequately addressed. Several procedures have been designed to "open" the valve angle. One such procedure is the M-plasty. This procedure, outlined in **Fig. 39.8,** resects some of the caudal end of the upper lateral cartilages and a medial triangle of the upper lateral cartilage. This resection allows widening of the valve angle.

Other methods used to open the valve angle include the use of permanent flaring sutures in the upper lateral cartilages. These sutures are applied in a vertical mattress fashion across both upper lateral cartilages to flare them out laterally, thus opening the valve angle. Spreader grafts, placed between the septum and the upper lateral cartilages, can also be used via an open or closed rhinoplasty approach to widen the valve angle and increase dimensions of the valve area.

Harvesting Cartilage

When patients have cartilage or bone remaining in the septal space, this material can be used for reconstructive purposes. However, in revision cases, adequate tissue is often not available. Ear cartilage can be harvested for this purpose and should be discussed with the patient preoperatively. Conchal cartilage makes excellent grafting material, and its donor site leaves no significant cosmetic deformity. This is performed either through a postauricular incision or an anterior approach with the incision placed just medial to the antihelical fold. The dissection is carried down through the cartilage, and the flaps are elevated on both

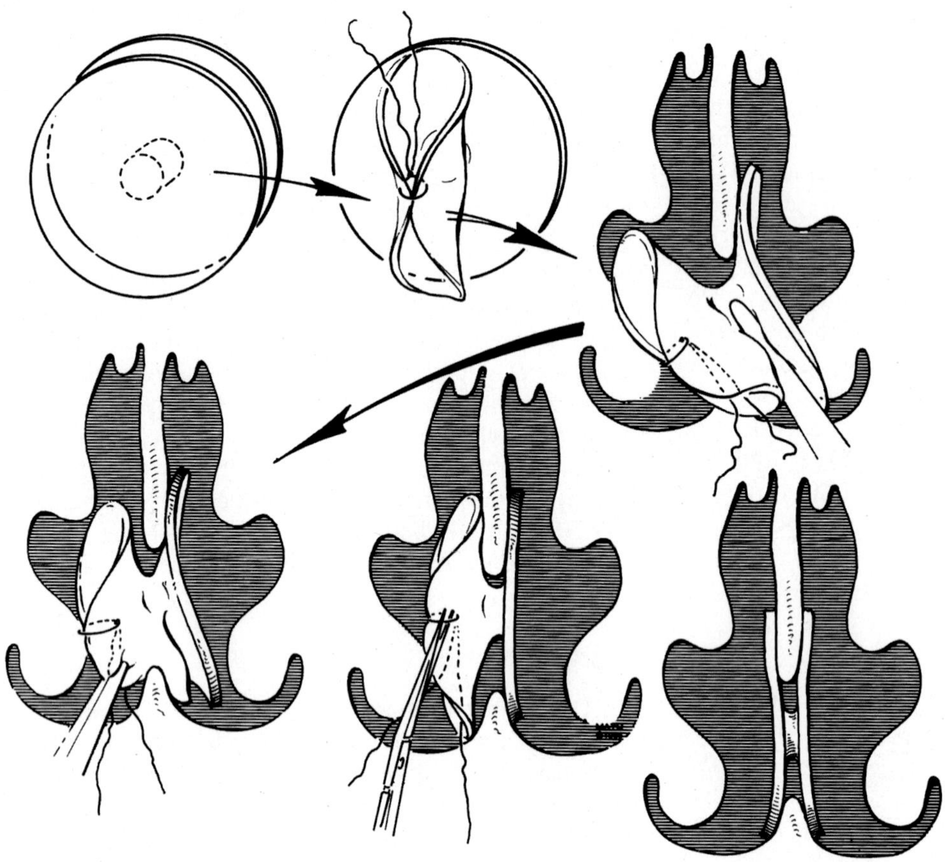

Fig. 39.7 The placement of a septal button. **(A)** The button is custom made to fit the dimensions of the perforation. **(B)** One flange is sutured together to aid placement. **(C,D)** This flange is placed into the defect and advanced into position. **(E)** The suture is cut, and **(F)** buttoned in place. Excess Silastic can be trimmed at this time.

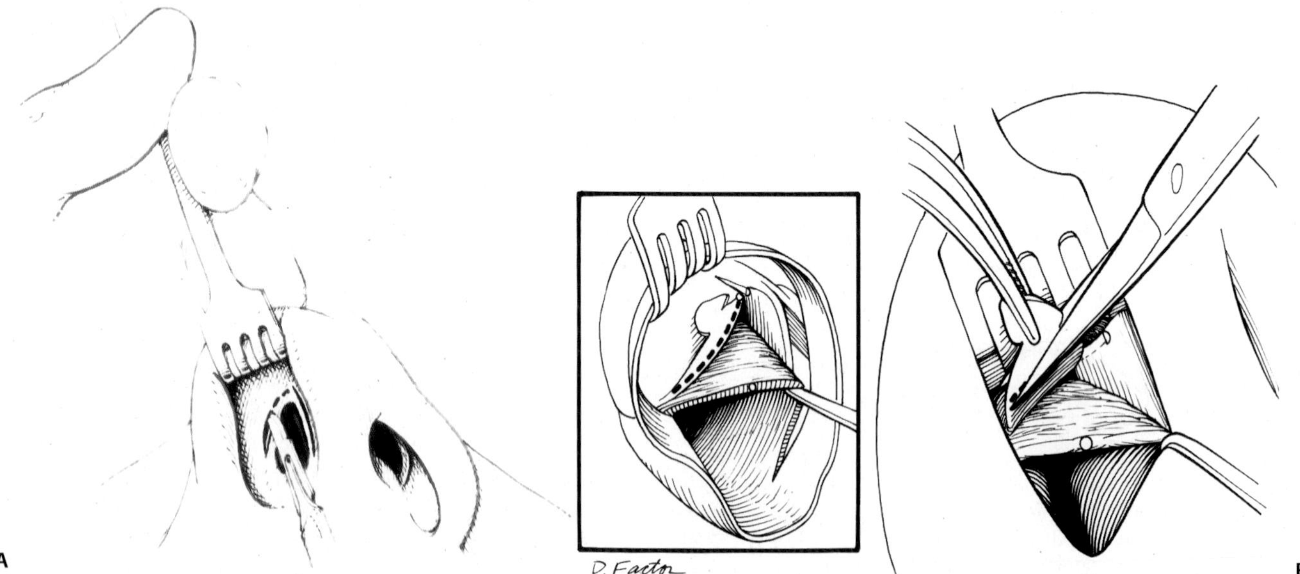

Fig. 39.8 An M-plasty to correct the nasal valve. **(A)** The upper lateral cartilage is exposed via an intercartilaginous incision that is made contiguous to the hemitransfixion incision (making a T incision). **(B)** The upper lateral is sharply separated from the septum, and a triangle, with its base directed medially, is trimmed from the cartilage.

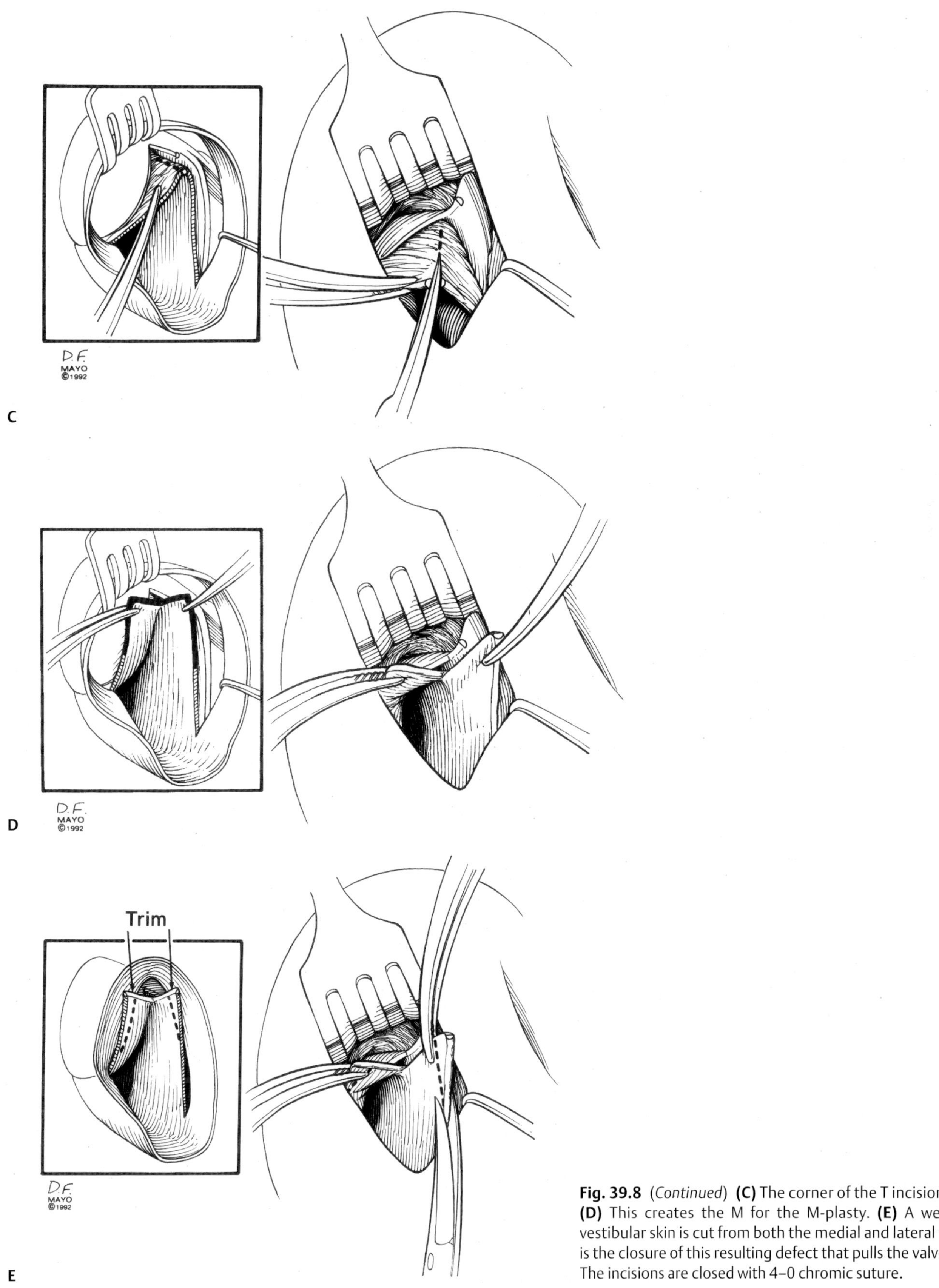

Fig. 39.8 (*Continued*) **(C)** The corner of the T incision is cut.
(D) This creates the M for the M-plasty. **(E)** A wedge of
vestibular skin is cut from both the medial and lateral flaps. It
is the closure of this resulting defect that pulls the valve open.
The incisions are closed with 4–0 chromic suture.

sides of the cartilage (**Fig. 39.9**). The entire concha cavum and cymba can be removed. Tie-over bolsters are sutured in place and removed on postoperative day 5.

For patients needing additional material or stronger support, rib cartilage is an excellent alternative. This material is stronger and less likely to warp, although morbidity is higher with significantly greater postoperative pain. Rib cartilage is especially useful for large defects, such as a saddle deformity, due to its inherent strength and the length of tissue available. This is harvested via an incision overlying the lower ribs. Dissection is performed in a subperichondrial plane to avoid damaging the pleura, freeing the rib circumferentially and harvesting as needed for reconstruction (**Fig. 39.10**).

Others have reported using exogenous or alloplastic materials for resurfacing work or for closing perforations.

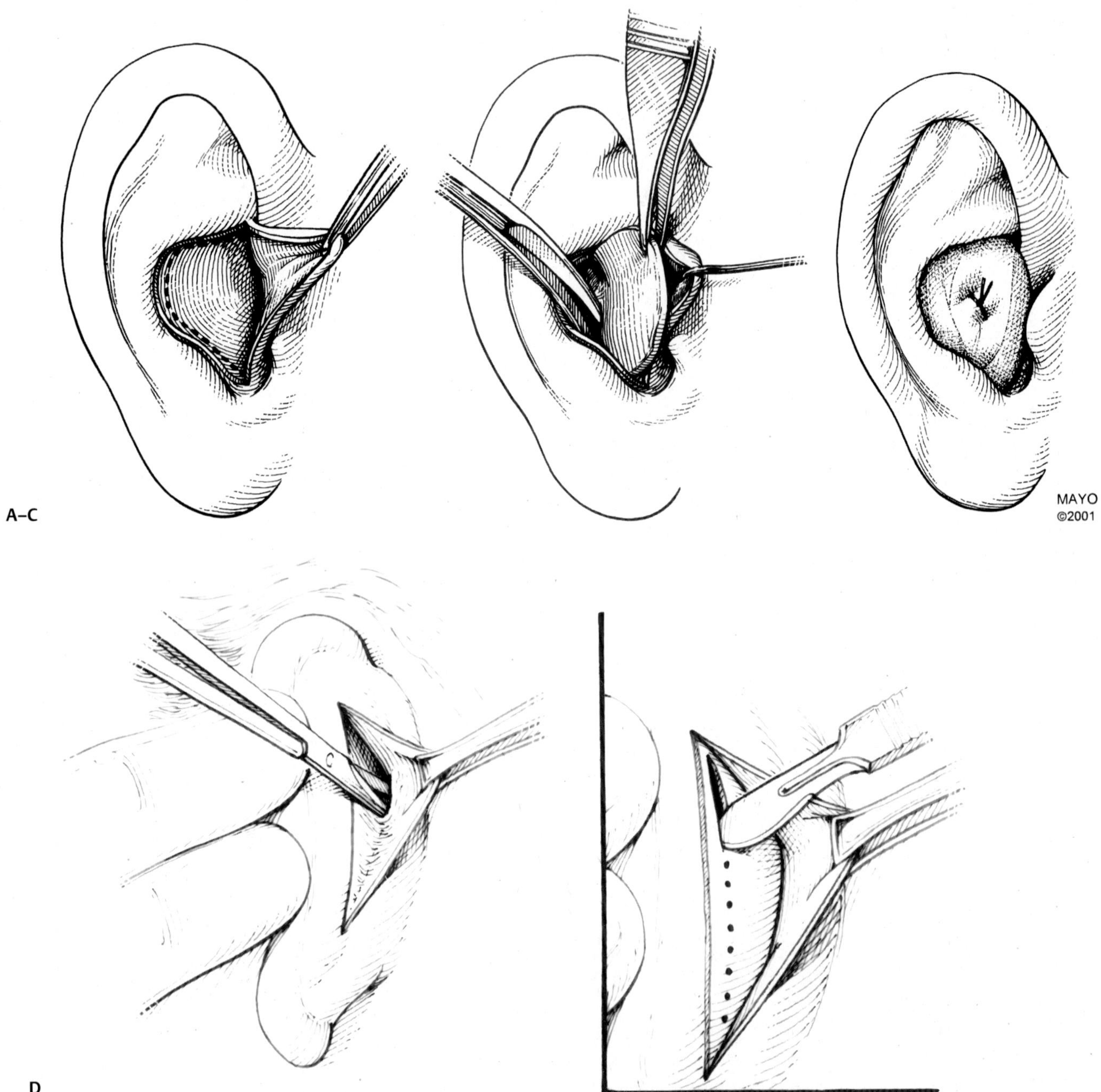

Fig. 39.9 Harvesting conchal cartilage. **(A)** An anterior conchal incision is made, and a supraperichondrial flap is raised. **(B)** The cartilage is incised and harvested. Both the concha cavum and the cymba are harvested; care is taken, however, to preserve the root of the helix and the antihelical rim. **(C)** The skin is closed in a single layer after meticulous hemostasis, and a bolster is placed to prevent hematoma formation. The bolster can be removed after 5 days. **(D)** Alternatively, the posterior approach can be used.

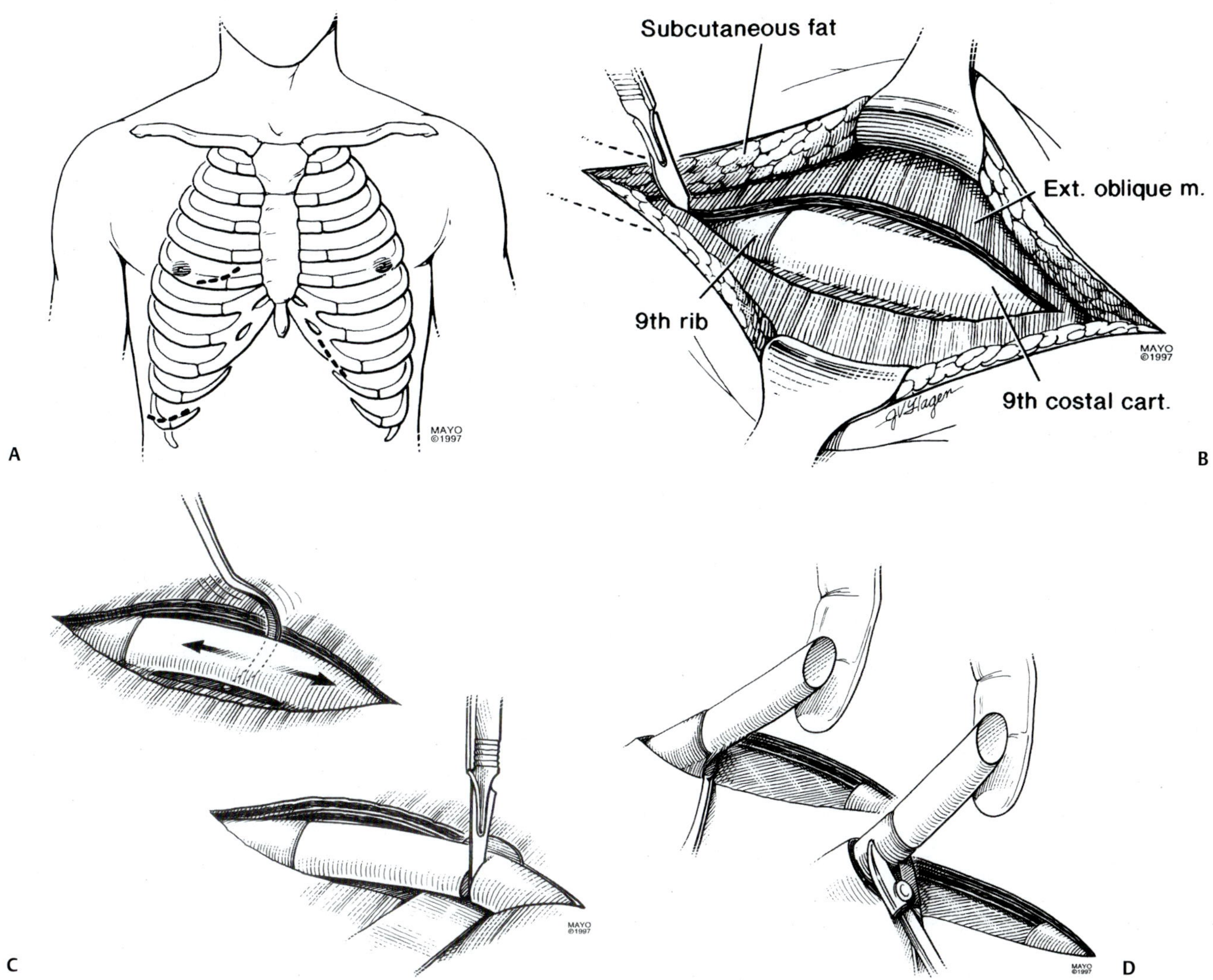

Fig. 39.10 Harvesting rib cartilage. **(A)** Common sites for incisions to harvest rib. **(B)** The muscle and subcutaneous tissues are divided. Spreading between muscle fibers, which avoids cutting the muscle, minimizes postoperative discomfort. **(C)** The cartilage is dissected in a subperichondrial plane, which avoids damaging the pleura. **(D)** The rib is harvested.

These materials present a risk of infection, resorption, or extrusion. The advantage of autogenous materials is the reduction of these risks and no extra costs. The disadvantages include donor site morbidity, lack of availability, and increased operative time.

Closure

Before closing, the intraseptal space is inspected, ensuring correct graft placement. Tears in the mucosa are sutured closed using a 4–0 chromic suture on a Castro-Viejo needle driver. Once the incisions are closed, proper intranasal dressings and stents are suggested. Various authors have advocated different types of dressings. However, the goals are the same: to help reapproximate the septal flaps, maintain proper flap and cartilage positioning, and discourage hematoma formation. Quilting sutures or internal packings achieve these goals. Stents are also used for these purposes and help discourage synechia formation. An external nasal dressing maintains proper position of the soft tissue as well as the nasal bones and cartilage and helps avoid postoperative trauma to the nose externally.

Results

The complications of revision septal surgery are essentially the same as in primary surgery. Scarring, due to misplaced incisions and tears in the mucoperichondrial flaps, can lead to further postoperative obstruction. Septal perforations can occur as well. Failure to adequately alleviate symptoms of nasal obstruction may be due to failure to diagnose its etiology. External nasal deformities can result from improper removal of cartilage and bone or from long-term resorption of either, with resultant scar tissue contracture. Use of meticulous surgical techniques in a bloodless field, adequate diagnosis and approach, and avoidance of mucosal tears will minimize these complications.

Patients should be informed of the expected recovery time. Postoperative edema can last for several weeks, and the healing process usually takes over a year to complete, during which time the nose may change its shape. Thus, patients should be encouraged to wait many months before assessing the final adequacy of surgical results, although most improvement should be noticeable early.

Conclusion

Patients needing revision surgery for nasal airway obstruction with difficulty breathing are usually a major challenge. Of critical importance is the accurate diagnosis of the cause for the persistent obstruction. The goal of the surgery is to reestablish the normal anatomical relationships to improve the nasal airway. The fundamental principles of primary septal surgery still apply, and special techniques for revision surgery have been discussed. By correctly diagnosing the problems and surgically reconstituting "normality," the surgeon can frequently alleviate the patient's significant airway symptoms.

Suggested Reading

Arbour P, Bilgen E. Understanding aerodynamics in the correction of the narrow nose. Rhinology 1986;24:41–47.

Beekhuis GJ. Nasal obstruction after rhinoplasty: etiology, and techniques for correction. Laryngoscope 1976;86:540–548.

Blomfield B. A plea for the discontinuance of the submucous resection of the septum operation. J Otolaryngol Soc Aust 1972;3:432–434.

Constantian MB, Clardy RB. the relative importance of septal and nasal valvular surgery in correcting airway obstruction in primary and secondary rhinoplasty. Plast Reconstr Surg 1996;98:38–54.

Cottle MH, Loring RM, Fischer GG, Gaynon IE. The "maxilla-premaxilla" approach to extensive nasal septum surgery. Arch Otolaryngol 1958;68:301–313.

Courtiss EH, Goldwyn RM. The effects of nasal surgery on airflow. Plast Reconstr Surg 1983;72:9–19.

Daniel RK. Rhinoplasty and rib grafts: evolving a flexible operative technique. Plast Reconstr Surg 1994;94:597–611.

Dommerby H, Rasmussen OR, Rosborg J. Long term results of septoplastic operations. ORL J Otorhinolaryngol Relat Spec 1985;47:151–157.

Goldman IB. Rhinoplastic sequelae causing nasal obstruction. Arch Otolaryngol 1966;83:151–155.

Haraldsson PO, Nordemar H, Anggard A. Long-term results after septal surgery: submucous resection versus septoplasty. ORL J Otorhinolaryngol Relat Spec 1987;49:218–222.

Johnson NE. Revision surgery of nasal septum. N Y State J Med 1971;71:2300–2302.

Kerth JD, Bytell DE. Revision in unsuccessful rhinoplasty. Otolaryngol Clin North Am 1974;7:65–74.

Lipton RJ, Kern EB. Nasal septal reconstruction. In: Pillsbury HC, Goldsmith MM, eds. Operative Challenges in Otolaryngology–Head and Neck Surgery. Part II: Nasal and Sinus Surgery. Chicago: Year Book Medical Publishers; 1990.

Mina MMF, Downar-Zapolski Z. Closure of nasal septal perforations. J Otolaryngol 1994;23:165–168.

Pirsig W, Kern EB, Verse T. Reconstruction of anterior nasal septum: back-to-back autogenous ear cartilage graft. Laryngoscope 2004;114(4):627–638.

Schonsted-Madsen U, Stoksted PE, Outzen KE. Septorhinoplastic procedures versus submucous resection of the septum, using septum perforation as an indicator. Rhinology 1989;27:63–66.

Slavit DH, Bansberg SF, Facer GW, Kern EB. Reconstruction of caudal end of septum: a case for transplantation. Arch Otolaryngol Head Neck Surg 1995;121:1091–1098.

Stucker FJ, Hoasjoe DK. Nasal reconstruction with conchal cartilage: correcting valve and lateral nasal collapse. Arch Otolaryngol Head Neck Surg 1994;120:653–658.

Sulsenti G, Palma P. Complications and sequelae of nasal base and tip surgery. Facial Plast Surg 1997;13:25–43.

Tzadik A, Gilbert SE, Sade J. Complications of submucous resections of the nasal septum. Arch Otorhinolaryngol 1988;245:74–76.

Revision Sinus Surgery of the Ethmoid Sinuses

David R. Edelstein

The effective, long-term treatment of patients with chronic rhinosinusitis represents one of the greatest challenges facing otolaryngologists. With chronic sinusitis becoming the leading chronic disease in the United States today, the issues associated with treating these patients have increased.[1] Each patient with chronic sinusitis poses a very challenging quality of life issue for the physician.[2,3] The improved effectiveness of diagnostic tools, such as rapid computed tomography (CT) scanning and endoscopic examination of the nose and paranasal sinuses, has led to more surgery. This rise in surgical volume, unfortunately, has also led to more failures, underscoring the need for doctors to understand both how to treat the long-term sinusitis sufferer and how to approach revision sinus surgery. The goal of any revision surgery should be to cure disease, to ameliorate symptoms, and to avoid complications.

The significant failure rate experienced after initial sinus surgery is attributable to several different factors. First, sinusitis is not a monolithic disease but five different diseases grouped under one name. There is an anatomical form, an infectious form, an immunologic form, a ciliary dyskinesia form, and a mucus disorder form. Some forms of sinusitis are more amenable to effective cure by surgery than others. For example, the anatomical form of sinusitis, where there may be a septal deflection blocking the middle meatus outflow tract, is generally very curable through nasal and sinus surgery. However, most patients suffer from more than one type of this disease, leading to mixed surgical results.

Second, the anatomy of the ethmoid sinuses makes them susceptible to initial surgical failures.[4] Commonly called a labyrinth, the ethmoid sinuses are divided into three major sets of cells with several subsets and adjunctive cell groups. The ethmoids are made up of the infundibular cells, the bullar cells, and the posterior cells. Most ethmoid surgery involves the anterior two sets, the infundibular and the bullar cells, which drain through the middle meatus. Endoscopic sinus surgery drains these cells best through an anterior approach. A common source of surgical failure is the inability of many sinus surgeons to identify readily the middle and posterior drainage patterns through the superior meatus. The ground lamellar, which is the attachment of the middle turbinate to the lateral wall, may impede the drainage of bullar cells into the middle meatus. Thus, attention should be paid to opening the superior meatus, the "forgotten meatus."[5] Indeed, the sphenoethmoid recess is more important to the eventual success of severe ethmoid sinusitis cases than most surgeons realize. Although an anterior endoscopic approach to the posterior cells is possible, and makes it easy to visualize these cells postoperatively, they cannot drain unless they have easy dependent drainage, which is usually not possible to achieve through an anterior approach. Haller, Onodi, agger nasi, and sinus lateralis cells may also need to be identified preoperatively and intraoperatively to achieve full ethmoid sinus drainage.

Finally, sinus surgery itself is not uniform. There are many variations in the types of sinus surgery performed depending on the physician's background, training, philosophy toward the use of technology, and his or her perspective on miniature openings for sinus ostia.[6,7] Depending on the approach taken in the initial procedure, the extent to which revision surgery may be required and its effectiveness can vary widely. For example, many patients who underwent sinus procedures before the advent of endoscopic sinus surgery had traditional inferior meatal openings, with the more natural middle meatal ostia being left untouched and blocked. Patients who underwent such Caldwell-Luc procedures without opening the middle meatus may now present with abnormal ciliary linings of the maxillary sinus due to the complete stripping of the natural respiratory mucosa, which was a common result of the older forms of maxillary surgery. Other patients may have had destructive middle turbinectomies as part of older intranasal sphenoethmoidectomies, which will reduce the effectiveness of the newer endoscopic approaches and thus limit long-term results. Some of these patients may have formed scarring or synechiae in the sinus outflow tracts, requiring wide débridements.

Those patients who had only limited first-time surgery may need completion surgery. For example, some sinus surgeons choose to operate on only one side at a time, creating a need for revision surgery on the unoperated side. Other surgeons may have been loath to enter the frontal or sphenoid sinuses, leading to problems later on in the downstream ethmoid and maxillary sinuses.

Decision tree for chronic rhinosinusitis surgical failure

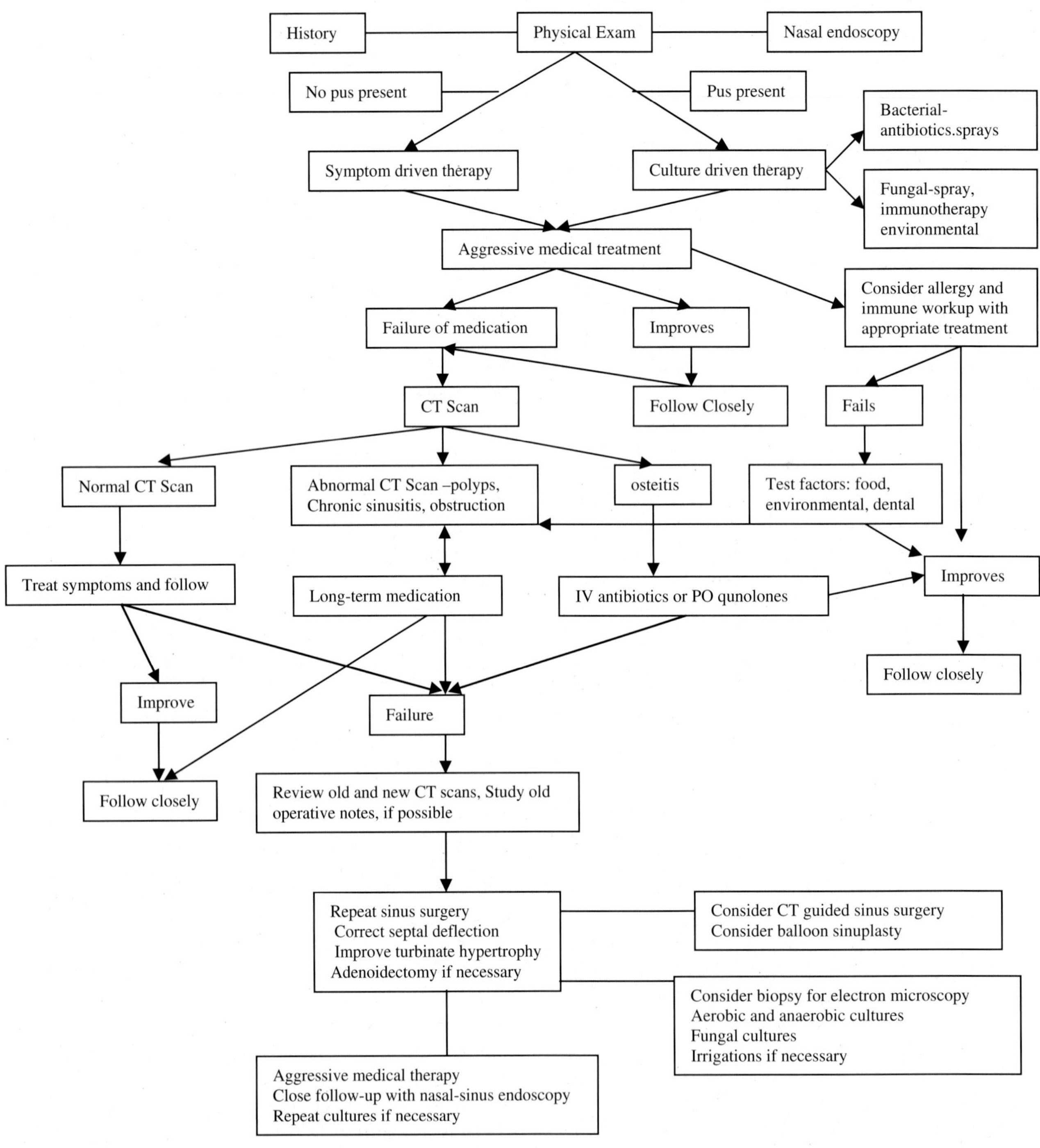

Finally, some surgeons never enter the more dangerous posterior ethmoid sinuses on the first surgery, hoping that the posterior cells will recover when the anterior ones clear. This variation in surgical approach makes evaluating the literature on failure rates somewhat difficult, given the need to understand authors' experiences, philosophies, and approaches to first-time cases.

Evaluation for Revision Cases

History

Taking a complete history is one of the most important parts of the evaluation process for any revision ethmoid sinus surgery. It is vital for the surgeon to understand the patient's history before the first procedure was performed to evaluate why the initial surgery did not succeed. The surgeon should inquire about such factors as prior medical and herbal therapies, antibiotics, sprays, allergy evaluation, and any other type of surgery. A full history may include information about, and tests of, the lower respiratory tract for asthma, pneumonia, and chronic bronchitis. This information may help point to causes of failure involving the mucosa or cilia. Allergies to aspirin and the presence of asthma can help in the diagnosis of Sampter syndrome, which has a very high recurrence rate. Prior sinus cultures may also be helpful to review. The presence of resistant staphylococcus and fungi may explain previous failure and help with postoperative planning if a second surgery is envisioned. It may be useful to ask for a computer printout from the patient's pharmacist of all medications taken over the past year or so. Many patients forget the type, dosage, and order of medications taken. It is possible that a common medication has been overlooked, which could help the patient avoid revision surgery or help improve the results of such surgery.

It is very important to review the records, including previous operative reports, of any other surgeon who has operated on the patient to have a road map of the success or failure of previous treatments. Before planning revision surgery, the conditions of areas such as the septum, middle turbinates, sinus meati, and special ethmoid cells should be carefully evaluated. Any complications to the fovea ethmoidalis or lamina papyracea as well as bleeding should be highlighted and identified. The patency of the sphenoid ostia and the frontal duct also should be investigated in the operative reports.[8] Unfortunately, operative dictations are not always complete or mention all areas of interest. Many surgeons, for example, do not note thinning of the lamina or report every breach of the orbit, even though they should.

Young sinus surgeons should be trained to spend time on their dictations and to develop a consistent style of reporting indications, findings, and surgical approaches accurately. Even if an area is not touched, for example, it should be mentioned in the operative report both to help with postoperative care and to record the fact that the surgeon thought about the possibility of unrecognized disease in that area. Every residency training program should periodically read, review, and grade the accuracy and reliability of surgical dictations to instill an understanding of the important role that accurate documentation plays in patient care (and surgical billing).

CT and MRI Evaluation

A fine-cut CT scan with 1 mm cuts is an essential element in the work-up of sinus surgical failures. The surgeon should ask for axial, coronal, and sagittal views, if available. Axial views provide an anteroposterior dimension. They can help the surgeon find the lateral wall of the posteriormost ethmoid cells and the sphenoid cells by helping to determine whether the lamina papyracea is flat or triangular in relationship to the orbital apex.[9] Coronal views help illuminate the ostiomeatal complex and the differences between the two sides. A coronal view can also help to identify higher cells on one side that may have been unopened during the first sinus surgery. This view will be essential if the frontoethmoid recess is to be opened at the time of revision surgery. Both axial and coronal views may help to identify areas of possible osteitis, particularly of the sphenoid sinus and orbital apex. Patients with suspected osteitis should be treated with either a course of long-term quinolone antibiotics or intravenous (IV) antibiotics prior to surgery.[10]

The sagittal view is underappreciated for its ability to help identify the drainage patterns of the posterior sinuses. In particular, sagittal views can aid the surgeon in determining the position of the ground lamella, which gives the insertion of the middle turbinate into the lateral wall. The superior meatus may lie anterior to the ground lamella or above it. Polyps growing from the posterior ethmoid sinuses may be appreciated blocking the superior meatus and only be identifiable on the sagittal views. To avoid complications of surgery in scarred bullar cells, it is essential to determine the position of the base of the skull and the down sloping of the middle ethmoid cells. Sagittal views also help to orient the revision sinus surgeon as to the dangerous angles and location of any infected cells at the base of the skull.

Comparing a current CT scan with a CT scan taken before the first surgery can also be helpful if the original preoperative scan is available. Such a comparison may help to differentiate between retained cells, scarring from the first surgery, and problem areas. A comparison of the two CT scans, for instance, can identify new areas of infection and areas of sinusitis inadvertently caused by the first surgery. It is essential to identify these areas to avoid making the same mistakes twice. Additionally, this comparison may highlight small but important deflections of the septum and floppy middle turbinates.

One of the classic mistakes made by inexperienced surgeons is to send a patient for a CT scan at an inopportune time. CT scanning should only be performed after maximal medical therapy, including antibiotics and topical steroid nasal sprays. The antibiotic course should be individualized from 10 days to 3 weeks, depending on the patient's problem and prior therapies. Allergy care should be included in the presence of immune or allergic disease. Another common mistake some physicians make is to have CT scans taken before the nose and sinuses have had a chance to heal completely after the initial sinus surgery. It may take more than 12 weeks for the mucosa of the sinuses to calm down. During this period, any scarring and mucosal disease should be treated by medication, such as steroids, or by office endoscopic manipulation in mini "touch-up" procedures. Performing a CT scan too soon after surgery may overemphasize recurrence and recidivism. CT scanning should be ordered by the rhinologist and not by an internist or family practitioner, who may not fully understand the timing or postoperative care issues. If possible, the same radiologist should be asked to compare the two CT scans. Earlier CT scanning should be performed only if there are any complications, such as visual disturbances or a suspected cerebrospinal fluid (CSF) leakage. Serial CT scanning is usually unnecessary, as a complete sinus procedure should provide ample exposure to the relevant sinuses by the use of rigid or flexible endoscopes.

A magnetic resonance imaging (MRI) scan has limited efficacy in identifying sinus surgery failures. Many patients with headaches are sent for MRIs, which can overstate the inflammation present in the nose and paranasal sinuses, particularly on T2-weighted images. Edematous mucosa and submucosa are hyperintense on T2-weighted images. After administration of gadolinium, the mucosa may enhance even more. Although retained secretions do not enhance on T1-weighted images after gadolinium, in chronically obstructed sinuses, the water may be absorbed and more proteinaceous, thereby appearing more intense on T1-weighted images. Patients are often told that they have recurrences following an evaluation of an MRI, when all that they truly have is viral inflammation or allergic mucosal disease.

An MRI may be helpful, however, in identifying an encephalocele or a meningoencephalocele. Orbital problems may be further highlighted through an MRI if there is possible disease in the orbital apex. Fat suppression techniques, for instance, may help the radiologist and surgeon differentiate between normal fat and an orbital abscess. An MRI may also be helpful in identifying the posterior extent of the frontal sinus, although it is of only limited use in outlining the essential ostiomeatal complex.

Finally, an MRI and MR angiogram of the sphenoid may help to differentiate mucosal disease from the carotid artery in revision cases.

Focused Examination

When examining a possible candidate for revision surgery, special attention should be paid to the nasal septum, the turbinates, the two major meati, the sphenoethmoid recess, the nasopharynx, the larynx, and the trachea. During the physical examination of the nose, measurements and angles may be taken to the base of the skull on both sides and to the face of the sphenoid. Although the use of CT-guided surgical techniques may make these measurements seem obsolete, this approach to the sinuses still helps to focus the surgeon's attention on the differences between, and problems individual to, each side of the nose. The angles required for introduction of the endoscope should be recorded to avoid anterior penetration of the skull base during surgery. Endoscopic identification of the lamina papyracea and of any related scars blocking its easy examination may help to pinpoint areas of recurrent disease and danger to the orbit. In addition, documenting the patient's gross visual acuity and extraocular movements may be helpful if there is any risk to the orbits or a prior history of diplopia or diminished visual acuity.

If the patient has been manipulated multiple times, examination with a soft, movable tip fiberoptic scope may be useful. Many revision patients have been extremely sensitized by rigid nasal endoscopes. The soft fiberoptic scope affords an adequate view into sinus recesses and the nasal cavity without touching the sensitive side walls. Children and the elderly may also benefit from this minimal touch technique. In addition, one may mobilize the end of a flexible scope around a small synechiae at the front of the middle turbinate. So long as there is normal sinus outflow identifiable by other means, revision cases do not have to be performed just to allow the introduction of a rigid scope.

Role of Cultures

Often, the surgeon is faced with recurrent drainage from the ethmoid sinuses that may be due to resistant bacteria. In such cases, early identification of an organism may reduce the need for revision surgery. Microculture techniques under endoscopic control can help avoid touching the nose before entering the sinuses through the middle meatus. Occasionally, resistant *Staphylococcus aureus* or *Pseudomonas* may be identified and necessitate the use of culture-directed antibiotics for short or long periods. Some highly resistant organisms may merit a course of IV antibiotics, although the medical literature is vague about their efficacy. However, patients who have undergone multiple revision surgeries may prefer the investigational use of IV antibiotics to repeated surgical manipulations.

Although fungal cultures are often obtained, identifying fungal infections can be difficult. Occasionally, fungal hyphae and a white "shag carpet" appearance can be seen in the ethmoid sinuses, making the diagnosis easier. Many etiologies have been proposed for fungal sinusitis, including direct fungal colonization of the nose, inflammatory response to fungus, invasive fungus, allergy to fungus, and immunoglobulin E (IgE)–related hypersensitivity to fungus.[11] The treatment of fungal sinusitis may include the use of topical corticosteroid or systemic steroids and the investigational use of topical antifungal agents. One useful hallmark in the treatment of recurrent fungus, particularly if the patient suffers from a hypersensitivity, is to try to control the environment of the patient's home or work spaces. Such a treatment regime would include the use of dehumidifiers and limitations on the patient's use of saline irrigations.

Causes of Sinus Surgery Failure

There are many causes of ethmoid sinus surgery failure (**Table 40.1**). The types of failure can be divided into five categories: scarring, incomplete disease removal, inadequate drainage pathways, recurrent disease, and alternate disease processes.

The most common places for scarring to occur include the area adjacent to the anterior tip of the middle turbinate, the frontoethmoid recess, and the superior meatus. Scar-related blockage of the anterior outflow of the middle meatus is very common. This may secondarily block the maxillary sinus outflow tract, causing recurrent infection and further inflammation, which can, in turn, promote progressive scarring.[12]

Choosing a Surgical Approach

Choosing the correct surgical approach for revision ethmoid surgery can be as difficult as choosing from among the many instruments on the sinus surgeon's instrument tray. Selection of the technique may be dependent on the surgeon's ability, access to instruments, patient choice, and availability of sufficient postoperative care.

First, the surgeon must decide whether revision septal surgery has to be performed. Proetz maintained that airflow should be directed into the nasal airway and away from the natural sinus ostia.[13] Proetz also found that the natural ostia have to be clear of disease. These principles should be remembered when evaluating nasal septal deviations and their effect on developing sinusitis

Table 40.1 Causes of Ethmoid Sinus Surgery Failure

1. **Anatomical**
   a. Deviated nasal septum
   b. Scarring and synechiae
   c. Lateralized middle turbinate
2. **Infectious**
   a. Bacteriologic: resistant
   b. Fungal
   c. Mixed flora
   d. Dental infections
   e. Osteitis/osteomyelitis
3. **Ciliary Dyskinesia**
   a. Primary dyskinesia
   b. Secondary dyskinesia
4. **Immunologic**
   a. Allergic
   b. Immune deficiency
5. **Mucus Disorder**
   a. Cystic fibrosis
   b. Inspissated mucus
6. **Iatrogenic**
   a. Incomplete débridement
   b. Insufficient follow-up
   c. Poor surgical timing
   d. Incomplete removal of polyposis
   e. Inexperience
   f. Retained foreign body
   g. Excessive removal of middle turbinate
7. **Patient related**
   a. Poor patient compliance
   b. Overirrigation of the nose and paranasal sinuses
8. **Syndromic**
   a. Sampter syndrome
   b. Midfacial maldevelopment
9. **Other**
   a. Gastric reflux
   b. Nasal-midfacial trauma
   c. Neoplasm
   d. Pollution, smoke, and chemical exposure

(**Fig. 40.1**). In addition, not all septal deflections are the same or have the same effect on secretory pressure, which may lead to sinusitis. For example, anterior abnormalities near the nasal valve have the greatest effect on airflow.

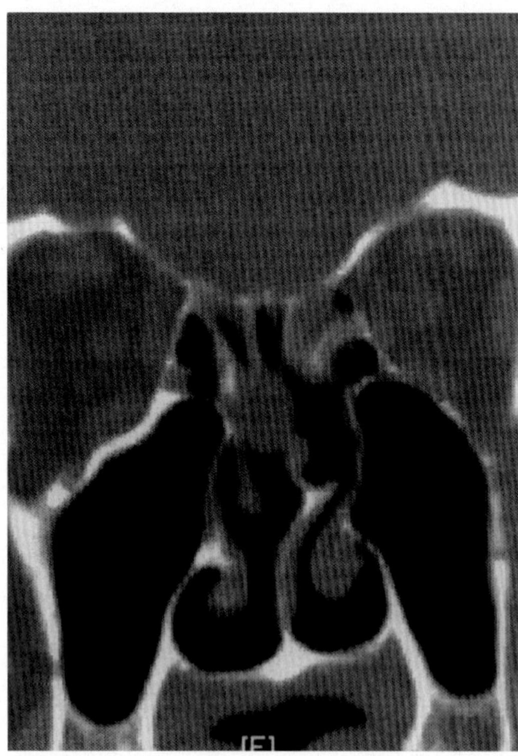

Fig. 40.1 Airflow directed toward the middle meatus violates Proetz's principles and promotes sinus disease due to disruption of the natural outflow pathways of the sinuses and mucus, with airborne allergens being directed into the ostiomeatal complex. This patient has a severe deviated nasal septum and excessive removal of the middle turbinate from the first surgery, which led to recurrent left ethmoid sinusitis.

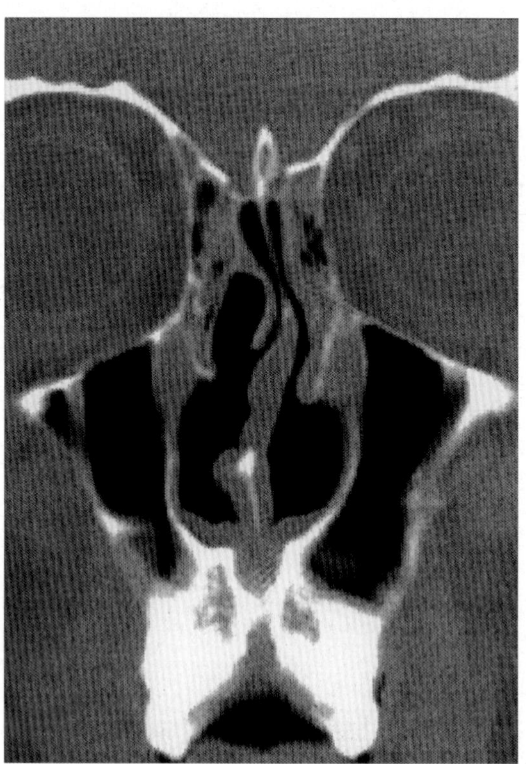

Fig. 40.2 Errors in judgment at the time of the primary surgery can predispose the patient to recurrent sinusitis. This patient had a poorly corrected deviated septum blocking the right ostiomeatal complex with excessive removal of the inferior turbinates. In addition, the concha bullosa on the right was partially opened, but it was not performed in a way that opened the ostiomeatal complex; therefore, the patient had recurrent bilateral ethmoid sinusitis.

The nasal valve is composed of the septum, the upper lateral cartilage, the nasal floor, and the anterior head of the inferior turbinate. Any of these structures may affect the nasal valve area and nasal air and mucus flow, which may predispose to stasis in the nose and resulting sinusitis. Secondarily, the flow patterns high near the middle turbinate affect the nasal resistance and the outflow patterns from the maxillary, anterior ethmoid sinus, and frontal sinuses (**Fig. 40.2**). A high, posterior deflection may abut the superior meatus and block the posterior ethmoid sinuses. Occasionally, a limited posterior deflection may be removed using an endoscopic approach without anterior incisions and elevations of scarred septal mucoperiosteum and mucoperichondrium.

Second, the surgeon should decide preoperatively whether a CT-guided system needs to be employed. Patients with significant nasal scarring, nasal polyposis, prior complications, or involvement of the posterior sinuses and the frontal sinus will benefit from the CT-guided technology that ensures a fine-cut 1 mm CT scan with almost unlimited data (**Fig. 40.3**). CT-guided systems also allow the surgeon to look at the nose and sinuses three-dimensionally before the procedure, enabling the physician to decide both

which instruments he or she needs to use and how to avoid dangerous anatomical sites adjacent to the orbit and base of the skull. CT-guided systems are particularly useful for mucoceles and single cell sinusitis cases as they help to confirm that the involved cells have been identified and opened properly (**Fig. 40.4**). They also serve as a wonderful teaching tool for inexperienced sinus surgeons and residents.

A variety of CT-guided systems are available, each with its own advantages and disadvantages. One should gain experience with one system and stick to it for complex cases. Using a single system will reduce the setup time for the operating room staff and the surgeon. CT-guided systems also afford the surgeon the ability to integrate the instruments with the system.

Third, the surgeon should decide whether or not the middle, inferior, or superior turbinates need to be shaved or reduced in any way. The turbinates are essential for the natural flow of mucus and air in the nose. They provide a vast air-conditioning vehicle for the nose and sinuses. They also carry a broad vascular flow to the nose containing necessary immune ingredients for protection from infection, such as immunoglobulin A (IgA). Nevertheless, the turbinates may suffer from the same mucosal disease as

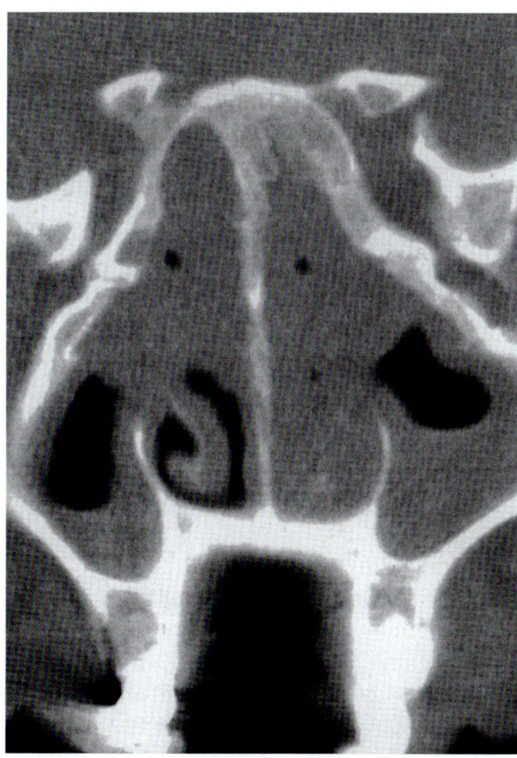

Fig. 40.3 Long-term ethmoid sinusitis may predispose a patient to developing osteitis of the base of the skull. This patient has had recurrent nasal polyps with severe ethmoiditis. The osteitis visible at the left base of the skull causes recurrent disease.

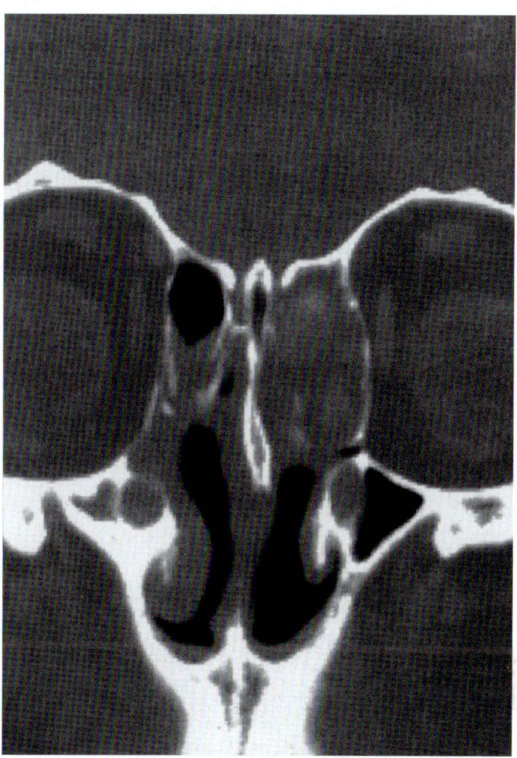

Fig. 40.4 Recurrent ethmoid sinus blockage and recurrent infection may develop into mucoceles. This patient has a history of recurrent nasal sinus polyposis with recurrent ethmoid mucoceles.

the sinuses and need to be reduced to remove polyps or to allow easy sinus outflow. The turbinates should not block the surgeon's view of the sinuses, necessary for the postoperative follow-up of the patient.

Fourth, the surgeon should determine whether there is disease in the adjacent sinuses that needs to be cleared. Traditional sinus surgeons opened the sphenoid recess as the initial stage of their intranasal ethmoidectomies. The posterior ethmoid sinuses are often involved along with the sphenoid due to the common recess. Polyp tissue in this area is often overlooked and may contribute to persistent ethmoid disease (**Fig. 40.5**). Frontal sinusitis may continually bathe the ethmoid sinuses with pus, causing an extensive inflammatory response. Maxillary sinusitis may also inflame the middle meatus secondarily and foster an environment that promotes polypoid blockage of the middle meatus and thus the ethmoid cells. Special cells such as the agger nasi, Haller cells, and supraorbital ethmoids may need to be specifically identified at the time of revision surgery.

Fifth, the surgeon needs to decide whether any special diagnostic or surgical techniques need to be used during the revision surgery. This includes taking special biopsies for electron microscopy to determine the competency of the sinus mucosa or the structural integrity of the

microcilia of the sinus lining.[14] This may also include orbital decompression if there is a mucocele in the ethmoid sinuses invading the orbit. Frontoethmoid drill-out procedures may also be required if the anterior ethmoid cells have scarred the frontal ducts. In extensive polyposis recurrences, the powered endoscopic instruments are often very useful. These instruments help to remove polyps without any tugging at the underlying tissue or bone, where the base of the polyps is unknown and may have been invaded by the previous surgeon. These microdébriders may also help to sculpt the middle turbinate to leave an adequate opening into the ostiomeatal complex without cutting out any turbinate tissue. Finally, these débriders help provide a bloodless field, as they have the advantage of continuous suction through their centers. Balloon catheter sinuplasty is a newer technique which may prove useful in our armamentarium of the future.[15]

Most of the open techniques, used as recently as the 1980s, are rarely employed today except in cases where there is significant orbital involvement or complications. For example, if there are orbital complications and CT guidance is unavailable or greater exposure is deemed necessary, an external ethmoidectomy with orbital retractors may be considered. Caldwell-Luc procedures may

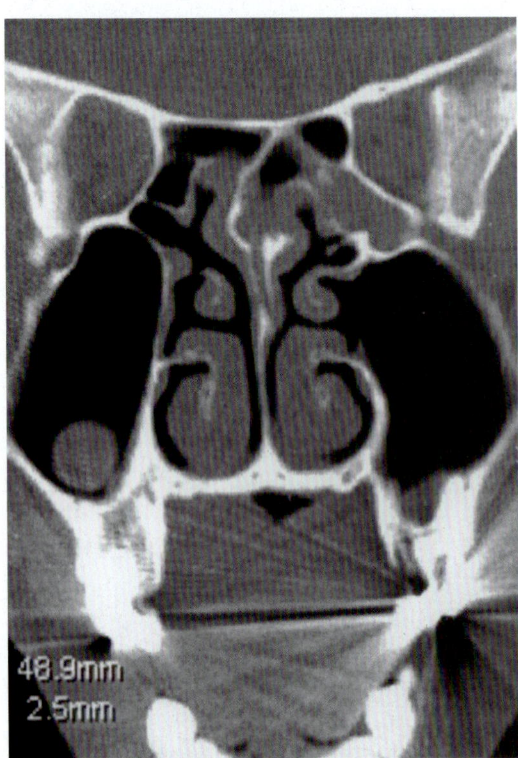

Fig. 40.5 Special ethmoid cells particularly in the posterior ethmoid region are often overlooked at the time of primary surgery. They are often the cause of recurrent symptoms and disease. At the time of revision surgery, the use of computed tomography guidance technology may be helpful in identifying and confirming that these cells are open. In this patient, a posterior Onodi cell on the left was retained, causing left eye pressure.

also be considered for recurrent lateral or inferior maxillary sinus polyposis. Osteoplastic flap obliteration of the frontal sinuses is still a good long-term treatment for recurrent frontal sinus disease where common endoscopic techniques have failed. Given their relatively high rate of complications, however, the decision to use one of these older techniques should only be made after careful consideration. Common complications include facial numbness, recurrent pain, dental sensitivity, and scarring.[16,17]

Finally, the revision surgeon must be cognizant of the need to avoid further scarring, which would predispose the patient to the cycle of additional disease. This may require prudent shaving of the anterior head of the middle turbinate or suturing a floppy middle turbinate to the midline septum. It may also include long-term stenting of the middle meatus with either inert materials, which need to be removed, or one of the dissolvable injectable materials now on the market. An essential part of any revision surgery is careful postoperative care and débridement. Sinus surgery patients are commonly followed weekly or every other week until the sinuses are healed. Although the average primary case needs between two and three débridements of scar and inflammatory tissue to ensure proper healing, more frequent débridements and more vigorous cleanings may be necessary to reduce scarring following revision surgery. Bhattacharyya, in 2004, highlights the fact that "revision endoscopic sinus surgery requires continued intense medical management."[18] Cohen and Kennedy suggest that medical management after sinus surgery should be continued until a stable cavity is achieved.[19] Recently, Desrosiers wrote that a rigorous postop treatment plan should include saline sprays or irrigations, oral or topical steroids, long-term macrolide antibiotics (if needed), aspirin desensitization (if applicable), careful examination of all postoperative cavities and revision surgery for select patients with difficult disease.[20]

Results of Revision Ethmoid Sinus Surgery and Prognostic Factors

One of the most difficult challenges facing the rhinologist is how to identify or predict the patient with the worst disease and the highest chance of recurrence. Recurrence can be defined as recidivistic disease or failure to resolve symptoms. Many factors have been proposed as predisposing patients to recurrent disease. These factors include the presence of reactive airway disease (asthma and bronchitis), a deviated septum, fungal nasal infections, middle meatal scarring, retained ethmoid disease, headaches, cystic fibrosis, dysmotility syndrome, immune disorders, and the "ASA triad" (aspirin sensitivity, asthma, and polyposis).[21,22] Of the many types of sinus disease, the anatomical form of sinusitis is most easily treated and has the lowest recidivism rate. The more physiologic forms of sinusitis with abnormalities in the respiratory lining tend to have lower success rates.

Over the past 30 years, recurrence rates have been reported as varying from 5 to 100%.[23–26] In the preendoscopic period, reported recurrence rates for traditional intranasal ethmoidectomies ranged from 22 to 33%.[27–29] During the early endoscopic intranasal ethmoidectomy period in the 1980s, Wigand reported a revision rate of 18%, Kennedy a rate of 38%, and Stankiewicz a rate of 100%.[26,30,31] As endoscopic sinus surgery became more prevalent and surgeons more experienced in the 1990s, the rates improved. Matthews, for example, reported a revision rate of 16%, and Gaskins reported a rate of only 4% due to scarring.[32,33] Schaitkin et al reported a rate of 34% with one revision and 8% after two revision surgeries.[34] Senior et al reported a rate of 18% in 1998 and Dursun and colleagues a rate of 28 to 6%, depending on the stage of disease.[35,36] McMains reported in 2005 an overall failure rate of 8% for patient undergoing revision surgery with all of the nasal polyposis patients failing revision endoscopic sinus surgery.[37]

Kennedy postulated that the extent of disease shown on a CT scan may predict the outcome of functional endoscopic sinus surgery (FESS), with involvement of more than the ethmoid sinuses being indicative of an increased failure rate.[38] Moses et al, in a 1998 study, however, did not find the radiographic extent of disease to be significant in predicting FESS failure.[39] Other authors, including Matthews et al, have found that CT findings must be correlated with symptoms to identify the toughest cases.[32] Recently, Smith suggested that preoperative CT scans may be a predictor of quality of life and endoscopic sinus surgery outcomes.[22]

The use of steroids by patients with severe disease may be correlated with worse outcomes.[39] This finding probably also correlates with asthmatics and bronchitics, who tend to need greater amounts of steroid medications. Steroids are also used more often by allergy patients, although Kennedy, Matthews et al, and Moses et al did not find any correlation between allergies and sinus surgery outcomes.[31,32,39] Furthermore, Waguespack has shown that allergy patients do not have any diminution of mucociliary clearance, which could predispose them to sinus disease.[40] Wynn found that higher recurrences occurred in allergic patients with asthma.[21]

Using rhinomanometry, Lund et al found no correlation between airflow patterns and sinus surgery results.[41] Anterior rhinometry, however, evaluates the nasal valve and not the ostiomeatal complex, which is more important for sinus outflow.

A local failure to open various sinuses can have a significant impact on sinus surgery success. For instance, Chambers et al found that scarring in the middle meatus and residual ethmoid air cell infection correlated with failed sinus surgery.[42] Hinohira identified maxillary sinus ostia stenosis as being the most common cause of sinus surgical failures, and Ramadan found that residual air cells in the frontal recess and ethmoid areas most often correlated with sinus surgery symptom failures.[43,44] A common factor underlying most of these failures was a lateralization problem caused by the position of the middle turbinate.

Complications of Revision Ethmoid Surgery

Complications of revision ethmoid surgery are equally prevalent as in primary cases. These complications include bleeding, ecchymosis, subcutaneous emphysema, dacryocystorhinitis, headaches, dural tears, CSF leakage, meningitis, pneumonia, diplopia, and blindness. Because bleeding tends to rise with increases in the amount of actively infected mucosa at the time of surgery, the prudent use of preoperative antibiotics may limit this problem. Any history of bleeding at the primary surgery should be pursued by a full hematologic history and appropriate work-up. Facial ecchymosis or emphysema occurs when there is a lamina papyracea violation and air is forced into the orbit by postoperative sneezing or nose blowing. If this occurred in the primary procedure, the patient should be warned that there is a high chance that it will occur again. At the time of the revision surgery, bleeding should be avoided and hemostatic agents should be used in the ethmoid sinuses, if necessary. In these cases, the nose should not be packed postoperatively or only packed very lightly to afford drainage into the nose from the sinuses and not into the eye or surrounding subcutaneous tissue.

Epiphora or excessive tearing may be a short- or long-term complication. The nasolacrimal duct runs anterior to the front of the middle turbinate. A wide maxillary ostium in this area should be avoided. Care to avoid taking more than the uncinate with a backbiter will avoid this complication. If this problem arises, then an endoscopic opening and drainage of the duct can be performed by experienced otolaryngologists with or without the aid of ophthalmologists.

Complications of the base of the skull and orbit can be avoided by rigorous adherence to the basic principles of the minimal touch technique. The use of CT-guided surgical units may also be helpful, if available. The surgeon should spend extra time in a revision case looking for known anatomical landmarks before exploring dangerous areas near the orbit or ethmoid roof.

Conclusion

Revision sinus surgery is one of the most challenging types of cases facing the rhinologist today. The decision tree for revision cases is elaborate because of the need to be more exact in making the diagnosis before the patient undergoes a second or third surgery. The demands on the revision surgeon are significantly greater because of both higher expectations on the part of the patient and the need to understand the success and failure of the primary surgeon. Complication rates for revision surgery can be reduced by taking a methodical approach: paying attention to details, identifying anatomical landmarks early in the procedure, using advanced technology such as powered débriders and CT guidance where available, and being aware of the possible outcomes and alternatives available at each point in the surgery. Revision surgeons should have all of the endoscopic and traditional sinus surgery techniques at their fingertips and fully understand the pros and cons of each maneuver. If properly performed, revision sinus surgery can be a successful adjunct to medical and environmental therapy for chronic rhinosinusitis.

References

1. National Academy on an Aging Society. Chronic and disabling conditions. 1999;1:1–6.
2. Gliklich RE, Metson R. The health impact of chronic sinusitis in patients seeking otolaryngologic care. Otolaryngol Head Neck Surg 1995;113:104–109.
3. Litvack JR, Griest S, James KE, et al. Endoscopic and quality-of-life outcomes after revision endoscopic sinus surgery. Laryngoscope 2007;117:2233–2238.
4. Stackpole SA, Edelstein DR. Anatomic variants of the paranasal sinuses and their implications for sinusitis. curr opin Otolaryngol Head Neck Surg 1996;4(1):1–6
5. Deloge R, Edelstein DR. Posterior ethmoid sinuses: the forgotten cells. Paper presented at: Annual Meeting of the American Rhinologic Society; September 6, 1997; San Francisco.
6. Kennedy DW, Senior BA. Endoscopic sinus surgery: a review. Otolaryngol Clin North Am 1997;30(3): 313–330.
7. Setliff RC III. The small-hole technique in endoscopic sinus surgery. Otolaryngol Clin North Am 1997;30:341–354.
8. Bradley DT, Koutoutakis SE. The role of agger nasi air cells in patients requiring revision endoscopic frontal sinus surgery. Otolaryngol Head Neck Surg 2004;131:525–527.
9. Edelstein DR, Arlis H, Bushkin S, Han JC. Posterior sinus anatomy: clinical correlations and pitfalls. In: Friedman M, ed. Operative Techniques in Otolaryngology–Head and Neck Surgery. Philadelphia: W.B. Saunders; 1991: 222–225.
10. Lee JT, Kennedy DW, Palmer JN, et al. The incidence of concurrent osteitis in patients with chronic rhinosinusitis: a clinicopathological study. Am J Rhinol 2006;20:278–282.
11. Ferguson BJ. Definitions of fungal rhinosinusitis. Otolaryngol Clin North Am 2000;33:227–235.
12. Musy PY, Koutakis SE. Anatomic findings in patients undergoing revision endoscopic sinus surgery. Am J Otolaryngol 2004;24:418–422.
13. Proetz AW. Essays on the Applied Physiology of the Nose. St. Louis: Annals Publishing; 1953:418.
14. Al-Rawi MM, Edelstein DR, Erlandson RA. Changes in nasal epithelium in patients with severe chronic sinusitis: a clinicopathologic and electron microscopic study. Laryngoscope 1998;108:1816–1823.
15. Bolger WE, Brown CL, Church CA, et al. Safety and outcomes of balloon catheter sinusotomy: multicenter 24-week analysis in 115 patients. Otolaryngol Head Neck Surg 2007;137:10–20.
16. Lofchy NM, Bumsted RM. Revision and open sinus surgery. In: Cummings C, ed. Otolaryngology–Head and Neck Surgery. 3rd ed. St. Louis: CV Mosby; 1996:1173–1188.
17. May M, Levine HL, Mester SJ, Schaitkin B. Complications of endoscopic sinus surgery: analysis of 2108 patients-incidence and prevention. Laryngoscope 1994;104: 1080–1083.
18. Bhattacharyya N. Clinical outcomes after revision endoscopic sinus surgery. Arch Otolaryngol Head Neck Surg 2004;130:975–978.
19. Cohen NA, Kennedy DW. Revision endoscopic sinus surgery. Otolaryngol Clin North Am 2006;39:417–435.
20. Desrosiers MY, Kilty SJ. Treatment alternatives for chronic rhinosinusitis persisting after ESS: what to do when antibiotics, steroids and surgery fail. Rhinology 2008;46:3–14.
21. Wynn R, Har-El G. Recurrence rates after endoscopic sinus surgery for massive sinus polyposis. Laryngoscope 2004; 114:811–813.
22. Smith TL, Mendolis-Loffredo S, Loehri TA, et al. Predictive factors and outcomes in endoscopic sinus surgery for chronic rhinosinusitis. Laryngoscope 2005;115:2199–2205.
23. Corey JP, Bumsted RM. Revision endoscopic ethmoidectomy for chronic rhinosinusitis. Otolaryngol Clin North Am 1989;22:801–808.
24. Bhattacharyya N. Computed tomographic staging and the fate of the dependent sinuses in revision endoscopic sinus surgery. Arch Otolaryngol Head Neck Surg 1999;125:994–999.
25. Sobol SE, Wright ED, Frenkiel S. One-year outcome analysis of functional endoscopic sinus surgery for chronic sinusitis. J Otolaryngol 1998;27:252–257.
26. Stankiewicz J. Complications of endoscopic intranasal ethmoidectomy. Laryngoscope 1987;97:1270–1274.
27. Eichel BS. Revision sphenoethmoidectomy. Laryngoscope 1985;95(3):300–304.
28. English GM. Nasal polypectomy and sinus surgery in patients with asthma and aspirin idiosyncrasy. Laryngoscope 1986;96:374–80.
29. Freedman H, Kern E. Complications of intranasal ethmoidectomy: a review of 1000 consecutive operations. Laryndoscope 1979;89:421–434.
30. Wigand ME. Transnasal endoscopical surgery for chronic sinusitis, III: Endonasal ethmoidectomy. HNO 1981;29: 287–293.
31. Kennedy DW. Functional endoscopic sinus surgery. Arch Otolaryngol 1985;111(10):643–649.
32. Matthews BL, Smith LE, Jones R, Miller C, Broodschmidt JK. Endoscopic sinus surgery: outcome in 155 cases. Otolaryngol Head Neck Surg 1991;104:244–246.
33. Gaskins RE. Scarring in endoscopic ethmoidectomy. Am J Rhinol 1994;8:271–274.
34. Schaitkin B, May M, Shairo A, Fucci M, Mester SJ. Endoscopic sinus surgery: 4-year follow-up on the first 100 patients. Laryngoscope 1993;103:1117–1120.
35. Senior BA, Kennedy DW, Tanabodee J, Kroger H, Hassab M, Lanza D. Long-term results of functional endoscopic sinus surgery. Laryngoscope 1998;108:151–157.
36. Dursun E, Bayiz U, Korkmaz H, Akmansu H, Uygur K. Follow-up results of 415 patients after endoscopic sinus surgery. Eur Arch Otorhinolaryngol 1998;255:504–510.
37. McMains KC, Koutakis SE. Revision functional endoscopic sinus surgery: objective and subjective surgical outcomes. Am J Rhinol 2005;19(14):344–347.
38. Kennedy DW. Prognostic factor, outcomes and staging in ethmoid sinus surgery. Laryngoscope 1992;102:1–18.
39. Moses RL, Cornetta A, Atkins JP Jr, Roth M, Rosen MR, Keane WM. Revision endoscopic sinus surgery: the Thomas Jefferson University experience. Ear Nose Throat J 1998;77(3):190–202.

40. Waguespack R. Mucociliary clearance patterns following endoscopic sinus surgery. Laryngoscope 1995;105(Suppl 71, Pt 2):1–40.
41. Lund VJ, Holmstrom M, Scadding GK. Functional endoscopic sinus surgery in the management of chronic rhinosinusitis: an objective assessment. J Laryngol Otol 1991;105:832–835.
42. Chambers DW, David WE, Cook PR, Nishioka GJ, Rudman DT. Long-term outcome analysis of functional endoscopic sinus surgery: correlation of symptoms with endoscopic examination findings and potential prognostic variables. Laryngoscope 1997;107:504–510.
43. Hinohira Y, Yumoto E, Hyodo M, Joko H. Revision endoscopic sinus surgery: long-term follow up and operative findings. Nippon Jibiinkoka Gakkai Kaiho 1995;98(8): 1285–1290.
44. Ramadan HH. Surgical causes of failure in endoscopic sinus surgery. Laryngoscope 1999;109:27–29.

Revision Surgery of the Maxillary Sinus

Charles P. Kimmelman

The goal of endoscopic maxillary sinus surgery for the treatment of chronic sinusitis is the restoration of the antral mucosa to a normal, noninflamed state with fully functioning mucociliary dynamics. The procedures are designed to restore ostial function by means of augmenting the size of the ostium and removing any obstacles to luminal ventilation and mucus egress. However, there are many impediments to a successful surgical result, including technical factors in the performance of the operation as well as systemic and local disorders suffered by the patient. Recognition of these factors allows surgeons to anticipate and avoid pitfalls before or during the initial surgery. In cases where revision surgery is indicated, identification and amelioration of the causes of failure in the prior operation should increase the likelihood of reversion to a normally functioning maxillary sinus.

Causes of Failure and Their Remedies

Technical Deficiencies

Placement of the Neo-ostium

The newly augmented maxillary ostium should incorporate the natural ostium. Thus, it is important to identify the natural ostium and enlarge it, rather than place a secondary opening in a different position.[1] Heterotopic ostia may not lie within the path of the flowing mucus blanket powered by cilia programmed to beat in the direction of the natural opening.[2] The resultant stasis of secretions can allow proliferation of microbes and/or more prolonged retention of inhaled toxins and pollutants. A similar mechanism also may lead to failure in previously operated antra with an inferior meatus antrostomy, in which the so-called recirculation sinusitis has been described. In this condition, infected mucus does not "drain" from the inferior antrostomy. Instead, it serves as an entry point for secretions that exit the natural os. Secretions are recycled instead of transported posteriorly into the nasopharynx.

Surgical Technique

Endoscopic surgery within the small, cramped space of the middle meatus favors contact of the delicate epithelium with instruments during their repeated insertion and removal. To limit injury to retained mucosal surfaces, the operator must adhere to a philosophy of extremely delicate handling of tissue. Small abrasions induce an inflammatory response that can at a minimum impair ciliary activity, and at worst avulse mucosa and induce synechiae and stenosis. The coating of instruments with viscoelastic substances, such as hylan B, can provide a measure of protection.[3] The presence of foreign material, such as free bone chips, or denuded bone (leading to an osteitis) can produce localized inflammation and subsequent scarring.[4] All foreign material must be removed and exposed bone covered or excised.

Failure to Recognize and Rectify Structural Anomalies

Anatomical anomalies, such as a hypersegmented sinus, Haller cells, persistent uncinate, septal deviation and perforation, and odontogenic processes (e.g., congenital cysts, apical cysts, oral antral fistula), allow foci of inflammation to persist or impair ostial function. Scarred sinus lumens from previous Caldwell-Luc procedures may entrap mucosa. These nascent mucoceles must be removed and exteriorized, a sometimes difficult task with a purely transnasal endoscopic approach.[5] Careful review of radiographs and complete inspection of the sinus should allow identification of unsuspected pathology. Depending on the anomaly, a canine fossa approach may be indicated. Dental disease should be evaluated in concert with an oral surgical colleague.

Elimination of Adjacent Sinus Disease

The antrum does not exist in a vacuum. Adjacent chronic inflammation and infection of the ostiomeatal complex involving the ethmoid labyrinth, the infundibulum, and the frontal recess must be identified and removed, or a recurrence of the maxillary sinus disease is possible.[4] All polypoid mucosal changes, granulation tissue, scarring, and stenosis should be removed in the region of the ostiomeatal complex.[6]

Postoperative Care

Postsurgical débridement of crusts and clots is considered a sine qua non of good technique, but how much débridement is enough? Overly vigorous and frequent manipulation

Decision tree for revision surgery of the maxillary sinus

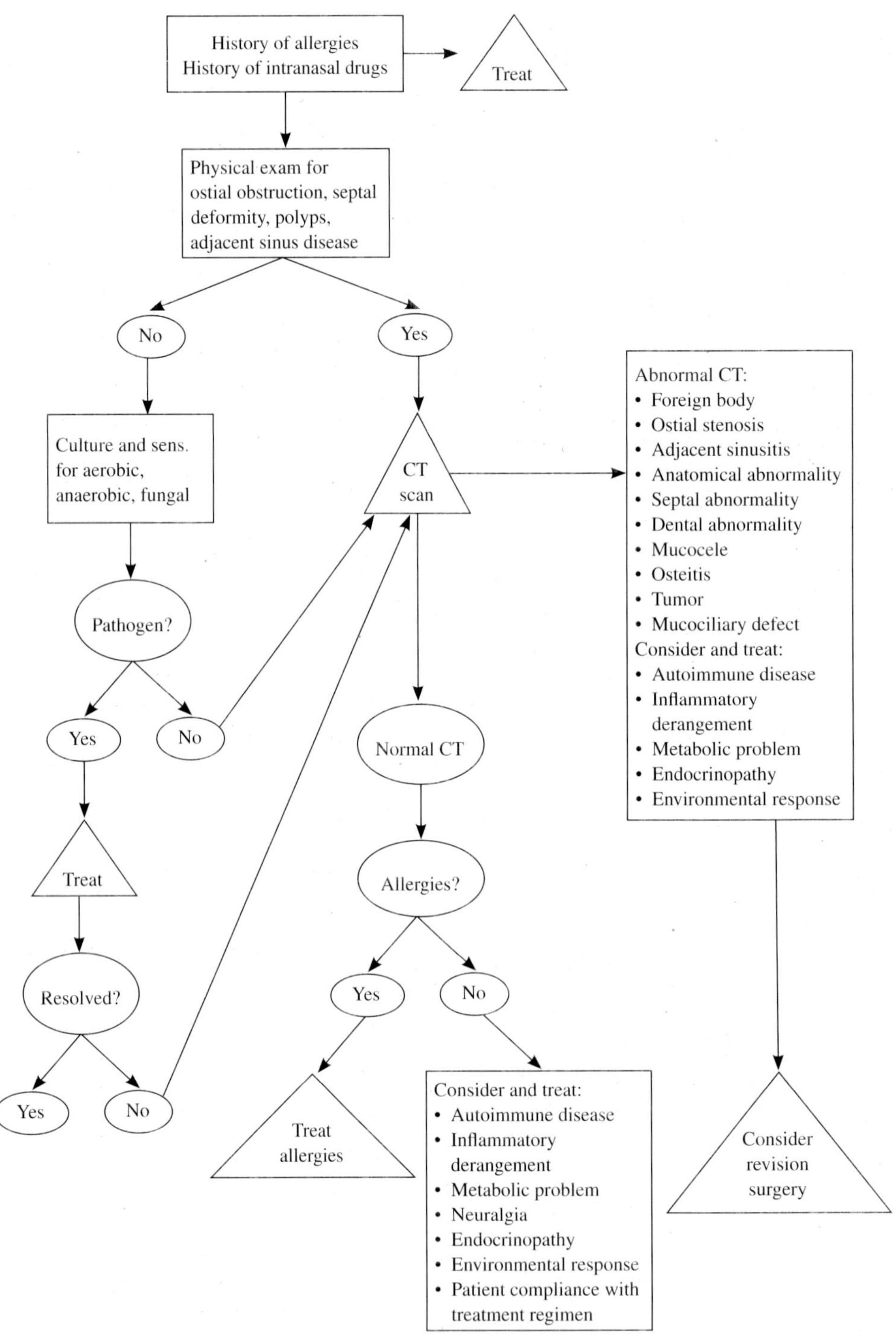

of the recently operated surfaces causes bleeding and may slow the resolution of inflammation. Too little débridement permits crusts and clots to form a substrate for infection, inflammation, and scarring. Gentle saline and/or hypertonic salt solution irrigation by the patient to reduce crusting is important in the postoperative regimen. Several days of topical oxymetazoline spray twice daily can reduce continued bleeding from raw surfaces. My preference is to conservatively débride the ostial site at weekly intervals for at least 3 weeks and at biweekly visits until crusts cease to form. Severe inflammation may warrant systemic antibiotics for longer than the standard 10-day period; the use of topical or systemic corticosteroids is also valuable in cases of more severe inflammation (granulation tissue) or early polyp formation. Physical barriers to the development of synechiae and stenosis are commonly employed. These range from the placement of packing materials, such as petrolatum gauze and Telfa, to the insertion of specialized stents. Unfortunately, these materials themselves are foreign bodies and can exacerbate inflammation and retention of secretions. A recent advance is the instillation of hylan B gel, which conforms exactly to the complex shape of the middle meatus. This biomaterial is nontoxic (it is 99% water) and reduces scarring and stenosis. Its transparency allows continued observation of the operative site, and it can be reapplied as needed.[3]

Extrinsic Factors

This category includes unfavorable factors thrust upon the maxillary sinus from the external environment.

Virulence of Infectious Agents

The resistance of bacteria and fungi to medical therapy will prolong an infection and may lead to chronicity. The prevalence of antibiotic use in the community selects resistant strains. Because patients with chronic sinusitis have already been on multiple courses of antibiotics, such resistance is even more likely. Furthermore, some microbes form protective biofilm barriers that prevent otherwise effective antimicrobials from entering their microenvironment. Potential remedies include accurate culture identification (aerobic, anaerobic, fungal) and sensitivity testing of organisms obtained under endoscopic guidance from sinus ostia, frequent endoscopic débridement and irrigation to remove necrotic exudate and biofilms, and, in severe cases, delivery of topical antibiotics or antifungals in irrigant or nebulized solutions.

Neoplasia

Although rare, the possibility of a neoplasm should always be kept in mind in the surgery for chronic sinusitis. Inverted papilloma, osteoma, and myxoma are benign tumors that can obstruct ostia and cause secondary inflammatory disease. Malignancies such as squamous cell carcinoma, adenoid cystic carcinoma, lymphoma, and metastases may also mimic chronic sinusitis. Unrecognized or incompletely treated tumors will often require revision surgery.

Trauma

Injury to the maxilla and dental structures may lead to a persistent focus of infection or contaminating fistula from the oral cavity. Bony sequestra and foreign bodies must be removed in order for the inflammation to resolve. Dental procedures, such as apicoectomy, root canal, and dental implant procedures, may damage the sinus mucosa and must be dealt with if chronic sinusitis is to resolve. Prior radiation therapy incorporating the maxilla can lead to osteoradionecrosis, synechiae with ostial obstruction, and desiccation of secretions, all of which may lead to chronic sinusitis.

Environmental Quality

The presence of inhaled irritants, allergens, and infectious agents is a risk factor for sinus disease. Crowded living conditions, cigarette smoke, and excessive dryness of ambient air are inimical to normal mucosal function and may be factors in the recurrence of disease. The surgeon must eliminate noxious physical environments to the extent possible.

Pharmacological Effects

Many commonly prescribed drugs have anticholinergic activity (antihistamines, anxiolytics, antidepressants) or dehydrating action (diuretics) that adversely impact mucocilary flow. Topical nasal agents (sympathomimetic amines, corticosteroids, anticholinergics, calcitonin) also impair nasal and ciliary function. Adrenergic beta-blocking drugs, either systemically administered or placed in the conjunctival sac and eliminated through the nose, may cause rhinitis. The long-term use of nasal cocaine destroys nasal epithelium and connective tissue and leads to chronic sinusitis that is often refractory to surgical amelioration. Failure to recognize the contribution of these drugs may jeopardize the success of maxillary sinus surgery.

Intrinsic and Systemic Factors

Mucociliary Defects

Abnormalities of ciliary morphology and dynamics lead to stasis of secretions with microbial proliferation and chronic sinusitis as a result. Derangements in the composition of nasosinal mucus may have the same effect. Chronic sinusitis in children should prompt consideration of cystic fibrosis and congenital ciliary defects (e.g., Kartagener syndrome). In such cases, electron microscopy of the epithelium removed at surgery may show characteristic anomalies in the ciliary microstructure.

Immune System Derangements

Allergy. Immunoglobulin E (IgE)–mediated allergic disease of the nose and sinuses is a commonly recognized cause of sinusitis and must be addressed in affected patients. Evaluation and treatment with topical and/or systemic corticosteroids, antihistamines, and anticholinergics may have to be supplemented with immunotherapy. Systemic mastocytosis can also be associated with chronic sinusitis.

Autoimmunity. Autoimmune disease, such as Wegeners granulomatosis, systemic lupus erythematosus, and scleroderma, may affect nasal and sinus function, leading to a chronic sinusitis. Wegener granulomatosis can be particularly insidious in its presentation as a chronic inflammation of the upper respiratory tract. These disorders should be considered if disease persists despite appropriate treatment.

Immunodeficiency. Congenital immunodeficiency syndromes commonly affect the sinonasal region. One of the most prevalent disorders is immunoglobulin A (IgA) deficiency, which, because of the role IgA plays in mucosal defense, is especially likely to foster the development of chronic sinusitis. What are not widely considered by otolaryngologists are defects of the innate immune system. Unlike the directed response of adaptive immunity (mediated by T and B lymphocytes) to specific antigens, the innate system consists of molecules that are destructive to a broad range of microbial invaders. A well-recognized example is the complex of complement molecules, but others, such as the mannose-binding proteins, also play a role in the body's defense. Lactoferrin, present in nasal mucus, is also an important agent. Absence or defects in these molecules may very well contribute to the development of chronic sinusitis, thus explaining some cases of persistent infection and inflammation that defy the physician's efforts. Acquired immunodeficiency syndrome (AIDS) is a well-known cause of chronic sinusitis and must be included in the differential diagnosis of recurrent maxillary sinusitis in individuals with the appropriate risk factors. Surgery has been recommended for AIDS patients with sinusitis.[7] However, until a permanent cure is found, recurrence of disease is likely to be inevitable, given the longer survival afforded by current medical treatments.

Defects in the control of inflammation. Excessive or prolonged inflammatory activity may play a role in the rapid return of disease after surgery. A classic example is triad asthma, in which a disorder of prostaglandin metabolism permits ongoing inflammation. Other potential disorders might involve elevated levels of inflammatory mediators or decreased activity of inhibitors of inflammation.

Endocrine-Metabolic Derangements

Hypothyroid states cause tissue edema that may encourage the development or persistence of sinusitis. Progesterones have a vasodilatory effect and may cause mucosal engorgement with ostial obstruction. Diabetes mellitus is associated with decreased phagocytic activity that may prolong or exacerbate sinusitis. Dietary deficiencies of vitamins A and C may rob the epithelium of important sustaining influences, leading to mucosal dysfunction.

Postoperative Neuralgia

The occasional patient will have a seemingly excellent postoperative result yet complain of persistent pain. A diligent search for overlooked inflammatory processes is negative. All ostia are open and patent, and the mucus is clear. Some of these poor outcomes may be due to neuralgia related to reflex sympathetic dystrophy from the preceding sinusitis or neural injury with neuroma formation from surgical trauma. These vexing cases may require a therapeutic trial with carbamazepine or other antineuralgics to confirm the diagnosis.

Patient Compliance

The active participation of the patient is critical to a successful sinus operation. There is much for the patient to do in the postoperative period, and continued care will be necessary for a long time thereafter, including the following: nasal irrigations, saline and/or corticosteroid sprays, visits to the doctor for endoscopy with or without débridement, and allergic follow-up, to name a few. These visits are time consuming, anxiety provoking, and, all too often, somewhat uncomfortable. Many patients will miss the occasional appointment; some return only at irregular intervals. A few are lost for long periods of time. Unfortunately, such lapses work adversely against a cure, as débridement, nasal hygiene, control of inflammation and allergy, and early management of infection are critical to success. Patient misuse and abuse of over-the-counter medications, which may lead to rhinitis medicamentosa, and the neurotic automanipulation or -instrumentation of the nose and sinuses further complicate follow-up. The role of the otolaryngologist as psychotherapist is particularly important in patients with chronic disease. The physician must be forthright concerning the likelihood of cure, the need for prolonged follow-up and repeated treatment, and the necessity for early evaluation and treatment of recurrent sinusitis.

Conclusion

The standard radical maxillary sinus operation, the Caldwell-Luc procedure, yielded to endoscopic maxillary sinus surgery because of the latter's retention of tissue and dedication to restoration of a normally functioning sinus. However, endoscopic approaches are not risk free or without failure.[8] There are many concurrent conditions and situations that can lead to recurrent disease or a dissatisfied patient. It behooves the rhinologist to consider these factors before embarking on both virgin and revision procedures to obtain the best result.

References

1. Parsons DS, Strivers FE, Talbot AR. The missed ostium sequence and the surgical approach to revision functional endoscopic sinus surgery. Otolaryngol Clin North Am 1996;29:169–183.
2. Schaefer SD. An anatomic approach to endoscopic intranasal ethmoidectomy. Laryngoscope 1998;108:1628–1634.
3. Kimmelman CP, Edelstein DR, Han JC. Sepragel sinus (hylan B) as a postsurgical dressing for endoscopic sinus surgery. Otolaryngol Head Neck Surg 2001;125:603–608.
4. Richtsmeier WJ. Top 10 reasons for endoscopic maxillary sinus surgery failure. Laryngoscope 2001;111:1952–1956.
5. Busaba NY, Salman SD. Maxillary sinus mucoceles: clinical presentation and long-term results of endoscopic surgical treatment. Laryngoscope 1999;109:1446–1449.
6. Ramadan HH. Surgical causes of failure in endoscopic sinus surgery. Laryngoscope 1999;109:27–29.
7. Sabini P, Josephson G, Reisacher W, Pincus R. The role of endoscopic sinus surgery in patients with acquired immune deficiency syndrome. Am J Otolaryngol 1998;19:351–356.
8. Penttila M, Rautiainen M, Pukander J, Kataja M. Functional vs. radical maxillary surgery: failures after functional endoscopic sinus surgery. Acta Otolaryngol Suppl 1997;529:173–176.

Decision tree for patient presenting with frontal region headaches or frontal sinusitis symptoms/signs

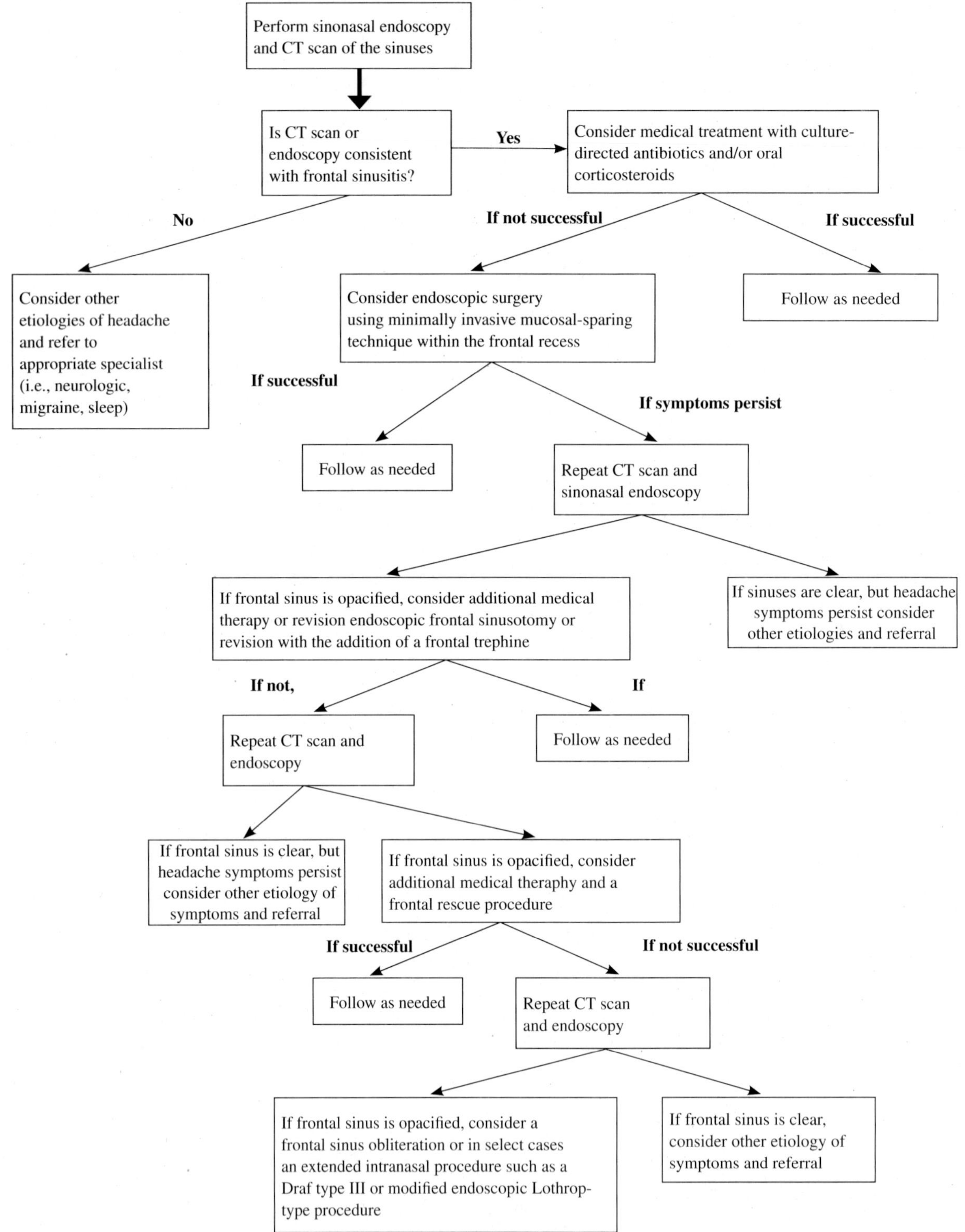

42 Revision Surgery of the Frontal Sinus

William E. Bolger and Stephanie A. Joe

Frontal sinus surgery has challenged otolaryngologists for more than a century. Today, modern endoscopic frontal recess surgery is widely considered to be one of the most difficult procedures otolaryngologists perform; revision frontal surgery is even more challenging. Adding to the difficulty, the underlying conditions are recalcitrant in nature, and patients are often exasperated, having subjected themselves to many medical and surgical treatments without substantial relief. The regional anatomy, technical aspects of frontal sinus surgery, and recalcitrant nature of sinusitis make caring for patients with frontal disease through surgery a formidable task. The trials and tribulations of frontal sinus surgery have been well documented and will not be reviewed here. The focus of this chapter will be revision surgery of the frontal recess in the modern endoscopic era.

Indications for Revision Frontal Sinus Surgery

Revision surgery of the frontal sinus is indicated for a variety of conditions. Common indications include persistent disease following incomplete initial surgery, iatrogenic disease due to scarring with osteoneogenesis, and recurrent chronic sinus disease. Typically, revision surgery is considered when a patient complains of significant symptoms, such as headache, facial pain, retro-orbital pain, nasal congestion, and postnasal drainage, which do not respond to medical therapy. Medical therapy includes antibiotics for infectious sinusitis and oral corticosteroid tapering regimens for inflammatory, allergic, and eosinophilic-type sinusitis conditions. The evaluation for revision surgery includes a thorough medical history, a detailed diagnostic sinonasal endoscopy, and a computed tomography (CT) scan. A CT scan can be especially useful in gaining insight into the cause of the frontal problem, such as frontal sinus outflow tract obstruction secondary to the presence of osteoneogenesis.

Management of Frontal Sinus Disease following Surgery

Prevention

Iatrogenic frontal sinusitis is a significant condition, one that is best prevented rather than treated. Prevention cannot be stressed enough, and it begins with an accurate diagnosis. If the diagnosis of sinusitis and the indications for surgery within each sinus are considered, the chance for unnecessary surgery and iatrogenic disease can be greatly reduced. Often when cases of iatrogenic frontal sinusitis are analyzed, it is evident that disease was limited initially to the osteomeatal complex and ethmoidal prerecess area, yet surgery was performed far up into or through the internal os of the frontal sinus; that is, the frontal sinus was radiographically normal, the patient had no or few symptoms referable to the frontal sinus, yet surgery was performed. This "while we are in there" approach to surgical indications for the frontal sinus can have lifelong deleterious consequences. Such an approach to surgery is not employed in other areas of the body. We would shudder if, while replacing a fully diseased knee, an orthopedist recommended a prosthesis for a normal or minimally diseased contralateral hip. Similarly, it would not be acceptable for a cardiac surgeon to replace a normal mitral valve during aortic valve replacement for advanced aortic valve disease. Iatrogenic frontal sinus disease can be prevented by carefully considering the indications for endoscopic frontal sinus surgery and the scope of the procedure.

Another critical area to consider is the individual patient's pathophysiology. Far too often we attribute sinus disease to "obstruction" and apply surgical principles to "relieve obstruction" and "facilitate drainage." Thereafter, in consultation for revision frontal sinus surgery, sinonasal tissue inflammation, not obstruction, is observed on endoscopy. A prolonged course of oral corticosteroids can bring about dramatic control of the primary disease process. The degree of disease resolution can be equal to or exceed that which is achieved with surgery. (This can be humbling to observe as a surgeon.) With continued follow-up, the disease recurs but can again be controlled with corticosteroid retreatment. Over time, it becomes clear that the disease is not related to ostial obstruction and does not require a "relief of ostial obstruction" solution. Rather, it is an inflammatory condition of the sinonasal membrane, a medical disease; hence, it responds to a medical solution. Unfortunately, our current medical armamentarium is largely limited to oral corticosteroids. These agents are not desirable on a long-term basis due to their side effects and potential adverse effects. Clearly, more acceptable medications need to be discovered. Until such time, surgery may be used as a last resort. However, it should be recognized that often surgery is recommended because of a lack of alternative treatment options, not a logical application based on the pathophysiology. If surgery is limited to disease sites that are refractory to medical therapy (antibiotics for bacterial disease, oral corticosteroids for eosinophilic inflammatory disease), and mucosal sparing surgical principles are maintained, patients can benefit from future discoveries in medical therapy. If aggressive surgery to relieve obstruction of the frontal recess is performed for mucosal membrane/medical disease and an iatrogenic obstruction results, the patient will not benefit from additional advances in medical care. The basic principle "First do no harm" has a central place in the surgical care of the frontal recess and sinus.

In addition to careful case selection, several technical considerations are important for preventing iatrogenic frontal sinusitis. Mucosal sparing within the recess is critical for avoiding postoperative stenosis and osteoneogenesis. Mucosal-sparing forceps, ostial seekers, and curets designed especially for the frontal recess allow disease and ethmoid septations to be removed without mucosal stripping. Fracture or partial resection of the middle turbinate can be associated with lateralization of tissue and frontal sinus obstruction. Lamina orbitalis (papyracea) removal can be associated with medialization of orbital fat across the frontal sinus and subsequent frontal obstruction.

Revision Frontal Sinus Surgery

Anatomical Considerations

An appreciation of adjacent structures is necessary before attempting operative dissection in the frontal recess. The superior portion of the uncinate process is intimately related to the frontal recess and sinus. This portion of the uncinate extends superiorly behind the attachment of the middle turbinate and commonly curves laterally to insert on the lamina papyracea. The air space just below this

insertion is termed the recessus terminalis, and the frontal recess is located superomedial to the uncinate insertion. The frontal sinus will drain and ventilate medial to the uncinate process. Less frequently, the uncinate inserts on the middle turbinate or the skull base. In these cases, the frontal recess communicates with the ethmoid infundibulum, and the frontal sinus drains lateral to the uncinate process.[1]

The medial extent of the frontal recess is usually formed by the vertical lamellar portion of the middle turbinate. The lateral extent of the frontal recess is the lamina orbitalis (papyracea). Its anterior limit is the agger nasi region. The posterior limit of the recess is variable, but in general, the posterior boundary is formed by the anterior wall of the ethmoid bulla.

The complexity of the frontal recess cannot be fully appreciated without consideration of the myriad of ethmoid cells that may pneumatize and drain into this area.[2] The agger nasi region, a prominence found superiorly in the lateral nasal wall just anterior to the insertion of the middle turbinate, is frequently pneumatized by an anterior ethmoid cell. When present, this cell (or cells) can significantly affect the shape of the anterior aspect of the frontal recess and form a portion of the anterior floor of the frontal sinus. Supraorbital ethmoid cells are ethmoid cells that ascend and pneumatize into the orbital plate of the frontal bone (pars orbitalis). They typically drain posterior to the frontal recess and sinus. On CT scan, supraorbital ethmoid cells can give the appearance of a duplicate frontal sinus and need to be considered carefully in both primary and revision surgery.[3] Another type of ethmoid cell affecting revision frontal sinus surgery is the frontal cell. This cell is located above the agger nasi cell and can extend into the frontal sinus to varying degrees. At times these cells also can give the appearance of a duplicate frontal sinus. They can contribute to frontal recess and sinus obstruction, and their bony walls may need to be addressed in revision frontal surgery.

Revision Endoscopic Frontal Sinusotomy

The goals in revision endoscopic frontal sinusotomy are restoration of normal frontal sinus function and sinus health. The narrow confines of the frontal recess present a technical challenge for the surgeon. Identifying the middle turbinate, agger nasi region, medial orbital wall, and skull base provides surgical orientation within the frontal recess. The skull base can be identified posteriorly in the ethmoid cavity and followed forward as it slopes upward into the frontal recess. Usually, the anterior ethmoid neurovascular bundle is located in the area where the skull base transitions from a horizontal orientation to a more vertical orientation in the frontal recess. The area of the frontal sinus ostium is identified and carefully widened. Attempts should be made to avoid circumferential dissection near the ostium to prevent circumferential stenosis.

Visualization and proper instrumentation are key elements in successful surgery. Because of its anterior location, dissection in the frontal recess requires the use of angled telescopes and forceps with curved shafts of suitable length to reach the frontal recess. Through-cutting forceps are recommended for mucosal preservation in the frontal recess. Endonasal microdébriders should be used cautiously to prevent inadvertent mucosal stripping during surgery. The orientation afforded by image guidance enhances endoscopic frontal sinus surgery and can facilitate a more complete procedure. However, image guidance should not be the major means of localization. Its use is not a substitute for knowing the anatomy or for meticulous, mucosal-sparing technique.

Weekly postoperative endoscopic examinations and débridement of clot, fibrinous material, and early scar are recommended for the first 4 to 6 weeks after surgery. The surgeon should be mindful that mucociliary clearance will remain impaired postoperatively for a significant length of time. As such, medical therapy is continued until the operative site has healed and local edema has resolved.

Revision endoscopic surgery can be performed for a host of conditions. One increasingly important condition is iatrogenic frontal sinusitis. The endoscopic approach can be used to remove scar tissue, osteoneogenesis, and residual ethmoid septations to relieve obstruction and restore the frontal sinus to health (**Figs. 42.1 and 42.2**). The endoscopic approach is a significant advance and has spared many patients from more morbid surgical procedures.

Combined Endoscopic Surgery and Trephine

When the endoscopic approach to the frontal sinus is exceedingly difficult, such as in revision surgery patients with scarring, osteoneogenesis, and loss of surgical landmarks, other approaches can be considered. One such complementary approach is a frontal sinus trephination. The advantages of a combined approach using an external frontal sinusotomy with the endoscopic transnasal approach are numerous.[4] This technique is extremely helpful in revision surgery where the surgical landmarks have been altered and mucosal preservation is critical. If the surgeon places the scope through the trephine, he or she can easily see the effect the surgical instrument is having on the surrounding mucosa of the frontal recess and sinus. Stripping of mucosa can be limited, and this can translate into quicker healing and improved postoperative results. Placing the scope though the trephine also avoids the problem of blood soiling the dependently positioned lens. From below, it can sometimes be difficult to see around the instrument shaft and view the mucosa while dissecting. These problems are avoided when visualizing through the trephine. With meticulous careful dissection and preservation of mucosa, scarring and osteoneogenesis can be reduced. The trephine technique is also useful when resecting frontal bullar cells that extend superiorly above the internal frontal ostium. In these patients, small instruments can also be placed through the trephine to remove parts of cells that are positioned beyond the reach of the currently available frontal sinus instruments.

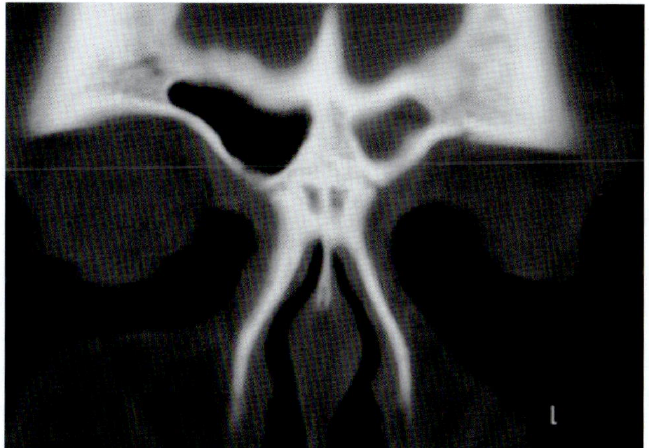

A

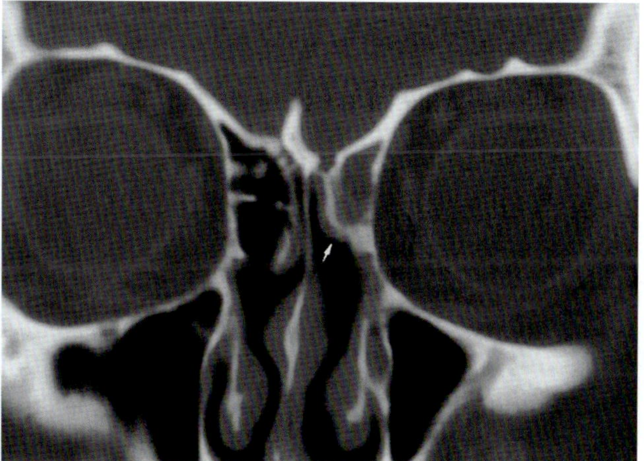

B

Fig. 42.1 (A) Iatrogenic left frontal sinusitis following endoscopic sinus surgery at another institution. Prior to surgery, the frontal sinus was normal. **(B)** The cut surface of the middle turbinate (*white arrow*) is scarred to the lamina orbitalis; osteoneogenesis is evident within the frontal recess and anterior ethmoid.

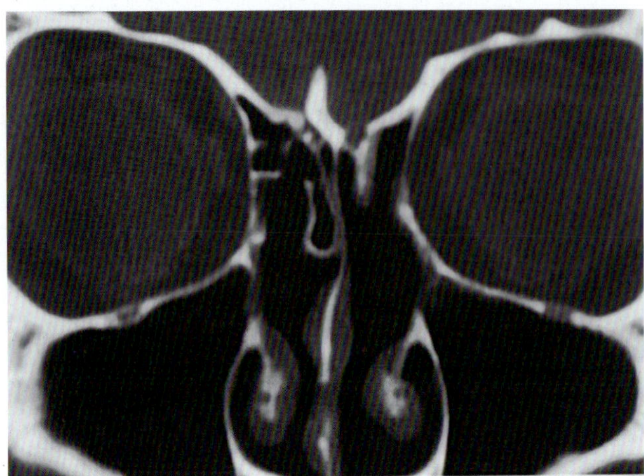

Fig. 42.2 Same patient as in **Fig. 42.1** following a revision endoscopic procedure at our institution. The frontal sinusitis has cleared, and the frontal recess/anterior ethmoid area is no longer obstructed. Bone and scar tissue were removed from the frontal recess, and a prolonged period of healing and postoperative débridement was needed for full recovery.

Frontal Sinus Rescue Procedure

The technique of mucoperiosteal flap advancement, or the "frontal sinus rescue procedure," has been used in cases of chronic frontal sinusitis after previous middle turbinate resection.[5] This technique is considered when the amputated remnant of the middle turbinate has scarred laterally across the frontal recess, leading to obstruction of the frontal sinus. A parasagittal incision is performed to release the middle turbinate "stub" from scar laterally. With the frontal recess now exposed, the mucosa is elevated off the lateral portion of the middle turbinate and carefully preserved, as this will become the mucoperiosteal advancement flap. The medial mucosa of the middle turbinate stub is removed along with the mucosa overlying the adjacent nasal roof to provide a recipient bed for the advancement flap (**Fig. 42.3**). The middle turbinate remnant bone is removed to the skull base. The mucoperiosteal flap is trimmed to fit and placed over the denuded roof. This procedure has the advantages

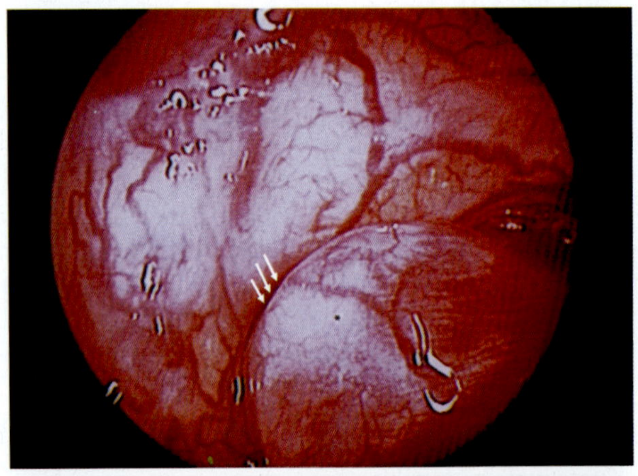

A

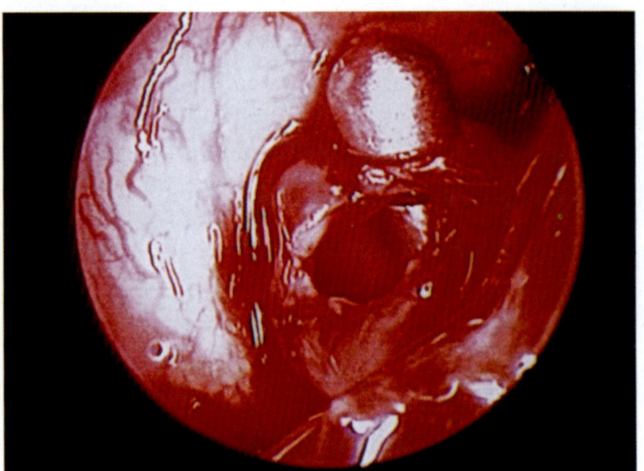

B

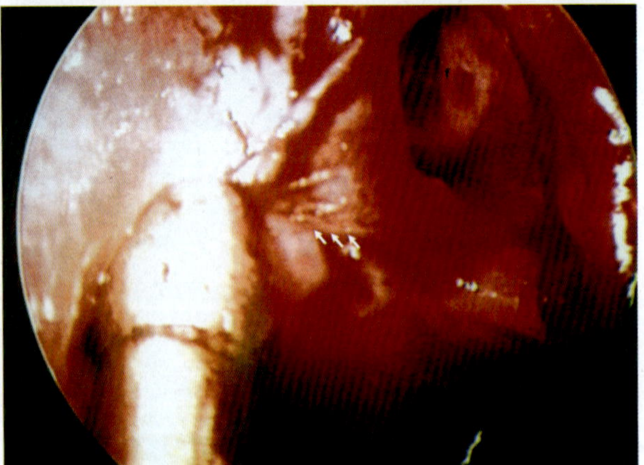

C

Fig. 42.3 (A) Endoscopic view through a left frontal sinus trephination viewing downward with a 30 degree endoscope. An invading frontal cell can be seen well above the internal frontal ostium (*asterisk*). Thickened secretions have been suctioned clear. The natural drainage passage is narrowed (*arrows*). **(B)** Endoscopic view through the frontal sinus trephination. A frontal sinus mushroom punch is seen removing the horizontal portion of the obstructing frontal cell. **(C)** Endonasal view of the patient in **A** and **B** through a 30 degree endoscope. The middle turbinate remnant has been removed to the skull base while preserving a medial flap of mucosa. This flap is being draped medially (*arrows*) with the suction to complete the frontal sinus "rescue" approach. The internal aspect of the frontal sinus can be seen through the newly opened frontal recess.

of preserving the natural sinus outflow tract and restoring mucociliary clearance. The mucosa at the frontal sinus ostium remains undisturbed. Furthermore, as the flap heals, adhesions form and pull the advancement flap medially, keeping the frontal sinus ostium patent. The potential for cerebrospinal fluid (CSF) leak exists with dissection adjacent to the lamella of the cribriform plate, the thinnest portion of the skull base.

Extended Endonasal Endoscopic Procedures

Frontal recess obstruction due to osteoneogenesis and scar limits the success of conservative endoscopic sinus surgery. Extended endonasal approaches relieve chronic frontal sinusitis and avoid the morbidity of frontal sinus obliteration.[6–8] Frontal recess stenosis is addressed by creating a wide central opening into the frontal sinus. A review of Dr. Wolfgang Draf's work in this field forms the foundation for additional consideration of these procedures. Draf describes three types of endoscopic drainage procedures.[5,9] The least invasive approach, a Draf type I frontal sinusotomy, or "simple drainage," is used for patients with mild frontal sinus disease. It consists of dissection in the frontal recess and removal of obstructing disease inferior to the frontal ostium. Draf types II and III are used in revision endoscopic sinus surgery cases. Draf type II, the "extended drainage," enlarges the natural frontal sinus drainage tract. Type IIA addresses ethmoid cells encroaching on the frontal sinus and creates a larger opening in the frontal sinus floor between the lamina papyracea and the middle turbinate. Type IIB extends

removal of the frontal sinus floor to the nasal septum with resection of the middle turbinate. "Median drainage" of the frontal sinus, or type III frontal sinusotomy, involves bilateral frontal recess surgery establishing common frontal sinus drainage. This is accomplished by resecting the superior nasal septum, removing the frontal sinus floor across the midline, and also removing part of the intersinus septum. In a review of several hundred cases in which these approaches were used, Weber, Draf, and colleagues reported an overall success rate ranging from 79.0 to 93.3% for the type II frontal sinusotomies and 91.5 to 95.0% for type III sinusotomies.[9] In these extended approaches, drilling is often employed to address osteoneogenesis and the spina nasalis interna.[10] Overlying scar tissue and residual mucosa are removed prior to and during drilling. Normal physiologic processes such as mucus production and mucociliary clearance can be interrupted, and significant local tissue trauma with prolonged edema and healing can occur. Local osteoneogenesis, circumferential scarring, and stenosis can arise despite the creation of a wide opening at the time of surgery.[6] Potential complications include an increased incidence of intraoperative CSF leak, as compared with the standard endoscopic frontal sinusotomy, and cosmetic deformity of the nasal dorsum. These approaches should be practiced with caution after consideration of all of the alternatives.

Caution is advised in linking these procedures to the specific pathophysiology of the patient. We have encountered several patients in postoperative referral who have had an endoscopic Lothrop procedure to improve frontal "drainage"; however, the pathophysiology of their sinusitis was clearly hyperplastic eosinophilic polypoid mucosal

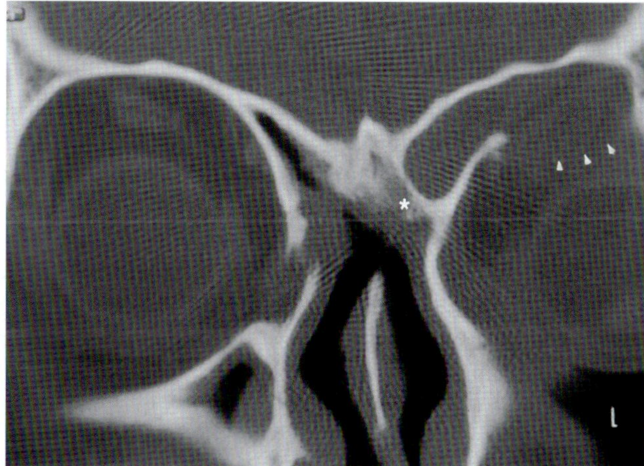

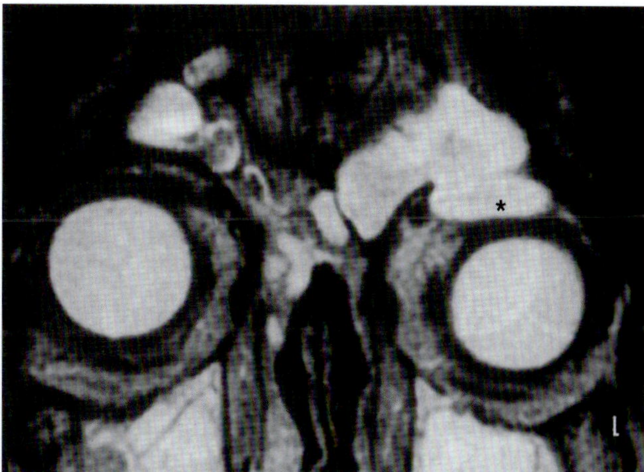

Fig. 42.4 (A) Computed tomography scan of a patient referred to our institution following an endoscopic Lothrop procedure. The improved drainage afforded by the Lothrop did not lead to resolution of disease. Rather, scarring and osteoneogenesis (*asterisk*) occurred along with the return of hyperplastic eosinophilic mucosal membrane disease. Obstruction of the left supraorbital ethmoid has led to a mucocele, erosion of the floor of the sinus, extension of the mucocele into the orbit (*arrowheads*), and proptosis. **(B)** Magnetic resonance imaging of the patient shows the mucocele extending into the orbit (*asterisk*).

membrane disease, not outflow tract obstruction. The Lothrop procedure failed to address the primary disease process, yet the patient was managed effectively with occasional courses of oral corticosteroids (**Fig. 42.4**). In contrast, the use of an extended approach to the frontal sinus to provide increased access for postoperative visualization and surveillance following endoscopic resection of an inverted papilloma of the ethmoid sinus that extended through the frontal recess into the lower aspect of the frontal sinus is well founded.

In summary, the value and role of this procedure are as yet not fully determined. The procedure is "required" at some institutions, but others manage very advanced cases of frontal sinusitis without needing to perform this procedure. A case-controlled series comparing this technique to endoscopic frontal sinusotomy with trephination and rescue and to osteoplastic flap with obliteration, for the various problems encountered, would be very helpful and revealing.

Frontal Obliteration

Prior to nasal endoscopy, several approaches have been tried in treating frontal sinusitis. Since the first report of a frontal sinus surgery in 1870, both intranasal and external approaches have been described.[11] A common theme is initial success followed by long-term failure, attributed to an inability to maintain a patent nasofrontal communication.[11,12] Limited intraoperative visualization of the frontal recess and skull base was a contributing factor. Poor or inconsistent results with these procedures set the stage for the osteoplastic approach.

Osteoplastic frontal sinus surgery was introduced in the United States by Goodale and Montgomery in 1958.[11,12] Though they involved more extensive dissection, osteoplastic procedures were associated with improved success rates as compared with other approaches such as the frontoethmoidectomy, Lynch, and Lothrop.[12] Due to what is felt to be its time-proven success, the osteoplastic approach to the frontal sinus became the standard against which all other procedures were judged. In the general treatment of chronic frontal sinusitis, osteoplastic frontal sinus obliteration is used by many rhinologists after other, less-invasive procedures fail. The procedure will not be described in detail here, as excellent descriptions exist elsewhere.[13,14] Successful obliteration depends on complete and thorough removal of the frontal sinus mucosal lining. The inner bony cortex of the sinus is drilled to remove mucosa from the vascular foramina of Breschet and expose the blood supply to the autologous graft. Mucosa is removed as far inferiorly as possible. The mucosal edges at the nasofrontal region are turned in toward the nasal cavity to prevent mucosal ingrowth into the frontal sinus

and subsequent mucocele formation. The choice of material for sinus obliteration varies among surgeons. Many materials have been used, including autologous fat, muscle, and bone, as well as hydroxyapatite.[11,15–17] Spontaneous osteoneogenesis with auto-obliteration of the sinus has also been tried.[11,16] Fat has been the most widely used and studied graft material. Revascularization of the graft has been shown as soon as 1 week after the procedure. Resorption occurs to a variable amount and is replaced by fibrous tissue.

One of the drawbacks in the use of frontal sinus obliteration is the incomplete ability to survey the sinus cavity for recurrence of disease. The radiographic evaluation for disease after frontal sinus obliteration can be difficult. Loevner et al performed a prospective study looking at the magnetic resonance imaging (MRI) findings after osteoplastic flap frontal sinus obliteration with fat autograft.[18] The 13 participants were either asymptomatic or had some resolution of their symptoms postoperatively. Endoscopic examination demonstrated the absence of frontal recess disease. Each patient underwent MRI studies between 9 months and 12 years after their procedure. Images obtained included T1-weighted pre- and postcontrast images and T2-weighted images. The T1 postcontrast and T2 images were performed with fat suppression techniques. The studies showed some degree of replacement of adipose tissue with lower signal soft tissue in all cases. Some amount of hyperintensity within the frontal sinuses on T2-weighted images and with contrast was also seen in all cases. Thus, these findings are nonspecific for the detection of inflammatory disease within an obliterated frontal sinus. The authors concluded that it is difficult to differentiate inflammation from the normal granulation process and/or scar. MRI is useful, however, for detecting mucocele formation in such cases.

Other disadvantages of frontal sinus obliteration include a large incision, neuralgias, paresthesias, headaches, and potential donor site morbidity. Intracranial complications such as CSF leak and sagittal sinus bleeding can occur, as well as infection of the fat graft or bone flap. Long-term follow-up is necessary to monitor for the development of late mucocele formation from the regeneration of retained sinus mucosa or ingrowth from the nasofrontal area.

A particularly difficult diagnostic problem is determining the etiology of headaches in patients who have undergone osteoplastic flap with fat obliteration. The differential diagnosis is broad and includes neuropathy, sinusitis, graft infection, and osteomyelitis. The trauma to the frontal bone part of the skull from surgery has also been implicated, as a percentage of skull fracture and craniotomy patients have headache symptoms. Distinguishing a postoperative neurologic symptom from sinusitis can be very difficult. As mentioned, imaging studies cannot completely evaluate for the presence of active sinus disease, even if a comprehensive panel including CT, MRI, bone scan, and tagged white blood cell (WBC) nuclear medicine scanning is employed. In 250 cases of osteoplastic frontal sinusotomy, Hardy and Montgomery reported a 6% incidence of persistent frontal pain or headache.[19] Approximately 1% of cases were attributed to postoperative neuralgia. The overall revision rate was 9.5%, with over 14 years of postoperative follow-p. Eight of the 20 patients who underwent later revisions did so for recurrent infection. Upon revision in six of the patients, no infection was found, with four resulting in negative reexplorations for persistent pain.[19]

Conclusion

Revision frontal sinus surgery is one of the most challenging surgical problems for otolaryngologists. Careful diagnosis and patient selection, along with meticulous surgical technique, can lead to successful outcomes in many patients. Endoscopy has provided new minimally invasive surgical options that have met with success in many patients. We look to the future for more technological advancements that can help more patients with this difficult condition.

References

1. Stammberger HR, Kennedy DW. Paranasal sinuses: anatomic terminology and nomenclature. Ann Otol Rhinol Laryngol Suppl 1995;167:7–16.
2. Bolger WE. Anatomy of the paranasal sinuses. In: Kennedy DW, Bolger WE, Zinreich SJ, eds. Diseases of the Sinuses: Diagnosis and Management. Hamilton, Ontario: BC Decker; 2000:1–11.
3. Owen RG, Kuhn FA. Supraorbital ethmoid cell. Otolaryngol Head Neck Surg 1997;116:254–261.
4. Kuhn FA. Surgery of the frontal sinuses. In: Kennedy DW, Bolger WE, Zinreich SJ, ed. Diseases of the Sinuses: Diagnosis and Management. Hamilton, Ontario: BC Decker; 2000:281–301.
5. Citardi MJ, Javer AR, Kuhn FA. Revision endoscopic frontal sinusotomy with mucoperiosteal flap advancement: the frontal sinus rescue procedure. Otolaryngol Clin North Am 2001;34:123–132.
6. Draf W. Endonasal micro-endoscopic frontal sinus surgery: the Fulda concept. Oper Tech Otolaryngol Head Neck Surg 1991;2:234–240.
7. Gross WE, Gross CW, Becker D, Moore D, Phillips D. Modified transnasal endoscopic Lothrop procedure as an alternative to frontal sinus obliteration. Otolaryngol Head Neck Surg 1995;113:427–434.
8. Lanza DC, McLaughlin RB, Hwang PH. The five year experience with endoscopic trans-septal frontal sinusotomy. Otolaryngol Clin North Am 2001;34:139–152.
9. Weber R, Draf W, Kratzsch B, Hosemann W, Schaefer SD. Modern concepts of frontal sinus surgery. Laryngoscope 2001;111:137–146.
10. Hosemann W, Gross R, Goede U, Kuehnel T. Clinical anatomy of the nasal process of the frontal bone (spina nasalis interna). Otolaryngol Head Neck Surg 2001;125:60–65.
11. Jacobs JB. 100 years of frontal sinus surgery. Laryngoscope 1997;107(Suppl):1–36.
12. McLaughlin RB. History of surgical approaches to the frontal sinus. Otolaryngol Clin North Am 2001;34:49–58.
13. Montgomery WW. Surgery of the frontal sinuses. Otolaryngol Clin North Am 1971;4:97–126.
14. Montgomery WW. State-of-the-art for osteoplastic frontal sinus operation. Otolaryngol Clin North Am 2001;34:167–177.
15. Snyderman CH, Scioscia K, Carrau RL, Weissman JL. Hydroxyapatite: an alternative method of frontal sinus obliteration. Otolaryngol Clin North Am 2001;34:179–192.
16. Javer AR, Sillers MJ, Kuhn FA. The frontal sinus unobliteration procedure. Otolaryngol Clin North Am 2001;34:193–210.
17. Shumrick KA, Smith CP. The use of cancellous bone for frontal sinus obliteration and reconstruction of frontal bony defects. Arch Otolaryngol Head Neck Surg 1994;120:1003–1009.
18. Loevner LA, Yousem DM, Lanza DC, Kennedy DW, Goldberg AN. MR evaluation of frontal sinus osteoplastic flaps with autogenous fat grafts. AJNR Am J Neuroradiol 1995;16:1721–1726.
19. Hardy JM, Montgomery WW. Osteoplastic frontal sinusotomy: an analysis of 250 operations. Ann Otol Rhinol Laryngol 1976;85:523–532.

Decision tree for recurrent epiphora or dacryocystitis

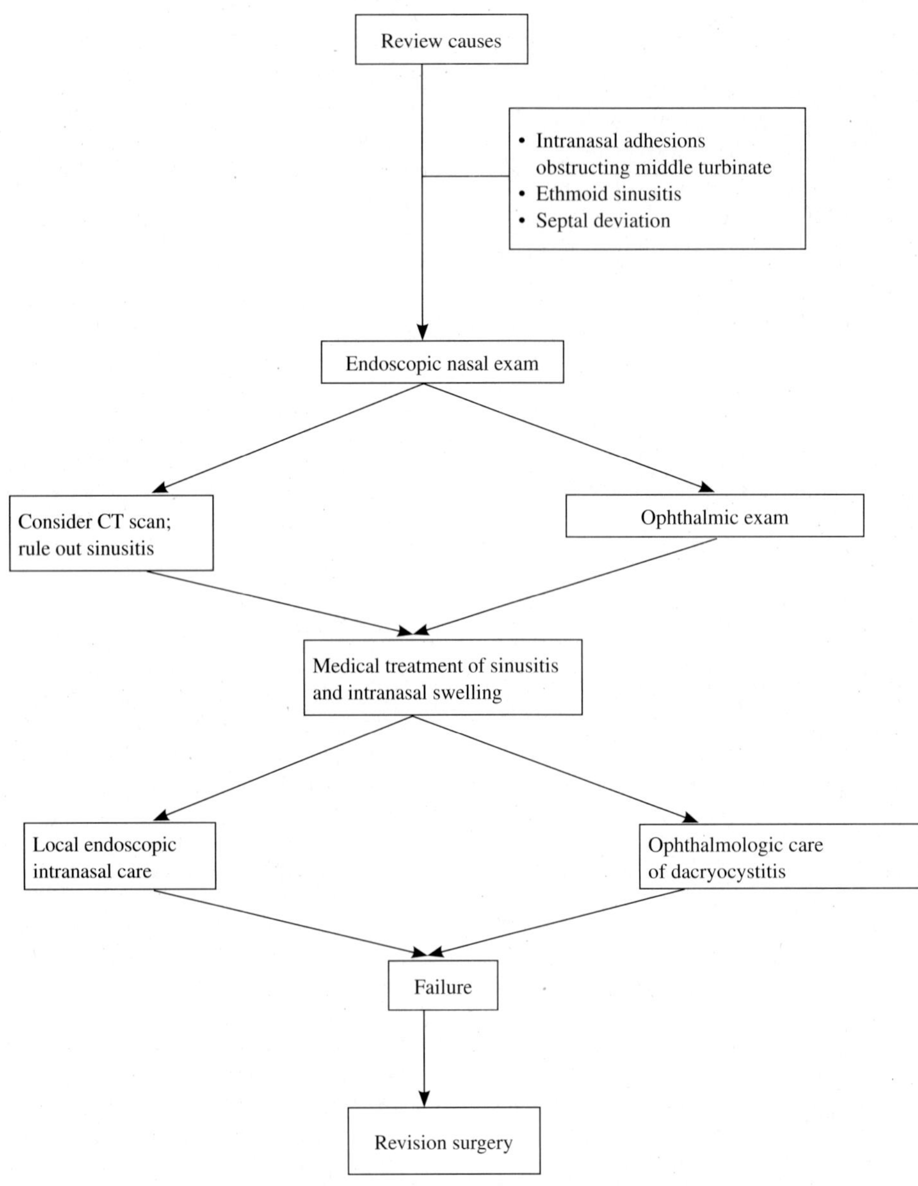

43 Revision Endoscopic Dacryocystorhinostomy

Ralph B. Metson and Mark Samaha

Revision endoscopic dacryocystorhinostomy (DCR) has proved to be an excellent treatment modality for the patient who develops recurrent epiphora or dacryocystitis after primary DCR.[1,2] Endoscopic instrumentation allows the surgeon to identify and correct the most common causes of DCR failure, which include intranasal adhesions, an obstructing middle turbinate, and occult disease of the ethmoid sinus.

In contrast to most surgical procedures, for endoscopic DCR, revision surgery is actually easier to perform than a primary procedure. The most technically challenging portion of lacrimal surgery is usually removal of thick bone along the lateral nasal wall overlying the lacrimal sac. Because this bone has already been removed in patients who have undergone previous DCR, revision endoscopic DCR is quite suitable for the surgeon who wishes to learn the technique of endoscopic DCR.

Surgical Technique

Revision endoscopic DCR may be performed under general or local anesthesia, depending on the patient's medical condition and the surgeon's preference. The patient is placed in the supine position with a slight reverse Trendelenburg position to decrease venous pressure at the operative site. Nasal packing strips soaked in 4% cocaine hydrochloride (HCL) solution are placed along the lateral nasal wall to provide decongestion. The nose and affected eye are draped in the operative field. A 4 mm diameter, 0-degree nasal endoscope is used for visualization for the majority of the procedure. A solution of 1% lidocaine HCL with epinephrine 1:100,000 is injected into the submucosa of the middle turbinate and the lateral nasal wall anterior to the attachment of the middle turbinate (**Fig. 43.1**).

The assistant surgeon passes a lacrimal probe through a canaliculus into the obstructed lacrimal sac. The tip of the probe can be observed with the endoscope as it tents the mucosa of the lateral nasal wall (**Fig. 43.2**). The surgeon then uses a sickle knife to make a crescent-shaped curvilinear incision ~1 cm anterior to the tip of the probe. There is occasionally extensive submucosal fibrosis from the primary surgery, which may need to be sharply elevated

with the sickle knife. The resulting posterior mucosal flap is then grasped with a straight Blakesley forceps and removed with a twisting motion to avoid avulsing the mucosa of the lateral nasal wall (**Fig. 43.3**). The mucosa adjacent to the opening created may need to be resected with similar bites with the Blakesley forceps to provide an opening of at least 10 mm.

If the sac has been entered after removal of the mucosa, the tip of the lacrimal probe will be visible. However, frequently there is additional scar tissue that needs removal before the sac can be entered. The intranasal opening is deepened with an angled Blakesley forceps directly laterally toward the sac (**Fig. 43.4**). Because scarring from previous surgery may obscure sac anatomy, it is important to use the probe that lies within the sac as a guide for tissue removal. Care is taken to remove only tissue

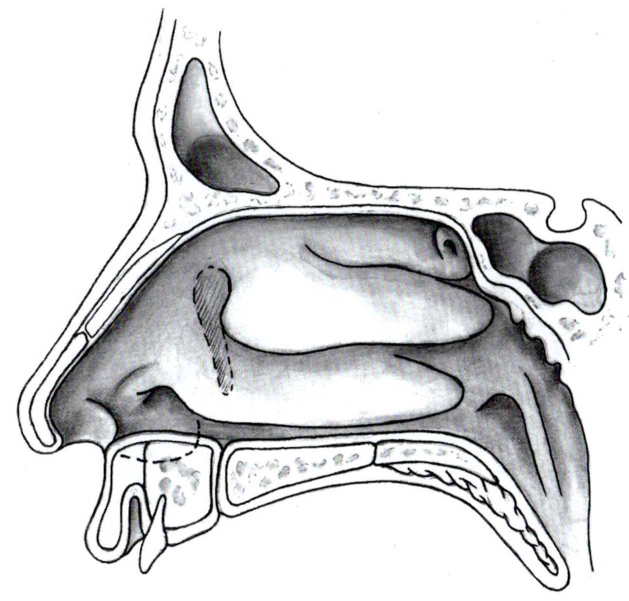

Fig. 43.1 View of the right lateral nasal wall demonstrates the relationship of the lacrimal sac and nasolacrimal duct to the turbinates. Note how a portion of the sac may extend beneath the middle turbinate, requiring turbinate resection for adequate exposure. (From Metson R. Endoscopic surgery for lacrimal obstruction. Otolaryngol Head Neck Surg 1991;104:473–479, with permission.)

411

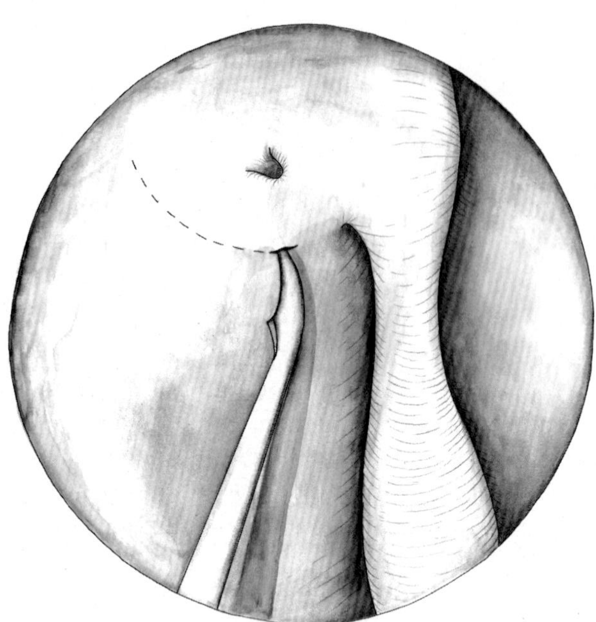

Fig. 43.2 Revision endoscopic dacryocystorhinostomy. A lacrimal probe passed through a canaliculus is seen tenting the nasal mucosa just anterior to the attachment of the middle turbinate. This probe indicates the location of the lacrimal sac. Nasal mucosa overlying the anterior edge of the sac is incised with a sickle knife. (From Metson R. The endoscopic approach for revision dacryocystorhinostomy. Laryngoscope 1990;100:1344–1347, with permission.)

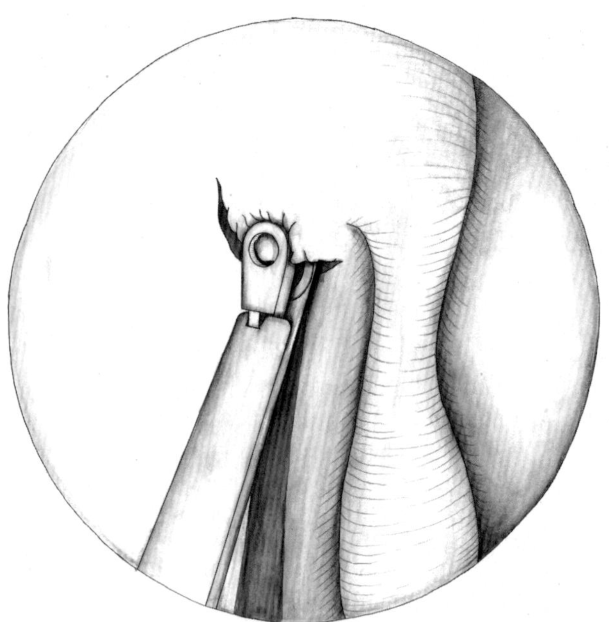

Fig. 43.3 The posterior flap of the nasal mucosa covering the lacrimal sac is grasped with biting forceps and removed. The mucosal opening is enlarged to a diameter of ~10 mm. (From Metson R. The endoscopic approach for revision dacryocystorhinostomy. Laryngoscope 1990;100:1344–1347, with permission.)

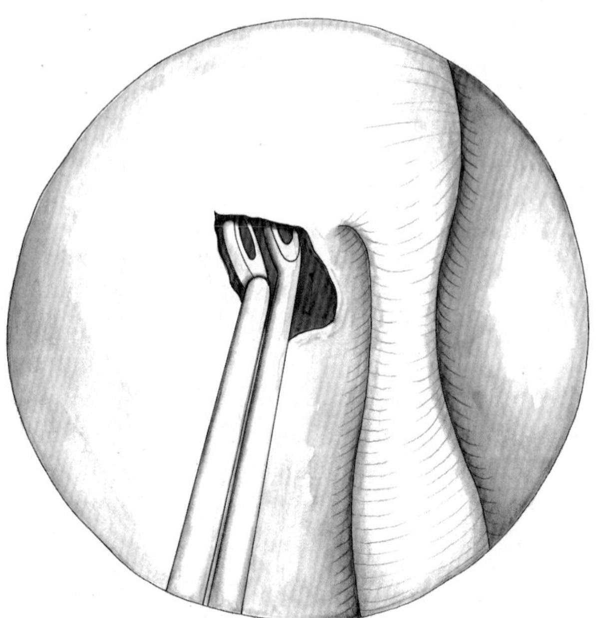

Fig. 43.4 Angled biting forceps are directed laterally to enlarge the opening into the lacrimal sac. An exposed lacrimal probe is used as a guide for tissue removal. After the opening into the lacrimal sac has been adequately enlarged, probes should pass freely into the nose from both superior and inferior canaliculi. (From Metson R. The endoscopic approach for revision dacryocystorhinostomy. Laryngoscope 1990;100:1344–1347, with permission.)

surrounding the probe to remain within the confines of the lacrimal sac and to avoid inadvertent entry into the orbit with exposure of periorbital fat. Once the intranasal opening has been sufficiently enlarged, the interior of the sac and internal common punctum are usually visible with a 30-degree endoscope. Occasionally, two separate internal puncta are visible in the sac interior. At this point, lacrimal probes should pass freely into the nose from the superior and inferior canaliculi. The lacrimal probe is then replaced by Silastic tubing that has its ends threaded over a rigid wire (Guibor Canaliculus Intubation Set, Medtronic ENT, Jacksonville, Florida). This tubing may be used instead of a lacrimal probe at the start of the case. The rigid ends of the tubing are passed through the superior and inferior canaliculi into the nose via the opening created in the lacrimal sac. The rigid ends protruding into the nasal cavity are then grasped individually with the Blakesley forceps (**Fig. 43.5**) and passed out of the nose. The rigid ends are then cut, and the Silastic tubing is trimmed and tied. The tubing forms a continuous loop that passes through the nasal cavity and canaliculi, and is thus unlikely to become dislodged (**Fig. 43.6**). The knot tying the Silastic tubing should not be under tension to avoid pressure injury to the canaliculi. The free ends of the Silastic tubing should be long enough to allow easy access for later tube removal, but short enough to not protrude outside the nasal cavity. Unless bleeding is a problem or a septoplasty is performed, nasal packing is unnecessary.

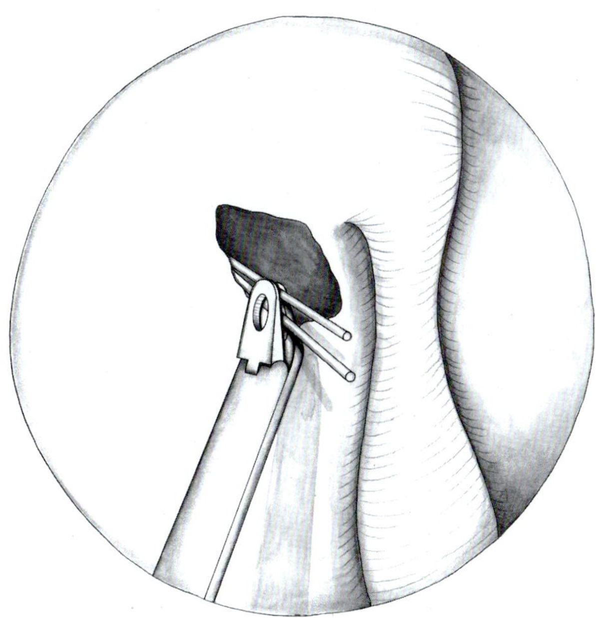

Fig. 43.5 The rigid ends of a Silastic intubation catheter are passed through the canaliculi and are grasped with the forceps, directed out of the nose, trimmed, and tied. (From Metson R. The endoscopic approach for revision dacryocystorhinostomy. Laryngoscope 1990;100: 1344–1347, with permission.)

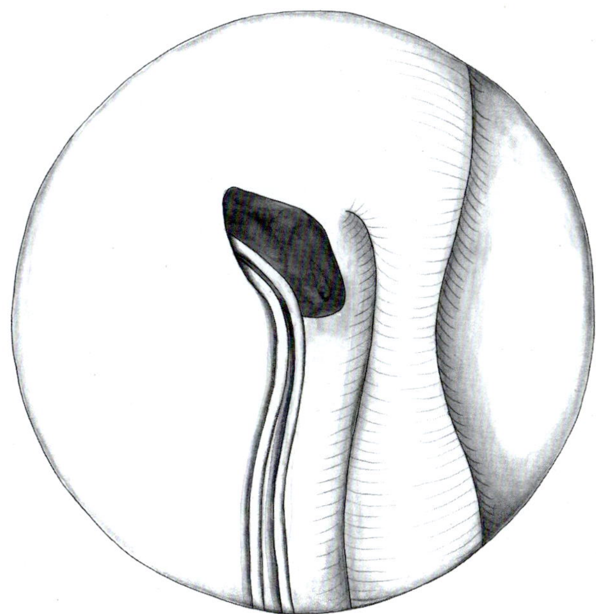

Fig. 43.6 View of Silastic catheters that stent the intranasal opening into the lacrimal sac during the healing period. (Used with permission from Metson R. The endoscopic approach for revision dacryocystorhinostomy. Laryngoscope 1990;100:1344–1347, with permission.)

Postoperative Care

Patients are discharged with a 1-week course of anti-staphylococcal oral antibiotics and instructions to begin twice daily nasal saline irrigation with a bulb syringe starting the day after surgery. Any remaining intranasal debris is removed on the first postoperative visit 1 week after surgery.

The Silastic tubing used to stent the surgical ostium is usually removed 2 months postoperatively by cutting the exposed loop of tubing at the medial canthus and withdrawing the tubing through the nose. If granulation tissue forms at the ostium around the tubing, it may be removed sooner. Alternatively, the tubing may be left for 6 months or longer in revision cases where scarring has been a problem. Patency of the lacrimal system is verified by irrigation of the canaliculi, as well as endoscopic observation of fluorescein dye flowing from the eye through the surgical ostium into the nose.

Surgical Results

Revision endoscopic DCR has been shown to be effective for those patients who have failed a primary conventional or endoscopic DCR.[1,2] Metson reported a 75% success rate for those patients who had persistent epiphora or dacryocystitis following external DCR.[3] Common causes of DCR

failures such as intranasal adhesions, concurrent ethmoiditis, an enlarged middle turbinate, and a septal deviation can be readily identified and corrected with the use of endoscopic instrumentation. In cases where patients fail repeated attempts at DCR, other causes of lacrimal obstruction, such as canalicular scarring, must be considered. Such cases may require conjunctivo cacryocystorhinostomy (CDCR).[3]

Complications

Endoscopic revision DCR should be performed only by those surgeons with extensive experience in endoscopic intranasal techniques. If excessive bleeding occurs during endoscopic revision DCR, the procedure should be terminated or converted to an external approach. Occasionally, orbital fat is exposed while removing bone to expose the lacrimal sac. This fat should not be disturbed or manipulated to avoid injury to intraorbital contents. Damage to the underlying medial rectus and superior oblique muscles can lead to diplopia. Direct optic nerve injury or laceration of intraorbital vessels with subsequent hemorrhage can both lead to blindness. Postoperative epistaxis severe enough to require nasal packing occurs in <5% of cases. When bleeding occurs, it is usually within 1 week after surgery and is caused by a branch of the sphenopalatine artery. Postoperative infection of the nasal cavity or orbit following endoscopic revision DCR is rare and can be treated with antistaphylococcal antibiotics.

Postoperative adhesions are one of the most common causes of surgical failure for both primary endoscopic[3] and external[4,5] DCR, and play a role in failure of revision endoscopic DCR. These adhesions usually occur between the lateral nasal wall and middle turbinate or septum and cause obstruction of the surgically created ostium. The incidence of this complication can be reduced by avoiding trauma to the mucosa of the middle turbinate, particularly on its lateral surface. Resection of the anterior portion of the middle turbinate, which is in proximity to the surgically created ostium, also minimizes the postoperative formation of adhesions between the two structures. Correction of a septal deviation and meticulous postoperative cleaning of debris in the operative site also decrease the likelihood of adhesion formation.

Conclusion

Endoscopic revision DCR is an effective treatment for patients who have failed primary external or endoscopic DCR. The use of endoscopic instrumentation provides excellent visualization for identification and treatment of the common causes of failure of the primary procedure. Revision endoscopic DCR is also technically easier to perform than the primary procedure. Therefore, it is a suitable procedure for surgeons who are acquiring experience with endoscopic surgery for lacrimal obstruction. Revision endoscopic DCR has the potential to reduce patient morbidity through greater utilization of local anesthesia, shorter hospitalization, and a less invasive surgical approach as compared with an external technique.

References

1. Metson R. The endoscopic approach for revision dacryocystorhinostomy. Laryngoscope 1990;100:1344–1347.
2. Orcutt JC, Hillel A, Weymuller EA Jr. Endoscopic repair of failed dacryocystorhinostomy. Ophthal Plast Reconstr Surg 1990;6:197–202.
3. Metson R. Endoscopic surgery for lacrimal obstruction. Otolaryngol Head Neck Surg 1991;104:473–479.
4. Welham RA, Henderson PH. Results of dacryocystorhinostomy analysis of causes for failure. Trans Ophthalmol Soc U K 1973;93:601–609.
5. Allen KM, Berlin AJ, Levine HL. Intranasal endoscopic analysis of dacryocystorhinostomy failure. Ophthal Plast Reconstr Surg 1988;4:143–145.

44 Epistaxis Control

Berrylin J. Ferguson and Barry M. Schaitkin

Epistaxis is common. Patients are often anxious and fearful that the bleeding represents infection, tumor, or impending stroke or that it may lead to exsanguination. Fortunately, epistaxis usually resolves with simple first aid measures such as anterior digital pressure or anterior packing. More problematic is epistaxis from a posterior site or beneath or behind a septal deflection. Death is rare, but morbidity is high, particularly in the older patient.[1,2] This review will discuss the analysis and control of predisposing conditions, nasal packing, and surgical interventions and embolization. The control of epistaxis is a stepwise series of increasingly elaborate interventions until control is achieved. Patients should be informed that there is no guarantee of control with a particular intervention but reassured that you will continue to be available to direct care until the bleeding stops.

Epidemiology

Epistaxis is a common problem afflicting both the young and old, with those over age 40 increasingly likely to require hospital admission. Patients ages 20 to 49 are more likely to be male; those over age 50 are equally distributed between the sexes. The decreased incidence of female epistaxis in the younger age group has been attributed to a premenopausal protective effect, although the mechanism is unknown.[1]

Directed History and Laboratory Examination

Risk factors for epistaxis include coagulopathies, septal perforations, hypertension, and nasal trauma.[2] Nasal trauma can range from nasal fracture to nose picking to the trauma of dry air administered through oxygen prongs. In the latter case, counseling the patient regarding nasal lubricants such as AYR gel (BF Ascher & Co., Lenexa, Kansas) and petroleum jelly or increased room humidity may prevent further bleeding.

The initial work-up for epistaxis includes a history (**Table 44.1**) followed by a physical examination, including all vital signs, with special attention on significant hypertension. Many patients will demonstrate some hypertension, which is secondary to the anxiety of the situation and not causal.

Laboratory studies are required only for recurrent or severe bleeding. These should include hematocrit, hemoglobin, and coagulation profiles. If bleeding is thought to be or has been profuse, then blood should be obtained for a type and cross. Patients initially packed and placed on a penicillin or a first-generation cephalosporin class of antibiotics may return with recurrent bleeding. In some cases, this is because this class of antibiotics can interfere with platelet function and may unmask a platelet abnormality in a patient who was previously compensated, thus leading to a perpetuation of bleeding, sometimes at additional, previously uninvolved sites. A repeat bleeding time and more elaborate coagulation work-up will aid in this diagnosis.

Control of Bleeding: Initial Encounter

The first step in the control of epistaxis is to protect the caregivers. This includes, at a minimum, gloves for all medical personnel and drapes for the patient. Face shields,

Table 44.1 Important Inclusions in History for Patient with Epistaxis

Factors that aid in localizing site
Side of bleeding, or predominant side
Mostly anterior, posterior, or both
Factors that predispose to bleeding
Hypertension
Coagulopathy
Family history of bleeding
Past episodes of bleeding
Medications (especially: aspirin and nonsteroidal anti-inflammatories, warfarin, vitamin E, or chemotherapy; see **Table 44.2** for a more complete listing)
Trauma—history of
Nasal steroid spray usage
Nose picking
Presence of septal perforation and date first noted
Onset of bleeding
Estimate of amount of blood loss

Decision tree for epistaxis

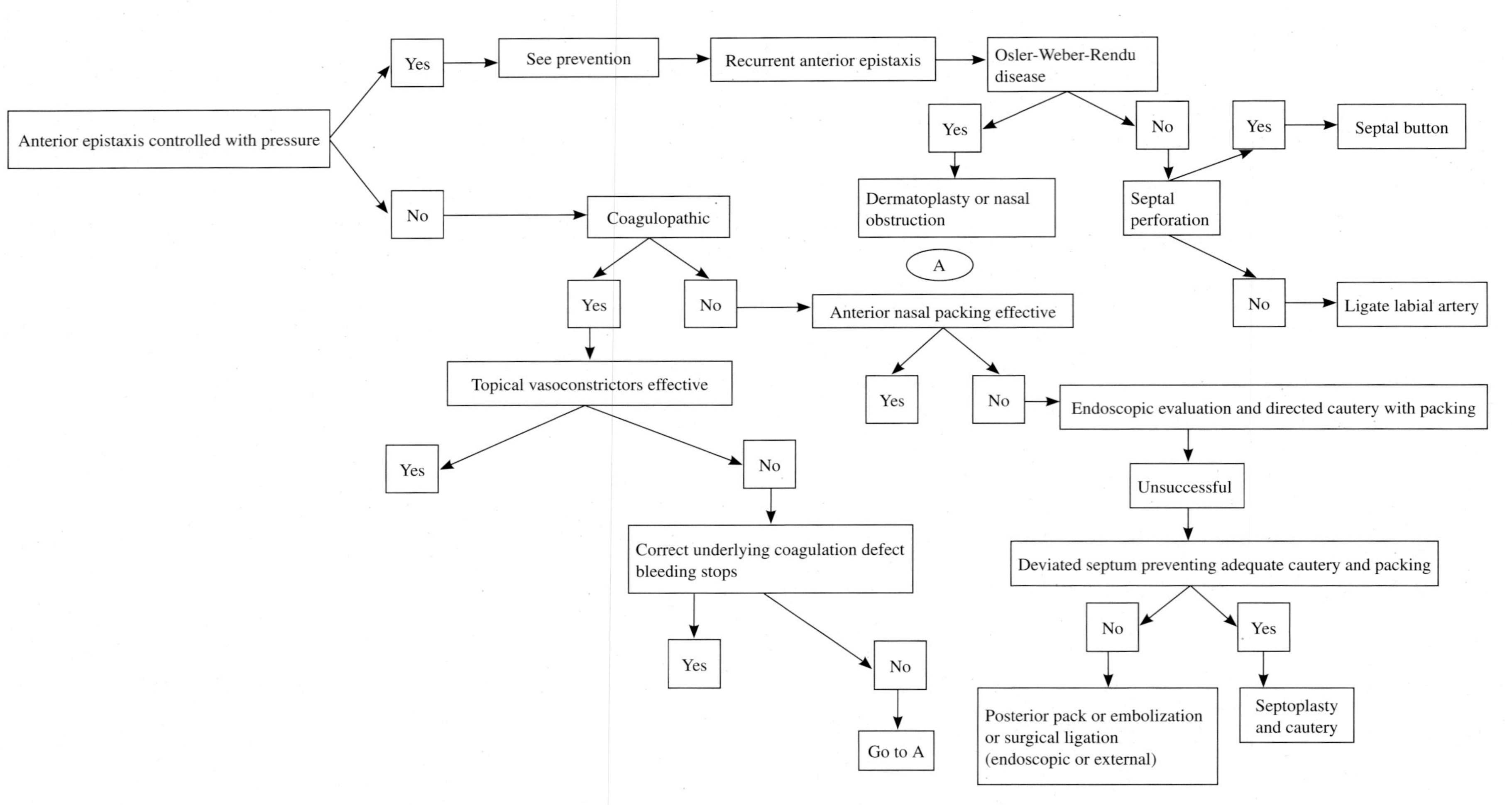

overgowns, and hair protection are required in some situations. Prepare all materials to control the bleeding, including pledgets soaked in an anesthetic (i.e., 4% Xylocaine) combined with a vasoconstrictor (a few drops of 1:1000 epinephrine or equal parts 4% oxymetazoline). Next, instruct the patient to gently blow his or her nose free of all blood clots. (Occasionally, this can be assisted with directed suction.) Then one or several pledgets soaked in Xylocaine and oxymetazoline are inserted into the nostrils under direct vision. In most cases, the vasoconstrictive effects of oxymetazoline combined with the pressure from the pledgets will slow the bleeding substantially within 10 minutes and allow inspection and painless cautery and, if required, packing.

In profuse anterior epistaxis, the injection of 1 to 2 mL of 1% Xylocaine with 1:100,000 epinephrine near the bleeding vessel only will increase vasoconstriction but also can slow bleeding by increasing the submucosal pressure on the vessel. Subsequently, electrocautery or chemical cautery with silver nitrate sticks can be applied.

Prevention

Patients with a history of anterior epistaxis should be taught first aid measures to employ if bleeding restarts, including appropriate anterior pressure, use of nasal lubricants, and avoidance of trauma, such as nose picking.

Patients using prescribed nasal sprays should be directed to aim them laterally and not toward the septum and to stop the sprays if bleeding occurs.[3] A Merocel (Xomed Inc., Jacksonville, Florida) sponge cut into several pieces and given to a patient with a history of anterior epistaxis may allow that patient to self-treat anterior epistaxis and avoid an emergency room visit. Recently, a device called NasalCEASE (Les Laboratoires Brothier, Nanterre Cedex, France), available in Europe as an over-the-counter product for 50 years, has become available in the United States. NasalCEASE is a specific calcium alginate product that has been shown to cause coagulation via platelet aggregation and plasmatic coagulation.[4] The patient places the sterile pack in the nose for a half hour and then removes it. To date there are no reports of toxic shock syndrome associated with the product. Patients who are prone to nosebleeds should be apprised of the medications that can cause coagulopathy and promote bleeding (**Table 44.2**).

Endoscopic Evaluation and Management

Patients with an easily seen anterior site of bleeding can be effectively treated with digital pressure, vasoconstrictors, and directed cautery and packing, if required. For patients with recurrent or posterior bleeding, endoscopic

Table 44.2 Medications That Can Prolong Bleeding

Advil	BC Cold Powder	Congesprinin
Alcohol	BC Powders	Cope
Aleve	Brufen	Coricidin
Alka-Seltzer	Buff-A-Com	Coumadin
Anacin	Buffadyne	Darvon with ASA
Anaprox	Bufferin	Darvon Compound
Anaproxn	Buffex	Daypro
Ansaid	Butalbital	Disalcid Tabs and Caps
Arthritis Pain Formula	Cama Arthritis Pain Reliever	Doan's Pills
Acetylsalicylic acid (ASA)	Cama-Inlay tabs	Dolia
Ascriptin	Caprin Capsules	Dolobid
Ascodeen-30	Casprin	Dristan
Aspercream	Cephagesic	Duradyne
Aspergum	Cheracol Caps	Duragesic
Aspirin	Children's aspirin	Easprin
Bayer Aspirin	Clinoril	Ecotrin
Baycol	Conaterol	Emprinin

(Continued on page 418)

Table 44.2 *(Continued)* **Medications That Can Prolong Bleeding**

Emprazil	Monacet with Codeine	Stendin
Equagesic	Momentum Muscle Back Formula	Stero-Darvon with Aspirin
Excedrin	Motrin	Supac
Feldene	Naprosyn	SX-65 Compound
Fiorinal	Norgesic	Synalgos Capsules
Flurbiprophen sodium	Nuprin	Synalgos DC
Four-Way Cold Tablets	Omega 3	Talwin
Ginkgo biloba	Pabirin Tablets	Tolectin
Goody's Extra Strength	Panadynes	Toradol
Ibuprofen	Panalgesic	Trandale
Indocin	Pepto-Bismol	Trental
Indomethacin	Percodan	Triaminicin
Lescol	Percodan-Demi	Trialgesic
Lipitor	Persantine	Trilisate
Magsal Tablets	Pravachol	Ursinus Inlay
Measurin	Quagesic	Vanquish
Meclomen	Relafen	Vitamin E
Medipren	Robaxisal	Vivo Med
Mevacor	Rufen	Voltaren
Midol Caplets	Simvastatin	Wesprin
Midol-200	Sine-Aid	Zactrin
Midol PMS	Soma Compound	Zorpin
Mobigesic Tablets	Stanback Powder/Max Powder	

assessment in an anesthetized and decongested state is optimal. The best chance of controlling epistaxis with the least intervention is the accurate visual localization of the bleeding before the nasal mucosa is traumatized with packing and cautery. Merocel packs can be trimmed to precise sizes to tamponade the bleeding and underlain with an absorbable collagen hemostatic material such as Helistat (Colla-Tech Inc., Plainsboro, New Jersey) or Avitene (Med Chem Products, Inc., Woburn, Massachusetts), which will not require removal. The mucosa will thus be protected from rebleeding when the nonabsorbable pack is removed. If the bleeding site can be accurately identified endoscopically, then cautery directed to the bleeding site is highly effective, and further packing may be unnecessary. The offending vessel may often be seen endoscopically as a raised bump protruding above the level of the mucous membrane. Gently touching it will produce bleeding, confirming this as the source. This may be accomplished in the office or emergency department; however, if endoscopically directed suction cautery

is required, then the patient is best taken to the surgical suite for general anesthesia, as it is quite difficult to achieve the level of anesthesia or instrumentation required for suction cautery outside the operating room.

Anterior Nasal Packing

Many materials are available for packing. The long, narrow ribbons of petroleum-impregnated gauze that require a layered placement from anterior to posterior and inferior to superior to prevent dislodgement down the nasopharynx and into the airway have been replaced in many centers with compressed synthetic material such as Merocel, which expands when inflated with liquid (blood, saline, oxymetazoline, or antibiotic solutions). Success rates with these types of materials are high, and even inexperienced clinicians can place these effectively, although such instrumentation should be discouraged by inexperienced clinicians in patients with coagulopathies.

Nasal packs (Rapid Rhino by Applied Therapeutics, Tampa, Florida) that are coated with a nonadherent gel knit (which activates platelet aggregation) and inflated with air once inserted and deflated prior to removal are more expensive (around $20 per device) but may be more comfortable. After packing, the oropharynx should be inspected. If blood is still running down the posterior pharynx, then the patient will require repacking, surgical or embolic intervention, or a posterior pack. Nonabsorbable packing is usually removed after 72 hours, and prophylactic antibiotics are generally given.

Posterior Nasal Packing

Fewer than 5% of all cases of epistaxis arise from a posterior source. Posterior packs are placed when an anterior pack is inadequate in controlling the bleeding and other options, such as embolization and surgical ligation, are not readily available. A posterior pack is made of rolled gauze secured with umbilical tape. Three long ties are attached to the pack. A slender catheter is inserted into each side of the nose, and this is grasped when it enters the oropharynx. Each catheter is secured to a tie on the posterior pack. The catheters are then backed out of the nose, bringing the attached posterior pack into position in the nasopharynx. The catheters are removed, and the ties are secured together around the columella. A pad should be placed to prevent pressure on the columella. The third tie is left long in the oropharynx and frequently brought out through the mouth and taped to the cheek to allow future removal of the pack. Posterior packs may be left in place for up to 3 to 5 days. Anterior packing is usually placed simultaneously. With the posterior pack in place, the danger of the anterior pack slipping backward into the nasopharynx and the airway is prevented. Patients require in-hospital observation during this period.

Long Merocel sponges can sometimes provide adequate posterior compression, as can balloon catheters. Balloon catheters can be slowly deflated and reinflated if bleeding restarts. Balloon catheters, including Foley catheters, often do not provide as precise a pressure as other packs.

Complications of Nasal Packing

Nasal packing, especially posterior packs, are associated with significant morbidity and sometimes death. Complications include the following:

1. Mucosal trauma and initiation of new sites of bleeding
2. Vagal response (bradycardia, hypotension, and apnea)
3. Dislodgement and aspiration of pack with airway obstruction
4. Infection and toxic shock syndrome
5. Hypoxia and worsening of sleep apnea

To minimize complications, packing should be placed carefully. Prophylactic antibiotics and supplemental oxygen should be given. Oversedation should be avoided, and a pulse oximeter in the patient with a posterior pack should be considered, especially in patients with other medical problems. Packing material less likely to cause toxic shock syndrome such as Merocel should be used rather than ribbon gauze. Toxic shock syndrome should be suspected if the patient develops a fever associated with rash, vomiting, diarrhea, and hypotension. Toxic shock syndrome is caused by an overgrowth of strains of *Staphylococcus aureus*, which produces the exotoxin toxic shock syndrome toxin-1 (TSST-1).

Coagulopathy

In the face of severe uncorrected coagulopathy, epistaxis interventions are frequently unsuccessful. The coagulation defect should be corrected, if possible. If this is not possible, then using absorbable packing with hemostatic properties, for example, FloSeal (Fusion Medical Technologies, Fremont, California), is recommended. Salt pork has been used for nasal packing in patients with thrombocytopenia. Salt pork contains an aqueous factor that induces platelet aggregation and is less irritating to the mucosa to remove than gauze packs. Pork nasal packs should not be used in patients who avoid pork for religious reasons. In coagulopathic patients, placing a nonabsorbable pack that must later be removed can lead to a cycle of bleeding from mucosal areas abraded by the pack. Before resorting to packing, apply topical vasoconstrictors such as oxymetazoline every 2 hours as needed. Saline sprays to minimize anterior nasal dryness are frequently employed to prevent continued bleeding from anterior nasal crusting. Although packs are seldom left in for more than 3 to 5 days because of concerns about infection, in the severely coagulopathic patient, packing can be left longer.

Hereditary Telangiectasia

Patients with repeated bleeding, a family history of bleeding, or telangiectasias of the tongue, lips, or fingertips may have hereditary telangiectasias, also known as Osler-Weber-Rendu disease. Treatment in these cases may involve argon laser cautery, although this is usually a temporary solution. Septal dermoplasty will provide longer relief. Surgeons working in the British health care system have advocated surgical nasal closure.[5] A reversible approach is alternating obstruction between the two sides of the nose with the use of cotton balls coated with petroleum jelly. These patients require further evaluation to rule out intestinal telangiectasia and pulmonary arteriovenous malformations.

Vascular Supply and Surgical Approaches

Either surgical ligation or embolization should be pursued in the patient with persistent epistaxis despite anterior and possibly posterior packing. The blood supply of the nose and the directed interventions are discussed anatomically in this section.

Both the internal and external carotid systems supply the nose. The sphenopalatine artery, a branch of the internal maxillary artery, which arises from the external carotid, is the main blood supply to the nose. The sphenopalatine artery enters through the sphenopalatine foramen at the posterior insertion of the middle turbinate and sends lateral nasal branches forward on both surfaces of the conchae (partly in bony canals), as well as a posterior septal arterial branch that crosses the back of the nasal cavity below the sphenoid sinus ostium and runs forward along the septum to anastomose with the nasopalatine artery, which enters through the incisive foramen. Surgical ligation or cautery of the sphenopalatine artery can be accomplished externally via a transantral (Caldwell-Luc) approach or endoscopically. In the external approach, an incision is made in the buccal mucosa overlying the maxillary sinus, and both the anterior and posterior bony walls of the maxillary sinus are removed. Behind the posterior bone of the maxillary sinus lie the internal maxillary artery and its divisions. A microscope facilitates the clipping of this tangled net of vessels. It is usually not possible to clearly distinguish the internal maxillary artery from its branches.

Recently, endoscopic clipping of the sphenopalatine artery as it exits the posterior maxillary sinus via the sphenopalatine foramen has greatly reduced the morbidity and time required to ligate this vessel.[6] Profuse bleeding, however, will make the endoscopic approach impossible.

The facial artery supplies the nasal cavity via three branches: (1) the septal branch of the superior labial artery, (2) small vessels from the lateral nasal artery that pierce the ala to supply the lateral vestibule, and (3) branches from the ascending palatine artery that serve the posterior lateral nasal cavity.

Over 90% of cases of epistaxis originate at the anterior nasal septum (Little's area) at the confluence of the labial, sphenopalatine, and ethmoidal arteries (Kisselbach's plexus). The vast majority of these are self-limited and respond to anterior pressure or packing. Bilateral ligation of the labial artery has recently been suggested as a treatment of refractory or recurrent cases of anterior epistaxis in the pediatric population. The labial artery enters the nose just anterior to the inferior turbinate and courses along the floor of the nose in the mucocutaneous junction of the vestibule, then branches onto the nasal septum in multiple directions. Under light general anesthesia in children, a 2–0 Vicryl suture is passed beneath the blood vessel in the mucocutaneous junction on the floor of the nose, followed by chemical or electrocautery of distal branches.[7]

The anterior and posterior ethmoidal branches of the ophthalmic artery enter the nasal cavity by way of the cribriform plate and supply the septum and lateral walls of the nose. Only these arteries are derived from the internal carotid; all others are from the external carotid. Iatrogenic injury during endoscopic sinus surgery to the anterior ethmoidal artery as it traverses intranasally from the ethmoidal foramen through the ethmoid sinus at the back of the frontal recess before entering the cribriform can also result in epistaxis. Retraction of the artery within the orbit can lead to orbital bleeding and require urgent orbital decompression. Surgical ligation of the anterior ethmoidal artery is usually accomplished with an external incision along the medial orbit to access the artery prior to its entrance into the ethmoidal foramen. A gull wing incision is made to minimize contracture, and the artery is identified 24 mm from the anterior lacrimal crest. The vessel is clipped and ligated under direct vision. Bleeding from the superior portion of the nose is suspicious for an ethmoidal artery origin. In some cases, if the site of bleeding cannot be identified, then simultaneous ligation of both the anterior ethmoidal artery and the internal maxillary artery may be appropriate. Ligation is recommended only when patients fail to stop bleeding with anterior nasal packing and/or nasopharyngeal packing or balloon tamponade.[8]

Embolization

Selective embolization of the internal maxillary artery with or without the facial artery is successful in 66 to 97% of cases.[9,10] Unilateral embolization is performed unless the side cannot be localized with certainty, in which case bilateral embolization can be performed. In some institutions embolization is more effective than external ligation, but overall, ligation is more effective. A literature review of external ligation showed an average failure rate of 10% compared with an embolization failure rate of 20% between 1965 and 1995. Embolization is less expensive and associated with fewer minor complications than external ligation techniques. The incidence of major complications between the two procedures is similar, at 4%. Major complications from external ligation include coma, myocardial infarctions, oral antral fistulas, and septal perforations. Major complications from embolization are more serious and include hemiplegia, facial nerve paralysis, and myocardial infarction. Embolization is sometimes used after failure to obtain control through ligation techniques and vice versa. The average age of failure with either ligation or embolization is 71 years, which is 10 to 15 years older than the average age of patients treated with ligation or embolization. The cause of failure in the older patient may be due to collateral flow. The major limitation to the use of embolization techniques is lack of availability of this option in most nontertiary medical centers.[11] Embolization is contraindicated in patients intolerant of radiographic dye or those in whom the source of bleeding is from a branch of the internal carotid system.

Conclusion

The treatment of epistaxis ranges from the simple to the complex, with potentially life-threatening complications. There is no one answer for any patient, and each must be approached thoughtfully in a stepwise fashion until control is achieved. Advances in hemostatic agents and endoscopic and radiographic embolization techniques are reducing the morbidity and failure rate in controlling epistaxis.

References

1. Tomkinson A, Roblin DG, Flanagan P, Quine SM, Backhouse S. Patterns of hospital attendance with epistaxis. Rhinology 1997;35(3):129–131.
2. Tan LK, Calhoun KH. Epistaxis. Med Clin North Am 1999; 83(1):43–56.
3. Ferguson BJ. Nasal steroid sprays and septal perforations. Ear Nose Throat J 1997;76(2):75–76.
4. Benninger MS, Marple BF. Minor recurrent epistaxis: prevalence and a new method for management. Otolaryngol Head Neck Surg 2004;131(3):317–320.
5. Lund VJ, Howard DJ. A treatment algorithm for the management of epistaxis in hereditary hemorrhagic telangiectasia. Am J Rhinol 1999;13(4):319–322.
6. Snyderman CH, Goldman SA, Carrau RL, Ferguson BJ, Grandis JR. Endoscopic sphenopalatine artery ligation is an effective method of treatment for posterior epistaxis. Am J Rhinol 1999;13:137–140.
7. Adornato SG. Epistaxis: new approach [letter to the editor]. Otolaryngol Head Neck Surg 2000;123:524.
8. Schaitkin B, Strauss M, Houck JR. Epistaxis: medical versus surgical therapy—a comparison of efficacy, complications, and economic considerations. Laryngoscope 1987;97(12): 1392–1396.
9. Moreau S, De Rugy MG, Babin E, Courtheoux P, Valdoazo A. Supraselective embolization in intractable epistaxis: review of 45 cases. Laryngoscope 1998;108:887–888.
10. Myssiorek D, Lodespoto M. Embolization of posterior epistaxis. Am J Rhinol 1993;7:223–226.
11. Cullen MM, Tami TA. Comparison of internal maxillary artery ligation versus embolization for refractory posterior epistaxis. Otolaryngol Head Neck Surg 1998;118: 636–642.

VI
Pediatrics

Decision tree for adenotonsillectomy

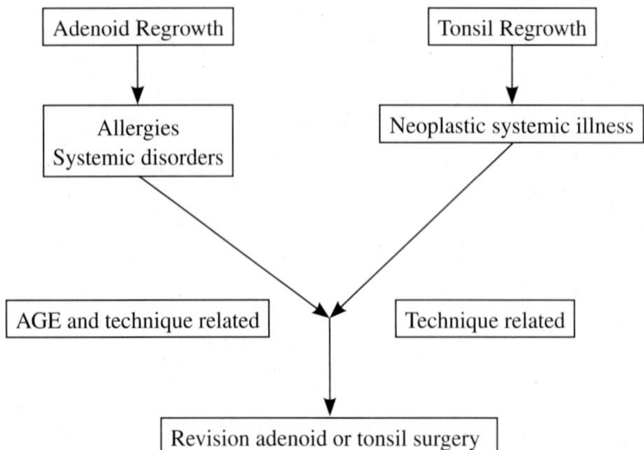

45 Revision Adenotonsillectomy

Ashutosh Kacker and Lianne M. de Serres

The need for revision adenotonsillectomy is not common, but it does occur on occasion. The failure of initial surgery may be related to patient or physician factors. To understand the regrowth of adenoids or tonsils, a comprehensive understanding of the anatomy of the nasopharynx, oropharynx, and Waldeyer ring, as well as the disease processes and surgical techniques, is required. Sometimes the recurrence of symptoms does not correlate with adenotonsillar hypertrophy.

Anatomy of the Nasopharynx, Oropharynx, and Waldeyer Ring

The nasopharynx lies between the soft palate and the nasal choanae and communicates with the nasal cavities, eustachian tube, and oropharynx. The boundaries of the nasopharynx are the free edge of the soft palate anteriorly, posteriorly by the pharyngeal wall, and laterally by the palatopharyngeal arches. In the newborn, the nasopharynx is short and follows a gentle curve (small anteroposterior diameter), whereas the nasopharynx and oropharynx form an angle of almost 90 degrees by puberty. The adenoids are located in the roof of the nasopharynx at the skull base.

The oropharynx is the posterior continuation of the oral cavity beyond the tonsillar pillars. The anterior palatine pillar is formed by the palatoglossus muscles, the posterior palatine pillar by the palatopharyngeus muscles. Between the two arches are the palatine tonsils. At birth, the base of the tongue and the larynx are high in the neck, with the epiglottis overlapping the soft palate. The base of the tongue and the larynx descend with growth and reach the adult location by age 4, when the base of the tongue and the lingual tonsils form a part of the anteroinferior wall of the oropharynx. The oropharynx is lined with stratified squamous epithelium. The lamina propria contains connective tissue, seromucinous glands, and numerous neutrophils, lymphocytes, and plasma cells.

A ring of lymphoid tissue, called the Waldeyer ring, encircles the proximal end of the aerodigestive tract. This structure is comprised of three major lymphoid aggregates (pharyngeal tonsils and adenoids, palatine tonsils, and lingual tonsils) and four minor lymphoid aggregates (tubal tonsils, lateral pharyngeal bands, pharyngeal granulations, and lymphoid tissue in the laryngeal ventricle).

The pharyngeal tonsil tissue (adenoids) is located in the roof of the nasopharynx, is noncapsulated, and is covered with respiratory epithelium. The adenoids increase in size after birth and usually atrophy by puberty. The palatine tonsils are oval lymphoid masses that lie in the tonsillar fossae, capsulated by the pharyngobasilar fascia, and lined by stratified squamous epithelium. The lingual tonsil tissue located in the base of the tongue is last to develop and persists into adult life.

Examination of the Nasopharynx

Conventionally, adenoidal size has been assessed using high kilovoltage lateral soft tissue films of the neck (**Fig. 45.1**), but flexible fiberoptic examination of the nasopharynx has become the gold standard (**Fig. 45.2**). Assessing the degree of adenoidal hypertrophy involves consideration of the size of the adenoid relative to the choanal openings. An obstruction of the nasopharynx > 50% or an adenoid-to-choana ratio > 0.6 is usually associated with symptomatic obstruction.[1–3] Flexible fiberoptic endoscopy helps to rule out other causes of nasal/nasopharyngeal obstruction, such as choanal narrowing, polypoid disease, posterior turbinate hypertrophy, and nasopharyngeal neoplasms that may be missed on traditional radiographs.

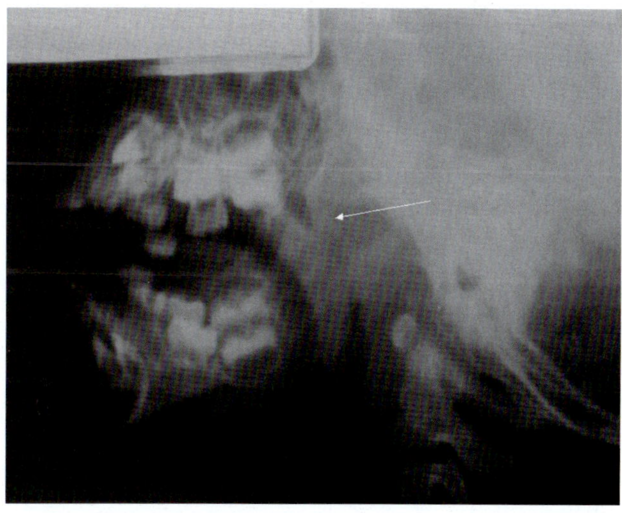

Fig. 45.1 X-ray showing adenoidal hypertrophy.

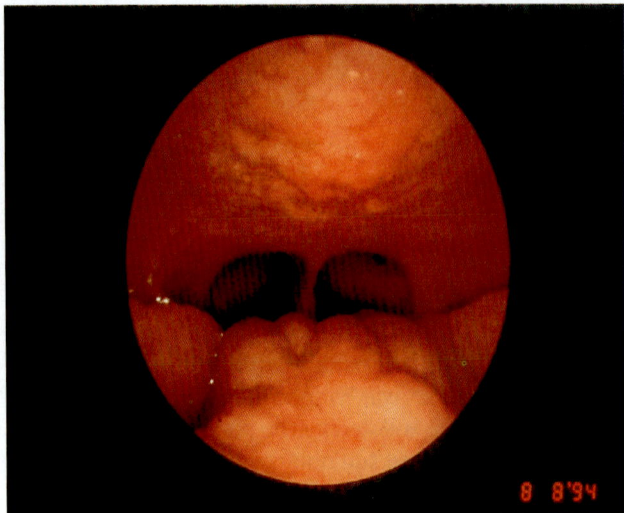

Fig. 45.2 Endoscopic picture showing adenoidal hypertrophy.

Adenoid Regrowth

Adenoid regrowth should be suspected in patients with recurrent symptoms of nasal obstruction, that is, snoring, mouth breathing, and/or hyponasal speech. The incidence of symptomatic adenoidal regrowth is unknown, but it is felt to be very low. In the study by Buchinsky et al, only 1 in 175 (0.6%) patients developed adenoidal regrowth after adenoidectomy that required revision surgery.[4] In the same study, 46 had at least one symptom suggestive of nasopharyngeal obstruction, out of which 35 underwent a flexible fiberoptic nasopharyngeal examination that revealed < 40% nasopharyngeal obstruction in all patients.

Adenoid regrowth can occur, secondary to patient factors or surgical technique at the primary procedure. Age may contribute to adenoid regrowth, as very young children have a very small nasopharynx, and both visualization and complete excision can be difficult. Patients who are on an immunosuppression regimen after solid organ transplantation or are immunodeficient (human immunodeficiency virus (HIV) or acquired immunodeficiency syndrome (AIDS) positive) mount a nonspecific response to antigens leading to lymphoid hypertrophy.[5] Biopsy or complete removal of these tissues is recommended to rule out a lymphoproliferative disorder. Once the diagnosis of lymphoma is excluded, patients on immunosuppression are treated with reduction in immunosuppressive medications, and immunodeficient patients are treated for the underlying disease.

Patients with hypertrophy of minor lymphoid aggregates may require surgical excision of this tissue. Patients with severe allergies can also present with lymphoid hypertrophy, particularly of choanal adenoidal tissue, which may be managed initially with nasal steroids and control of allergies.[6] Surgical excision is required if symptoms persist despite an adequate medication trial.

Adenoid regrowth can also occur after a superior or partial adenoidectomy has been performed. This procedure is typically performed in patients in whom there is a concern for postoperative hypernasality, such as patients who have had a cleft palate repair, patients with a submucous cleft of the palate, and patients who have a history of nasal regurgitation or preoperative hypernasality.[7]

In these instances, only the superior adenoids around the torus tubarius are removed. These patients can require revision adenoidectomy if the lower portion of the adenoid pad hypertrophies further.

Tonsillar Regrowth

Regrowth of the palatine tonsils is less common than the adenoids because the palatine tonsils are encapsulated. The incidence of palatine tonsil regrowth is also not known. The most common reason for tonsillar regrowth is incomplete removal at the time of the initial surgical procedure. An inferior pole remnant can hypertrophy over time, and if this remnant is large enough, it could be a source of recurrent tonsillitis and, less commonly, a source of recurrent pharyngeal obstruction. The inferior tonsillar pole may be incompletely removed because the boundaries between the inferior palatine tonsil pole and lingual tonsil can be indistinct. Surgeons may choose to be more conservative in this region to avoid the very vascular base of the tongue region,

Table 45.1 Surgical Techniques

Adenoidectomy
Curet adenoidectomy
Adenotome
Bovie adenoidectomy
Laser-assisted adenoidectomy
Endoscope-assisted adenoidectomy
Power-assisted adenoidectomy
Tonsillectomy
Cold tonsillectomy (knife/snare techniques)
Bovie tonsillectomy
Laser tonsillectomy
Harmonic scalpel
Partial adenoidectomy
Superior adenoidectomy for palatal abnormalities
Tonsillotomy/partial tonsillectomy
Tonsils are debulked in a subcapsular fashion using powered instrumentation (microdébrider)

Table 45.2 Causes of Adenoid and Tonsillar Regrowth

Patient factors
Age
Post-transplantation lymphoproliferative disorder
Hypertrophy of minor lymphoid aggregates
Immune deficiency syndromes (e.g., HIV disease)
Atopy
Surgical techniques
Unintentional incomplete removal
Partial adenoidectomy
Partial tonsillectomy

particularly when operating for obstructing hypertrophic tonsils and absolute removal of the tonsil is less important.

Tonsillar regrowth may be seen more frequently with a newer procedure for tonsillectomy. Intracapsular partial tonsillectomy recently has been introduced as a means to remove obstructing tonsillar tissue. This procedure involves removal of tonsillar tissue by means of a microdébrider, leaving the tonsillar capsule intact and a very thin layer of residual tonsillar tissue. Early experience with this procedure reveals improvement in postoperative pain over standard methods because the pharyngeal musculature is left unexposed. However, there have been a few instances in which residual tonsillar tissue has regrown, necessitating revision subcapsular tonsillectomy (personal communication, Peter Koltai, M.D., September 2001). Long-term follow-up of patients will be required to ascertain the rate of symptomatic tonsillar regrowth using this technique (**Tables 45.1, 45.2, and 45.3**).

Surgical Management of Adenoidal and Tonsillar Regrowth

Tonsillar regrowth usually is managed by routine tonsillectomy as per the experience of the treating otolaryngologist. This can be accomplished using the electrocautery, cold knife, CO_2 laser, or, as recently described, harmonic scalpel. Revision adenoidectomy may require modification

Table 45.3 Management of Adenoid and Tonsillar Regrowth

Medical management
Control of environmental allergy
Reduction of immunosuppression in transplant patients
Surgical management
Revision adenoidectomy
Revision tonsillectomy

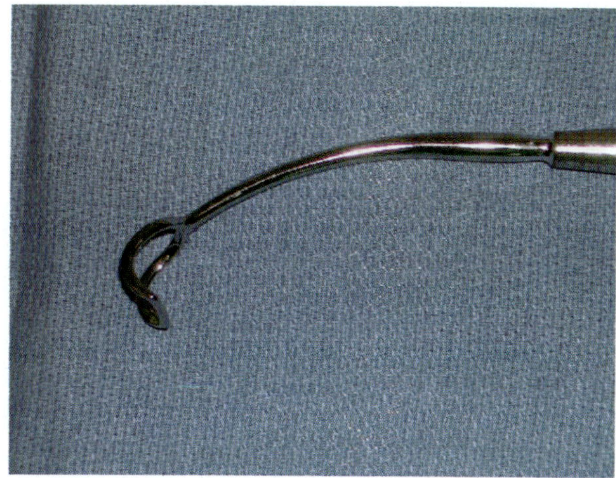

Fig. 45.3 Adenoidectomy curet.

of the surgical technique to adequately address the regrowth of tissue (**Figs. 45.3, 45.4**).

The use of endoscopes may provide improved visualization, especially in the region of the nasal choanae and the pharyngeal recess.[8] In addition, the use of powered instrumentation may enhance complete excision, although there are no data supporting the superior nature of this technique.[9,10]

Conclusion

Adenotonsillar regrowth is uncommon, although adenoidal regrowth is more common. Common reasons for regrowth include incomplete surgical excision at the initial procedure, young age, and immunosuppresion/immunodeficiency syndromes. Revision adenoidectomy may require modification in surgical technique to adequately clear the nasopharynx of obstructing tissue.

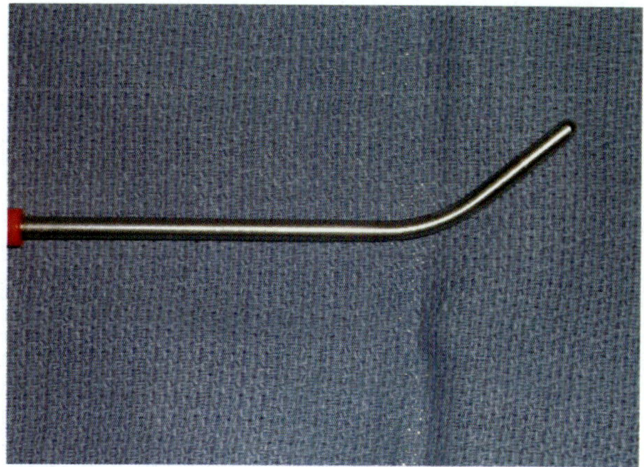

Fig. 45.4 Microdébrider blade for adenoidectomy.

References

1. Wormald PJ, Prescott CA. Adenoids: comparison of radiological assessment methods with clinical and endoscopic findings. J Laryngol Otol 1992;106:342–344.
2. Kemaloglu YK, Goksu N, Inal E, Akyildiz N. Radiographic evaluation of children with nasopharyngeal obstruction due to the adenoid. Ann Otol Rhinol Laryngol 1999;108:67–72.
3. Elwany S. The adenoidal-nasopharyngeal ratio (AN ratio): its validity in selecting children for adenoidectomy. J Laryngol Otol 1987;101:569–573.
4. Buchinsky FJ, Lowry MA, Isaacson G. Do adenoids regrow after excision? Otolaryngol Head Neck Surg 2000;123:576–581.
5. Huang RY, Shapiro NL. Adenotonsillar enlargement in pediatric patients following solid organ transplantation. Arch Otolaryngol Head Neck Surg 2000;126:159–164.
6. Demain JG, Goetz DW. Pediatric adenoidal hypertrophy and nasal airway obstruction: reduction with aqueous nasal beclomethasone. Pediatrics 1995;95:355–364.
7. Kakani RS, Callan ND, April MM. Superior adenoidectomy in children with palatal abnormalities. Ear Nose Throat J 2000;79:303–305.
8. Cannon CR, Replogle WH, Schenk MP. Endoscopic-assisted adenoidectomy. Otolaryngol Head Neck Surg 1999;121:740–744.
9. Stanislaw P Jr, Koltai PJ, Feustel PJ. Comparison of power-assisted adenoidectomy vs adenoid curette adenoidectomy. Arch Otolaryngol Head Neck Surg 2000;126:845–849.
10. Yanagisawa E, Weaver EM. Endoscopic adenoidectomy with the microdebrider. Ear Nose Throat J 1997;76:72–74.

Decision tree for initial presentation

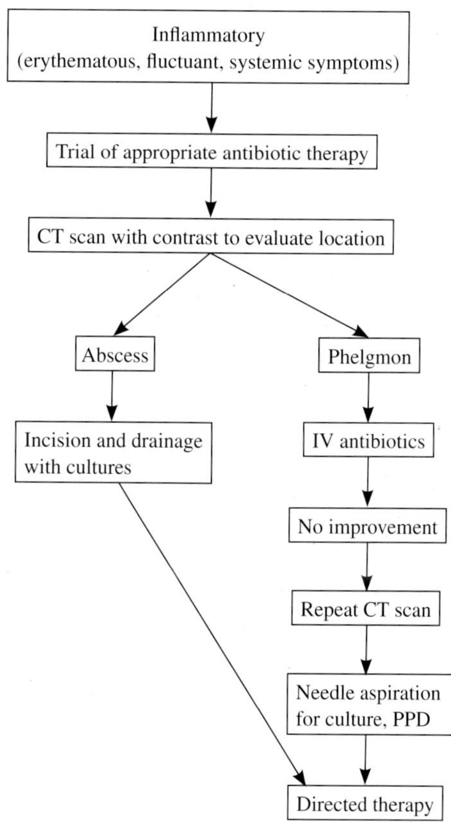

Decision tree for recurrent neck mass

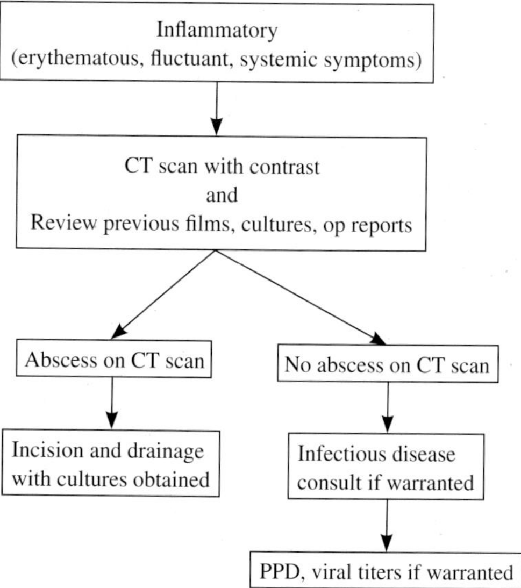

Decision tree for initial presentation

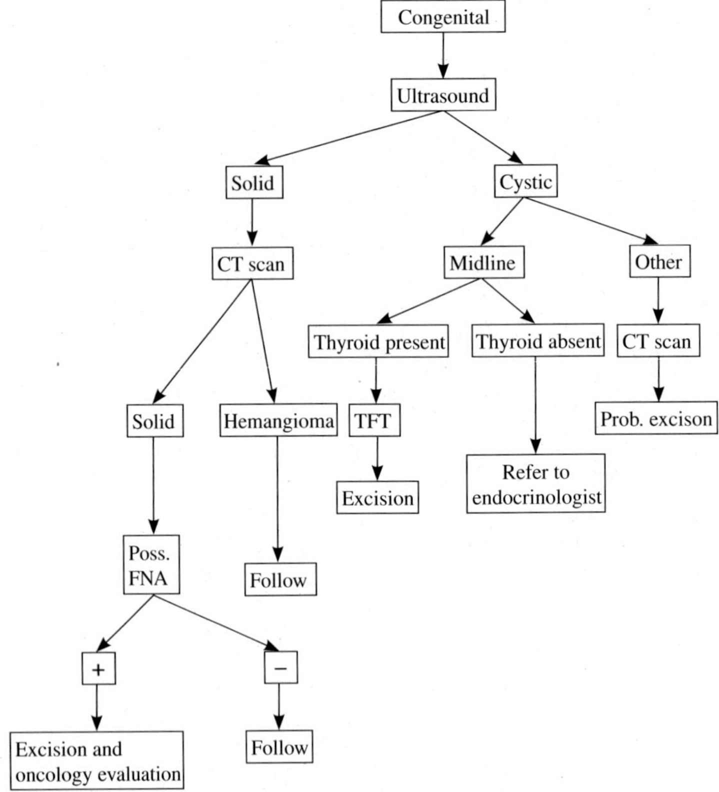

Decision tree for recurrent neck masses

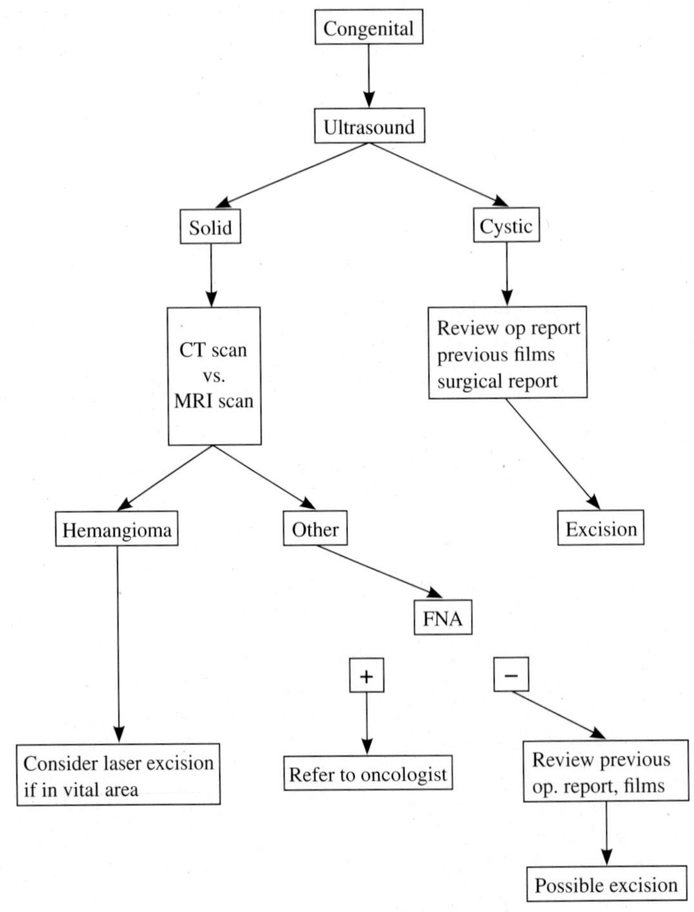

46 Recurrent Neck Masses in Children

Jacqueline E. Jones

The management of recurrent neck masses in children can be difficult. One must weigh the concerns of malignancy against the possibility of overtreatment of these lesions, which will overwhelmingly be benign. This chapter uses four sample case studies to examine the main types of masses: inflammatory, congenital, and malignant.

It is estimated that 50% of all 2-year-old children have palpable cervical adenopathy.[1] Inflammatory masses are usually associated with signs of an upper respiratory tract infection, such as fever, rhinorrhea, and tenderness over the mass. The mass can be warm to the touch with associated overlying erythema and edema. Congenital lesions are usually slower growing and on appearance are soft. Malignant lesions show persistent growth and are commonly fixed and hard to palpation. In the surgical management of neck masses, care should be taken to preserve landmarks that may be useful if the masses reoccur. In evaluating recurrent neck masses in the postoperative period, a thorough evaluation should be obtained to rule out complications of surgery as compared with a recurrence (i.e., a seroma or stitch abscess that may mimic a recurrent mass).

Inflammatory Neck Masses

Palpable lymphadenopathy in the neck is a common finding. Any lymph node > 10 mm is characterized as cervical adenopathy.[2] The most common cause of cervical adenopathy in children is a viral infection of the upper respiratory tract. Most viral infections run their course within 7 to 10 days, and cervical adenopathy will usually resolve with the resolution of the virus. In a smaller number of cases the lymphadenopathy will remain for weeks to months, prompting visits to the physician for consultation. The more common viruses causing lymphadenopathy are Epstein-Barr virus, enterovirus, adenovirus, and human immunodeficiency virus (HIV).

Bacterial infections of the upper respiratory tract are also associated with cervical adenopathy. Bilateral cervical adenopathy is a frequent finding in children with group A β-hemolytic strep pharyngitis. *Streptococcus pneumoniae, Haemophilus influenzae,* and *Moraxella catarrhalis* are the most common organisms causing otitis media and sinusitis. Unilateral or bilateral cervical adenopathy can be associated with these infections as well. *Staphylococcus aureus* and group A *Streptococcus* are implicated in 60 to 85% of cases of unilateral cervical adenitis in children.[3] These infections usually occur when infection drains into a lymph node from a proximal site in the head and neck. These nodes are warm to the touch, soft, and painful. Cervical adenitis from these two organisms can be seen more commonly in neonates and young children.[4]

Unilateral cervical adenopathy can also be due to mycobacterium infections, cat scratch fever, and toxoplasmosis. Atypical mycobacterium infection is more commonly associated with unilateral cervical adenitis. These nodes are usually slow growing, with overlying erythema and thinning of the skin. If left untreated, fistula formation may occur.

The diagnostic work-up for children with recurrent neck masses requires a thorough history and physical exam. The findings of infection in other sites of the head and neck point to the primary cause of cervical adenitis, and appropriate culture and treatment should be undertaken. For children who have failed antibiotic therapy, a thorough laboratory evaluation for other infectious etiologies should be undertaken. This should include an evaluation for Epstein-Barr virus, cytomegalovirus (CMV), toxoplasmosis, and HIV. A computed tomography (CT) scan or magnetic resonance imaging (MRI) should be performed to more completely evaluate the mass and plan medical and, if needed, surgical therapy. If possible, the original CT and/or MRI should be obtained and compared with the postoperative films in the evaluation of recurrent masses. In the immediate postoperative period (i.e., the first 3 months), an ultrasound may be helpful to rule out a postoperative seroma.

Case 1

A 15-month-old female was presented to her pediatrician with a 4-day history of temperature to 104°F (40°C) and left neck swelling. She was diagnosed with cervical adenitis and started on antibiotics. The swelling worsened, and the child was admitted for intravenous (IV) antibiotics. Urine, blood, and cerebrospinal fluid (CSF) cultures were all negative. Her white blood cell (WBC) count was 10.9, and a chest x-ray was negative. Her condition worsened, and she was transferred to a tertiary care hospital for further evaluation. Upon admission she was noted to have

Decision tree for initial presentation

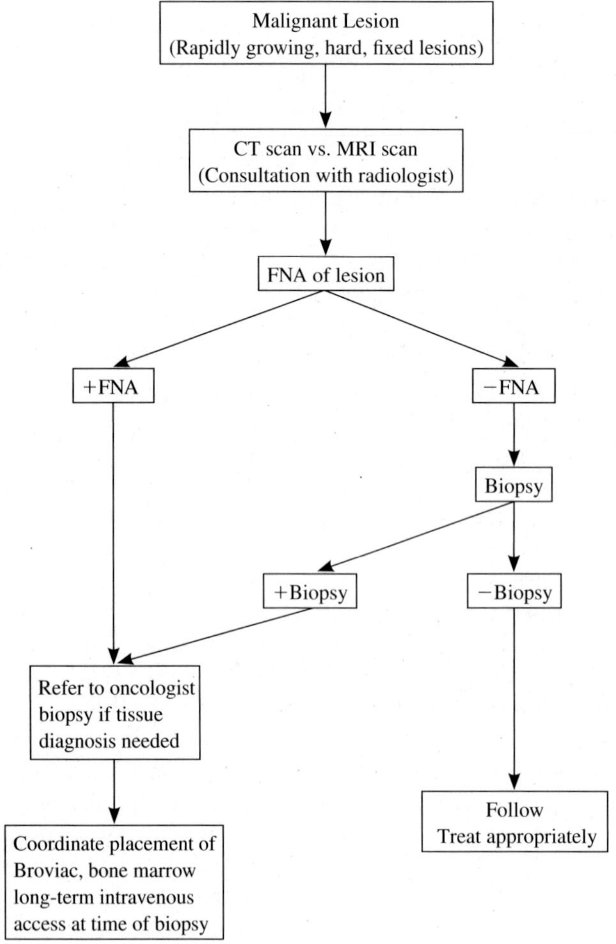

profound neck and facial swelling with respiratory distress from swelling in the floor of the mouth. She was brought to the operating room, where direct laryngoscopy revealed significant laryngeal edema. A tracheotomy was performed as well as incision and drainage of her neck abscesses. The patient was begun on clindamycin and cefuroxime. A CT scan was performed. Initial cultures grew only *S. aureus,* and the purified protein derivative (PPD) was negative. The patient was returned to the operating room 1 week later for extensive débridement of her neck. She was maintained on IV antibiotics and slowly improved. She was decannulated 1 month after admission and discharged to home.

Case 2

A 2-year-old female was transferred to a tertiary care hospital with persistent fevers and neck swelling following incision and drainage of a right lateral neck mass. The patient had a 4-day history of an upper respiratory tract infecction with fever and progressive neck swelling. She was started on oral antibiotics by her pediatrician with continued progression of her fevers and neck swelling. The child was admitted to a local hospital, where she was brought to the operating room, and incision and drainage of her right neck mass was performed. Postoperatively, she continued with fevers to 104°F (40°C) and an elevated WBC count. She was transferred to a tertiary care hospital for evaluation. Upon admission her WBC was 23,000, and she was febrile to 100.4°F (38°C). The right neck revealed a healing incision but was indurated and erythematous. A CT scan revealed a deep neck abscess as well as a continued small collection at the site of the previous incision. The patient was brought to the operating room, where neck exploration and drainage of the neck abscess with placement of a Penrose drain in the site occurred. She was maintained on a 10-day course of IV antibiotics, and the drain was removed on the 3rd postoperative day. Her fevers defervesced, and she was discharged home on postoperative day 10.

Congenital Neck Masses

The most common congenital lesions of the head and neck are lymphangiomas, hemangiomas, thyroglossal duct cysts, and branchial cleft cysts. Hemangiomas are the most common tumor of infancy. They have three phases of growth: rapid proliferation (3–9 months), a quiescent period of variable length, and a spontaneous, slow involution phase (18 months–10 years). MRI is extremely useful in confirming the diagnosis of hemangiomas.[2] Treatment of hemangiomas is required only if they impinge on vital structures (i.e., the subglottic space or orbit), as the vast majority will resolve without intervention. Venous malformations are located in the head and neck in 40% of cases. They are considered to belong to a group of benign vascular tumors that form in the head and neck. Physical examination reveals a soft, compressible mass that is red to bluish in color. Venous malformations do not undergo spontaneous involution as compared with hemangiomas. Diagnosis can be made by the use of MRI and CT. Treatment of these lesions requires a multimodality approach, including surgery, sclerosing agents, and medical therapy.[2]

Approximately 75% of lymphatic malformations occur in the neck. They are postulated to develop from sequestered lymphatic sacs that fail to communicate with peripheral drainage channels. Lymphangiomas are usually present at birth but can appear as late as 2 years of age.[3] Physical examination reveals a soft, compressible lesion that enlarges as the child grows. CT is helpful in delineating the extent of the lymphatic malformation and is an essential tool for preoperative planning. Treatment of lymphangiomas includes surgical excision or the injection of sclerosing agents into macrocystic lesions.[4] Because these lesions are benign, the sacrifice of vital structures in the surgical excision of these lesions is not advised.

Thyroglossal duct cysts are the most common midline neck masses in children. They arise from the thyroid anlage, which descends from the foramen cecum at the base of the tongue. The tract descends from the foramen cecum to pass in close proximity to the developing hyoid bone and terminates in the pyramidal lobe of the thyroid. A cyst may form anywhere along the path of its descent.[3] Thyroglossal duct cysts may occur at any time from early in childhood until adulthood. On examination they present as a midline neck mass that moves on protrusion of the tongue. An ultrasound may be helpful in differentiating these lesions from a reactive cervical lymph node. Because these lesions can become recurrently infected, surgical excision is recommended. Ultrasound is also useful in confirming the presence of the thyroid gland in the neck prior to the excision of a thyroglossal duct cyst. Failure to excise the midportion of the hyoid bone can lead to a 30% incidence of recurrence.

Branchial cleft cysts arise from remnants of the branchial apparatus. The vast majority of branchial cleft anomalies arise from the second branchial cleft system.[5] Physical examination reveals a cystic lesion of the anterior neck. These cysts are located most commonly on the left side in the anteroinferior cervical triangle. They enlarge slowly and may not present until later in life. Branchial cleft cysts that occur in childhood are usually associated with an acute infection of the cyst. Third and fourth branchial cleft cysts can occur in the neck but are infrequently seen. Branchial cleft sinuses and fistulas can present as draining lesions in the anterior neck. Secondary

Decision tree for recurrent neck masses

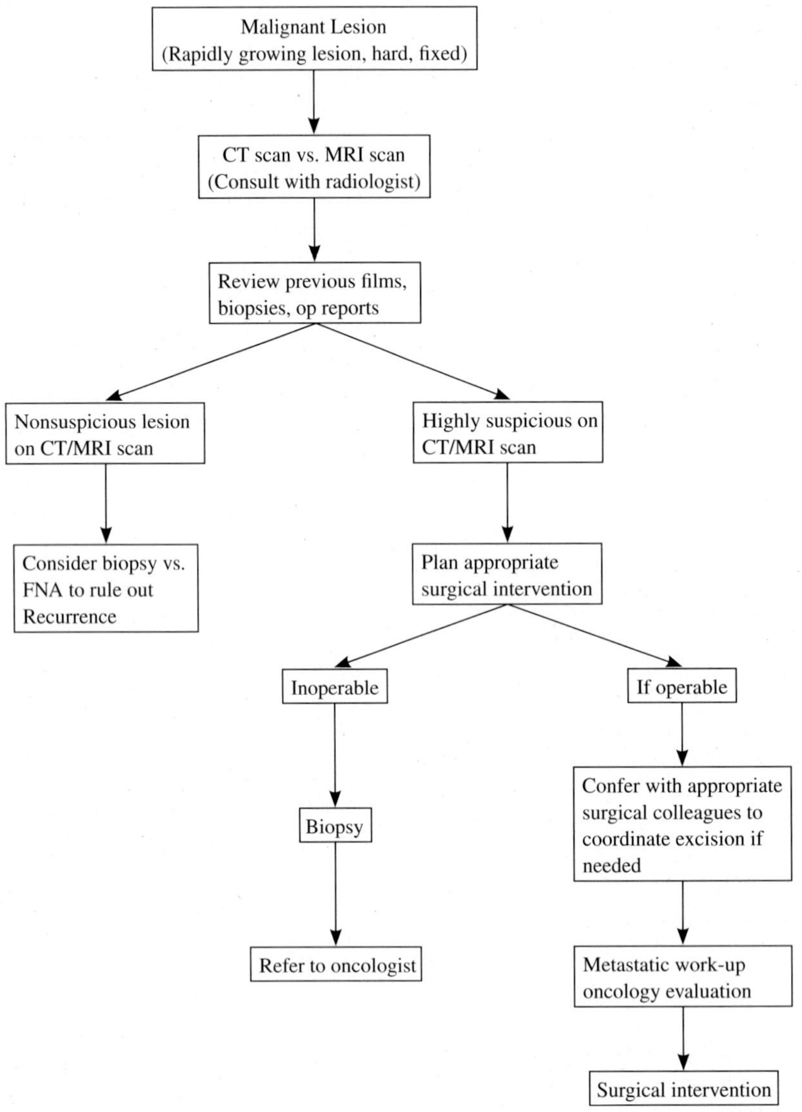

infections of these lesions can lead to erythema and edema of the fistula or sinus tract. MRI or CT scan can be useful in evaluating these lesions preoperatively to plan surgical excision. In rare cases a fistulogram may be required to delineate the course of a branchial cleft sinus or fistula. A barium swallow may help to identify the opening of a third branchial cleft abnormality in the pyriform sinus.[6] Failure to excise the entire tract will lead to a significant rate of recurrence. In evaluating recurrent lesions, a CT or MRI is of vital importance to plan appropriate surgical excision. In cases that are chronically infected, the use of IV antibiotics both pre- and postoperatively should be considered.

Other less common causes of congenital neck masses are the sternocleidomastoid tumor of infancy and cervical thymic cyst. Children with a sternocleidomastoid tumor of infancy usually present during the first 2 months of life with torticollis and a hard mass located within the sternocleidomastoid muscle. This mass is thought to result from contusion of the sternocleidomastoid muscle during delivery. However, such tumors can appear after cesarean section, and abnormal position in utero may play a role. CT scan or MRI confirms the presence of a fibrous mass within the sternocleidomastoid muscle. These tumors usually resolve by 1 year of age. Physical therapy for the resultant torticollis is helpful in preventing muscle contraction.

The cervical thymic cyst develops from the thymic primordia. The thymic primordia starts its descent at the pyriform sinus running through the thyroid membrane, emerging between the common carotid artery and the vagus nerve to descend posterior to the glossopharyngeal nerve and lateral to the thyroid membrane into the mediastinum. Once the thymic primordia merges at the midline, the thymic epithelium develops into lobules separated by mesenchymal septa.[7] Thymic cysts can form anywhere along the path of descent of the thymic primordia into the mediastinum. The typical clinical presentation is of a unilateral, slowly enlarging mass, which is painless. These lesions usually present by 10 years of age. Though benign in nature, they can cause compression of the trachea or esophagus with enlargement. Treatment is surgical excision.

Radiologic evaluation of congenital neck masses should include a CT or MRI for all lesions that are not midline in nature. Consultation with the radiologist should be obtained prior to obtaining a film in recurrent cases. Because sedation is commonly required in young children to obtain an adequate study, consultation with the radiologist will minimize the need for additional radiologic studies. Although few studies have documented the complication rate of revision surgery in children, experienced surgeons are aware that these cases can have a more difficult postoperative recovery with a higher complication rate.

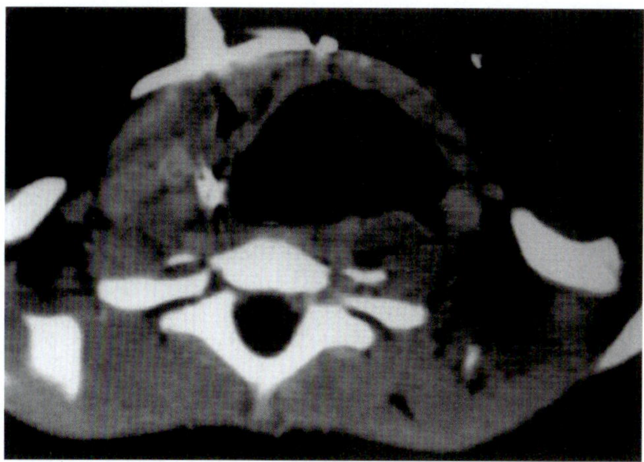

Fig. 46.1 Computed tomography scan of the neck showing a large, tubular, multiloculated cystic mass extending from the oropharynx to the superior mediastinum.

Case 3

A 3-year-old male was admitted due to an enlarging neck mass. He had been followed by his pediatrician for a "cyst" in the neck for the past several months. Over the previous 2 weeks his mother had noticed increasingly noisy breathing with decreased oral intake. Physical examination at the time of admission revealed a 16 cm painless mass located in the left neck, posterior to the sternocleidomastoid muscle. The trachea was deviated to the right. The patient was in extreme respiratory distress and was brought to the operating room, where an emergency tracheostomy was performed. A postprocedure CT scan (**Fig. 46.1**) revealed a large tubular, multiloculated mass extending from the oropharynx to the superior mediastinum. A fine needle aspiration biopsy was performed, which revealed benign cells. The patient underwent surgical excision of the mass (**Fig. 46.2**) and tolerated the procedure well. The pathology was

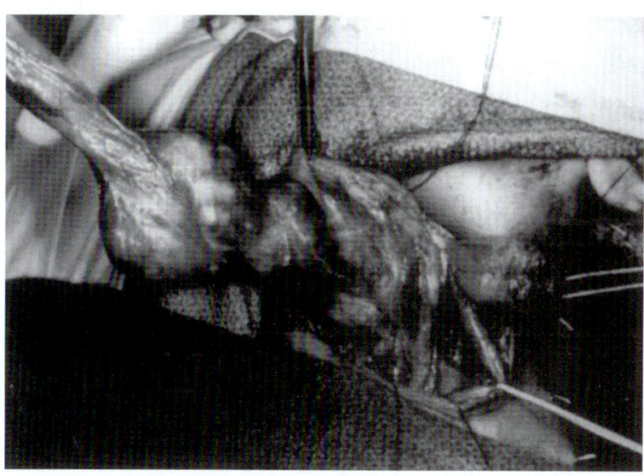

Fig. 46.2 Surgical excision of a large cystic mass from the right neck.

Decision tree for physical exam, laboratory evaluation, radiologic evaluation

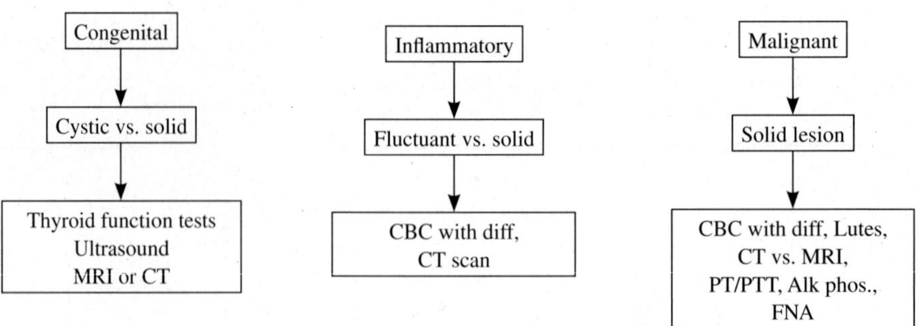

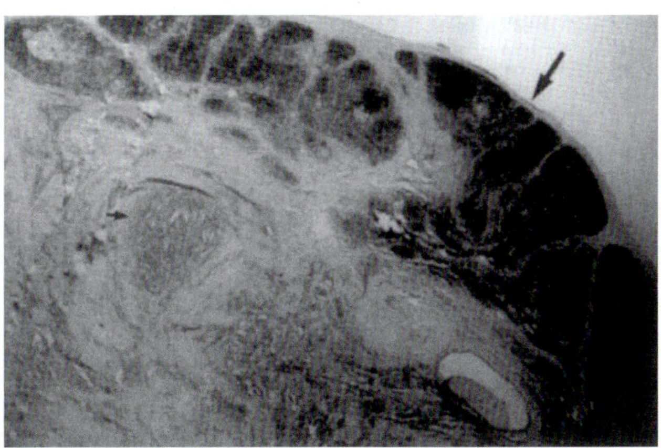

Fig. 46.3 Pathologic examination revealed cells consistent with a thymic cysts showing the characteristic findings of thymic tissue with Hassall corpuscles and cholesterol clefts in the cyst wall.

consistent with a thymic cyst (**Fig. 46.3**). The patient underwent a CT scan 3 months later that revealed no recurrence of the cyst.

Malignant Neck Masses

The vast majority of neck masses in children are benign in nature; however, the clinician must maintain a high level of suspicion so as not to delay the diagnosis in the rare case of malignancy. Following accidental death, cancer is the second most common cause of death in children. It is estimated that 27% of childhood malignancies present in the head and neck.[3] The most common malignant tumors found in the neck are lymphoid tumors such as Hodgkin disease and non-Hodgkin lymphoma.[8] These lymphoid malignancies account for 55% of all childhood cancer.[3] Lesions usually present as enlarging neck masses and can be associated in 30% of patients with constitutional symptoms, such as fever, malaise, night sweats, and weight loss.[8] These masses are usually seen in multiple locations in the neck. They are nontender and firm to the touch. A thorough examination of other sites such as the axilla and groin for evidence of pathologic adenopathy should be undertaken. Examination of the spleen and liver for hepatosplenomegaly should be performed. A CT scan will show the presence of multiple enlarged lymph nodes throughout the neck. Needle aspiration can be used in young children; however, cooperation in children younger than 10 years of age can be difficult. The risks of complications from attempting aspiration on an uncooperative child may outweigh the benefits of needle aspiration in the office. In revision cases where only a small mass may be present and may be difficult to locate in scar tissue,

CT-guided needle biopsy under general anesthesia should be considered. An open biopsy is generally required to confirm the pathologic diagnosis in younger or uncooperative children. When planning this initial biopsy, consideration should be given to the need for further surgical intervention. The incisions should be planned and landmarks retained that will be conducive to further surgery.

Rhabdomyosarcoma is the most common solid tumor of the head and neck in children. It can occur in any muscle tissue in the body but can also be found in sites where striated muscle is not commonly seen, such as the urinary bladder.[8] Presentation in the head and neck can be in such sites as the nasopharynx, orbit, and ear. The presentation of persistent pain, epistaxis, and rhinorrhea associated in some cases with serous otitis media should necessitate evaluation of the nasopharynx for a possible sarcoma. In 35% of cases of rhabdomyosarcoma of the nasopharynx, infiltration of the skull base occurs.[8]

Leukemia can also present with painless lymphadenopathy of the neck. The most common leukemia in children is acute lymphoblastic leukemia. Abnormalities on hematological evaluation reveal anemia in 80% of cases, elevated WBC count in 50%, and thrombocytopenia.[8] A biopsy of the mass confirms the diagnosis.

Neuroblastoma accounts for 10% of malignancies in children. It is derived from primordial neural crest cells and can present in the head and neck. The most frequently seen area is the olfactory bulb, where it extends from the neurepithelium into the nasal cavity. Metastatic disease is seen in <10% of cases.[8]

Although the vast majority of malignant pediatric head and neck tumors are treated with radiation and chemotherapy, careful planning at the time of initial biopsy will spare a child a second general anesthesia. If suspicion is high that the tumor will prove to be malignant, consultation with a pediatric oncologist should be obtained. A bone marrow biopsy and possible placement of a Broviac catheter can be performed at the time of the initial biopsy. Surgical excision of malignant neck masses in children follows the principles of cancer surgery employed in adults. In biopsy-proven malignant tumors in which total excision of the lesion is warranted (i.e., squamous cell cancer), the excision of the tumor with wide margins and removal of regional lymph nodes should be undertaken. In cases where a stoma is created (i.e., a laryngectomy) or if growing bone is excised (i.e., mandibulectomy or maxillectomy), consideration of the growth of the child should be considered.

Case 4

An 18-month-old female presented to her pediatrician with a 1-week history of fever, lethargy, and poor oral intake. Physical examination revealed bilateral cervical adenopathy.

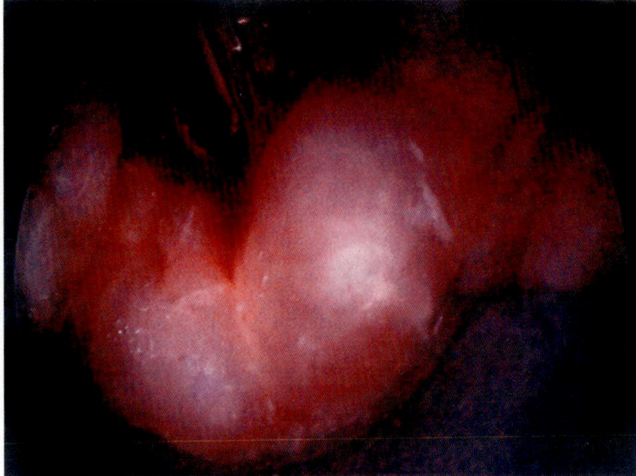

Fig. 46.4 Intraoperative photo showing edema of the larynx secondary to acute lymphoblastic leukemia.

The diagnosis of a viral upper respiratory infection with cervical adenitis was made, and the child was discharged home on antibiotics. Over the next 24 hours she developed worsening fever and neck swelling and presented to the emergency room for evaluation. On examination, she presented with severe respiratory distress. There was circumferential swelling of the neck as well as laryngeal edema. The child was brought to the operating room, where her airway was secured. Direct laryngoscopy revealed significant edema of the airway without erythema (**Fig. 46.4**). A CT scan revealed extensive cervical adenopathy (**Fig. 46.5**).

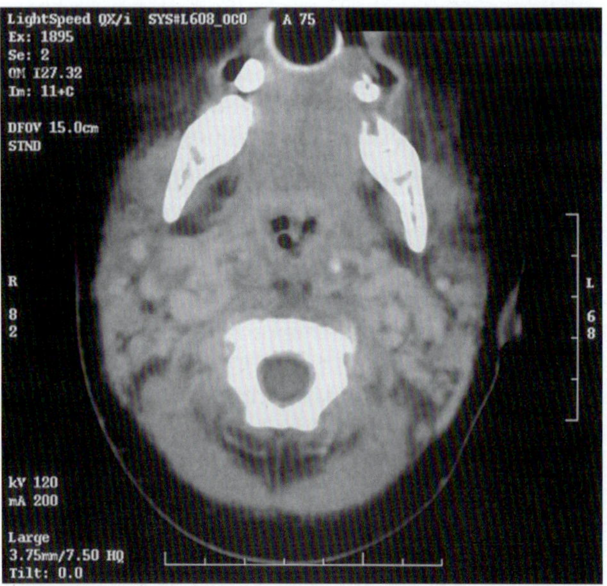

Fig. 46.5 Computed tomography scan of the neck in a patient with acute lymphoblastic leukemia.

Table 46.1 Neck Masses in Children

Congenital masses:

Hemangioma

Lymphatic malformation

Thyroglossal duct cyst

Branchial cleft cyst

Sternocleidomastoid tumor of infancy

Inflammatory neck masses:

Cervical adenitis (viral or bacterial)

Suppurative adenitis

Mononucleosis

Cervical tuberculosis

Malignant neck masses:

Lymphosarcoma

Hodgkin disease

Neuroblastoma (more common 1–6 years of age)

Leukemia (more common 1–6 years of age)

Rhabdomyosarcoma (more common 1–6 years of age)[6]

Thyroid cancer (more common 7–13 years of age)[6]

Epidermoid cancer (more common 14–21 years of age)[6]

A biopsy of the neck mass was consistent with acute lymphoblastic leukemia (ALL).

Conclusion

The management of recurrent neck masses in children requires a thoughtful evaluation of the patient. The vast majority of neck masses are benign in etiology, with the largest percentage secondary to infectious causes (**Table 46.1**). Examination of the child with special attention to the time course, location, appearance, and feel of the mass will assist in the diagnosis. Inflammatory masses are the most rapidly growing and are warm to the touch, with overlying erythema of the skin. Malignant masses have persistent enlargement and are most commonly firm to the touch and nontender. Congenital masses are slow growing unless acutely infected and can be firm to cystic on palpation. CT, MRI, and biopsy are helpful in elucidating the primary diagnosis and assisting with treatment. A thorough review of the previous radiologic and pathology specimens prior to revision surgery will assist in successfully treating recurrent neck masses in children.

References

1. Nelson R. Textbook of Pediatrics. 5th ed. Philadelphia: WB Saunders; 1950:1027–1029.
2. Toma R, Umberto GR. Pediatric ultrasound, II: Other applications. Eur Radiol 2001;15.
3. May M. Neck masses in children: diagnosis and treatment. Ear Nose Throat J 1978;57:136–158.
4. Greinwald JH, Burke DK, Sato Y, et al. Treatment of lymphangiomas in children: an update of Picibanil (OK-432) sclerotherapy. Otolaryngol Head Neck Surg 1999;121(4):381–387.
5. Bloom DA, Adler BH, Forsythe RC, et al. Congenital piriform fossa sinus tract presenting as an asymptomatic neck mass in an infant. Pediatr Radiol 2003;33:360–363.
6. Chandler JR, Mitchell B. Branchial cleft cysts, sinuses and fistulas. Otolaryngol Clin North Am 1981;14(1):175–186.
7. Jones JE, Hession B. Cervical thymic cysts. Ear Nose Throat J 1996;75(10):678–680.
8. Han G, Kazemian P. A relatively common childhood cancer. U Toronto Med J 2001;79(1):46–51.

Decision tree for recurrent otitis media/revision tympanostomy tubes

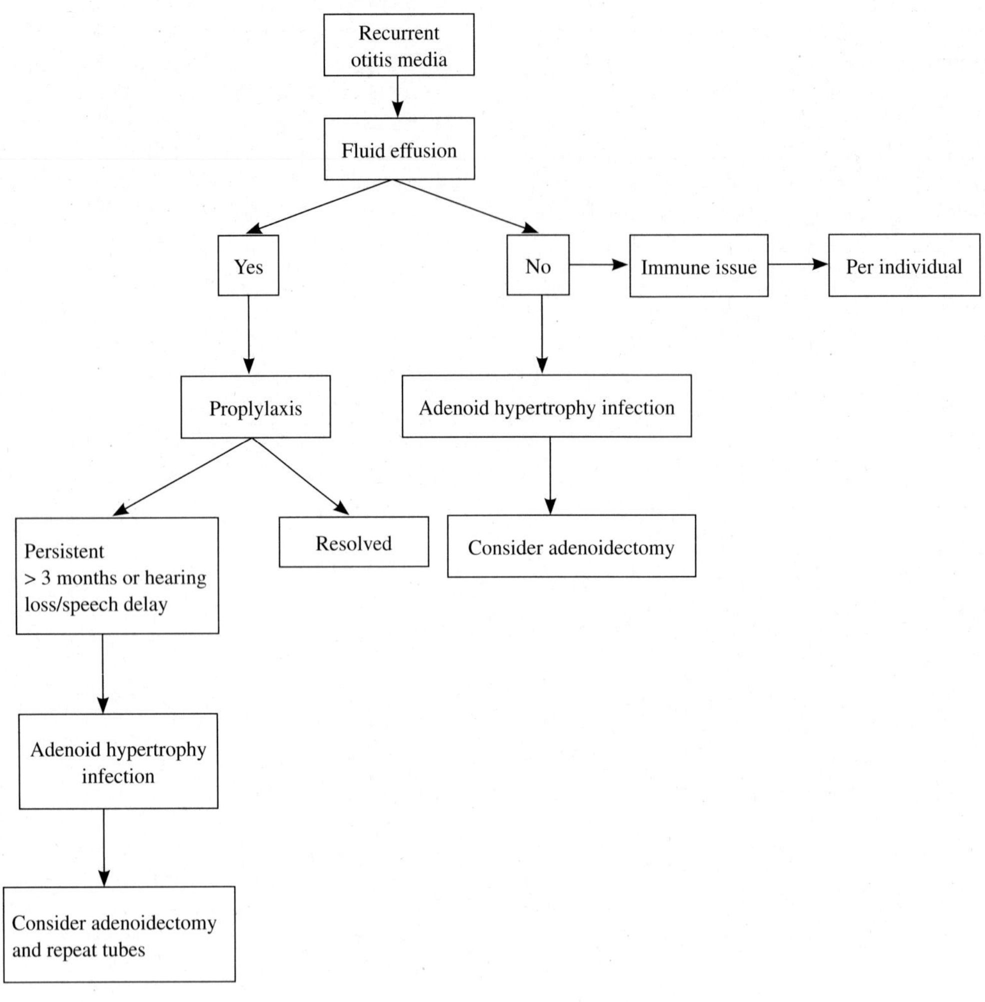

47 Otitis Media and Revision Tympanostomy Tubes

Sarah A. Stackpole

Otitis media and upper respiratory infection are the two most common conditions seen by pediatricians in the United States.[1] Otitis media occurs in children in a bimodal pattern, peaking during infancy and again at grammar school entry. Rates of infection have risen with changing socioeconomic and environmental conditions. Investigators have correlated these increases with rising rates of day care attendance and atopic allergy. Both trends seem likely to continue, thereby maintaining a high rate of otitis media and its sequelae in our patient population.

Most children experience the peak of acute ear infections prior to age 2, but a substantial minority will continue to experience recurrent acute infections or chronic effusions. Myringotomy and tube placement have been shown in many studies to be extremely effective for both otitis media with effusion and recurrent acute otitis media.[1–4] Patients requiring repeated tube insertions for prolonged otitis, however, represent 22.0 to 35.2% of this overall otitis population.[5,6] Evaluation of this more chronic otitis-prone subgroup requires consideration not only of the tube insertion procedure but also of the underlying contributing factors.

Preoperative Evaluation

Infectious Considerations

Nasopharyngeal Culture

Persistent otitis media may manifest as recurrent acute infections or chronic middle ear effusion. The nasopharynx may serve as a source of initial infection from upper respiratory tract infection or repeated colonization from bacteria harbored in the adenoid tissue. Nasopharyngeal culture may yield bacteriologic identification to direct antibiotic therapy, as the bacteriology correlates well with middle ear cultures in 62% of patients.[7] Negative nasopharyngeal culture results are strongly correlated with sterile middle ear cultures, with negative predictive values ranging from 94 to 100% for the main pathogens *Haemophilus influenzae*, *Streptococcus pneumoniae*, and *Moraxella catarrhalis*.[7,8]

Prophylaxis

Prophylactic antibiotics have been shown to be effective for prevention of acute infection and increased resolution of middle ear effusion. Polymerase chain reaction techniques have demonstrated bacterial activity in a middle ear considered to be sterile by traditional bacteriologic culture. Thus, initial treatment of acute infection may have to be followed by a more prolonged course of antibiotic treatment at a lower dosage. Although investigators vary somewhat in treatment duration, amoxicillin remains the antibiotic of choice for prophylaxis.[9] The increasing rates of antibiotic resistance in multiple pathogens lead researchers to urge for "more selective use of this mode [antibiotics] of prevention."[9,10] Nonantibiotic methods such as antiviral vaccines and environmental changes can impact on prevention, but tympanostomy tubes remain a mainstay of treatment in the current arsenal for otitis media, offering the only substantial option to antibiotic therapy. Oral steroids have not proven efficacious in resolving chronic effusions.

Anatomical Considerations

Adenoidectomy

The nasopharynx is believed to be a reservoir of potential contamination for the middle ear. Infected secretions may enter into an inflamed or fluid-filled middle ear and cause ongoing infection. Adenoidectomy has been advocated with revision tube placement to remove this tissue as a source of infection. Removal of enlarged adenoid tissue is also felt to decrease obstruction at the nasopharyngeal lumen. Adenoidectomy has been demonstrated in multiple trials to decrease the likelihood of reinsertion of subsequent tubes when performed in association with initial tubes.[11,12] However, Paradise et al[13] failed to show a clear reduction in otitis media with adenoidectomy or adenotonsillectomy without tube placement. Therefore, these additional surgeries should not replace repeat tube insertion, but rather be done in appropriate patients in conjunction with revision tube placement. Finally, tonsillectomy alone has not been clearly demonstrated to have a direct effect on otitis media; the decision for tonsillectomy should be based on standard criteria for infectious or obstructive indications.

Craniofacial Anomalies

Developmental anomalies that affect the palate or skull base are strong indicators for tube placement and replacement. Midline clefting disorders such as Pierre Robin syndrome result in severe eustachian tube dysfunction. Submucous cleft palate and bifid uvula are also associated with poor eustachian tube function, as are other craniofacial disorders that may involve the skull base without frank clefting, including Down, Crouzon, Treacher Collins, Apert, Goldenhar, and Turner syndromes. Patients with such anomalies will likely continue with severe middle ear problems and are thus candidates for rapid tube replacement.

Sinonasal Conditions

Associated sinonasal disease such as polyposis or chronic sinusitis may be associated with chronic otitis media. A detailed history should be obtained and further investigation conducted in appropriate patients. Evaluation of the posterior nasal cavity and nasopharynx is easily accomplished with a flexible endoscope. This may yield important information regarding the underlying etiology of eustachian tube dysfunction, such as an antrochoanal polyp or Tornwaldt cyst. The nasopharynx should be routinely evaluated in all adults with otitis media to assess for nasopharyngeal malignancy. Early nasopharyngeal carcinoma or lymphoma may have few other overt findings beyond middle ear fluid, and failure to examine the nasopharynx may cause a delay in diagnosis. In young children, radiologic assessment of obstruction may be substituted for direct endoscopy preoperatively, as appearance of the nasopharynx can be confirmed at the time of tube placement. However, nasopharyngeal films may not fully correlate with potential nasopharyngeal obstruction. The removal of even mildly enlarged adenoids may result in improvement in recurrent otitis that cannot be fully explained, but it presumably reflects removal of the source of contamination.[11–13]

Immunologic Considerations

Allergy

A history of allergic and immune problems should also be sought. Classic allergic congestion of the sinonasal mucosa can involve the lining of the eustachian tube and middle ear mucosa.[14] Elevated levels of eosinophilic cationic protein

have been demonstrated in 87.5% of patients sampled with chronic sterile middle ear effusions. Allergic evaluation should be conducted at the time of consideration for revision tubes. This may be done by serologic testing (radioallergosorbent test [RAST] panel) or by skin testing. In some allergic patients, a clinical trial of oral antihistamine therapy may prove effective in resolving middle ear effusion in conjunction with appropriate antibiotic treatment. Longer-term therapy can then be maintained.

Immune Disorders

Nonallergic immune dysfunction should also be evaluated in individuals with no other identifiable risk for recurrent otitis. Immunoglobulin subsets can be evaluated quantitatively. Human immunodeficiency virus (HIV) infection may manifest initially as middle ear effusion and may progress toward further stages of chronic otitis media.[15] If not previously treated, some HIV patients may resolve a middle ear effusion with appropriate antiviral therapy. Other disorders affecting local immunity and defenses, such as immotile ciliary disorders and mucopolysaccharidoses, may also contribute to chronic sinusitis and otitis. Patients with suggestive histories should be appropriately evaluated.

Otologic and Hearing Issues

Conductive Hearing Loss

Prolonged conductive hearing loss in the setting of otitis media with effusion is a common indication for tube placement.[2,16] Criteria vary somewhat between reports, ranging from a 10 to 20 dB threshold for the air–bone gap. A conductive loss in the presence of other communication issues such as speech or developmental delay will present a very strong indication for early tube replacement.[16–18] Patients with a permanent underlying sensorineural hearing loss will also benefit from surgical resolution of an overlying conductive fluid component. They can then benefit from the maximal appropriate amplification, without the additional conductive overlay.

Complications of Otitis Media

Revision tube placement should be strongly considered for patients who have experienced complications of otitis media, as they may be at risk for recurrence of that complication or for worsening of otologic function. Such complications include otogenic facial nerve paralysis, labyrinthitis, mastoiditis, petrositis, cholesteatoma, meningitis, and intracranial abscess.[4,19,20] These sequelae of otitis media are still seen regularly in underdeveloped countries where antibiotics and tube placement are not routinely available.[21] Long-term tube replacement should also be strongly considered for ears in which early adhesive changes have begun. Early intervention and maintenance of good middle ear ventilation may prevent further retraction, atelectasis, and ossicular erosion in vulnerable ears.

Cochlear Implant Patients

Acute otitis media can cause mastoiditis in a cavity previously opened for cochlear implantation, which may result in labyrinthitis or even meningitis. Gantz et al[22] reported an 8-year series of cochlear implant patients in which 5.6% of children developed otitis media, which progressed to mastoiditis in 1%. Three of these five cases lost implant function, and one developed acute labyrinthitis. A trial of prospective tube placement in young cochlear implant candidates showed no cases of progression to mastoiditis and no loss of implant function in otitis-prone children.[23] Therefore, tympanostomy tube insertion should be considered prior to or at the time of cochlear implantation in otitis-prone patients.

Special Populations

Individuals with special needs for excellent eustachian tube function may require tympanostomy tube placement despite the absence of effusion. Such candidates include persons who suffer from severe barotrauma and patients receiving hyperbaric oxygen therapy.[24] Such persons may experience pain, pressure, hearing loss, fluid effusion, and even middle and inner ear hemorrhage from difficulties with pressure equalization during compression and decompression.[25] This may occur during air flight or from the hyperbaric chamber. Patients requiring tube placement for air flight are quite rare, as most can be managed with medical decongestant therapy. However, 20 to 30% of patients receiving hyperbaric treatment will not tolerate the middle ear effects and will benefit greatly from tube placement.[25]

Surgical Considerations

Tube Selection

The rate of perforation after tympanostomy tube placement varies significantly with the size of the tube, being much greater with larger bore tympanostomy tubes designed for long-term retention.[26–28] Selection of the type of tube should therefore be predicated upon the anticipated duration of needed ventilation. Many children will gradually outgrow poor eustachian tube function, although adults requiring multiple insertions are less likely to improve spontaneously. Therefore, tympanostomy tubes should be avoided unless there are other indications for prolonged ($>$ 12 months) ventilation.

Studies of complications of various types of tubes have distinguished several differences between grommets and tympanostomy tubes (**Table 47.1**). The large inner flanges of tympanostomy tubes retard the rate of extrusion substantially: at 24 months, Weigel et al[26] noted a 69% retention rate in Goode tympanostomy tubes versus 34% or less in grommets. The extrusion rates were not statistically different between various styles within the grommet group. The size of the tube inner diameter, however, adversely correlates with obstruction. The small inner diameter of the Reuter-Bobbin was associated with a 74% rate of obstruction in that series,[26] significantly higher than the other styles, whether grommet or tympanostomy tube.

Table 47.1 Differences between Grommets and Tympanostomy Tubes

Tube Type	Duration of Average Retention (months)	Rate of Obstruction (%)	Rate of Perforation (%)
Grommets			
Shepherd[26]	9.8	11.0	0.0
Armstrong[26]	10.7	25.0	0.0
Reuter-Bobbin[26]	17.2	75.0	0.0
Shepherd[27]	8.4	8.9	2.7
Armstrong[27]	9.6	0.0	11.8
Paparella I[27]	11.6	8.2	3.4
Standard polyethylene[28]	8.4		2.2
Tympanostomy Tubes			
Goode[26]	20.7	36.0	12.0
Goode[28]	32.8		14.5
Paparella II[27]	16.7	13.7	10.4

The material of the tube or coating applied may also affect the tube retention or obstruction. Karlan et al[29] demonstrated differences in the surfaces of commercially available tubes, with fluorocarbon being notably smoother than silicone. Greater roughness results in greater bacterial adhesion. Their finding correlated with a nearly 3-fold increase in short- and long-term infections: 28% for silicone versus 11% for fluorocarbon. Additional experimental treatments of the tube material have been directed at these infection issues. Silver oxide coating may offer some reduction in long-term otorrhea, and ionization has been shown to decrease bacterial adhesion.[30,31]

Surgical Techniques

Tympanostomy tube placement is generally performed using magnification. Many tubes are placed in children under general anesthesia, but some surgeons prefer a papoose technique.[32,33] Tubes are typically placed in adults using local anesthesia only; however, general anesthesia may be indicated in selected circumstances. Although sterile preparation of the external canal is recommended if a middle ear culture is to be obtained, standard povidone-iodine is not effective in reducing postinsertion otorrhea.[34] Myringotomy and tube insertion have been demonstrated to not cause systemic bacteremia[35]; therefore, no intravenous or preoperative oral antibiotics are routinely recommended for this purpose. Antibiotic prophylaxis may, however, be indicated in high-risk individuals or in conjunction with other, more invasive procedures, such as adenoidectomy. Oral administration of antibiotics during the immediate postoperative period may also substantially reduce short-term otorrhea.

Tube placement is recommended in the anterior quadrant of the tympanic membrane. This avoids placement close to the incudostapedial joint and round window membrane. The incision may be performed with the myringotomy knife or with the CO_2 laser.[36,37] If myringotomy is to be performed without tube placement, laser myringotomy has been shown to provide a substantially longer period of patency.[38] However, this prolongation of patency did not translate into a significant reduction in the later prevalence of effusion. Therefore, tube placement remains indicated. When the incision is performed with the myringotomy knife, it may be oriented in either a radial or circumferential direction, as neither has been demonstrated to affect long-term healing.[39]

Mitomycin C

Reports of topical mitomycin application to extend myringotomy patency suggest a possible role for mitomycin as an alternative to tube placement in selected patients.

Mitomycin C is an antineoplastic aminoglycoside that has been used extensively to prevent adhesions in ophthalmic surgery.[40] Investigators have studied its application topically after myringotomy and found substantial prolongation of patency.[40–42] The average prolongation of patency ranged from 3.5[42] to 9.5[41] weeks, a substantial advantage over the short closure time of 2 or 3 days for standard myringotomy.

Topical Antibiotics

Topical application of antibiotic drops after tube placement reduces the short-term incidence of postoperative otorrhea.[43,44] A single dose administered at the time of procedure reduced the rate of otorrhea from 12.0 to 8.8%,[43] but the greatest reduction was seen with more prolonged administration, from 2 to 5 days postoperatively. This was particularly evident in patients with purulent or mucoid effusions, reducing the rate of otorrhea from 29% in controls (no drops) to 17% in a 48-hour treatment group.[43] The rate of otorrhea is highly associated with the findings in the middle ear: ears with dry taps or serous effusions rarely developed otorrhea, whereas ears with purulent or mucoid effusions had very high rates. The choice of drops includes mixtures such as Neosporin/polymyxin, aminoglycosides, sulfonamides, and quinolones. Quinolones avoid the potential for ototoxicity associated with aminoglycoside solutions and have excellent antipseudomonal activity as well as gram-positive activity.

Vasoconstrictors

Other topical agents may also reduce postoperative bleeding and otorrhea. Topical application of vasoconstrictors such as xylometazoline hydrochloride[45] and phenylephrine hydrochloride[46] have been shown to reduce postoperative tube obstruction. Xylometazoline alone reduced obstruction from 10.5 to 0%,[45] and phenylephrine (in conjunction with antibiotic drops) reduced obstruction from 8.6 to 2.3%.[46] Both compounds are believed to reduce bleeding from the wound edges.

Anesthetics

Topical anesthetic drops may also reduce postoperative pain after tympanostomy tube placement and may be as effective as oral analgesics.[32] However, studies of topical lidocaine as well as tetracaine have also reported postoperative vertigo and facial nerve weakness, suggesting medication penetration into the inner ear.[34,47] Anesthetic drops applied prior to actual myringotomy incision reduce subsequent pain and are less associated with inner ear penetration. They must typically be applied for an extended period of time (> 30 minutes) for maximal effect. Phenol may also be used as a local anesthetic. It produces temporary blanching of the tympanic membrane with anesthesia in the affected region. No permanent tympanic membrane changes from local agents have been reported from experimental models, including phenol, tetracaine, and lidocaine/prilocaine.[48]

Acoustic Trauma

Suction aspiration has been suggested as a cause of possible acoustic trauma. Temporary auditory brainstem response (ABR) threshold shifts have been reported, with resolution at 1 month postoperative testing.[49] A randomized series for myringotomy and tube placement with and without suctioning of the middle ear effusion found no evidence of acoustic trauma and no increased difficulty of tube insertion or increased rate of subsequent otorrhea.[50] These studies suggest that fluid may be suctioned from the middle ear when necessary.

Complications

Otorrhea

The most common complications of tympanostomy tubes are otorrhea and permanent perforation. Otorrhea may occur at any time after myringotomy and may be associated with a recurrent acute otitis media or with granulation tissue. Reports of frequency range from 0[26] to 66%,[6] varying with type of effusion as well as type of tube (**Table 47.2**). Otorrhea and granulation can often be treated successfully with oral and topical antibiotics, thus avoiding the need for premature tube removal. Occasionally the tube itself may

seem to act as a foreign body, generating a granulation response: if a prolonged trial of antibiotic therapy is ineffective, removal of the tube may allow resolution of otorrhea.

Water Exposure

Contamination of the middle ear by water exposure has long been reviled as a cause of chronic otorrhea. However, an excellent study by Hebert et al[51] demonstrated clean tap water is unlikely to penetrate completely through the tube at surface pressures. However, changes in water viscosity with soap, as well as increased water pressure with depth (e.g., dunking or diving), allowed contamination to occur. Practical water exposure guidelines can thus minimize risk for otorrhea while allowing patients to pursue limited desired water activities.

Perforation

Residual perforations persisting after tube extrusion or removal occur infrequently, ranging from 0 to 14.5% (**Table 47.2**). Perforations are much more commonly seen with large bore, T-style tubes. These tubes have a larger diameter of the tube, longer flanges, and prolonged retention in the tympanic membrane. These factors contribute to more permanent scar formation, rather than the improved healing seen with smaller, shorter-acting tubes. Perforations may be repaired by patch tympanoplasty, or with operative repair and grafting if patching is not successful.

Tympanosclerosis

Tympanosclerosis is a common sequela of both otitis media and tympanostomy tube insertion. Careful reporting

Table 47.2 Comparison of Complications Associated with Tympanostomy Tubes

Study	Tube	Number of Ears	Otorrhea (%)	Perforation (%)	Cholesteatoma (%)
Valtonen et al[6]	Shah	281	66.5	2.3	*
Weigel et al[26]	Armstrong	26	17.0	0.0	*
	Reuter	26	42.0	0.0	*
	Shepherd	23	0.0	0.0	*
	Goode T-tube 75	50	12.0	12.0	*
Klingensmith[27]	Paparella I	232	26.6	3.4	0.4
	Shepherd	119	16.1	2.7	0.8
	Armstrong	23	15.0	11.8	0.0
	Paparella II (T)	226	37.9	10.4	1.3
Golz[28]	Grommet + T	2604	15.9	3.06	*

* Not recorded.

of this finding is uncommon in operative series, but two long-term studies reported rates of 40.0 and 48.6%.[52] Sclerosis within the layers of the tympanic membrane was markedly increased in laboratory rats treated with myringotomy versus those with experimental acute otitis media treated with antibiotics alone.[53] Hyalinization and calcification occur in the collagen layer of the tympanic membrane; these processes may be accelerated by trauma and inflammation, as well as by the increased oxygen concentration in the middle ear afforded by the ventilation of the tube.[54]

Medial Tube Displacement

An uncommon result of tympanostomy tubes is medial displacement of the tube beyond an intact drum, rather than extrusion into the external canal. This has been reported with both grommet and T-tube designs.[27] The mechanism for this atypical migration is postulated to be trapping of the rim of the tube flange causing medial rather than external migration. These trapped tubes will often act as a foreign body and are typically removed surgically.

Cholesteatoma

Cholesteatoma occurs rarely after tube placement, ranging from 0.8% in grommets to 1.3% with tympanostomy tubes (**Table 47.2**). In cholesteatoma series, however, a history of prior tube insertion is extremely common: one

pediatric study reported a 48% rate of prior tubes, with 19% having had multiple tube insertions.[55]

Middle or Inner Ear Injury

Serious injuries to middle or inner ear structures are exceedingly rare with myringtomy. Bleeding may occur from damage to anomalous vascular structures in the middle ear during incision.[56] The most common vascular anomaly in the anterior middle ear is an aberrant internal carotid artery. Dehiscence of the jugular bulb is most common inferiorly. Some vascular injuries may be controlled with local tamponade and supportive care, but others may require aggressive intervention to control the feeding vessel. Vestibular and neurologic sequelae are also exceedingly rare, including perilymphatic fistula and facial nerve weakness.[57] Anterior placement of the incision site minimizes risk to the ossicles, round window membrane, and intratympanic facial nerve.

Conclusion

Otitis media remains a prevalent problem, particularly in the pediatric population. Detailed assessment of the otitis-prone individual is essential in managing these patients to avoid the sequelae of chronic otitis media and multiple tympanostomy reinsertions. Tympanostomy tubes remain essential to patient management, particularly as an effective option to prolonged antibiotic therapy in this era of rising resistance.

References

1. Daly KA, Giebink GS. Clinical epidemiology of otitis media. Pediatr Infect Dis J 2000;19:S31–S36.
2. Franklin JH, Marck PA. Outcome analysis of children receiving tympanostomy tubes. J Otolaryngol 1998;27:293–297.
3. Klein JO. Management of otitis media: 2000 and beyond. Pediatr Infect Dis J 2000;19:383–387.
4. Bluestone CD. Clinical course, complications and sequelae of acute otitis media. Pediatr Infect Dis J 2000;19:S37–S46.
5. Riley DN, Herberger S, McBride G, et al. Myringotomy and ventilation tube insertion: a ten-year follow-up. J Laryngol Otol 1997;111:257–261.
6. Valtonen H, Qvarnberg Y, Nuutinen J. Tympanostomy in young children with recurrent otitis media: a long-term follow-up study. J Laryngol Otol 1999;113:207–211.
7. Gehanno P, Lenoir F, Barry B, et al. Evaluation of nasopharyngeal cultures for bacteriologic assessment of acute otitis media in children. Pediatr Infect Dis J 1996;15:329–332.
8. Faden H, Stanievich J, Brodsky L, et al. Changes in nasopharyngeal flora during otitis media of childhood. Pediatr Infect Dis J 1990;9:623–626.
9. Klein JO. Clinical implications of antibiotic resistance for management of acute otitis media. Pediatr Infect Dis J 1998; 17:1084–1089.
10. Klein JO. Preventing recurrent otitis: what role for antibiotics? Contemp Pediatr 1994;11:44–60.
11. Coyte PC, Croxford R, McIsaac W, et al. The role of adjuvant adenoidectomy and tonsillectomy in the outcome of the insertion of tympanostomy tubes. N Engl J Med 2001; 344:1188–1195.
12. Gates GA. Otitis media: the pharyngeal connection. JAMA 1999;282:987–989.
13. Paradise JL, Bluestone CD, Colborn DK, et al. Adenoidectomy and adenotonsillectomy for recurrent acute otitis media. JAMA 1999;282:945–953.
14. Ogra PL. Mucosal immune response in the ear, nose and throat. Pediatr Infect Dis J 2000;19:S4–S8.
15. Kohan D, Giacchi RJ. Otologic surgery in patients with HIV-1 and AIDS. Otolaryngol Head Neck Surg 1999;121:355–360.
16. Bluestone CD. Role of surgery for otitis media in the era of resistant bacteria. Pediatr Infect Dis J 1998;17: 1090–1098.
17. Gravel JS, Wallace IF. Language, speech, and education outcomes of otitis media. J Otolaryngol 1998;27(Suppl 2): 17–25.
18. Paradise JL. Otitis media and child development: should we worry? Pediatr Infect Dis J 1998;17:1076–1083.

19. Elliott CA, Zalzal GH, Gottlieb WR. Acute otitis media and facial paralysis in children. Ann Otol Rhinol Laryngol 1996; 105:58–62.

20. Goldstein NA, Casselbrant ML, Bluestone CD, et al. Intratemporal complications of acute otitis media in infants and children. Otolaryngol Head Neck Surg 1998;119:444–454.

21. Rutka J, Lekagul S. No therapy: use, abuse, efficacy, and morbidity—the European versus the third-world experience. J Otolaryngol 1998;27(Suppl 2):43–48.

22. Kempf HG, Stover T, Lenarz T. Mastoiditis and acute otitis media in children with cochlear implants: recommendations for medical management. Ann Otol Rhinol Laryngol Suppl 2000;185:25–27.

23. Luntz M, Teszler CB, Shpak T, et al. Cochlear implantation in healthy and otitis-prone children: a prospective study. Laryngoscope 2001;111:1614–1618.

24. Bent JP, April MM, Ward RF. Atypical indications for Otoscan laser-assisted myringotomy. Laryngoscope 2001;111: 87–89.

25. Vrabec JT, Clements KS, Mader JT. Short-term tympanostomy in conjunction with hyperbaric oxygen therapy. Laryngoscope 1998;108:1124–1127.

26. Weigel MT, Parker MY, Goldsmith MM, et al. A prospective randomized study of four commonly used tympanostomy tubes. Laryngoscope 1989;99:252–256.

27. Klingensmith MR, Strauss M, Conner GH. A comparison of retention and complication rates of large-bore (Paparella II) and small-bore middle ear ventilating tubes. Otolaryngol Head Neck Surg 1985;93:322–330.

28. Golz A, Netzer A, Joachims HZ, et al. Ventilation tubes and persisting tympanic membrane perforations. Otolaryngol Head Neck Surg 1999;120:524–527.

29. Karlan MS, Skobel B, Grizzard M, et al. Myringotomy tube materials: bacterial adhesion and infection. Otolaryngol Head Neck Surg 1980;88:783–795.

30. Biedlingmaier JF, Samaranayake R, Whelan P. Resistance to biofilm formation on otologic implant materials. Otolaryngol Head Neck Surg 1998;118:444–451.

31. Gourin CG, Hubbell RN. Otorrhea after insertion of silver oxide-impregnated silastic tympanostomy tubes. Arch Otolaryngol Head Neck Surg 1999;125:446–450.

32. Derkay CS, Wadsworth JT, Darrow DH, et al. Tube placement: a prospective, randomized double-blind study. Laryngoscope 1998;108:97–101.

33. Brodsky L, Brookhauser P, Chait D, et al. Office-based insertion of pressure equalization tubes: the role of laser-assisted tympanic membrane fenestration. Laryngoscope 1999;109:2009–2014.

34. Baldwin RL, Aland J. The effects of povidone-iodine preparation on the incidence of post-tympanostomy otorrhea. Otolaryngol Head Neck Surg 1990;102:631–634.

35. Brown OE, Manning SC, Phillips DL. Lack of bacteremia in children undergoing myringotomy and tympanostomy tube placement. Pediatr Infect Dis J 1995;14:1101–1102.

36. Silverstein H, Kuhn J, Choo D, et al. Laser-assisted tympanostomy. Laryngoscope 1996;106:1067–1074.

37. Cohen D, Schechter Y, Slatkine M, et al. Laser myringotomy in different age groups. Arch Otolaryngol Head Neck Surg 2001;127:260–264.

38. Szeremeta W, Parameswaran MS, Isaacson G. Adenoidectomy with laser or incisional myringotomy for otitis media with effusion. Laryngoscope 2000;110:342–345.

39. Guttenplan MD, Tom LW, DeVito MA, et al. Radial versus circumferential incision in myringotomy and tube placement. Int J Pediatr Otorhinolaryngol 1991;21:211–215.

40. Jassir D, Buchman CA, Gomez-Marin O. Safety and efficacy of topical mitomycin C in myringotomy patency. Otolaryngol Head Neck Surg 2001;124:368–373.

41. Estrem SA, Baker TJ. Preapplication of mitomycin C for enhanced patency of myringotomy. Otolaryngol Head Neck Surg 2000;122:346–348.

42. Estrem SA, VanLeeuwen RN. Use of mitomycin C for maintain myringotomy patency. Otolaryngol Head Neck Surg 2000;122:8–10.

43. Scott BA, Strunk CL Jr. Post-tympanostomy otorrhea: a randomized clinical trial of topical prophylaxis. Otolaryngol Head Neck Surg 1992;106:34–41.

44. Garcia P, Gates GA, Schechtman KB. Does topical antibiotic prophylaxis reduce post-tympanostomy tube otorrhea? A meta-analysis. Ann Otol Rhinol Laryngol 1994;103:54–58.

45. Jamal TS. Avoidance of postoperative blockage of ventilation tubes. Laryngoscope 1995;105:833–834.

46. Altman JS, Haupert MS, Hamaker RA, et al. Phenylephrine and the prevention of postoperative tympanostomy tube obstruction. Arch Otolaryngol Head Neck Surg 1998;124: 1233–1236.

47. Hoffman RA, Li CJ. Tetracaine topical anesthesia for myringotomy. Laryngoscope 2001;111:1636–1638.

48. Gnuechtel MM, Schenk LL, Postma GN. Late effects of topical anesthetics on the healing of guinea pig tympanic membranes after myringotomy. Arch Otolaryngol Head Neck Surg 2000;126:733–735.

49. Mason JDT, Mason SM, Gibbon KP. Raised ABR threshold after suction aspiration of glue from the middle ear: three case studies. J Laryngol Otol 1995;109:726–728.

50. Egeli E, Kiris M. Is aspiration necessary before tympanostomy tube insertion? Laryngoscope 1998;108:443–444.

51. Hebert RL II, King GE, Bent JP III. Tympanostomy tubes and water exposure. Arch Otolaryngol Head Neck Surg 1998;124:1118–1121.

52. Maw AR. Development of tympanosclerosis in children with otitis media with effusion and ventilation tubes. J Laryngol Otol 1991;105:614–617.

53. Mattsson C, Magnuson K, Hellstrom S. Myringotomy: a prerequisite for the development of myringosclerosis? Laryngoscope 1998;108:102–106.

54. Mattsson C, Marklund SL, Hellstrom S. Application of oxygen free radical scavengers to diminish the occurrence of myringosclerosis. Ann Otol Rhinol Laryngol 1997;106: 513–518.

55. Edelstein DR, Parisier SC, Ahuja GS, et al. Cholesteatoma in the pediatric age group. Ann Otol Rhinol Laryngol 1988; 97:23–29.

56. Jacobsson M, Davidsson A, Hugosson S, et al. Aberrant intratympanic internal carotid artery: a potentially hazardous anomaly. J Laryngol Otol 1989;103:1202–1205.

57. Jensen JH. Perilymph fistulas caused by myringotomy. ORL J Otorhinolaryngol Relat Spec 1986;48:293–296.

Decision tree for cleft lip and palate repair recurrences

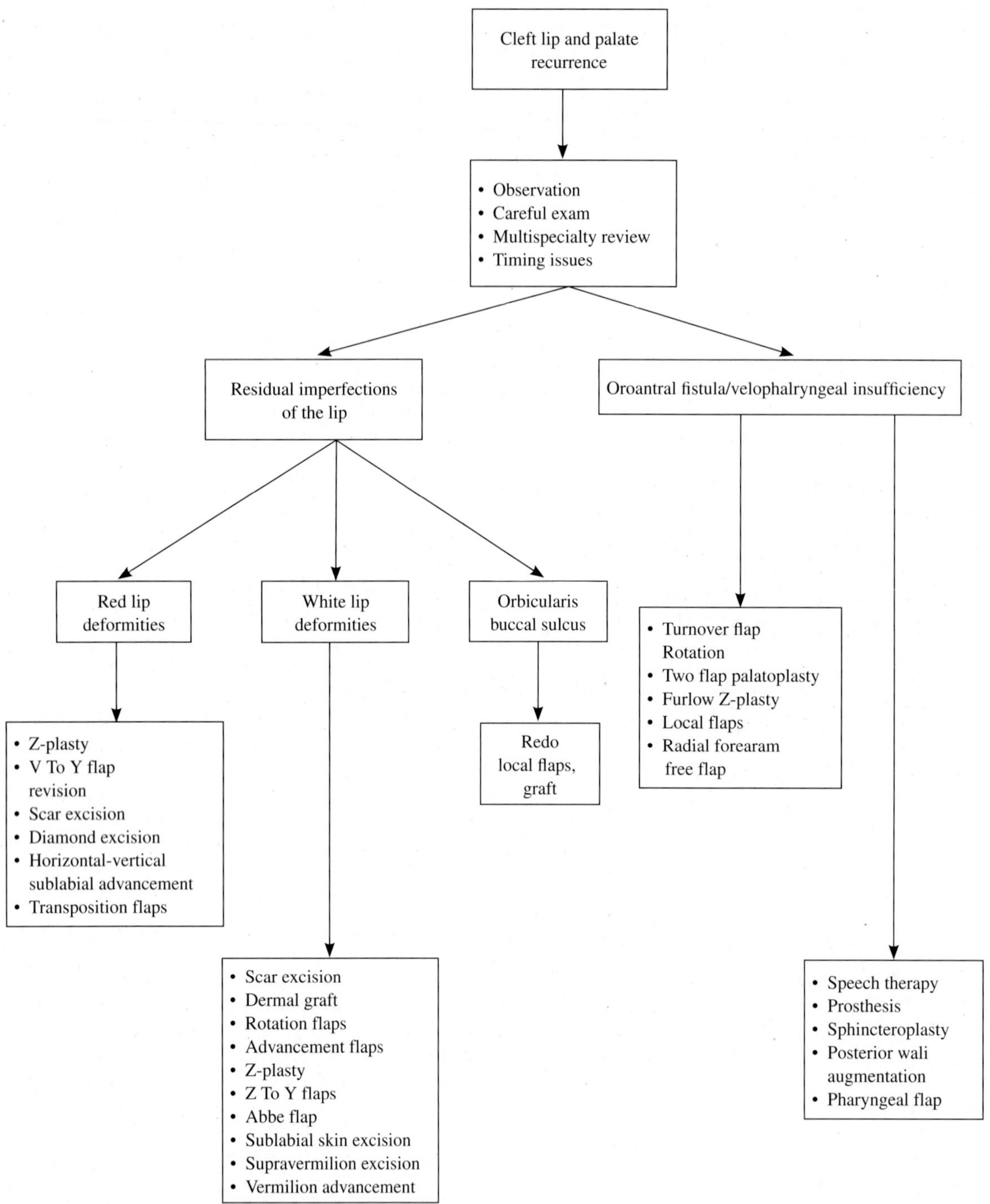

Revision Cleft Lip and Palate Surgery

Patrick J. Byrne and James D. Sidman

Cleft lip and palate surgery represents an intervention on complex, three-dimensional interrelated abnormalities that undergo continued growth and development postoperatively. Residual imperfections and imbalances of the lip are very common; in fact, they may be considered the rule rather than the exception. Likewise, cleft palate surgery has a significant incidence of oronasal fistula formation and velopharyngeal insufficiency. The key to successful management of secondary deformities of the cleft lip and palate lies in an accurate diagnosis of the abnormality present. The surgeon must have an assortment of treatment choices in his or her armamentarium and choose the appropriate one thoughtfully. This chapter will begin with an outline of the essential treatment options for the primary repairs. This is followed by a listing of the common secondary deformities that may persist (or manifest as growth and development continue), with the treatment options available for each. A more thorough discussion of the secondary deformities and the treatment options available then follows. An attempt is made to provide the most useful techniques for the most common problems, keeping in mind that a vast array of techniques have been described for each historically. The cleft lip nasal deformity will only be briefly touched upon.

I. Primary unilateral cleft lip repair
   A. Straight line closure
   B. Millard rotation advancement repair
   C. Tension-Randall triangular flap repair
II. Primary bilateral cleft lip repair
   A. Veau straight line repair
   B. Millard straight line muscle repair with worked flaps
III. Primary cleft palate repair
   A. V to Y pushback/two-flap palatoplasty
   B. Furlow double-reverse Z-plasty
IV. Secondary deformities of unilateral and bilateral cleft lip
   A. Red lip deformities
      1. Vermilion deficiency ("whistler's deformity")
      2. Vermilion excess
      3. Vermilion border deformities
   B. White lip deformities
      1. Irregularities of the philtrum
      2. Short upper lip
      3. Tight upper lip
      4. Long white lip
      5. Columellar abnormalities

   C. Orbicularis
   D. Buccal sulcus abnormalities
V. Secondary deformities of cleft palate
   A. Palatal fistula
   B. Velopharyngeal insufficiency (VPI)
VI. Correction of secondary cleft lip deformities
   A. Red lip deformities
      1. Z-plasty
      2. V to Y mucosal advancement
      3. Revision of lip repair
      4. Excision of scar
      5. Diamond excision
      6. Horizontal versus vertical vermilion excision
      7. Sublabial buccal mucosal advancements
      8. Transposition flaps
   B. White lip deformities
      1. Scar excision
      2. Dermal grafts, subcutaneous rotation flaps
      3. Redo lip repair with rotation-advancement flaps
      4. Z-plasty
      5. V to Y advancement flaps
      6. Abbe flap
      7. Subalar skin excisions
      8. Supravermilion excisions
      9. Vermilion advancement
   C. Orbicularis deformities
      1. Take down repair, reapproximate muscle
   D. Buccal sulcus abnormalities
      1. Local rotation or advancement flaps
      2. Grafts: oral mucosa, split thickness, palatine mucoperiosteal
VII. Correction of secondary cleft palate deformities
   A. Oronasal fistula
      1. Observation
      2. Turnover flaps
      3. Rotation flaps
      4. Redo two-flap palatoplasty
      5. Furlow double-reverse Z-plasty
      6. Local flaps: nasolabial, buccinator, tongue
      7. Radial forearm free flap
   B. Velopharyngeal insufficiency
      1. Speech therapy
      2. Prosthesis
      3. Sphincteroplasty
      4. Posterior pharyngeal wall augmentation
      5. Pharyngeal flap

Secondary Deformities of Unilateral and Bilateral Cleft Lip

The primary treatment of unilateral cleft lip differs considerably from the treatment of bilateral clefts. In general, the bilateral cleft lip patient represents a significantly greater challenge to the facial plastic surgeon. However, the secondary deformities that present later with unilateral and bilateral cleft lips are often similar. Therefore, these two distinct entities will be considered together for the purposes of discussing the correction of secondary deformities. The cleft lip nasal deformity will not be included in this text.

Evaluation

The key to successful outcomes with revision surgery lies in the accurate diagnosis of the deformity. One must be both thorough and precise. The patient must be observed carefully in both animation and repose. The scar is only one aspect of the lip evaluation. The entire lip must be analyzed critically. This includes the white lip, the orbicularis muscle function, the vermilion border, Cupid's bow, the philtral columns, the white roll, the columella, and the sulcus. The lip is inspected in all three dimensions. This careful evaluation of the entire lip is then performed in animation, as the patient smiles and puckers. Next, the lip is palpated. The integrity of the orbicularis oris is determined at rest and in motion. The distensibility of the lip is checked. Measurements are made of the landmarks. It may be helpful to consider the lip as if it had not been operated on before, to evaluate the entire lip and not simply focus on what seems initially to be the deformity. Photodocumentation is performed.

Timing

Multiple factors influence the timing of the secondary procedure. Initially, it is best to be conservative and allow time for the initial procedure to fully heal. The patient may be mature enough at this point that he or she is aware of an abnormality that exists and wishes it corrected. This must be taken into consideration, as significant psychological stress may be associated with the deformity. Because the treatment of the cleft lip and plate is a multistage process, it may be possible to perform the revision surgery at the time of another procedure.

Red Lip Deformities

Vermilion Deficiency

Deficiencies of the red lip, which include the classic "whistler's deformity" (a central notching defect) of the bilateral cleft lip, are relatively common after cleft lip repair.[1] In the case of the unilateral cleft, this often takes the form of a Cupid's bow deficiency. The vermilion deficiency may be the result of the overaggressive resection of the mucosa or secondary to poor alignment of the orbicularis oris. Another manifestation includes asymmetry of the vermilion.

The patient with evidence of vermilion deficiency must be carefully examined to determine if the problem is secondary to inadequate orbicularis approximation versus excessive resection of mucosa. This is commonly seen after the rotation-advancement technique when excessive scar contracture occurs. Failure to recognize the former will lead to inadequate correction.

Treatment Options

The vermilion deficiency of either unilateral or bilateral cleft lip may be treated with a V to Y mucosal advancement flaps, Z-plasties, transposition flaps, free grafts, or cross lip flaps (Abbe flaps). Initially, inspection will reveal if the defect is secondary to a tethering band in the sulcus. If so, this can be released and elongated with a Z-plasty.

The V to Y advancement flap is often useful. In this case, the V incision is made with the apex toward the sulcus, extending superiorly to the vermilion border. Including the orbicularis muscle in the flap adds fullness to the reconstruction. The mucosa is advanced superiorly and closed as a Y to fill in the deficient area.

A Z-plasty may correct the deficiency adequately. This can be performed on either the wet or dry lip; however, transposition of the wet lip into dry lip, or vice versa, is to be avoided if possible. Larger central deficiencies may be corrected by making a longer incision along the entire labial sulcus and advancing the buccal flaps inferiorly toward the vermilion-cutaneous junction. This is often difficult due to scarring in the sulcus from previous repair.

Vermilion Excess

The excessive upper lip hang of vermilion excess is due to either imprecise alignment or inadequate excision of tissue at the time of initial repair. It is often most noticeable in the lateral segment. This may be corrected in several ways. A horizontal ellipse excised from the wet lip is effective and prevents a visible scar. Inrolling of the outer vermilion with trial sutures may be used to ensure symmetry. If the dental incisors are aligned, they can be used as background to ensure proper leveling. It is important to note any vertical indentation present along the line of the previous repair. If so, then a vertical excision of this scar is preferred to advance the edges properly with eversion to achieve an even outer contour of the lip.

Vermilion Border Irregularities

Misalignment of the superior edge of the vermilion is one of the most common lip deformities. This anatomical area is quite unforgiving to the primary surgeon: vermilion border irregularities are obvious due to the color mismatch of vermilion to cutaneous lip. They result from technical error or at times are secondary to the soft tissue deficiency of the primary deformity.

If the rest of the lip repair is satisfactory, then localized procedures at the region of the step-off are effective. A diamond excision can realign the border and simultaneously narrow any widening of the lower end of the philtral scar that may be present. Z-plasty is also effective.

Cupid's bow asymmetries can be treated with either full-thickness skin excision (just above the white roll) or de-epithelialization with vermilion advancement.

White Lip Deformities

Irregularities of the Philtrum

The central dimple and philtral columns are the characteristic feature of the upper lip. The loss of philtral definition is one of the most common lip landmark abnormalities after primary repair. The secondary deformity may be a loss of the prominence, a widening of the scar, discoloration, or improper location of the scar outside the proper location. Revision of the philtral scar is often performed concurrently with nasal or vermilion revisions. Once again, proper analysis is crucial prior to the procedure. Obicularis dehiscence must be identified and corrected if present. Straight line excision is preferred to re-create the desired column. Superficial scars may be treated with cutaneous excision alone. Dermal and subdermal scar may even be used to add bulk or closure. Dermal grafts may be used as well. A central dimple can be created with a deep suture from the dermis to the premaxilla periosteum.[1] In bilateral clefts, the repaired philtrum is often too wide, and narrowing of the philtrum can be used to lengthen the columella.

Short Upper Lip

Short upper lip, or vertical deficiency, may have many causes. Often, a temporary reduction in vertical height is seen after the rotation advancement repair of a unilateral cleft lip. This is due to scar contracture, with subsequent relaxation, and resolves over a 6-month period. A permanent vertical deficiency may be caused by vertical scar contracture. Technical errors include inadequate dissection, repositioning, and fixation of the orbicularis, inadequate rotation, and failure to extend the incision across

the base of the columella. Once again, all layers may be involved, making precise diagnosis critical. In the case of a superficial scar contracture, simple excision may suffice. Often, however, a major revision with reopening of the entire lip is necessary. Typically, this involves a rotation advancement, with care taken to perform an adequate backcut (at 45 degrees to the horizontal) as necessary to achieve the desired rotation. Additional length of the advancement flap may be achieved from the nasal sill. Another technique to correct less significant vertical deficiency is a Z-plasty of the upper scar, so as to hide the incisions in the shadow of the nostril.

Tight Upper Lip

The normal upper lip is full and protrudes slightly in front of the lower lip. When excessive soft tissue is removed at the time of the original repair, then an indrawn upper lip is created, stretched across the teeth and lying behind the lower lip. This appearance is accentuated in the presence pf maxillary retrusion.

The correction of this deformity is best treated by addressing the underlying bony deficiency. Reconstruction of the hypoplastic maxilla will often achieve the best results. This is usually done during the teenage years. However, when this is not an issue, an Abbe flap may be necessary. This cross lip flap is placed in the midline to re-create the philtrum and Cupid's bow regardless of the original repair performed. The texture and color differences of the upper and lower lip make this procedure undesirable.

Long White Lip

Long upper lip, or vertical excess, is uncommon. Excessive rotation of the rotation-advancement flap may produce such a deformity. This is a difficult problem to correct. Typically, the lip needs to be reopened. The scar is excised, and the lip is derotated and de-advanced. An anchoring suture from the lateral lip to the pyriform aperture can help to retain position. Another option is the excision of an ellipse of skin and muscle from just beneath the nasal sill or ala. Careful inspection may reveal that the vertical excess is actually a relative lengthening of the lip lateral to the repair with cranial displacement of the alar base secondary to insertion of the C-flap under the base. This is corrected by excising the C-flap and advancing the alar base inferiorly.

Orbicularis Abnormalities

Some of the many manifestations of inadequate dissection, release of, and approximation of the orbicularis at the time of the original repair have been mentioned. It is critical to identify these when considering secondary surgery. They include widening of the cutaneous scar, vermilion deficiencies, thinning of the lip, and short lip. Functionally, inadequate muscle reconstruction results in a lip that functions improperly during speech, facial expression, whistling, and mastication. In addition, the alar base of the nose is often displaced laterally. Simple procedures that do not correctly align and approximate the orbicularis oris will likely fail. The orbicularis is generally approached transcutaneously, as with the above described techniques. In the unusual case of an adequate cutaneous scar without the need for revision, the muscle may be approached fro m the mucosal surface.[1] Three 4–0 Vicryl sutures are used in the repair of the orbicularis, and a Z-plasty may be employed to provide additional length.

Buccal Sulcus Abnormalities

A deficient buccal sulcus most commonly occurs in bilateral cleft cases. Lip function is compromised, and orthodontic procedures may be difficult due to the lack of space. Error in technique is the common cause. Revision requires excision of the band of scar tissue. The defect is then closed with grafts of full-thickness skin, oral mucosa, or mucoperiosteum, or local mucosal rotation flaps. Placement of an acrylic splint or stent may be performed to maintain the height of the sulcus during the healing process. This is left in for 3 weeks. This appliance may represent a compliance challenge to the younger patient. For this reason, it may be best to wait until the child is 4 to 6 years of age before performing the correction of a blunted sublabial sulcus.

Secondary Deformities of Cleft Palate

Palatal Fistula

The incisive foramen divides the primary (hard palate anterior to the incisive foramen) from the secondary (hard and soft palate posterior to the foramen) palate. Fistulas are more common after repair of complete clefts of the primary and secondary palate repair of an isolated secondary palate cleft.[2] Alveolar clefts are usually not repaired at the time of the initial surgery. These are thus residual clefts rather than fistulas. They may occur anywhere along the line of closure, and are particularly common at the junction of the hard and soft palate. This may result after inadequate mobilization of the palatal musculature off the hard palate at the time of the original repair. True fistulas are also caused by excessive wound tension, infection, hematoma, flap necrosis, and faulty suturing technique. Fistulas after repair of cleft palate have a reported incidence in the range of 20%.[2] Smaller fistulas may

be asymptomatic. In such cases, the repair may be delayed until a future procedure or simply not done. Symptomatic patients complain of food or liquid passing into the nasal cavity. Hypernasal speech may also be present.

Diagnosis

The diagnosis is usually obvious, but on occasion a fistula may require careful inspection to locate. A lacrimal probe may be used to palpate along the repaired cleft to localize the fistula. The hypernasal speech of velopharyngeal insufficiency may be related to the fistula or to an inadequacy of the soft palate. Plugging the fistula with a piece of dental wax or gum may help elucidate this during speech testing.

Treatment

Treatment options for a palatal fistula include observation, prosthetic rehabilitation, local flap closure, revision of the palatal closure, and distant flaps.

Observation is an acceptable choice for asymptomatic fistulas or in cases of extenuating circumstances, which may press the surgeon to hold off on further surgery. Waiting until a planned future procedure is often reasonable.

A prosthesis may play a role in certain circumstances. Patients with large fistulas who have undergone failed attempts at closure previously, with significantly scarred palates, may be best treated with a prosthesis. These can be difficult to maintain in younger children and will require refitting as the child grows. Leakage can also continue around the prosthesis.

Local rotation flap closure is appropriate for many defects, particularly those of the hard palate, or at the junction of the hard and soft palate. Single-layer closures such as freshening of the edges and closure are to be avoided because of the likelihood of failure. Thus, two-layered mucoperiosteal flap closure is often the best technique for treating palatal fistulas. The design of the flap must adhere to certain principles. The first is the size of the flap. This must be designed significantly larger than the defect. The surgeon must keep in mind the inflexible nature of scarred mucoperiosteum and design the rotation to allow sufficient mobility to cover the defect without tension. Finally, the closure must be performed in two layers.

Incisions are made ~5 mm from the edge of the fistula, and turn-in flaps of mucoperiosteum are created. Undermining of the nasal layer of these flaps can aid in mobilization. The larger the fistula, the greater the distance these circumferential incisions must be made from the edge of the fistula to span across the diameter of the defect. Next, the mucoperiosteal rotation flap for oral layer closure is made. This is to be $1^{1}/_{2}$ to 2 times larger than the size of the defect. Closure is thus performed in two layers with 4–0 Vicryl, without overlap of the oral and nasal layer suture lines.

When the fistula is large and in the mid- to anterior portion of the soft palate, then revising the repair with a modification of the Von Langenbach palatoplasty with lateral relaxing incisions may be effective. A Furlow double-reverse Z-plasty may also be used, particularly when additional length of the palate is desired.

Very large fistulas are rare. When they do occur, they represent a significant challenge. Options for repairing such defects are tongue flaps, buccal flaps, and radial forearm free laps. The tongue flap is an anteriorly based flap that was first described by Guerero-Santos and Altamirano in 1966.[1] The nasal closure is achieved by creating mucoperiosteal flaps hinged on the edge of the defect. The tongue flap is then raised with an appropriate width and length. Some muscle is included in the flap to protect the submucosal plexus. The dead space may be obliterated by passing the long ends of the turning flap through the tongue flap. The patient is maintained on nasogastric tube feedings for a minimum of 1 week. The flap is divided in 10 to 21 days.

Very large defects may require a radial forearm free flap. The vascular pedicle of the flap is passed through the cleft and tunneled through the cheek to be anastomosed to the facial vessels. Turnover flaps are created for the nasal layer if possible. Otherwise, the flap may be turned on itself for a split-thickness skin graft applied to the undersurface.

Velopharyngeal Incompetence

Hypernasality occurs when there is the perception of excessive nasal resonance on vowel and vocalic consonants; hyponasality is the lack of nasal resonance. Poor velopharyngeal function may be secondary to neurogenic etiologies, developmental mislearnings, or structural problems of the velopharyngeal port. A complete work-up requires not only a complete speech evaluation but also nasopharyngoscopy or videofluoroscopy. The nasopharyngoscopy is best performed with the patient awake, to allow visualization of the velopharynx during varied speech. The palatal closure is assessed in this manner.

Treatment options include speech therapy. In mild or inconclusive cases, a trial of speech therapy is indicated. Should this fail to achieve the desired result, surgical options are considered. Revision of the palatal closure may be considered. For example, a Furlow technique may provide additional palatal length to allow improvement. However, more commonly an additional procedure will be necessary.

Pharyngoplasty

Sphincter pharyngoplasty in the context of velopharyngeal surgery refers to the creation of superiorly based lateral

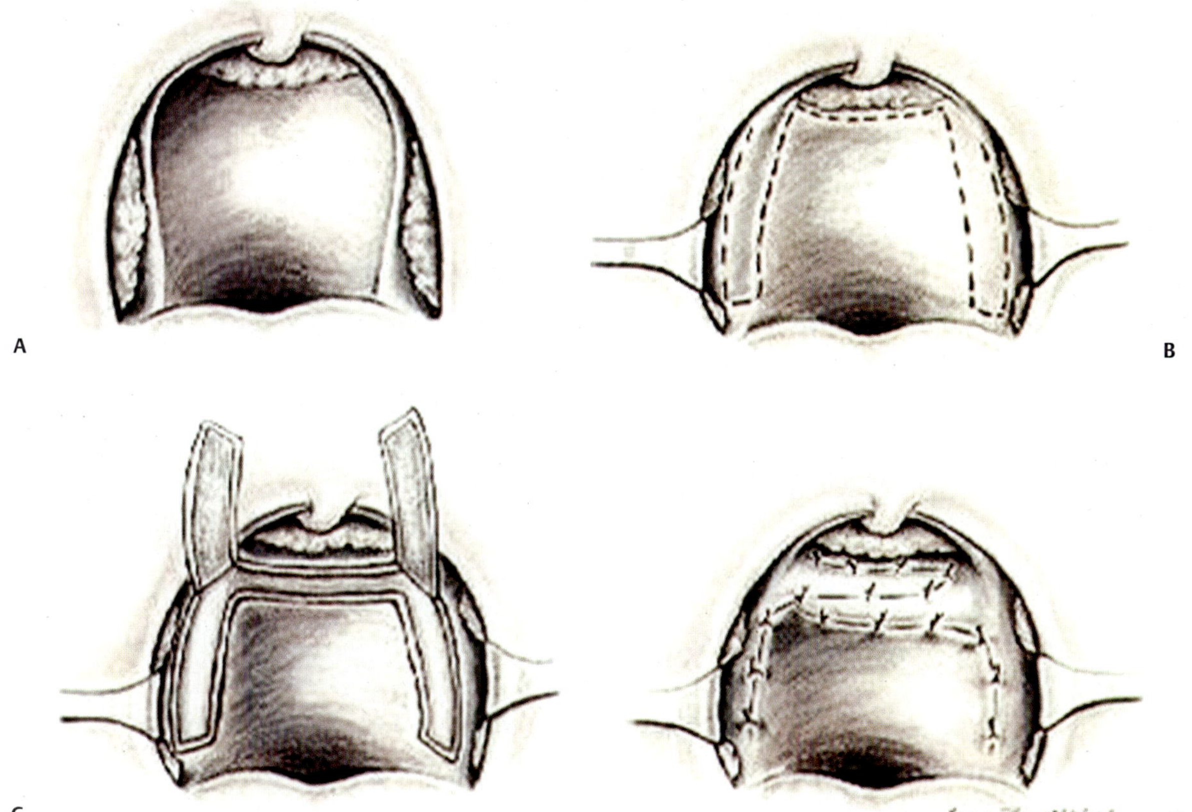

Fig. 48.1 Sphincteroplasty. **(A–D)** Outline of closure of flaps.

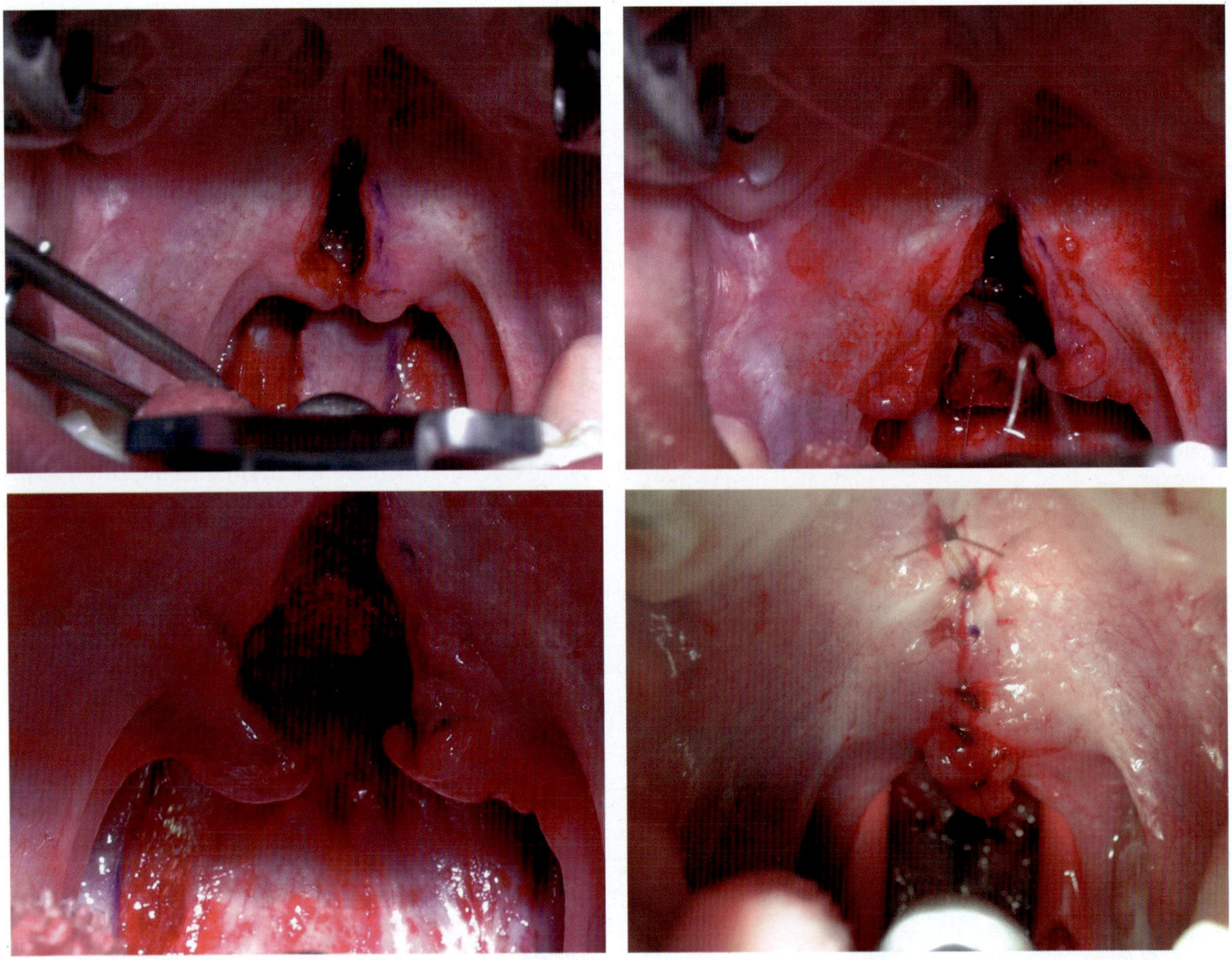

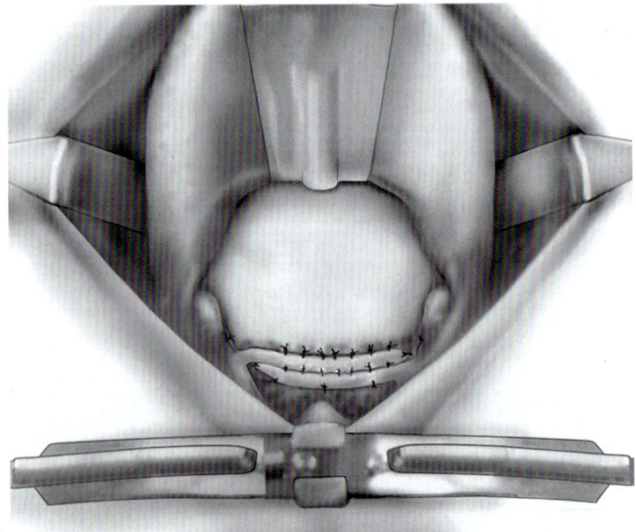

Fig. 48.2 Sphincteroplasty. **(A–D)** Photos show palatal incisions.

pharyngeal flaps. These are sewn along the posterior na-sopharyngeal wall to create a sphincter mechanism. This accomplishes both the closure of lateral gaps secondary to poor lateral wall motion and the closure of gaps along the posterior pharyngeal wall by the shelf of transposed tissue.

The level of the placement of the flaps is determined. This should be placed somewhat higher than what appears to be the level of velopharyngeal closure (**Figs. 48.1, 48.2, and 48.3**). It should be superior enough so as not to be visible through the oral cavity. The superiorly based lateral flaps are developed. The incision is made initially inferiorly at the inferior border of the posterior tonsillar pillar. The dissection is a muscle-mucosal flap, as palatopharyngeus muscle is included as part of the flap. This is performed bilaterally. A horizontal incision is made at the desired level of placement in the posterior pharyngeal wall, and a 5 mm slot is created. The bilateral flaps are then transposed into the space created. The flaps may be either sutured end to end or layered to provide greater bulk. In this case, the mucosa

Fig. 48.3 Sphincteroplasty. Two-layer closure of the palatal fistula with augmentation.

of one flap is oriented superiorly, and the other inferiorly. These are sutured in place with 4–0 Vicryl.

Pharyngeal Flaps

Pharyngeal flaps are relatively commonly performed. There is some debate as to the relative merits of the pharyngeal flap versus the pharyngoplasty (or sphincteroplasty) in the treatment of velopharyngeal incompetency. However, the pharyngeal flap is a reliable method of treating this problem. In this procedure, the flap of posterior pharyngeal tissue is usually pedicled superiorly, although inferiorly and laterally based flaps have been described. It is especially well suited for the closure of centrally located defects. Ideally, the patient for whom a pharyngeal flap is chosen has good lateral wall motion but inadequate motion anteriorly of the soft palate. This is determined by endoscopy or fluoroscopy.

The area of the flap is injected with local anesthetic with epinephrine. The flap is raised as a musculo-mucosal flap. The dissection is continued superiorly enough to allow closure of the velopharynx. A central incision is made in the palate to receive the flap. Two-layer closure with careful approximation of the mucosa is performed. The procedure divides the nasopharynx into two separate lateral ports.

Snoring is common postoperatively. Although sleep apnea is rare, a period of observation for this is required.

Conclusion

The treatment of the cleft lip and palate patient is a significant challenge. Although the surgical techniques have advanced considerably, in recent decades it is the emergence of the multispecialty team approach to the care of these patients that has significantly improved the quality of their care. Likewise, outcome has improved. However, the need for revision surgery is so common as to be an expected component of their comprehensive long-term care. This is especially true for bilateral cleft lips.

Essential to the effective management of secondary deformities of the cleft lip and palate patient is an accurate diagnosis. Due diligence in identifying the pathology allows a thoughtful and appropriate choice of treatment.

References

1. MacCarthy JG. Cleft lip and palate and craniofacial anomalies. In: McCarthy J ed. Plastic Surgery. Vol. 4. Philadelphia: WB Saunders; 1990:2771–2877.

2. Sadove AM, Eppley B. Correction of secondary cleft lip and nasal deformities. Clin Plast Surg 1993;20(4): 793–801.

Decision tree for revision laryngotracheal surgery in children

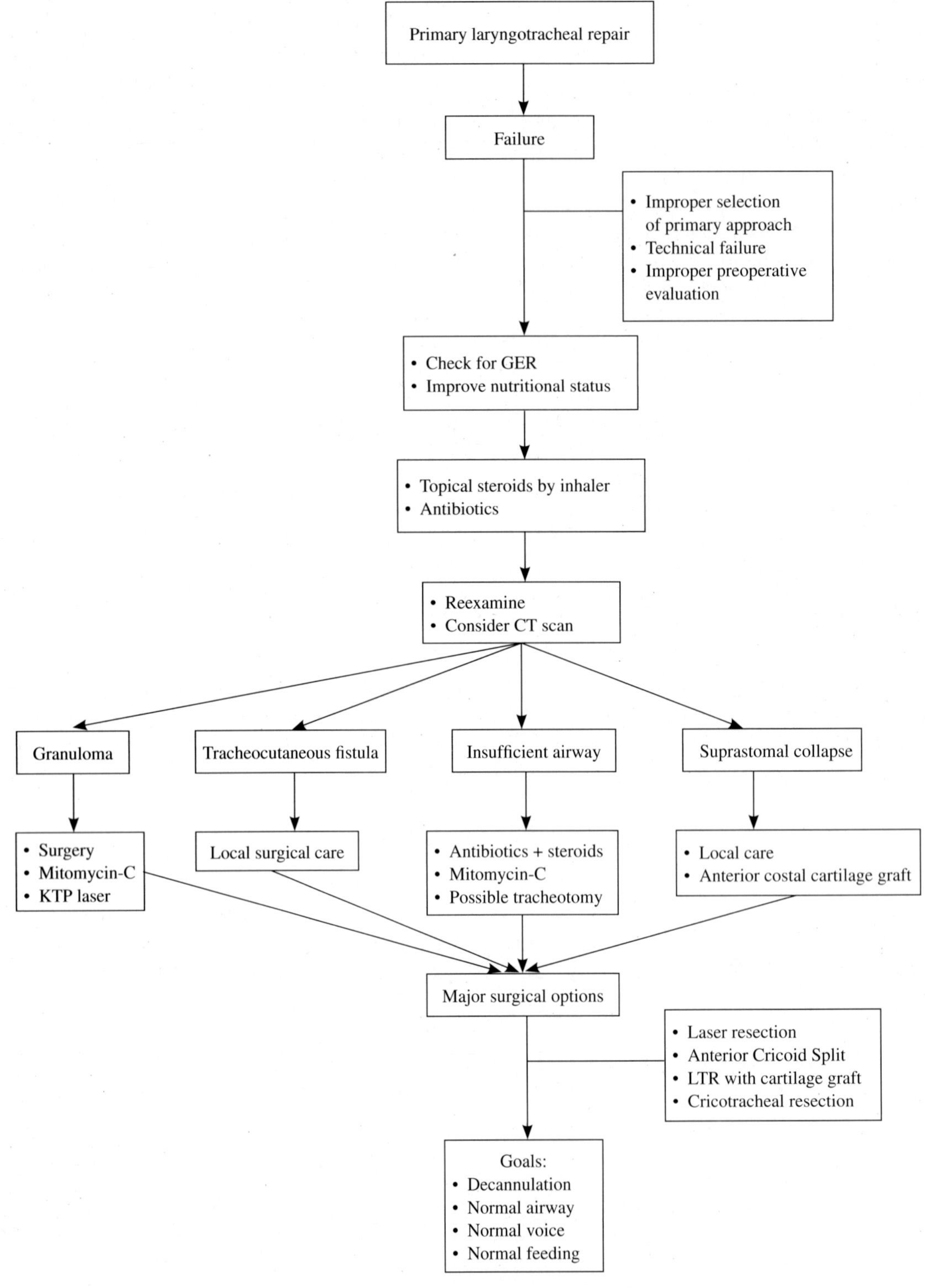

Laryngotracheal Revision Surgery in Children

Richard Nicollas and Jean Michel Triglia

Major reconstructive procedures on the airway, such as laryngotracheal reconstruction, will not always provide a good airway without any further therapy. It is important for the discussion to distinguish between the "usual cares" which are considered to be adjunctive measures and failures or postoperative problems that need revision surgery. The aim of this chapter is to describe failures and revision surgery.

Many pathologies such as laryngeal dyskinesia and vocal cord paralysis (in neonates), or subglottic stenosis, subglottic hemangioma, and even tumors (in children), can be responsible of laryngeal dyspnea. This chapter is devoted to examining this particular problem in the revision management of pediatric subglottic stenosis, which is the most frequent pathology needing a revision surgical procedure.

Even in the hands of the most experienced surgeons, primary laryngotracheal surgery can result in a less than satisfactory outcome in the short term with respect to the correction of the airway. Failure in the correction of the laryngotracheal lumen after primary laryngotracheal reconstruction by an external or endoscopic approach or the reappearance of a dyspnea following a successful surgery results in the option to perform laryngotracheal revision surgery. Short- and long-term failures occur despite a multitude of improvements and refinements that have been accomplished in pediatric laryngotracheal surgery since its inception.

The goals of laryngotracheal surgery in children are to eliminate primary disease, choose the best operative procedure for the individualized case to prevent recurrent disease, restore the theoretical airway diameter, andrestore serviceable voice and feeding.

General Considerations

When surgery for a laryngotracheal pathology fails, it usually can be ascribed to either improper selection of the technical procedure and/or technical failures or improper preoperative evaluation. Gastroesophageal reflux (GER) is a common occurrence in children,[1] especially when they have a breathing problem.[2] Experienced authors recom-

mend reflux investigation and treatment before operating for subglottic stenosis.[1,3,4] Antireflux treatment is always given before and after laryngeal surgery because, first, reflux is very common, and, second, it has been shown that patients with uncontrolled GER have a higher rate of failure in laryngotracheal reconstruction.[4]

It is very important to determine the patient's nutritional status prior to revision surgery. Several postoperative complications, such as healing defects, often occur in malnourished children.

In all cases, topical steroids given by aerosol technique and antimicrobial agents (oral or intravenous) are used postoperatively, as proposed by several authors.[4]

Subglottic Stenosis Revision Surgery

At the present time, laryngotracheal reconstruction via augmentation with graft cartilage is the mainstay of treatment. Cricotracheal resection is becoming the alternative option for managing subglottic stenosis. For Ochi et al, in a 10-year experience, ~30% of laryngotracheal reconstruction cases required revision surgery to achieve decannulation, implying that insufficient airway was obtained.[3] The various problems that can occur after reconstruction procedures will be evaluated from the less to the most important. For each one, prevention and management will be described.

Granulomas

Granulomas are very usual and can be considered as one of the events that need further therapy in the initial plan. They often occur in the suprastomal region and can interfere with decannulation.

Prevention

Many factors can induce granulomas. Whatever the surgical procedure—cricotracheal resection or laryngotracheal reconstruction—suturing has to be performed under the mucosa. The use of stenting can generate granulomas because the stent represents a foreign object. In most cases, granulomas are caused by the vocal cords or false cords trying to close over the stent. The same phenomenon can occur if the epiglottis is scarred. Long-term stenting has to be placed through the false and true vocal cords without contact with the epiglottis. When possible, it is better to perform a single-stage procedure because of need for short-term stenting.

Treatment

Granulomas can be treated by surgical removal with or without mitomycin-C in topical agents.[1,5] This product is an antineoplastic antibiotic that acts as an alkylating agent by inhibiting deoxyribonucleic acid (DNA) and protein synthesis. Surgery can be performed under telescope or microscope with microsurgical instruments or laser. In children, potassium titanyl phosphate (KTP) laser has been used successfully and easily with 400 μm fiber and 0-degree telescope.[6] This procedure allows for very precise removal in anatomical regions that are often difficult to reach. Mitomycin-C is used by topical application of a 20% solution in saline during 2 to 4 minutes at the surgical site.

Tracheocutaneous Fistulas

Tracheocutaneous fistulas are frequent but minor problems in the epithelialization of the tracheostomy tract.

Prevention

Tracheocutaneous fistulas occur in ~50% of patients with tracheotomy, but most of them have been decannulated in the third year.[7] Preventing fistulas requires short-term tracheotomy when possible, along with occlusive and compressive bandaging after decannulation. For this period, the child is restricted from swimming, and parents have to be careful during bathing.

Treatment

Surgical closure is indicated if the fistula persists 6 months after decannulation.[7] It begins with removal of the epithelialized tract from the skin to the trachea. The tracheal opening is sutured, and subhyoidian muscles are stitched to each other on the midline. The skin is sutured. A compressive bandage is then made.

Suprastomal Collapse

Suprastomal collapse is not common, but it may interfere with decannulation.

Prevention

Suprastomal collapse may be due to the type of stenting used.[7] After a "two-stage" laryngotracheal reconstruction, the area between the Silastic roll and the tracheostomy tube is unsupported. This area often becomes weakened because of the inward pressure caused by the tracheostomy tube and collapses into the lumen. During reconstruction, the cartilage graft has to enlarge the stenosis region and be long enough to support the suprastomal trachea.[8]

Treatment

If the suprastomal trachea collapses into the lumen, it may respond to decannulation and disappear. If decannulation remains impossible, a surgical solution can be proposed. One solution is to suture the collapsed trachea anteriorly to the strap muscles on each side.[7] The intubation is left for at least 2 days. Thus, the collapsed trachea is both supported by the tube and "extracted" by sutures. A treatment by steroids (intravenous followed by oral) will avoid airway inflammation. If this solution fails, laryngotracheal reconstruction with an anterior costal cartilage graft can be performed.[1,4] Its goal is to make the anterior part of the trachea more rigid.

Insufficient Airway

Insufficient airway in the operated area is, in fact, the real failure after subglottic stenosis surgery. The airway is considered sufficient when the subglottic lumen admits a bronchoscope that is no more than one size smaller than normal for the patient's age.[7] Failure can be acute, caused by inflammatory process, or midterm, provoked by fibrosis. Acute stenosis must be considered as a postoperative incident, whereas secondary stenosis will be considered and managed as new stenosis.

Inflammatory Stenosis

Prevention

Investigation and treatment of GER must be done preoperatively. If medical therapy fails, surgical correction can be indicated. Uncontrolled GER will lead to a higher rate of failure, especially if a laryngeal stent is present.[4] It has been shown that 71% of idiopathic subglottic stenosis cases have positive pH probe study in the pharynx.[9] A nasogastric tube is forbidden during the stenting period because it can provoke GER.

Wide-spectrum antimicrobial therapy is always started on the day of surgery and continued postoperatively for 7 to 10 days.[4]

Treatment

When a new inflammatory stenosis appears, surgical aggression such as another external approach must be avoided. Conservative methods are indicated; their goal is to correct inflammation and/or infection. General and topical (with aerosol) antibiotics and steroids are given. If the patient has been decannulated, a tracheotomy can be necessary with the same adjunctive therapy. Sometimes, stenting can be useful. Topical mitomycin-C is also indicated in such cases of hyper-reactive mucosa, as suggested by several authors.[1,5]

Mid- or Long-Term Stenosis

Prevention

In the following discussion, we will evaluate preventive steps that can be taken before, during, and after each particular surgical procedure.

Laser Resection   This technique is done through an endoscopic approach. It is indicated when stenosis is anterior and noncircular and when its vertical size is <1 cm.[10] During the procedure, it is important to deliver the least amount of energy as possible to avoid secondary stenosis induced by perichondrial lesions. Postoperatively, an aerosol with steroids and antibiotics are useful to prevent local infections and inflammation.[10]

Anterior Cricoid Split   This technique is indicated for neonatal subglottic stenosis without other obstruction and with good pulmonary reserve. Seven criteria have been established for patient selection:

Extubation failures on at least two occasions secondary to subglottic pathology

Weight >1500 g

No ventilator support for at least 10 days

Less than 30% supplemental oxygen

No congestive heart failure for at least 1 month

No acute respiratory tract infection

No antihypertensive medication for at least 1 month

During the surgical procedure, the mucosa must be carefully treated. Postoperatively, antimicrobial medication must be given, and an oral diet is forbidden. The nasotracheal tube has to be removed 7 to 10 days after the surgical procedure.

Laryngotracheal Reconstruction

This technique using a cartilage graft should be considered the standard in subglottic stenosis treatment.[11] The graft can be anterior or posterior, depending on the stenosis extension. For lateral stenosis or high-grade stenosis, grafts can be anterior and posterior. Either a single-stage or "traditional" two-stage approach can be taken. Associated airway pathologies such as broncho- and tracheomalacia increase the single-stage failure rate, whereas prior surgical procedures do not.[12] During surgery, great care must be taken to protect the mucosa. Perichondrium must be placed into the lumen of the respiratory tract. Cartilage grafts must be firmly sutured and must expand over the entire stenosis region and the suprastomal trachea. Postoperatively, it is better to immobilize the child's head and neck for 15 days to avoid rotation of the grafts. If a traditional two-stage procedure is done, an oral diet is allowed 2 days later; in a single-stage procedure, an oral diet can be allowed when stenting is removed. Endoscopic examination must be performed once or twice a week to control laryngotracheal healing. Extubation is performed in the operating room during an endoscopy.

Cricotracheal Resection   The concept behind this technique is to eliminate disease and to perform an end-to-end anastomosis between two safe parts of the respiratory tract. This procedure can be indicated as soon as the posterior part of the cricoid is free and can be stitched safely to the tracheal ring. As in laryngotracheal reconstruction, associated bronchopulmonary pathologies can induce failure, as reported by Triglia et al.[13] During the procedure, the surgeon must be careful with the recurrent laryngeal nerve; sutures must be made submucosally to avoid granulomas and dehiscence. Postoperatively, the measures are the same as those following laryngotracheal reconstruction.

Treatment

Secondary stenosis has to be managed as primary stenosis with few particularities. In case of failure after an anterior cricoid split, a cartilage graft can be necessary.

A fibrous web after laryngotracheal reconstruction can be treated endoscopically by laser and/or mitomycin-C. Laser is used to perform radiate incisions. In these cases, KTP laser is more appropriate than CO_2 laser for two reasons: first, it is easier to manipulate in the subglottis; second, it helps with healing.[14] After a cricotracheal resection, a circular stenosis or a lateral fibrous web can appear (< 0.5 cm thick) and can be operated on in the same way.

A new stenosis after laryngotracheal reconstruction can be treated either by further reconstruction or by cricotracheal resection. In cases of reconstruction failure, lateral cuts can be made together with anterior and posterior enlargement.[15] If this technique is performed, a single-stage procedure cannot be done, and stenting is left in place for

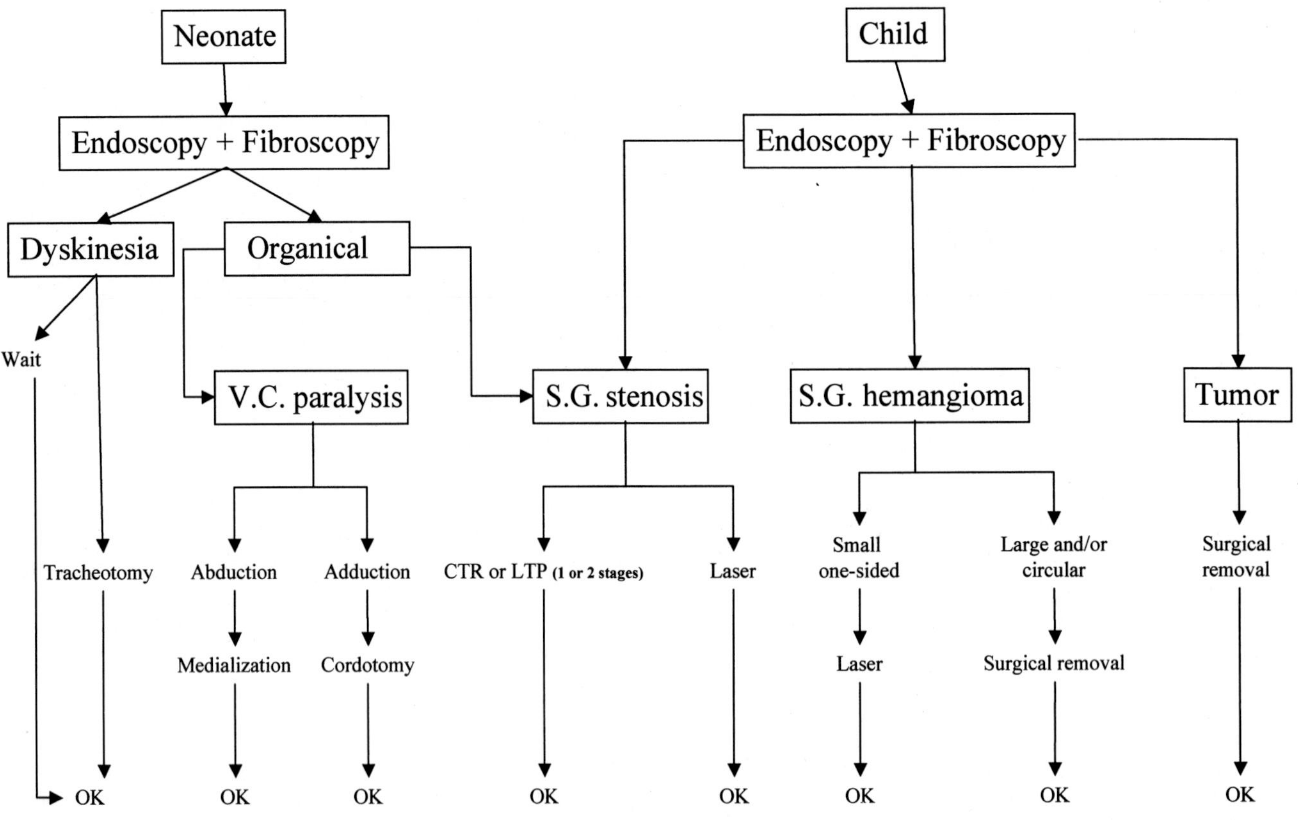

Fig. 49.1 Laryngeal dyspnea in neonates and children: primary surgical management.

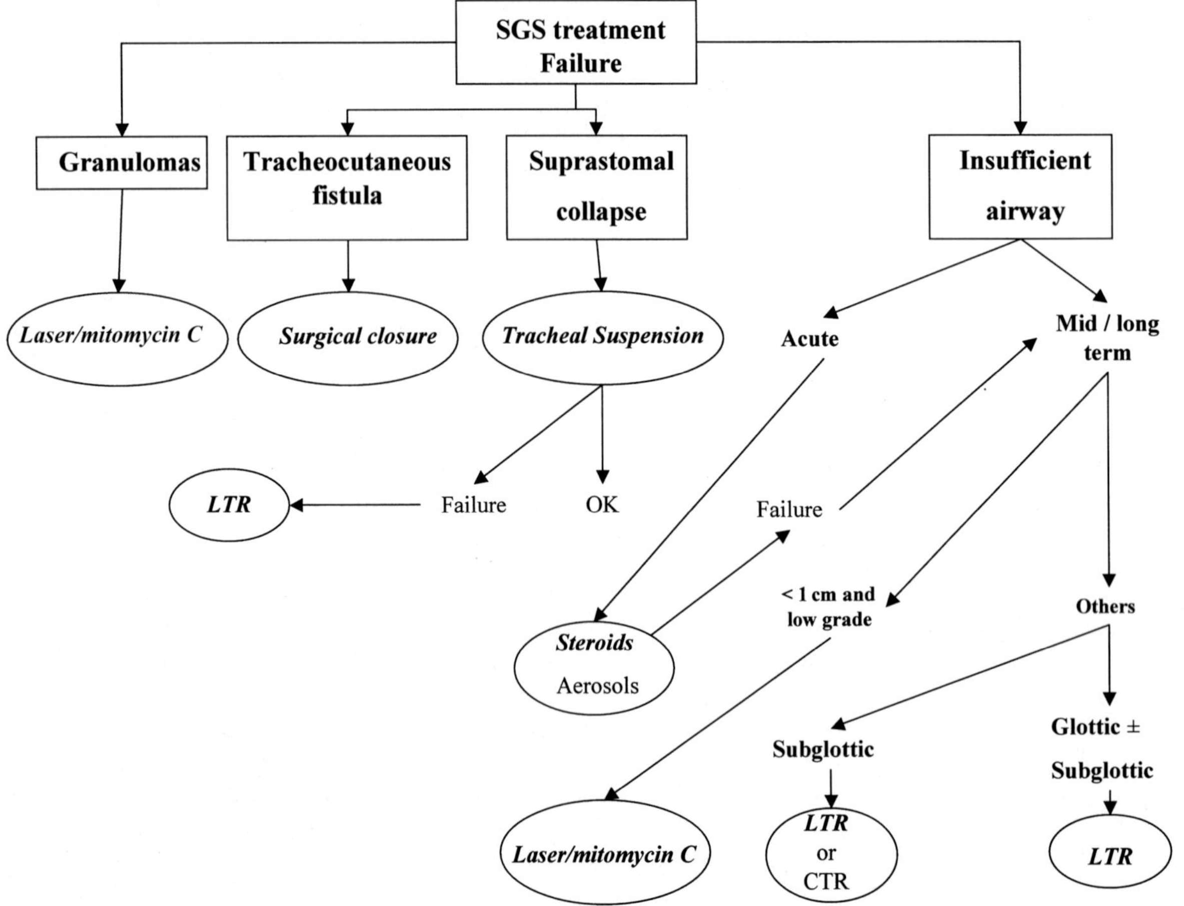

Fig. 49.2 Revision management of subglottic stenosis.

3 to 6 months. Rutter et al showed that 48% of cricotracheal resections were performed because of laryngotracheal reconstruction failures.[11]

Results reported in the literature are better with cricotracheal resection than with other procedures for similar indications and stenosis grade.[1] In case of failure after resection, the main techniques as reported by Rutter et al can be used.[11] Posterior cricoid splits and/or grafts, arytenoidopexy, arytenoidectomy, and expansion laryngotracheal reconstruction can be proposed.

The main goal of laryngotracheal stenosis management is decannulation, which is the last major step of the procedure and reflects the ultimate success of the "mission." The first major moment is the preoperative evaluation, which allows for individualized treatment. Investigation and management of associated patholo-gies such as GER and cardiopulmonary abnormality are initially required. After any kind of laryngotracheal reconstruction, minor surgical procedures may be needed.

Several authors, including Ochi et al, showed that patients requiring revision surgery after a laryngotracheal reconstruction tended to have worse stenosis upon presentation and tended to come from the higher-grade stenosis categories.[3] In those cases, a multioperated larynx will be much more inflammatory, and the mucosa will be more reactive. On the other hand, the consensus from reviews of revision laryngotracheal surgery cases has shown that revision surgery is less successful than primary procedures. Subglottic stenosis revision surgery has to be individualized because of the different ways children heal (**Figs. 49.1 and 49.2**).

References

1. Cotton RT. Management of subglottic stenosis. Otolaryngol Clin North Am 2000;33:111–130.
2. Holinger LD, Konior RJ. Surgical management of severe laryngomalacia. Laryngoscope 1989;99:136–142.
3. Ochi JW, Evans NG, Bailey CM. Pediatric airway reconstruction at Great Ormond Street: a ten-year review. Revisional airway reconstruction. Ann Otol Rhinol Laryngol 1992;101:595–596.
4. Gray S, Miller R, Myer CM, Cotton RT. Adjunctive measures for successful laryngotracheal reconstruction. Ann Otol Rhinol Laryngol 1987;96:509–513.
5. Ward RF, April MM. Mitomycin-C in the treatment of tracheal cicatrix after tracheal reconstruction. Int J Pediatr Otorhinolaryngol 1998;44:221–226.
6. Nicollas R, Giovanni A, Triglia JM, Geigle P, Bonneru JJ. Le Laser KTP dans les voies aériennes supérieures de l'enfant. Etude préliminaire á propos de 23 cas. Ann Otolaryngol Chir Cervicofac 1998;115:54–58.
7. Ochi JW, Evans NG, Bailey CM. Pediatric airway reconstruction at Great Ormond Street: a ten-year review. Decannulation and suprastomal collapse. Ann Otol Rhinol Laryngol 1992;101:656–658.
8. Triglia JM, Nicollas R, Roman S. Management of subglottic stenosis in infancy and childhood. Eur Arch Otorhinolaryngol 2000;257:382–385.
9. Maronian NC, Azadeh H, Waugh P, Hillel A. Association of laryngopharyngeal reflux disease and subglottic stenosis. Ann Otol Rhinol Laryngol 2001;110:606–612.
10. Nicollas R, Triglia JM, Belus JF, Bonneru JJ, Marti JY. Le laser CO$_2$ en laryngologie infantile. Ann Otolaryngol Chir Cervicofac 1996;113:243–249.
11. Rutter MJ, Hartley BEJ, Cotton RT. Cricotracheal resection in children. Arch Otolaryngol Head Neck Surg 2001;127:289–292.
12. Cotton RT, Myer CM, O'Connor DM, Smith ME. Pediatric laryngotracheal reconstruction with cartilage grafts and endotracheal tube stenting: the single-stage approach. Laryngoscope 1995;105:818–821.
13. Triglia JM, Nicollas R, Roman S. Primary cricotracheal resection in children: indications, technique and outcome. Int J Pediatr Otorhinolaryngol 2001;58:17–25.
14. Kyzer MD, Aly AS, Davidson JM, Reinisch L, Ossof RH. Sub ablation effects of the KTP laser on wound healing. Lasers Surg Med 1993;13:62–71.
15. Cotton RT, Gray SD, Miller RP. Update of Cincinnati experience in pediatric laryngotracheal reconstruction. Laryngoscope 1989;99:1111–1116.

Decision tree for pediatric sinusitis

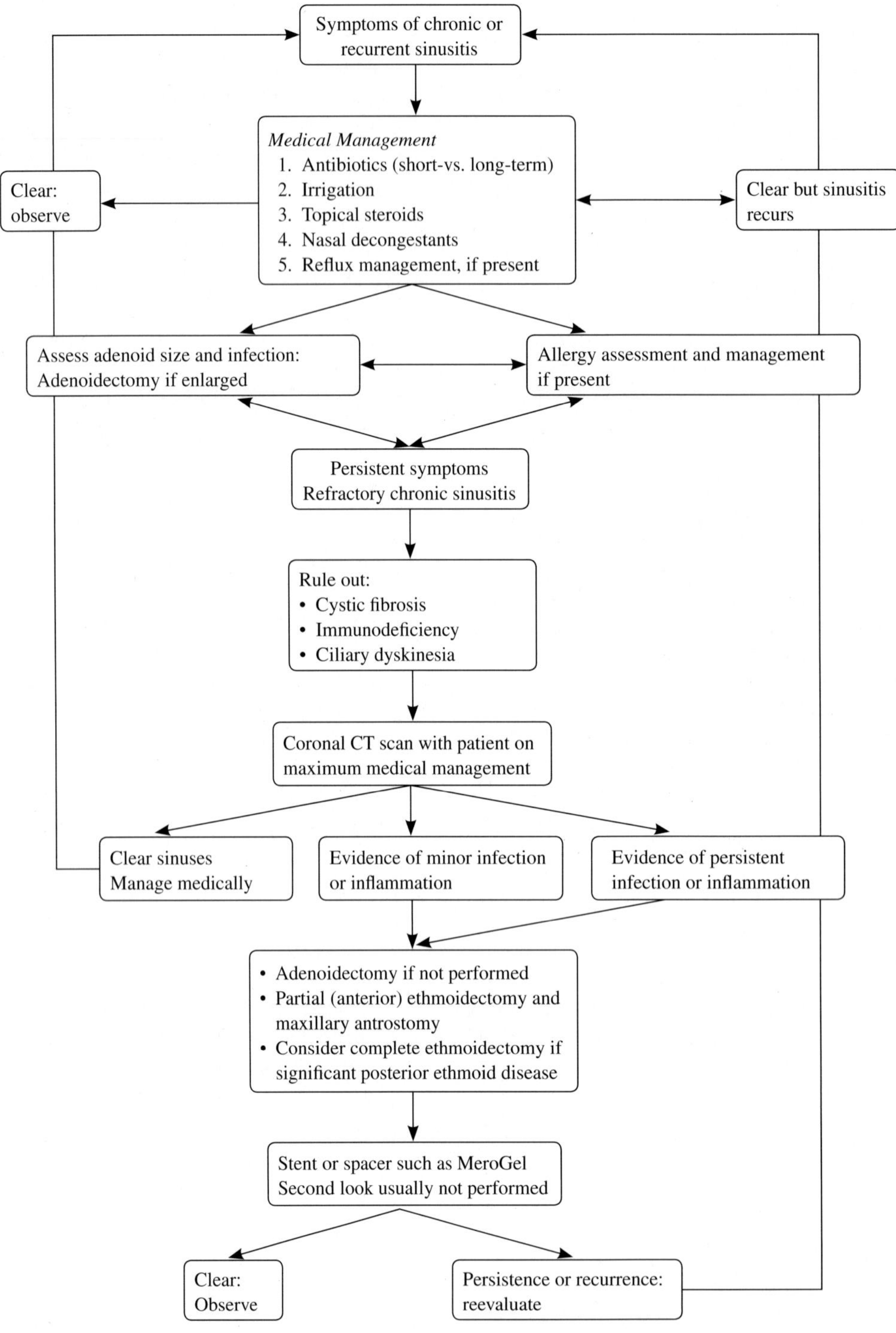

Pediatric Sinusitis Revision Surgery

Rodney P. Lusk

There remain significant controversies regarding the diagnosis and management of pediatric sinusitis. Pediatric sinusitis is estimated to complicate ~5 to 10% of upper respiratory infections in early childhood.[1,2] Because children average six to eight upper respiratory illnesses per year, this makes sinusitis a very common problem. In a quality of life assessment, Cunningham found that sinusitis had a more significant impact on children and their families than asthma, juvenile rheumatoid arthritis, and other chronic disorders.[3]

Pathophysiology of Chronic Rhinosinusitis

Age is clearly one of the most significant factors in pediatric sinusitis.[4] Children have an immature immune system; therefore, they are more likely to develop upper respiratory tract viral infections and associated acute sinusitis. There is a strong association between sinusitis and respiratory viral infections.[5] The viral infections cause mucosal edema and ciliary disfunction, which obstructs the ostium and increases the chance of establishing a bacterial infection of the sinuses.[6,7] Because the infundibulum is one of the narrowest drainage sites, it would be expected that the adjacent anterior ethmoid sinuses and maxillary sinuses would be the most likely to be involved with sinusitis. Viral infections are thought to cause significant ciliary dysfunction by decreasing the ciliary beat frequency[8] or destroying the ciliary blanket.[9] This sets up the appropriate conditions for a bacterial infection. As the ciliary function improves, the sinuses clear, and the infection resolves. This likely accounts for the high incidence of spontaneous resolution of acute sinusitis.

One of the more dramatic discoveries in recent years has been the presence of biofilms within the crypts of the adenoid tissue. Biofilms have been noted to cover as much as 50% of the surface in children with chronic sinusitis and 2% in children with obstructive sleep apnea.[10] Biofilms have been noted in the crypts of chronically infected tonsils and adenoids.[11] The infected adenoid tissue may be the nidus for recurrent or chronic sinusitis. Biofilms are independent of the size of adenoid tissue and this may account for the improvement in symptoms of sinusitis when even small adenoids are removed.

The role of allergy in chronic sinusitis remains controversial. Rachelefsky[12–14] was the first to point out an association between allergic symptoms and sinusitis in children. It is said that bacterial sinusitis occurs often in patients with allergic rhinitis, but this correlation has not yet been confirmed. Huang[15] studied this issue for 5 years in children with perennial allergic rhinitis (PAR) and seasonal allergic rhinitis (SAR) and found that the prevalence of sinusitis was significantly higher among patients with PAR than among those with SAR regardless of age or season. The patients with mold allergy PAR had a higher risk than those with nonmold allergies. Huang concluded that mold allergy is an important risk factor for sinusitis. There does appear to be a strong correlation between the allergic response and fungal infections in some patients. This is commonly referred to as allergic fungal sinusitis. The presentation of pediatric patients with allergic fungal sinusitis is different from that in adults, because children have more malleable bones and therefore a greater incidence of obvious abnormalities of the facial skeleton; also, the disease appears to be more unilateral.[16] Computed tomography (CT) scans show an equal amount of bony erosion.[4,17]

There are numerous studies that show that ~50% of children with sinusitis also have allergies, but the cause and effect has not been definitively demonstrated.[18–20] There has been a long-standing association between asthma, allergies, and chronic sinusitis. Riccio et al, for example, found that allergic asthmatic children with chronic rhinosinusitis have a typical T helper type 2 (Th2) cytokine pattern, but also that nonallergic asthmatic children share a similar pattern.[21] They indicated that these findings suggest the existence of a common pathophysiological mechanism shared by upper and lower airways, which is consistent with the concept of unified airways disease, and has been increasingly recognized.[22]

Without a doubt, there is increasing resistance of bacteria to antibiotics, especially *Streptococcus pneumoniae*, which has made medical management of chronic sinusitis more difficult.[23] The aerobic pathogens in pediatric chronic sinusitis include bacteria typical of acute sinusitis as well as organisms more characteristic of chronic disease. Chronic sinus infections, however, have a significant role of antibiotic-resistant aerobes, including multiply resistant *S. pneumoniae*.

Gastroesophageal reflux (GER) may be associated with chronic sinusitis.[24] The incidence of GER in children is not known, but Bothwell et al maintain that GER is present in a majority of children with chronic sinusitis.[25] Chambers et al found that GER was the only reliable historical symptom that predicted a bad outcome in adults.[26] There is, however, conflicting information in the literature. Phipps et al found a higher incidence of GER (63%) in children with sinusitis, and 79% improved their symptoms with medical management of GER.[27] Suskind et al studied patients undergoing antireflux surgery and who had failed medical management.[28] In this severe but very young group of patients (< 2 years old), only two patients (14%) had severe chronic sinusitis and otitis media. Yellon et al also found an incidence of sinusitis in only 10% of patients with biopsy-proven esophagitis.[29] These two studies may lead one to conclude that sinusitis is not associated with GER. Without out a doubt, however, there are some children with sinusitis and GER. Reflux may be intermittent and not identified with a 24-hour pH probe study. If present, it should be treated with proton pump inhibitors, which could prevent surgery.

Imaging

It is now clear that plain films do not adequately image pediatric sinuses.[30] In the acute setting we would expect these studies to be positive, and therefore of little use, because the infection is not limited to the nasal cavity.[7] Gwaltney's and Glasier et al's work showed a high incidence of opacification of the anterior ethmoid and maxillary sinuses with acute rhinovirus infections.[7,31] The coronal CT is currently the imaging method of choice for assessing the status of the sinuses. In general, sinusitis is a clinical diagnosis, and radiographic imaging is not necessary in children to confirm the diagnosis. CT scans should be obtained when both the parents and the surgeon feel surgical intervention is warranted. The CT scan is used primarily to look for anatomical abnormalities that would increase the risk of surgical complications. It should be obtained after a trial of maximum medical management that includes broad-spectrum antibiotics and topical nasal steroid sprays for at least 4 weeks. It is important not to be trapped, by an anxious or frustrated parent, into operating on a child with minimal disease on a CT.

Culture

In general, cultures of the nasal cavity have not been readily used in the pediatric population. The literature is mixed regarding the efficacy of directed cultures. Jiang et al[32] showed that the bacteriology of the middle meatus was different from that found in the ethmoid bulla. They therefore concluded that the bacteriological findings in the middle meatus may not reflect the real bacteriology

in chronic sinusitis and are therefore not valid. Other studies have shown a high correlation with antral punctures.[33,34] In the cooperative patient, endoscopically directed cultures of the middle meatus may be very useful, particularly in communities with increased resistance.

Medical Management

Because antibacterial therapy is most often empirically chosen to treat the disorder, knowledge of the typical etiologic agents and awareness of the antibacterial susceptibility profiles in a given community are of paramount importance. There is now recognition of the importance of nontypable *Haemophilus influenzae* that is unresponsive to first-generation cephalosporins, tetracyline-resistant grampositive cocci, and the increasing emergence of β-lactamase-positive respiratory pathogens such as *H. influenzae* and *Moraxella catarrhalis.* These realities mandate the more conservative use of antibiotics in upper respiratory tract infections and the use of newer therapeutic agents for acute and chronic sinusitis.

There is much that is unknown about antibiotic therapy and chronic sinusitis. There is one subject in recent publications on pediatric sinusitis on which most authors agree, however, and that is that the public cannot continue to expect to receive antibiotics on demand solely because of purulent nasal discharge, and that clinicians cannot continue to prescribe broad-spectrum and expensive antibiotics for minimal indications. Antibiotics are often used to treat viral upper respiratory tract infections, even though they are usually ineffective. The inappropriate use of antibiotics contributes to the emergence of drug-resistant bacterial pathogens. It is frequently difficult to assess if the infection is viral or complicated by a bacterial infection that would be improved with antibiotic therapy. Reviews in the literature emphasize the need for primary medical management and not surgical intervention. In the most resistant cases, however, surgery can perform a significant therapeutic role, as subsequently outlined.

Chronic sinusitis is associated with more resistant bacteria and therefore will need to be treated with broader spectrum antibiotics. For the most resistant strains of pneumococcus, File et al found the newer form of amoxycillin/clavulanate (AMX/CA) 2000/125 mg and the fluoroquinolones were highly active against these cultured isolates from community-acquired respiratory tract infection patients.[35,36] These drugs, however, should be saved for the most resistant infections.

There are proponents of the use of long-term, low-dose therapy with erythromycin in patients who do not respond to aggressive medical management.[37] Don et al recommended intravenous (IV) antibiotic therapy as an alternative to endoscopic sinus surgery.[38] They felt this was warranted because of the risk of interference with facial skeletal growth and complications of endoscopic sinus surgery. There is now conclusive evidence that endoscopic sinus surgery does not interfere with facial growth, and the risks of endoscopic sinus surgery is small.[39] In the study by Don et al, 89% of patients had complete resolution of symptoms following IV therapy with selective adenoidectomy, and 11% failed IV therapy and required endoscopic surgery.[38] Their criteria for performing selective adenoidectomy are not clear, and they report significant complications with IV therapy as well. IV therapy is, however, a potential modality of therapy in resistant cases.

Some investigators have recommended topical aerosolized antibiotics, but others have found it to be ineffective.[40] At this time a firm recommendation about its use cannot be made.

Prospective studies are lacking in the use of antihistamines and decongestants. In theory, decongestants would decrease the amount of edema and open the ostia. This has not been proven, however. Topical steroids have been shown to decrease edema within 2 weeks and may be of modest benefit. Topical steroids have been shown to be safe and not interrupt growth.[41,42]

Some investigators have used IV immune serum globulin (IVIG) to treat patients who do not have immune deficiencies but do have chronic sinusitis.[43] They concluded that IVIG was successful in improving the medical management of chronic sinusitis. They also thought the mechanism by which IVIG may be helpful is probably not based on the concept of immune replacement therapy, but more likely is an immune or inflammatory modulating agent.

Surgical Management

There is little doubt that chronic sinus symptoms occur in children with large obstructive adenoid pads. If the obstructive adenoid pad is not removed, the nasal cavity cannot become healthy. There are several studies that indicate adenoidectomy improves the signs and symptoms of sinusitis.[44,45] We now know this is likely due to the removal of adenoid tissue infected with biofilms therefore the size of the adenoid pad may not be a factor. Removal of the infected tissue will clear approximately 50% of children with recurrent or chronic sinusitis.[46] Good prospective studies assessing the efficacy of adenoidectomy in well-documented cases of sinusitis have yet to be performed.

Endoscopic sinus surgery is the primary method of treatment for chronic sinusitis now. The indications for endoscopic sinus surgery remain controversial. The Consensus Panel preferred to divide their indications into absolute and possible indications.[47]

Absolute indications include complete nasal airway obstruction in cystic fibrosis due to massive polyposis or closure of the nose by medialization of the lateral nasal wall, antrochoanal polyp, intracranial complications, mucoceles and mucopyoceles, orbital abscess, traumatic injury to the optic canal, dacryocystorhinitis due to sinusitis and resistant to medical treatment, fungal sinusitis, some meningoencephaloceles, andsome neoplasms.

Relative or possible indications, which cover the vast majority of patients, are chronic rhinosinusitis that persists despite optimal medical management and after the exclusion of any systemic disease and optimal management that includes 2 to 6 weeks of adequate antibiotics and treatment of any concomitant diseases. The Consensus Panel felt that only a small fraction of all children suffering from chronic sinusitis will require surgery but this accounts for the majority of patients.[47]

Some researchers feel that endoscopic surgery is rarely indicated.[48,49] With more experience, many surgeons have modified their surgery to be less aggressive.[50,51] Many investigators have now found that endoscopic ethmoidectomy can be performed safely in children and has an efficacy of around 80%.[45,51–57] Extensive spheno-ethmoidectomy is usually not justified in children unless they have symptomatic polyps secondary to cystic fibrosis or allergic fungal sinusitis.

Functional endoscopic sinus surgery (FESS) has become an effective tool in treating chronic sinusitis that is refractory to medical therapy. Reported success rates, defined mainly on the basis of improvement over preoperative symptoms, have been encouraging and ranged between 71 and 93%. Bent performed a meta-analysis that revealed a success rate of 88.4% with surgical management in children who had failed medical management.[57]

The technique has evolved over time. Most surgeons perform a limited procedure that involves an anterior ethmoidectomy and maxillary antrostomy. There continues to be some controversy over the size of the maxillary antrostomy. Many surgeons have become more conservative in the size of their antrostomy.[58,59] My personal preference is to remove the entire uncinate process, up to but not including the area of the root of the middle turbinate. It is important to leave the mucosa in this area to prevent scarring in the frontal recess. If I can see into the ostium with a 30-degree telescope, then I do not enlarge it. If, however, there is evidence of a polypoid mucosa in the ostium of the maxillary sinus or if it is edematous and can only be identified with a seeker, then I enlarge it posteriorly with through-biting instruments. With the advancement of instrumentation, microdébrider, and sharp through-biting instruments, we are now able to preserve the mucosa along the lamina papyracea and basal lamella most of the time and thereby prevent scarring and promote better healing. On occasion, usually less than 30% of the time, the posterior ethmoid sinuses will need to be entered. It is quite unusual, less than 10% of the time, that the sphenoid sinus or frontal sinuses will need to be entered. The frontal recess is the source of the frontal sinuses, which are not developed in children; therefore, instrumentation of this area should be performed very carefully.

Early on it was felt that a second look and cleaning of the cavity were necessary.[60] In the pediatric population, this meant a second anesthetic. Ramadan found that treatment with IV dexamethasone during endoscopic sinus surgery was safe and was helpful in reducing scarring and swelling noted during the second-look procedure.[61] Use of corticosteroids was particularly helpful in children with asthma, lower CT scores, and no exposure to smoking and in children older than 6 years. Walner et al then found that not performing a second look did not increase the incidence of revision surgery.[62] Based on their findings, Fakhri et al concluded that second-look endoscopy did not decrease the incidence of revision surgery; therefore, the second look was of no benefit following routine FESS.[63] It has now become common practice to use some type of absorbable stenting material in children and not perform the second look. The stenting material I currently prefer is MeroGel (Medtronic Xomed, Jacksonville, Florida).

Many areas of surgical management of sinusitis need further investigation, but none are more important than the impact on facial growth. There are piglet models that show interruption of facial growth on the side of endoscopic surgery, but the animals clinically did not show evidence of abnormal growth.[64,65] Lund et al had evidence that very aggressive surgical management of midface lesions is not associated with interruption of facial growth.[66] Wolf et al did not note any evidence of interruption of facial growth; however, these two studies did not perform accurate measurements of the facial skeleton.[67]

Bothwell et al sought to determine whether FESS performed in children with chronic rhinosinusitis alters facial growth.[37] Sixty-seven children with a mean age of 3.1 years at presentation were evaluated for facial growth 10 years later (mean age 13.2 years). In this group, 46 children underwent FESS, and 21 did not undergo FESS. Quantitative anthropomorphic analysis was performed using 12 standard facial measurements on both groups. A facial plastic expert performed blinded qualitative facial analysis on standardized photographs. Both quantitative and qualitative analyses showed no statistical significance in facial growth between children who underwent FESS as compared with those who had chronic sinusitis but did not undergo FESS. Their data showed there were no deviations, or trends toward deviation, from the standard norms in children. They concluded there was no evidence that FESS affected facial growth in children.

Research in the area of pediatric sinusitis will continue to be difficult because of the multifactorial nature of the disease. Large clinical studies are going to be required to further elucidate the pathophysiology, as well as the medical and surgical management of chronic sinusitis. It is also likely that these studies will not be performed because of their expense and complexity.

References

1. Wald ER. Sinusitis in children. N Engl J Med 1992;326: 319–323.
2. Gooch WM III. Antibacterial management of acute and chronic sinusitis. Manag Care Interface 1999;12(2):92–94.
3. Cunningham JM, Chiu EJ, Landgraf JM, Gliklich RE. The health impact of chronic recurrent rhinosinusitis in children. Arch Otolaryngol Head Neck Surg 2000;126(11): 1363–1368.
4. Nguyen KL, Corbett ML, Garcia DP, et al. Chronic sinusitis among pediatric patients with chronic respiratory complaints. J Allergy Clin Immunol 1993;92:824–830.
5. Daele JJ. Chronic sinusitis in children. Acta Otorhinolaryngol Belg 1997;51(4):285–304.
6. Guo Y, Majima Y, Hattori M, Seki S, Sakakura YA. Comparative study of the ciliary area of the maxillary sinus mucosa and computed tomographic images. Eur Arch Otorhinolaryngol 1998;255(4):202–204.
7. Gwaltney JM Jr, Phillips CD, Miller RD, Riker DK. Computed tomographic study of the common cold. New Engl J Med 1994;330:25–30.
8. Joki S, Toskala E, Saano V, Nuutinen J. Correlation between ciliary beat frequency and the structure of ciliated epithelia in pathologic human nasal mucosa. Laryngoscope 1998;108(3):426–430.
9. Guo Y, Majima Y, Hattori M, Seki S, Sakakura Y. Effects of functional endoscopic sinus surgery on maxillary sinus mucosa. Arch Otolaryngol Head Neck Surg 1997;123(10): 1097–1100.
10. Coticchia J, Zuliani G, Coleman C, et al. Biofilm surface area in the pediatric nasopharynx: chronic rhinosinusitis vs. obstructive sleep apnea. Arch Otolaryngol Head Neck Surg 2007;133:110–114.
11. Galli J, Ardito F, Calo L, et al. Recurrent upper airway infections and bacterial biofilms. J Laryngol Otol 2007;121: 341–344.
12. Rachelefsky GS, Katz RM, Siegel SC. Chronic sinusitis in children with respiratory allergy: the role of antimicrobials. J Allergy Clin Immunol 1982;69:382–387.
13. Rachelefsky GS, Katz RM, Siegel SC. Chronic sinusitis in the allergic child. Pediatr Clin North Am 1988;35: 1091–1101.
14. Rachelefsky GS. Sinusitis in children: diagnosis and management. Clin Rev Allergy 1984;2:397–408.
15. Huang SW. The risk of sinusitis in children with allergic rhinitis. Allergy Asthma Proc 2000;21(2):85–88.
16. McClay JE, Marple B, Kapadia L, et al. Clinical presentation of allergic fungal sinusitis in children. Laryngoscope 2002;112(3):565–569.

17. Manning SC, Mabry RL, Schaefer SD, Close LG. Evidence of IgE-mediated hypersensitivity in allergic fungal sinusitis. Laryngoscope 1993;103:717–721.
18. Furukawa CT. The role of allergy in sinusitis in children. J Allergy Clin Immunol 1992;90:515–517.
19. Liu CM, Shun CT, Song HC, Lee SY, Hsu MM, How SW. Investigation into allergic response in patients with chronic sinusitis. J Formos Med Assoc 1992;91:252–257.
20. Savolainen S. Allergy in patients with acute maxillary sinusitis. Allergy 1989;44:116–122.
21. Riccio AM, Tosca MA, Cosentino C, et al. Cytokine pattern in allergic and non-allergic chronic rhinosinusitis in asthmatic children. Clin Exp Allergy 2002;32(3):422–426.
22. Venarske DL, deShazo RD. Sinobronchial allergic mycosis: the SAM syndrome. Chest 2002;121(5):1670–1676.
23. Nelson JD. Changing trends in the microbiology and management of acute otitis media and sinusitis. Pediatr Infect Dis 1986;5(6):749–753.
24. Barbero GJ. Gastroesophageal reflux and upper airway disease. Otolaryngol Clin North Am 1996;29(1):27–38.
25. Bothwell MR, Parsons DS, Talbot A, Barbero GJ, Wilder B. Outcome of reflux therapy on pediatric chronic sinusitis. Otolaryngol Head Neck Surg 1999;121(3):255–262.
26. Chambers DW, Davis WE, Cook PR, Nishioka GJ, Rudman DT. Long-term outcome analysis of functional endoscopic sinus surgery: correlation of symptoms with endoscopic examination findings and potential prognostic variables. Laryngoscope 1997;107(4):504–510.
27. Phipps CD, Wood WE, Gibson WS, Cochran WJ. Gastroesophageal reflux contributing to chronic sinus disease in children: a prospective analysis. Arch Otolaryngol Head Neck Surg 2000;126(7):831–836.
28. Suskind DL, Zeringue GP III, Kluka EA, Udall J, Liu DC. Gastroesophageal reflux and pediatric otolaryngologic disease: the role of antireflux surgery. Arch Otolaryngol Head Neck Surg 2001;127(5):511–514.
29. Yellon RF, Coticchia J, Dixit S. Esophageal biopsy for the diagnosis of gastroesophageal reflux-associated otolaryngologic problems in children. Am J Med 2000;108:131S–138S.
30. McAlister WH, Lusk RP, Muntz HR. Comparison of plain radiographs and coronal CT scans in infants and children with recurrent sinusitis. [See Comments.] AJR Am J Roentgenol 1989;153:1259–1264.
31. Glasier CM, Ascher DP, Williams KD. Incidental paranasal sinus abnormalities on CT of children: clinical correlation. AJNR Am J Neuroradiol 1986;7:861–864.
32. Jiang RS, Lin JF, Hsu CY. Correlation between bacteriology of the middle meatus and ethmoid sinus in chronic sinusitis. J Laryngol Otol 2002;116(6):443–446.
33. Gold SM, Tami TA. Role of middle meatus aspiration culture in the diagnosis of chronic sinusitis. Laryngoscope 1997;107(12, Pt 1):1586–1589.
34. Ozcan M, Unal A, Aksaray S, Yalcin F, Akdeniz T. Correlation of middle meatus and ethmoid sinus microbiology in patients with chronic sinusitis. Rhinology 2002;40(1):24–27.
35. File TM Jr, Jacobs MR, Poole MD, Wynne B. Outcome of treatment of respiratory tract infections due to *Streptococcus pneumoniae*, including drug-resistant strains, with pharmacokinetically enhanced amoxycillin/clavulanate. Int J Antimicrob Agents 2002;20(4):235–247.
36. Pfaller MA, Ehrhardt A, Jones RN. Frequency of pathogen occurrence and antimicrobial susceptibility among community-acquired respiratory tract infections in the respiratory surveillance program study: microbiology from the medical office practice environment. Am J Med 2001;111:4S–12S.
37. Cervin A, Kalm O, Sandkull P, Lindberg S. One-year low-dose erythromycin treatment of persistent chronic sinusitis after sinus surgery: clinical outcome and effects on mucociliary parameters and nasal nitric oxide. Otolaryngol Head Neck Surg 2002;126(5):481–489.
38. Don DM, Yellon RF, Casselbrant ML, Bluestone CD. Efficacy of a stepwise protocol that includes intravenous antibiotic therapy for the management of chronic sinusitis in children and adolescents. Arch Otolaryngol Head Neck Surg 2001;127(9):1093–1098.
39. Bothwell MR, Piccirillo JF, Lusk RP, Ridenour BD. Long-term outcome of facial growth after functional endoscopic sinus surgery. Otolaryngol Head Neck Surg 2002;126(6):628–634.
40. Desrosiers MY, Salas-Prato M. Treatment of chronic rhinosinusitis refractory to other treatments with topical antibiotic therapy delivered by means of a large-particle nebulizer: results of a controlled trial. Otolaryngol Head Neck Surg 2001;125(3):265–269.
41. Skoner DP, Gentile D, Angelini B, Kane R, Birdsall D, Banerji D. The effects of intranasal triamcinolone acetonide and intranasal fluticasone propionate on short-term bone growth and HPA axis in children with allergic rhinitis. Ann Allergy Asthma Immunol 2003;90(1):56–62.
42. Allen DB, Meltzer EO, Lemanske RF Jr, et al. No growth suppression in children treated with the maximum recommended dose of fluticasone propionate aqueous nasal spray for one year. Allergy Asthma Proc 2002;23(6):407–413.
43. Ramesh S, Brodsky L, Afshani E, et al. Open trial of intravenous immune serum globulin for chronic sinusitis in children. Ann Allergy Asthma Immunol 1997;79(2):119–124.
44. Vandenberg SJ, Heatley DG. Efficacy of adenoidectomy in relieving symptoms of chronic sinusitis in children. Arch Otolaryngol Head Neck Surg 1997;123(7):675–678.
45. Rosenfeld RM. Pilot study of outcomes in pediatric rhinosinusitis. Arch Otolaryngol Head Neck Surg 1995;121(7):729–736.
46. Lusk R. Pediatric chronic rhinosinusitis. Curr Opin Otolaryngol Head Neck Surg 2006;14:393–396.
47. Clement PA, Bluestone CD, Gordts F, et al. Management of rhinosinusitis in children: consensus meeting, Brussels, Belgium, September 13, 1996. Arch Otolaryngol Head Neck Surg 1998;124(1):31–34.
48. Poole MD. Pediatric endoscopic sinus surgery: the conservative view. Ear Nose Throat J 1994;73(4):221–227.
49. Otten FW, van Aarem A, Grote JJ. Long-term follow-up of chronic maxillary sinusitis in children. Int J Pediatr Otorhinolaryngol 1991;22(1):81–84.
50. Lusk RP. The surgical management of chronic sinusitis in children [Review]. Pediatr Ann 1998;27(12):820–827.

51. Parsons DS, Phillips SE. Functional endoscopic surgery in children: a retrospective analysis of results. Laryngoscope 1993;103:899–903.

52. Lusk RP. Endoscopic approach to sinus disease [Review]. J Allergy Clin Immunol 1992;90(3, Pt 2):496–505.

53. Gross CW, Gurucharri MJ, Lazar RH, Long TE. Functional endonasal sinus surgery (FESS) in the pediatric age group. Laryngoscope 1989;99:272–275.

54. Lazar RH, Younis RT, Long TE. Functional endonasal sinus surgery in adults and children. Laryngoscope 1993;103:1–5.

55. Lusk RP, Muntz HR. Endoscopic sinus surgery in children with chronic sinusitis: a pilot study. Laryngoscope 1990; 100:654–658.

56. Manning SC, Wasserman RL, Silver R, Phillips DL. Results of endoscopic sinus surgery in pediatric patients with chronic sinusitis and asthma. [See Comments.] Arch Otolaryngol Head Neck Surg 1994;120(10):1142–1145.

57. Hebert RL, Bent JP III. Meta-analysis of outcomes of pediatric functional endoscopic sinus surgery. Laryngoscope 1998;108(6):796–799.

58. Setliff RC. The small-hole technique in endoscopic sinus surgery. Otolaryngol Clin North Am 1997;30(3):341–354.

59. Davis WE, Templer JW, LaMear WR, Davis WE Jr, Craig SB. Middle meatus anstrostomy: patency rates and risk factors. Otolaryngol Head Neck Surg 1991;104(4):467–472.

60. Lusk RP. Surgical management of sinusitis. In: Lusk RP, ed. Pediatric Sinusitis. New York: Raven Press; 1992:77–127.

61. Ramadan HH. Corticosteroid therapy during endoscopic sinus surgery in children: is there a need for a second look? Arch Otolaryngol Head Neck Surg 2001;127(2): 188–192.

62. Walner DL, Falciglia M, Willging JP, Myer CM III. The role of second-look nasal endoscopy after pediatric functional endoscopic sinus surgery. Arch Otolaryngol Head Neck Surg 1998;124(4):425–428.

63. Fakhri S, Manoukian JJ, Souaid JP. Functional endoscopic sinus surgery in the paediatric population: outcome of a conservative approach to postoperative care. J Otolaryngol 2001;30(1):15–18.

64. Mair EA, Bolger WE, Breisch EA. Sinus and facial growth after pediatric endoscopic sinus surgery. Arch Otolaryngol Head Neck Surg 1995;121(5):547–552.

65. Carpenter KM, Graham SM, Smith RJ. Facial skeletal growth after endoscopic sinus surgery in the piglet model. Am J Rhinol 1997;11(3):211–217.

66. Lund VJ, Howard DJ, Wei WI, Cheesman AD. Craniofacial resection for tumors of the nasal cavity and paranasal sinuses: a 17 year experience. Head Neck 1998;20(2): 97–105.

67. Wolf G, Greistorfer K, Jebeles JA. The endoscopic endonasal surgical technique in the treatment of chronic recurring sinusitis in children. Rhinology 1995;33(2): 97–103.

Index